TCH CARDIOLOGY

HEARTS AND HEART-LIKE ORGANS

Volume 2

TCH CARDIOLOGY

Contributors

Russell T. Dowell

Allan M. Lefer

William M. Manger

Germano Marchetti

P. R. Moret

Henry I. Russek

Linda G. Russek

H. Sandler

Hans Selye

Robert C. Smallridge

H. Lowell Stone

George J. Trachte

Åke Wennmalm

TCH CARDIOLOGY

HEARTS AND HEART-LIKE ORGANS

Volume 2
Physiology

Edited by

GEOFFREY H. BOURNE

Saint George's University
School of Medicine
Grenada, West Indies

Academic Press 1980
A Subsidiary of Harcourt Brace Jovanovich, Publishers
New York   London   Toronto   Sydney   San Francisco

ACADEMIC PRESS, INC.
111 Fifth Avenue, New York, New York 10003

United Kingdom Edition published by
ACADEMIC PRESS, INC. (LONDON) LTD.
24/28 Oval Road, London NW1 7DX

Library of Congress Cataloging in Publication Data
Main entry under title:

Hearts and heart–like organs.

  Includes bibliographies.
  CONTENTS:
v. 2. Physiology.
    1. Heart. I. Bourne, Geoffrey Howard, Date.
QP111.4.H4   591.1'16   80–18121
ISBN 0–12–119402–7 (v. 2)

TCH CARDIOLOGY

Contents

4 Catecholamines and the Heart
WILLIAM M. MANGER

5 Emotion and the Heart
HENRY I. RUSSEK and LINDA G. RUSSEK

6 The Nature of Stress and Its Relation to Cardiovascular Disease
HANS SELYE

List of Contributors

Numbers in parentheses indicate the pages on which the authors' contributions begin.

Russell T. Dowell (419), Department of Physiology and Biophysics, University of Oklahoma Health Sciences Center, Oklahoma City, Oklahoma 73190

Allan M. Lefer (1), Department of Physiology, Jefferson Medical College, Thomas Jefferson University, Philadelphia, Pennsylvania 19107

William M. Manger (161), Associate Professor of Clinical Medicine, National Hypertension Association, Inc., New York University Medical Center, New York, New York 10016

Germano Marchetti (525), Gruppo Lepetit S.p.A., Via Durando, 38 Milan, Italy

P. R. Moret (333), University of Geneva, Center of Cardiology Hospital, Geneva, Switzerland

Henry I. Russek (263), One North Ocean Boulevard, Boca Raton, Florida 33432

Linda G. Russek (263), One North Ocean Boulevard, Boca Raton, Florida 33432

H. Sandler (435), Biomedical Research Division, National Aeronautics and Space Administration, Ames Research Center, Moffett Field, California 94035

Hans Selye (289), International Institute of Stress, 2900 boul. Edouard-Montpetit, Montreal, Quebec H3C 3J7, Canada

Robert C. Smallridge (93), Division of Medicine, Walter Reed Army Institute of Research, Washington, D.C. 20012

H. Lowell Stone (389), University of Oklahoma Health Sciences Center, Oklahoma City, Oklahoma 73190

George J. Trachte (1), Department of Physiology, Jefferson Medical College, Thomas Jefferson University, Philadelphia, Pennsylvania 19107

Åke Wennmalm (41), Department of Clinical Physiology at Karolinska Institutet, Huddinge University Hospital, S-141 86 Huddinge, Sweden

Preface

The exchange of oxygen between the atmosphere and living tissues was a problem for the first life on earth. This problem of respiration became mechanically complex once multicellular organisms evolved. The more complicated such organisms became, the more difficult logistically the problem became. Eventually in animals, a specialized fluid capable of carrying oxygen was developed, together with a series of pipes to convey it to the most distant tissues and with a centrally-placed pump to push the fluid to its destination. Some animals developed one pump and some depended on several. The originally simple pump became more complex as air breathing added to the respiratory problems. The original straight tubular heart evolved into a two, a three, and eventually a four-chambered heart, reaching the apex of its development in mammals.

Many factors in civilized life affect the normal functioning of the heart in modern humans, and heart attacks afflict one million people a year in the United States alone. Of these, less than half survive. The structure and function of the heart are therefore central themes in the orchestration of medical research and practice, which incorporates knowledge and discoveries from diverse disciplines.

The present series of volumes has been designed to give biological and biomedical researchers anatomical and physiological perspectives of the heart from invertebrates to humans. It has not been possible to be comprehensive (I cannot even guess how many volumes that would take), but at least we have picked out the highlights in the areas covered.

Volume 1 traces the heart through the invertebrates and the lower vertebrates to humans. Volume 2 deals with the physiology of the heart, its evolution, the effects of hormones, exercise, stress, bedrest, hypoxia, and the control of the coronary system. Volume 3 takes up the area of pathology and surgery of the heart, viruses of the heart, and the status of cardiac surgery and cardiac transplantation. In this volume, especially, only a limited number of fields can be covered, but we hope in later volumes (still being planned) specifically to cover heart attacks and the fundamentals of the structure and functioning of the cardiac cell.

This treatise is intended to provide a basis for the continued study of the heart for a greater understanding of its complexities and to help generate ideas for further research on this vital organ.

Geoffrey H. Bourne

Contents of Other Volumes

Volume 1: Comparative Anatomy and Development

Volume 3: Pathology and Surgery of the Heart

1

Effects of Hormones on the Heart

Allan M. Lefer and George J. Trachte

I. General Concepts

In reviewing the effects of hormones on the heart, one is impressed with the diversity of types of humoral agents that influence cardiac function. The heart appears to be a significant target organ for a wide variety of humoral agents, including many hormones. Several of these important relationships are covered in other chapters of this treatise (i.e., prostaglandins and the heart, the thyroid and the heart, and catecholamines and the heart). Therefore we will not duplicate these efforts. We will discuss the effects of four major groups of hormones that exert prominent cardiac actions. These are the corticosteroids (i.e., adrenal cortical steroids), anterior and posterior pituitary hormones, pancreatic hormones, and the major components of the renin–angiotensin system. In the case of the adrenal cortex, the active hormones are steroids, whereas all the other groups of hormones considered in this chapter are polypeptides of various molecular weights ranging from the small heptapeptide (e.g., angiotensin III) to adrenocorticotropic hormone (ACTH), which comprises 39 amino acid residues.

We will discuss each hormone in terms of three major effects: (1) inotropic (i.e., effect on contractile mechanisms), (2) chronotropic (i.e., effect on heart rate), and (3) coronary vasoactivity (i.e., effect on the caliber of the coronary vasculature). With these three critical parameters the reader will be able to obtain a reasonably comprehensive picture of the overall effects of a given hormone on the status of cardiac performance. This will be of value in ascertaining the overall effect of a hormone in situations in which hormone therapy may be considered for a circulatory disturbance. Thus if the inotropic, chronotropic, and coronary vascular effects are known, one could determine whether a given hormone would be a good candidate to protect the ischemic myocardium against the extension of infarct size.

In the case of myocardial ischemia, one would prefer an agent that did not have significant positive or negative inotropic activity (e.g., increased inotropic activity increases myocardial oxygen demand, whereas cardiodepression could impair the noninvolved portion of the myocardium). Obviously any agent that increased heart rate would also increase myocardial oxygen demand, whereas a modest bradycardia may be somewhat beneficial by improving cardiac efficiency. In the case of coronary vasoactivity, coronary vasoconstriction would be dangerous because it would further restrict blood flow to the myocardium, whereas a modest vasodilation might be beneficial, although a profound vasodilation might result in systemic hypotension or a redistribution of coronary blood flow so as to produce subendocardial ischemia.

II. Corticosteroids

A. Effects in Isolated Cardiac Tissue

Many investigators have found that relatively low concentrations of corticosteroids exert cardiotonic actions on isolated heart preparations. Although some preparations are more sensitive to corticosteroids than others, only rabbit atria appear to be unresponsive to corticosteroids (Briggs and Holland, 1959; Levy and Richards, 1962, 1964).

1. Mineralocorticoids

Aldosterone, the most potent naturally occurring mineralocorticoid, has been shown to exert a positive inotropic effect in papillary muscles isolated from cats (Lefer, 1967a,b; Loubatières and Sassine, 1963; Loubatières *et al.*, 1964; Sayers *et al.*, 1966; Tanz, 1960), guinea pigs (Sayers *et al.*, 1966), and monkeys (Nayler, 1965). This cardiotonic effect occurs at concentrations on the order of 10^{-9} M. Aldosterone was found to be ineffective over a wide range of concentrations in isolated frog hearts (Gross, 1960; Hajdu, 1957), and in rat trabeculae carneae (Ullrick and Hazelwood, 1963). This unresponsiveness is probably not due to a temperature effect, because aldosterone was shown to exert a slightly greater positive inotropic effect in mammalian cardiac tissues at 27° than at 37°C (Lefer, 1967b). Sayers and Solomon (1960) found a similar lack of temperature specificity with other corticosteroids in the rat heart–lung preparation.

In the blood-perfused rat heart–lung preparation, physiological concentrations of aldosterone enabled the heart to perform two to four times as much work as that performed without aldosterone (Ballard *et al.*, 1960). However, this effect may not have been due solely to an inotropic action, since one cannot exclude beneficial effects on the pulmonary vasculature in this preparation. In contrast, aldosterone (Areskog, 1962; Imai *et al.*, 1965) failed to exert a positive inotropic effect in the blood-perfused dog heart–lung preparation. This lack of response in the dog heart–lung preparation was probably not due to a concentration effect. More likely, aldosterone may exert a restorative effect only on the corticosteroid-deficient myocardium and may be ineffective in the presence of normal corticosteroid concentrations, since it was ineffective when perfused with normal blood (Areskog, 1962; Imai *et al.*, 1965) but was effective when perfused with corticosteroid-depleted blood (Ballard *et al.*, 1960).

Aldosterone exerts a maximum positive inotropic effect of only 20–35%, a value considerably less than that exerted by cardiac glycosides or catecholamines (Sayers *et al.*, 1966; Tanz and Kerby, 1961) under comparable experimental conditions. Therefore the modest cardiotonic effect of aldosterone should not be considered a substitute for cardiac glycosides or other inotropic agents in cardiac failure.

Other mineralocorticoids also exert positive inotropic effects in isolated cardiac tissue. Deoxycorticosterone (DOC) stimulates the isolated frog heart (Hajdu, 1957; Hajdu and Szent-Györgyi, 1952; Hoffmann, 1954; Loynes and Gowdey, 1952) and the dog heart–lung preparation (Areskog, 1962). Low doses of DOC have been reported to stimulate beating rat and chick heart fragments in tissue culture (McCarl *et al.*, 1965), but high doses of DOC are depressant in these preparations (Cornman and Gargus, 1957;

Cornman *et al.*, 1957). Similar biphasic effects occur in perfused guinea pig hearts (Hoffmann, 1954) and in isolated cat papillary muscles (Emele and Bonnycastle, 1956). In general, DOC in moderate doses (e.g., 10^{-8} to 10^{-7} M) exerts a small positive inotropic effect. High doses of DOC are generally depressant, although in some cases this depressant effect may be due to the steroid vehicle.

The potent synthetic mineralocorticoid 9α-fluorocortisol (9αFF) is also a cardiotonic steroid. Nayler (1957) found that 9αFF increased the work and efficiency of the isolated toad heart, but to a lesser extent than cardiac glycosides. Tanz and collaborators (1956, 1957) reported that 9αFF protected the cellular integrity of isolated cardiac muscle cells subjected to electrical stimulation in an isolated tissue bath. However, 2α-methyl-9α-fluorocortisol, which has mineralocorticoid potency similar to that of aldosterone, did not exert a significant inotropic effect in isolated cat papillary muscles (Lefer, 1967c). In this case the ethanol as a vehicle may have masked a potential inotropic effect. Several of these studies emphasize the importance of careful controls for the steroid vehicle, which may have direct cardiodepressant effects independent of the steroid molecules.

Most mineralocorticoids appear to exert positive inotropic effects that are modest when compared to the much larger inotropic effects observed with cardiac glycosides or catecholamines tested under the same conditions as the mineralocorticoids. There is a relatively long latent period for the inotropic effect of mineralocorticoids (i.e., about 20–60 min for attainment of the peak effect). This latency is similar to that observed with aldosterone in the intact animal and may represent a period of enzyme induction (Edelman *et al.*, 1963) or tissue binding (Hollander *et al.*, 1966) that may be obligatory for the action of these steroids. The inotropic effect of mineralocorticoids is probably not directly mediated by sodium and potassium transport or by coronary blood flow changes, since it can occur in the absence of these changes. The inotropic effect is enhanced under conditions of cardiac hypodynamia, a feature shared with many other inotropic agents (e.g., ouabain, norepinephrine) (Blinks and Koch-Weser, 1963).

2. Glucocorticoids

The two major naturally occurring glucocorticoids, corticosterone and cortisol, have not been shown to exert a significant inotropic effect. Several investigators have failed to find any significant inotropic activity of cortisol in the isolated frog (Hajdu and Szent-Györgyi, 1952), cat, or guinea pig heart (Sayers *et al.*, 1966); in the dog heart–lung preparation (Imai *et al.*, 1965); or in isolated papillary muscle preparations (Emele and Bonnycastle, 1956; Sayers *et al.*, 1966). Cortisol has been shown to stimulate the rate of embryonic chick heart fragments (Cornman and Gargus, 1957; Cornman *et al.,* 1957), the endurance of rat heart–lung preparations (Sayers and Solomon, 1960), and the overall performance of acidotic dog heart–lung preparations (Nobel-Allen *et al.,* 1973), but no direct inotropic measurements were made in any of these studies. Thus the beneficial or cardiotonic action of cortisol may have been due to a metabolic or cellular action independent of an inotropic effect.

Corticosterone did not stimulate the frog heart (Hajdu, 1957; Hajdu and Szent-Györgyi, 1952) or the dog heart–lung preparation (Areskog, 1962), and a cardiodepressant effect of corticosterone was reported in isolated rat hearts (Nasmyth, 1957) and in embryonic chick heart fragments (Cornman and Gargus, 1957). However, corticosterone was a potent cardiotonic agent in the rat heart–lung preparation (Sayers and Solomon, 1960; Solomon *et al.,* 1959). In these same experimental preparations, high doses of corticosterone clearly depressed the heart. Thus the evidence does not favor the view that corticosterone exerts a direct positive inotropic effect, even though it may improve cardiac function indirectly by other actions.

Several other glucocorticoids have been tested for inotropic activity in isolated heart preparations. Cortisone, in low to moderate concentrations, exerts a small cardiotonic effect in several mammalian preparations (Cornman *et al.,* 1957; Hoffmann, 1954; Tanz, 1960; Tanz and Kerby, 1961), but not in the isolated frog heart (Hajdu and Szent-Györgyi, 1952), whereas high doses of cortisone uniformly depressed the heart (Emele and Bonnycastle, 1956; Tanz, 1960). Prednisolone (Areskog, 1962; Lefer, 1967b; Tanz and Kerby, 1961), methylprednisolone, dexamethasone, and betamethasone (Lefer, 1967b) appear to have no significant inotropic activity in a variety of cardiac preparations.

Thus glucocorticoids exert little or no inotropic effects at moderate concentrations and only modest negative inotropic effects at high concentrations. The inotropic action of these steroids may be partially due to the mineralocorticoid effects exerted by these steroids at high doses. In this regard several of the more potent synthetic glucocorticoids that lack salt-retaining properties (e.g., prednisolone and methylprednisolone) are devoid of inotropic activity. Despite the lack of prominent inotropic effects, glucocorticoids may be essential for the maintenance of normal cardiac function by some other action, since glucocorticoids may be essential for the maintenance of normal cardiac performance in adrenalectomized animals.

B. Effects in Whole Animals

The cardiac effects of corticosteroids are more difficult to interpret in the whole animal. The rate of inactivation of corticosteroids is more rapid in the intact animal than in isolated systems because of the presence of the liver, kidneys, and other metabolic systems (e.g., plasma enzymes and blood cells). Furthermore, one cannot be sure of the directness of the effect in the whole animal unless cardiac or peripheral factors are rigidly controlled. Thus one must interpret effects in the whole animal with some degree of caution.

Loubatières and co-workers (1962, 1964; Loubatières and Sassine, 1963) studied the inotropic activity of a variety of corticosteroids in intact dogs and found that almost all the steroids tested demonstrated positive inotropic effects of greater magnitude than that observed in isolated heart preparations. Dexamethasone (Bouyard, 1965; Bouyard and Klein, 1963; Loubatières *et al.*, 1964) exerted a 70–80% increase in cardiac contractile force, whereas methylprednisolone, betamethasone, and triamcinolone exerted a 40–50% increase in contractile force (Bouyard, 1965; Bouyard and Klein, 1963; Loubatières *et al.*, 1964) in the anesthetized dog. These investigations also showed that small doses of aldosterone exerted a 15–25% increase in contractile force in anesthetized (Loubatières *et al.*, 1962) and in conscious dogs (Loubatières and Sassine, 1963). All these steroids were injected intravenously, so that systemic pressor effects (e.g., change in outflow resistance of the heart) may have modified the cardiac effects in these studies. The large magnitude of these changes is also surprising in view of the much smaller inotropic effects usually observed in isolated cardiac tissue. However, the responses were reported in percentage increases with no absolute values reported, and if the hearts were depressed from the anesthetic or the surgery, one would expect a relatively larger response than in normal animals. Moreover, these large effects have not been duplicated elsewhere (Lefer, 1967a,b; Novak *et al.*, 1970), even in dogs subjected to bilateral vagotomy and carotid sinus denervation (Jefferson *et al.*, 1971) in order to remove the neural regulatory mechanisms, which could mask potential myocardial or peripheral vascular effects, or both.

Cortisol usually is either inactive or only very weakly inotropic in the whole animal (Dalton *et al.*, 1968; Jefferson *et al.*, 1971; Kadowitz and Yard, 1970; Lefer, 1967a; Small *et al.*, 1959). However, Bouyard (1965) reported that moderate doses of cortisol exerted a negative inotropic effect in the dog heart. Since the aqueous form of cortisol was employed, the depressant effect obtained could not be attributed to a vehicle effect. Thus, as in isolated heart preparations, glucocorticoids are only very weakly cardiotonic or are ineffective. This, of course, does not rule out possible actions of these steroids on other aspects of cardiac function (i.e., myocardial metabolism).

C. Coronary Vascular Effects

Very few studies have been published on the coronary vascular effects of corticosteroids. These few studies all concern the effects of glucocorticoids. Vyden and co-workers (1974) reported that methylprednisolone (50 mg/kg) administered to dogs in acute myocardial ischemia resulted in a coronary vasodilation of about 20%. This effect occurred several hours after administration of the steroid and no vehicle controls were used. Moreover, it was really a reduction in the rate of decline in coronary flow rather than an absolute increase in flow. Previously, Spath *et al.* (1973) showed that methylprednisolone exerts a "vasodilator effect" in the pancreatic vasculature, but this effect was small, transient, and found to be due solely to the benzyl alcohol in the vehicle.

Vinas *et al.* (1977) recently reported that methylprednisolone (30 mg/kg) increased coronary blood flow in dogs undergoing cardiopulmonary bypass, but the flow in the control group was quite low. Therefore, in all probability, methylprednisolone prevented the decline in coronary flow observed in control dogs (i.e., cardiopulmonary bypass dogs not given steroid). Again, no vehicle controls were used, which also could have contributed to this effect, as was shown by Nayler and Seabra-Gomes (1976) in the perfused hypoxic rat heart.

In a well-controlled study, Beardsley *et al.* (1976a) studied the coronary vascular and inotropic action of isolated cat hearts perfused at constant coronary perfusion pressure. Moreover, this preparation was studied in control as well as in hearts subjected to myocardial ischemia. No significant coronary vascular or inotropic effect occurred over the 2-hr observation period at concentrations of methylprednisolone and dexamethasone up to $1 \times 10^{-3} M$. It is therefore unlikely that glucocorticoids exert any significant coronary vasoactive effect acutely.

D. Uptake of Corticosteroids by the Heart

Several important studies have appeared in recent years on the uptake of corticosteroids by cardiac tissue. Funder *et al.* (1973) showed that dexamethasone binds specifically to cardiac cytosol in the rat and dog. The higher-degree affinity was similar in both species and is suggestive of a cardiac receptor for glucocorticoids. Aldosterone also was taken up by hearts of both species; the process was not indicative of mineralocorticoid specific receptors in the heart. Beardsley *et al.* (1976b) extended these findings to cat cardiac tissue and reported a dramatic uptake of both dexamethasone and methylprednisolone under a variety of experimental conditions. Glucocorticoid uptake was temperature and pH dependent, being optimal at 37°C and pH 7.3–7.4. Maximal uptake occurred within 60 min and was independent of energy-requiring processes. Recent studies also indicate similar effects in the mouse heart (Coutard *et al.*, 1978) and the pig heart (Bottoms *et al.*, 1969).

Additional work has been conducted on the tissue uptake of [³H]methylprednisolone (Lefer *et al.*, 1977; Okuda and Lefer, 1977) and [³H]dexamethasone (Young *et al.*, 1977) in acute myocardial ischemia. Surprisingly, after the liver, kidney, and pancreas, the heart was the next highest organ extracting glucocorticoids both in normal and ischemic cats. Myocardial uptake was rapid, being essentially complete by 60 min. Moreover, myocardial tissue metabolized only about 15% of the ³H-labeled steroid taken up after 2 hr. This very low rate of metabolism of corticosteroids by myocardial tissue confirms the earlier finding of Travis and Sayers (1958), who reported a 10% degradation of cortisol by the rat heart over 90 min. These findings are consistent with an important role of glucocorticoids in cardiac tissue.

Okuda and associates (1976) studied the cellular localization of tritiated dexamethasone and methylprednisolone in the normal and ischemic cat heart. Although lesser amounts of steroid were taken up by ischemic hearts compared with nonischemic cardiac tissue, considerable amounts of steroid accumulated in ischemic tissue. Cardiac homogenates were subjected to sucrose-density gradient centrifugation to localize the organelles taking up the steroids. Most of the glucocorticoid was associated with a plasma membrane fraction and with a lysosomal fraction. These two fractions accounted for 90% of the label taken up by the heart. These data are consistent with a membrane stabilizing action of the glucocorticoids both in nonischemic and ischemic hearts and help explain the beneficial action of glucocorticoids in preserving ischemic myocardial tissue in the absence of significant inotropic, chronotropic, or coronary vasodilator effects.

E. Glucocorticoids in Myocardial Infarction

In recent years increasing attention has been given to pharmacological means of modifying the degree of ischemic damage in acute infarction. In 1965 Ebaid and co-workers reported that large doses of cortisol in patients and in dogs reduced S-T segment elevation of the electrocardiogram. These results were extended by Libby *et al.* (1973), who showed that cortisol given intravenously at a dose of 50 mg/kg shortly after occlusion of the left anterior descending coronary artery effectively reduced electrocardiographic, histological, and enzymatic indices of infarct extension.

In 1974 Spath *et al.* found that the synthetic glucocorticoid methylprednisolone, at a dose of 30 mg/kg, prevented the spread of ischemic damage in the cat subjected to acute myocardial ischemia. Methylprednisolone was even more effective when given 1 hr after the onset of ischemia than when it was given before ischemia. These workers also provided firm evidence that stabilization of lysosomal membranes may be one of the major mechanisms of its protective effect. These findings were also confirmed using dexamethasone (Spath and Lefer, 1975) in the same experimental model, which also stabilized lysosomes in the ischemic portion of the myocardium.

In the last few years, many papers on the effect of glucocorticoids in myocardial ischemia in man and in experimental animals (Beardsley *et al.*, 1976a; Busuttil *et al.*, 1975; Da Luz *et al.*, 1976; Hoffstein *et al.*, 1976; Masters *et al.*, 1976; Morrison *et al.*, 1975, 1976; Osher *et al.*, 1976; Roberts *et al.*, 1976; Shatney *et al.*, 1976; Toyama and Reis, 1975) have been published. Most of these indicated that steroids exert a beneficial effect. Two prominent clinical studies showed data indicating a preservation of jeopardized myocardial tissue with one or two doses of methylprednisolone (Morrison *et al.*, 1975, 1976). In these important clinical series, the steroid was given acutely and resulted in a decreased mortality as well as a reduction in infarct size. This protective action of methylprednisolone was challenged by Roberts *et al.* (1976), who reported that multiple doses of glucocorticoid (i.e., every 6 hrs for 48 hrs) were deleterious to patients with myocardial infarction. Unfortunately, these investigators waited at least 7 hr after the first elevation in plasma creatine phosphokinase before initiation of treatment. These results indicate that care must be taken in giving an appropriate dose of glucocorticoid very soon after the onset of myocardial ischemia and that administration of the glucocorticoid should not be prolonged beyond about 8 hr after the first dose. Another group of investigators failing to observe a beneficial effect of methylprednisolone observed the effects of this steroid for only 2 hr after its administration (Osher *et al.*, 1976), which may not have been long enough to observe a protective effect on myocardial performance and integrity.

Other studies have helped clarify the mechanism of the protective effect of glucocorticoids in myocardial ischemia. Busuttil and co-workers (1975) reported that methylprednisolone preserves myocardial lysosomal integrity and modulates cyclic GMP levels in myocardial ischemia. Moreover, the interrelationship between cyclic GMP and cyclic AMP may be important in the regulation of lysosomal membrane integrity (Busuttil *et al.*, 1975). Additional evidence for the preservation of myocardial lysosomal integrity by methylprednisolone in ischemia was provided by Hoffstein and co-workers (1976), who showed ultrastructurally that lysosomal disruption is an early consequence of ischemia and that this can be prevented by methylprednisolone. Similarly, Nayler and Seabra-Gomes (1976) showed methyl-prednisolone to prevent the loss of intracellular enzymes, including creatine phosphokinase in the hypoxic perfused rat heart consistent with a cellular protective effect.

Recently Toyama and Reis (1975) reported that cortisol can significantly reduce the decrease in myocardial compliance observed in myocardial ischemia. This would prevent impairment of ventricular performance and enable the jeopardized myocardium to function more normally. Other investigators have proposed metabolic actions as the mechanism of the protective effect of glucocorticoids in myocardial ischemia (Da Luz *et al.*, 1976; Masters *et al.*, 1976). In this regard, methylprednisolone has been thought to improve coronary collateral flow or to enhance carbohydrate metabolism (i.e., producing a positive lactate balance or enhancing cardiac glucose uptake). However, these effects of glucocorticoids are neither well established nor are they able to account completely for the protective effect in myocardial ischemia. Thus carefully obtained data suggest that glucocorticoids are ineffective in improving collateral flow in the coronary bed during ischemia (Eckstein, 1954).

One of the most important recent studies of glucocorticoids in myocardial ischemia was reported by Shatney and collaborators (1976). These investigators measured infarct volume in the dog heart with a combination of histochemical and morphological techniques, and they clearly showed that methylprednisolone reduces the size of the developing infarct. Furthermore, the optimal time for methylprednisolone administration was found to be 1 hr after the onset of the ischemic event. This agrees closely with earlier studies that 1-hr post-ischemia is appropriate for glucocorticoid administration (Spath *et al.*, 1974; Spath and Lefer, 1975).

It now appears clear that pharmacological administration of glucocorticoids early in the infarction process is of definite benefit to the jeopardized myocardial tissue and helps to prevent the extension of the infarcted myocardium. This beneficial effect occurs in man as well as in experimental animals (e.g., cat, dog). Although the mechanism of the protective effect of glucocorticoids is not fully known, several groups of investigators have suggested hemodynamic, metabolic, and membrane stabilization as their major mode of action. Present data favor lysosomal and cell membrane stabilization as an important phase of the protective effect, although other mechanisms may be involved. Clearly, additional work on this important subject is necessary to resolve these questions.

No direct data are available on the effects of mineralocorticoids in myocardial ischemia. However, based on their physiological properties (e.g., positive inotropic effect) the relative lack of cardiac receptors for them, and their failure to stabilize lysosomal and cellular membranes, it would be unlikely that they would be of benefit in acute myocardial ischemia. Similar conclusions have been drawn between the efficacy of the glucocorticoids and mineralocorticoids in circulatory shock (Lefer and Spath, 1977).

Table 1 summarizes the cardiac effects of glucocorticoids and mineralocorticoids and their actions in the ischemic myocardium.

III. Pancreatic Hormones

The pancreas secretes three hormones: glucagon, insulin, and somatostatin. Glucagon and insulin function in the regulation of blood glucose concentration and metabolism, whereas somatostatin is known to inhibit both glucagon and insulin release from the endocrine pancreas. In addition to their basic metabolic actions, glucagon and insulin produce cardiac effects at pharmacological levels and these actions may be of potential interest in certain cardiovascular disorders.

A. Glucagon

Glucagon, the pancreatic hyperglycemic factor, has been extensively examined for cardiac actions. It is a polypeptide hormone consisting of 29 amino acid residues and has a molecular weight of 3485 daltons (Bromer *et al.*, 1975). Farah and Tuttle (1960) demonstrated positive inotropic and chronotropic responses to glucagon in a variety of species. Subsequently, other investigators have confirmed cardiac activity of glucagon and have attempted to establish the mechanism of action and potency of the cardiac action of this hormone.

Farah and Tuttle's initial work (1960) revealed an increased force of contraction in isolated atria from rats, dogs, cats, and guinea pigs at glucagon concentrations ranging from 3 to 170 nM. Physiological concentrations of glucagon fluctuate around 57 pM (200 pg/ml) (Goodner *et al.*, 1977), indicating that cardiac stimulation occurs at concentrations three orders of magnitude greater than those present *in vivo*. Therefore physiological actions of glucagon do not include alteration of cardiac contractile strength, but pharmacological doses of this agent can produce significant positive inotropic effects.

Many investigators also found substantial positive inotropic effects of glucagon on ventricular tissue. Farah and Tuttle (1960) observed an increase in contractility of the dog heart–lung preparation at a final circulating glucagon concentration of 15 nM. Isolated right ventricular cat papillary muscles increased active tension development 0–50% in response to gluca-

TABLE I

Cardiac Effects of Corticosteroids

Hormone	Inotropic effect	Chronotropic effect	Coronary vasoactive effect	Comments	Action on ischemic myocardium
Mineralocorticoids	Moderate positive effect	None	None	Moderate uptake, no membrane stabilization	Unknown, but unlikely to protect
Glucocorticoids	None	None	None directly, may help preserve vasculature	Large uptake, stabilizes lysosomal and cell membranes	Preserves myocardial integrity

gon in the concentration range from 14 nM to 14 μM (Marcus *et al.*, 1971; Glick *et al.*, 1968). Glucagon also elicited elevations in contractile activity of isolated perfused rat hearts (Mayer *et al.*, 1970) and intact canine hearts (Glick *et al.*, 1968), the latter experiencing a 73% increase in the first derivative of left ventricular pressure development (dP/dt max) after a bolus dose of 50 μg/kg glucagon. These studies firmly established inotropic activity attributable to glucagon.

Investigators attempting to determine the potency of glucagon often compared its inotropic actions to those of epinephrine. Mayer *et al.* (1970) found glucagon and epinephrine to increase contractility equally in isolated perfused rat hearts at concentrations from 30 to 300 pM, but higher concentrations of epinephrine continued to increase contractile activity, whereas glucagon did not (Mayer *et al.*, 1970). Maximal responses to the two agents revealed epinephrine to elevate contractility double the extent of glucagon. Regan and co-workers (1964) also noted similar increases in left ventricular dP/dt max in dogs with 14 nmoles glucagon or 28 nmoles epinephrine. Thus glucagon is a moderately potent inotropic agent, with its maximal stimulation of the heart being less than that elicited by catecholamines.

The mechanism by which glucagon stimulates the myocardium was initially believed to be mediated by β-adrenergic receptors, because dichloroisoproterenol, a β-adrenergic antagonist, prevented cardiac actions (Farah and Tuttle, 1960). Reserpine, a catecholamine depleting agent, did not reduce the glucagon response (Farah and Tuttle, 1960), and therefore, glucagon was assumed to stimulate the β-adrenergic receptor directly rather than act via a catecholamine releasing action. However, subsequent studies using more effective β-adrenergic antagonists, such as propranolol, did not reduce cardiac responsiveness to glucagon (Glick *et al.*, 1968; Lucchesi, 1968). These reports indicated that glucagon is devoid of β-adrenergic agonistic properties and does not require the release of catecholamines to stimulate cardiac tissue.

Cardiac actions of glucagon were also found to be independent of changes in blood sugar, which result from glucagon administration. Farah and Tuttle (1960) subjected the dog heart–lung preparation to low (9 mg/dl) and high (280 mg/dl) glucose concentrations and found unaltered inotropic responses to glucagon. Inotropic actions of glucagon, therefore, cannot be attributed to alterations in blood sugar.

The basis for the cardiac activity of glucagon is now presumed to be related to its well-known ability to stimulate adenyl cyclase, which increases cyclic AMP production. Brunt and McNeill (1978) recently reported increased cyclic AMP levels preceding contractility responses to glucagon in the isolated perfused rat heart. These investigators also found low doses of theophylline, a phosphodiesterase inhibitor, to potentiate the inotropic responses to glucagon (1978), as have others (Marcus *et al.,* 1971). Lucchesi (1968), employing higher levels of theophylline (10 mg/kg) in dogs, eliminated inotropic actions of glucagon. These results implicate cyclic AMP as the mediator of glucagon-induced contractility responses, because high doses of theophylline eliminated glucagon responses, whereas lower doses potentiated them. These two agents, therefore, appear to act via a common mechanism of action, with theophylline being the more potent agent.

Nevertheless, cyclic AMP has not gained universal acceptance as the basis for the cardiac activity of glucagon (Mayer *et al.,* 1970). These investigators demonstrated a separation of inotropic and cyclic AMP responses to glucagon in the isolated rat heart. After treatment with dichloroisoproterenol, glucagon increased cyclic AMP levels without changes in contractility. These investigators also found the initiation of the inotropic response to glucagon in normal tissue to precede cyclic AMP increases, thus making a cyclic AMP mediation of the inotropic response unlikely because of the temporal sequence of events (Mayer *et al.,* 1970). Despite this challenge, activation of adenyl cyclase remains the most attractive explanation of the cardiac actions of glucagon.

Although the exact relationship between glucagon, cyclic AMP, and contractility has not been clearly established, one agent known to be essential for the contractile activity of glucagon is calcium. Visscher and Lee (1972) demonstrated increased inotropic responses to glucagon, as external calcium was reduced in isolated perfused cat heart preparations. No inotropic effect of glucagon was observed in calcium-free perfusate where the heart was arrested. Entman *et al.* (1969) revealed a cyclic AMP stimulation of calcium uptake by isolated microsomal fractions of dog hearts. Glucagon stimulated adenyl cyclase to increase calcium uptake by these fractions. Actions of glucagon required more time than those of cyclic AMP, thus supporting the role of cyclic AMP as a second messenger (Entman *et al.,* 1969). This increase in sarcoplasmic binding of calcium is also in agreement with Visscher and Lee's work (1972), since they could not detect an increase in calcium accumulation by hearts after glucagon treatment. Glucagon, therefore, may act to alter intracellular calcium distribution in producing its inotropic actions.

Other cardiac effects of glucagon include an increased heart rate and coronary vasodilation. The chronotropic action has been observed in a variety of species (Farah and Tuttle, 1960), including man (Dhingra *et al.,* 1974). Chronotropic responses to glucagon were sustained after wide variations in extracellular glucose levels (Farah and Tuttle, 1960). The chronotropic action of glucagon, therefore, is unrelated to adrenergic mechanisms or blood sugar alterations, but it is believed to result from elevation of cyclic AMP.

The chronotropic activity of glucagon discussed previously referred to glucagon effects on the sinoatrial node, the primary pacemaker of the heart. Chronotropic effects of glucagon are not restricted to this node but also influence other pacemaker tissue in the heart. Lucchesi and others (1969) demonstrated a 300% increase in heart rate when glucagon (4 μg/kg) was administered to dogs after their sinoatrial nodes were crushed. Glucagon has also been shown to enhance canine atrioventricular (A-V) conduction (Lipski *et al.,* 1972) and was capable of eliminating A-V block in some studies in dogs (Steiner *et al.,* 1969) and in humans (Kones, 1971), thereby suggesting it as a possible therapeutic agent for conduction abnormalities. Glucagon, then, affects the cardiac conduction system to increase the frequency of action potentials in nodal tissue and to stimulate the conduction of impulses from the atria to the ventricles.

Glucagon increases coronary perfusion in dogs (Nayler *et al.,* 1970) and man (Manchester *et al.,* 1970). Goldschlager and associates (1969) and Nayler *et al.* (1977), however, noted parallel elevations in coronary flow and oxygen utilization in humans and dogs. This relationship between flow and oxygen demand suggests that the glucagon-induced coronary dilation resulted from increased oxygen demand rather than from a direct action of glucagon. Moir and Nayler (1970) confirmed this supposition in the potassium-arrested isolated perfused dog hearts. Glucagon had no effect on coronary flow in the arrested heart, whereas other dilators (e.g., isoproterenol and nitroglycerin) retained their effectiveness. Glucagon, therefore, is an indirect dilator of the coronary circulation, the dilation stemming from increased oxygen demand produced by its inotropic action.

In summary, glucagon produces significant increases in cardiac contractility and modest increases in rate, and only indirectly dilates coronary vasculature. Inotropic and chronotropic actions are not related to glucose concentrations, adrenergic receptors, or endogenous catecholamine release. The cardiac actions of glucagon probably result from a stimulation of adenylate cyclase to increase cyclic AMP levels, which may increase calcium storage in the sarcoplasmic reticulum. Calcium has been firmly established as a requisite cofactor for the inotropic action of glucagon.

These marked cardiac effects of glucagon have made it a potential therapeutic agent for selected cardiovascular disorders. The inotropic effects of glucagon stimulated interest in its applicability to conditions of heart failure and myocardial infarction. However, the inotropic action of glucagon in experimental heart failure has been reported to be inconsistent, being either absent (Gold *et al.,* 1970; Winokur *et al.,* 1975) or present under a variety of experimental conditions (Cornman *et al.*, 1957; Nobel-Allen *et al.*, 1973). Although heart failure was induced by identical procedures in those studies reporting glucagon inotropic activity, hearts were examined *in vivo*, and in those hearts not responding to glucagon, they were tested *in vitro*. The data on glucagon in chronic heart failure, therefore, is inconclusive, although glucagon remains a possibility for treatment of this disorder.

Glucagon has been examined in cases of myocardial infarction by a host of investigators. Diamond and associates (1971) revealed an increase in contractility in humans suffering from myocardial infarction, as have Puri and Bing (1969) in dogs. The benefit of increasing myocardial contractility remains doubtful, though, because glucagon increases oxygen demand in conjunction with increases in contractility. The elevated requirement for oxygen could further jeopardize the ischemic myocardium. Alternatively, subinotropic concentrations of glucagon have been found to improve recovery of isolated perfused rat hearts subjected to brief hypoxic episodes (Busuttil *et al.*, 1976). Reduced cyclic GMP concentrations were cited by these investigators as the basis for the salutary action of glucagon. Although the inotropic activity of glucagon appears to be of little value in treatment of myocardial infarction, its influence on cell biochemistry may be beneficial. The myocardial actions of glucagon and their applicability to ischemic states are listed in Table II.

The most successful clinical application of glucagon to a cardiac abnormality is in myocardial conduction defects. In addition to abolishing a complete A-V block in man (Kones, 1971), it has also been shown to be effective in dogs after A-V block of different etiologies. After blockade of the A-V node with formalin, glucagon (50 μg/kg) increased ventricular rate by 33%, indicating a stimulation of ventricular pacemaker tissue (Hurwitz, 1971). A reversal of depressed conduction produced by propranolol again indicated no β-adrenergic receptor involvement in cardiac actions of glucagon and also exhibited another potential clinical application for glucagon in instances of propranolol overdoses (Whitsitt and Lucchesi, 1968). Myocardial clinical uses of glucagon, then, primarily center around treatment for depressed or blocked conduction of electrical impulses. Alternative possibilities include treatment of chronic heart failure, and in small doses glucagon may improve recovery from ischemic injuries of short durations.

B. Insulin

Insulin is the major hormone secreted by the pancreas. Insulin produces cardiac actions of a lesser magnitude than does glucagon, and thus has generated less interest than glucagon. Insulin, however, is essential for

TABLE II

Cardiac Effects of Pancreatic Hormones

Hormone	Inotropic effect	Chronotropic effect	Coronary vasoactive effect	Comments	Action on ischemic myocardium
Glucagon	Large positive effect	Increases heart rate	Modest dilation	Lysosomal labilization	Does not protect in ischemia
Insulin	Moderate positive effect	None	Slight dilation	Stimulates glucose uptake	Does not protect directly in ischemia
Somatostatin	None	Not known	No clear-cut effect	Has not been well studied	Not known

normal myocardial function and is also considered to have therapeutic potential.

Insulin has been reported to produce modest positive inotropic actions in isolated tissues in piglets, cats (Lee and Downing, 1976), and rabbits (Snow, 1976; Sassine *et al.*, 1975) and *in vivo* in lambs (Downing *et al.*, 1977) and piglets (Nudel *et al.*, 1977). Insulin increased tension development (i.e., *dP/dt* max) in these preparations by 20–40% at concentrations of 1 mU to 1 U/ml. Physiological concentrations of insulin are 20 μU/ml (Sherwin *et al.*, 1977), indicating cardiac stimulation at values two to four orders of magnitude greater than physiological concentrations. No contractile response to insulin was observed at concentrations lower than 100 μU/ml in isolated perfused rat hearts (Gmeiner *et al.*, 1974), emphasizing the requirement for extremely high insulin levels to obtain an inotropic action.

Insulin produced moderate increases in contractility without β-adrenergic receptor involvement; Nudel and co-workers (1977) reported the β-receptor antagonist, practolol, potentiated the inotropic action of insulin. Lee and Downing (1976) also reported no change in time to peak tension development after addition of insulin to cat papillary muscles, whereas catecholamines markedly decrease this parameter. Alterations in glucose concentrations also have no effect on cardiac responsiveness to insulin (Lee and Downing, 1976). Insulin, therefore, increases contractility of myocardial tissue independent of glucose alterations or catecholamine receptors.

However, insulin may affect cardiac contractility by altering responses to other humoral agents. Lee and Downing (1976) found insulin to depress contractility responses to norepinephrine, and a similar suppression of the inotropic activity of epinephrine was also observed (Nudel *et al.*, 1977). Additionally, Regan *et al.* (1963) reported the positive inotropic effect of acetylstrophanthidin to be reduced in the presence of insulin. Insulin actions on the heart, therefore, are not restricted to direct effects; they also include modulation of other hormonal actions, including those of catecholamines.

Insulin probably does not alter heart rate; most investigators have found no chronotropic action except in the presence of an epinephrinelike impurity (Puri and Bing, 1969). The increase in coronary perfusion by insulin in lamb hearts appears to be accompanied by a decrease in oxygen extraction (Downing *et al.*, 1977), and this finding has been confirmed in man (Rogers *et al.*, 1977). These data indicate the coronary vasodilator action of insulin to be unrelated to an increase in oxygen demand produced by its inotropic effect.

In summary, insulin has been demonstrated to produce a weak positive inotropic effect, increasing contractility in animal hearts maximally about

20–30% above control values. Insulin does not alter heart rate, but it dilates the coronary vasculature independently of a metabolic effect. Cardiac actions of insulin also include depression of other hormonal inotropic actions, insulin being capable of eliminating the responses to catecholamines and acetylstrophanthidin.

Other cardiac actions of insulin are of greater importance physiologically. Regan and co-workers (1974) found diabetic dog hearts to have an increased resistance to filling, possibly caused by increased glycoprotein content of the interstitium. Insulin (0.1 U/ml) increased protein synthesis in ribosomes of diabetic rat hearts (Stirewolt and Wool, 1966) and decreased protein degradation (Goodner *et al.*, 1977). The reduction in protein catabolism may involve an insulin action to lower the lysosomal enzyme content of hearts, as Wildenthal (1973) has described. Actions of insulin, as revealed by these studies, also include regulation of cardiac protein balance, with insulin increasing protein synthesis and inhibiting degradation.

Another prominent metabolic action of insulin and one that has received extensive clinical attention is its stimulation of myocardial glucose uptake (Morgan *et al.*, 1960; Gmeiner *et al.*, 1974; Regan *et al.*, 1974). Insulin stimulation of glucose uptake persists in anoxia, with anoxia and insulin acting together to accelerate glucose uptake greater than either factor alone (Gmeiner *et al.*, 1974). Morgan *et al.* (1960) also found insulin to increase transmembranal transport of glucose, whereas anoxia stimulated transport and intracellular phosphorylation. It was reasoned that insulin in combination with hypoxia, such as that encountered during coronary occlusion, would increase glucose uptake and stimulate glycolysis to result in increased high-energy phosphate production. However, Liedtke and co-workers (1976) revealed a worsened mechanical function of globally ischemic swine hearts receiving insulin than in those receiving no treatment. Hearts treated with insulin also survived for shorter periods despite an elevation in glocuse uptake (Liedtke *et al.*, 1976). All hearts rendered ischemic showed inhibition of glycolysis at the glyceraldehyde-3-phosphate dehydrogenase step, which indicates that insulin is not capable of elevating anaerobic glycolysis sufficiently to supply myocardial energy demands in low-flow conditions.

Another function of insulin thought to promote improved functioning of infarcted myocardium is a reduction in free fatty acid content of plasma (Ahmed *et al.*, 1978). Rogers and co-workers (1976) attributed a significant improvement in survival of patients with myocardial infarction to this reduction of free fatty acids. In contrast, Ahmed *et al.* (1978) found insulin to improve myocardial function and electrolyte distribution after coronary artery occlusion in dogs whether fatty acid levels were reduced or sustained at high levels. Beneficial actions of insulin in patients with coronary artery disease are not universal findings, however; Lesch and co-workers (1974) observed worsened signs of acute myocardial ischemia and elevated left ventricular end-diastolic pressures during atrial pacing in patients with coronary artery disease. Thus the benefit of insulin in ischemic heart disease is somewhat questionable, both positive and negative effects being noted in cardiac patients. The major cardiac actions of insulin and their applicability to ischemic heart disease are summarized in Table II.

C. Somatostatin (SRIF)

Somatostatin, the most recently discovered pancreatic hormone, has not been extensively investigated previously for cardiac actions. Trachte and Lefer (1979) examined effects of somatostatin in final bath concentrations of 1 ng/ml to 1.0 μg/ml on right ventricular cat papillary muscles and isolated cat coronary arteries perfused at a constant flow. Papillary muscles responded with a slight increase of $5 \pm 1.5\%$ in active tension development at the highest concentration utilized (i.e., 1 μg/ml). Coronary vessels did not react to somatostatin with a change in perfusion pressure at any concentration employed. These data reveal no marked effects of somatostatin on cardiac tissue, the inotropic effect being trivial when compared to other known inotropic substances.

IV. Renin–Angiotensin System

The renin–angiotensin system is a diffuse humoral system that generates several biologically potent vasoconstrictors (i.e., angiotensin II, angiotensin III). Renin is released by the kidneys and enzymatically cleaves angiotensinogen, which is produced by the liver, to the decapeptide angiotensin I. Angiotensin I is then converted to the biologically active octapeptide angiotensin II by converting enzyme (EC 3.4.15.1), with the pulmonary circulation containing the highest titer of this enzyme. Angiotensin II can be reduced to a heptapeptide with biologic activity, angiotensin III, by aminopeptidases. Two excellent reviews of this system have appeared recently (Reid *et al.*, 1978; Peach, 1977) and should be consulted further for clarification of this system. Each component of the system produces different degrees of cardiac stimulation and will be discussed separately.

A. Renin

Renin, the initiator of the system, is simply an endopeptidase that cleaves a decapeptide fragment (angiotensin I) from the angiotensinogen molecule. Renin produced no noticeable cardiac effects in the isolated perfused cat heart, according to Hill and Andrus (1940), which indicates an inability of renin to stimulate cardiac tissue directly.

B. Angiotensin I

Angiotensin I, which has some biologic activity in certain vascular beds, stimulates isolated rabbit atria to maximally increase tension development 60% at 10^{-6} M (Bonnardeaux et al., 1977). Right atrial myocardial tissue exhibited a greater sensitivity to the decapeptide than left atrial tissue (Bonndardeaux et al., 1977). The enhancement of contractility in these preparations was reduced after application of converting enzyme inhibition (CEI), revealing a dependency on conversion to angiotensin II for biologic activity (Ackerly and Peach, 1975). Inotropic actions of angiotensin I, however, were not reduced by converting enzyme blockade in isolated right ventricular cat papillary muscles, as is shown in Fig. 1 (Trachte and Lefer, 1979). Angiotensin I produced moderate increases in active tension development (maximal stimulation 50%), being the least potent angiotensin inotropically in ventricular myocardial tissue.

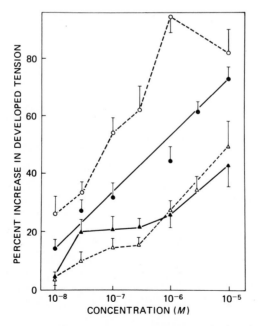

Fig. 1.   Biological activity of angiotensin in cat papillary muscle. △- - -△, angiotensin I (10); ▲—▲, CEI plus angiotensin I (6); ○- - -○; angiotensin II (6); ●—●, angiotensin III (12). The number in parenthesis is the number of entries studied.

Angiotensin I has been reported to have slight positive chronotropic activities (Bonnardeaux and Regoli, 1974) and is capable of constricting the coronary vasculature. However, both Gerlings and Gilmore (1973) and Britton and Di Salvo (1973) observed reduced coronary vascular responses to angiotensin I after converting enzyme blockade in dogs, indicating angiotensin II as the primary coronary constrictor. Recent data in isolated cat coronary arteries also show a reduction in constriction (i.e., smaller increase in pressure) in response to angiotensin I after converting enzyme inhibition (Trachte and Lefer, 1979). These data are depicted in Fig. 2. The results suggest a slight direct action of angiotensin I on the coronary vasculature with the majority of the decapeptide action being due to angiotensin II formation.

C. Angiotensin II

Angiotensin II is the most potent angiotensin regarding cardiac actions, as can be clearly seen in Figs. 1 and 2. Angiotensin II has been known to increase the contractility of cardiac tissue in a variety of preparations, in-

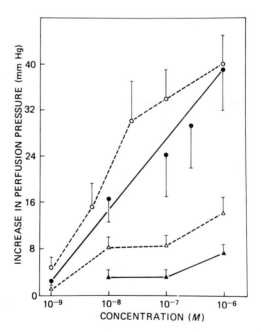

Fig. 2.   Biological activity of angiotensin in cat coronary arteries. △- - -△, angiotensin I (7); ▲—▲, CEI plus angiotensin I (14); ○- - -○, angiotensin II (9); ●—●, angiotensin III (7). The number in parenthesis is the number of entries studied.

cluding isolated cat hearts (Hill and Andrus, 1940), cat papillary muscles (Koch-Weser, 1964; Lefer, 1967), isolated cat (Koch-Weser, 1964) and rabbit atria (Bonnardeaux *et al.*, 1977), and dog heart–lung preparations (Mayer *et al.*, 1970). The increase in contractility produced by angiotensin II in papillary muscles can be seen in Fig. 1. The maximal stimulation occurred at 10^{-6} M and produced a 100% increase in active tension development. Koch-Weser (1964) found the maximal increase in contractility to angiotensin II to be less than that of norepinephrine (100% vs. 190%). Thus, although angiotensin II is a stronger inotropic stimulus than other angiotensins or pancreatic hormones, it is not as potent as the catecholamines in this respect.

Angiotensin II actions on the myocardium were initially suspected to result from release of catecholamines, an action of angiotensin known to occur at adrenal medullary (Peach, 1971) and nerve terminal sites (Peach, 1977). Koch-Wester (1965) demonstrated no catecholamine component of cardiac actions of angiotensin II. Neither β-blockade with nethalide nor catecholamine depletion with reserpine altered the contractile responses to angiotensin II (Koch-Weser, 1965). Additionally, Koch-Weser (1965) demonstrated a slight prolongation of the time required to develop peak tension after angiotensin, unlike catecholamines, which are known to shorten this period. Dempsey *et al.* (1971) also found intact angiotensin II responses after β-blockade with propranolol in cat papillary muscles. Thus, although angiotensin II can release catecholamines, inotropic effects appear to be exerted by a direct angiotensin action on the myocardium. This dual action of angiotensin II in cardiac tissue was recently clarified by Blumberg and co-workers (1975), who found angiotensin II to potentiate inotropic responses to tyramine (a catecholamine releasing agent) as well as to produce an inotropic effect through stimulation of angiotensin receptors. The predominant action of angiotensin II is probably its direct stimulation of angiotensin receptors, since catecholamine depletion or receptor blockade did not reduce its cardiac stimulation.

The threshold for inotropic responses to angiotensin is about 1 nM. Circulating physiological levels of angiotensin II, however, usually do not exceed 100 pM (Morton *et al.*, 1977), probably indicating no major role of angiotensin II in physiological regulation of cardiac contractility. However, during hemorrhage, circulating angiotensin II plasma concentrations exceed 1 nM (Morton *et al.*, 1977), a concentration greater than that required for myocardial activity. Therefore angiotensin II may influence cardiac contractility during certain situations, especially if these states also are characterized by increased sympathetic stimulation, such as in hemorrhage. In these instances angiotensin can influence cardiac contractility by potentiating sympathetic actions in addition to stimulating the heart directly.

The inotropic actions of angiotensin II appear to result primarily from stimulation of myocardial angiotensin II receptors. Catecholamine receptors are not involved, as was demonstrated by catecholamine depletion and β-adrenergic receptor blockade. Angiotensin II, however, can potentiate the release of catecholamines from nerve terminals and in this way can potentiate cardiac sympathetic responses. Maximal inotropic actions of angiotensin II were large but of a smaller magnitude than those of catecholamines.

Angiotensin II was observed to produce a decrease in heart rate when injected into intact dogs (Farr and Grupp, 1967); however, an increase in heart rate was noted with angiotensin II after baroreceptor denervation or buffering of blood pressure (Krasney et al., 1965). Sympathetic nervous blockade with bretylium tosylate or β-adrenergic blockade prevented the cardioaccelerator response to angiotensin II, revealing an adrenergic component to chronotropic actions of angiotensin II.

Krasney and co-workers (1965, 1967) observed no alteration of the chronotropic response to angiotensin II after adrenalectomy, thus eliminating catecholamines of adrenal origin from involvement in angiotensin II-induced heart rate changes. These results indicate that angiotensin II releases catecholamines at the level of the heart to produce increases in heart rate. Adrenal catecholamine release was shown not to be involved in this action. Positive chronotropic responses to angiotensin II were only observed in the absence of baroreceptor reflexes; a decrease in heart rate resulted when these reflexes were present.

Angiotensin II constricts all vascular beds, including the coronary vasculature. Lorber (1942) and Hill and Andrus (1940) noted a constrictor action of angiotensin II in isolated cat hearts, as did Gerlings and Gilmore (1973) in isolated dog hearts. Trachte and Lefer (1979) expanded on this work utilizing isolated perfused coronary arteries, and, as can be seen in Fig. 2, angiotensin II constricts these vessels in concentrations exceeding 1 ng/ml. The degree of constriction was similar to that of angiotensin III but was much more potent than that of angiotensin I.

The coronary constrictor activity of angiotensin II may be of significance in control of coronary blood flow in vivo. Gavras et al. (1978a) found an increased coronary blood flow after administration of an angiotensin converting enzyme inhibitor (i.e., teprotide) in sodium-depleted dogs. However, it had no effect in animals having normal sodium balance. Sodium depletion stimulates renin release, which increases angiotensin II production. The increased coronary flow after converting enzyme inhibition probably indicates a coronary constriction induced by angiotensin II in sodium-depleted animals (Gavras et al., 1978a). Interpretation of these results, however, is complicated by bradykinin-potentiating activities of teprotide, bradykinin being a vasodilator (Murthy *et al.*, 1977).

Cardiac actions of angiotensin II may be classified as positive inotropic and as coronary constrictor with variable chronotropic effects. The direct inotropic response is relatively large and is independent of catecholamines. Angiotensin II also influences cardiac tissue by potentiating the sympathetic nervous stimulation of contractility. Constrictor activity of angiotensin II is produced by direct stimulation of the angiotensin II receptor in coronary vascular smooth muscle. Chronotropic actions are mediated by nervous pathways, decreasing heart rate if pressoreceptors and reflex pathways are intact or increasing heart rate by catecholamine release if these pathways are interrupted.

These actions of angiotensin II make it highly unsuitable for use in ischemic heart disease. This agent decreases myocardial blood supply by constricting the coronary vasculature and increases myocardial oxygen demand by increasing contractility, two actions that would further compromise myocardial function in ischemic states. Angiotensin II also increases total peripheral resistance, which increases the amount of cardiac work required to pump blood. Gavras and others (1971) have found a prolonged infusion of angiotensin II to produce myocardial infarctions in rabbits, further emphasizing the negative actions of high levels on cardiac function.

Patients suffering from chronic heart failure have responded positively to inhibition of angiotensin-converting enzyme (Gavras *et al.*, 1978b). Many of these patients exhibited improved cardiac output and lowered left ventricular end-diastolic pressures after enzyme inhibition, indicating improved cardiac function. Saralasin, an angiotensin II receptor antagonist, also produced similar changes in 45% of the patients with chronic heart failure tested (Turini *et al.*, 1978). The improvement in cardiac function was attributed to reduced afterload, indicating that angiotensin II influences cardiac function by systemic as well as direct myocardial effects. Table III summarizes the undesirable effects of angiotensin II in myocardial ischemia.

D. Angiotensin III

Angiotensin III generally produces cardiac effects similar to those of angiotensin II. Bonnardeaux *et al.* (1977) observed angiotensin III to be equipotent to angiotensin II in increasing tension development in isolated rabbit atria. Trachte and Lefer (1979) found angiotensin III to be less potent than angiotensin II in isolated cat papillary muscles (Fig. 1). As can be seen, angiotensin III is intermediate in inotropic activity between angiotensin I

TABLE III

Cardiac Effects of the Renin–Angiotensin System

Hormone	Inotropic effect	Chronotropic effect	Coronary vasoactive effect	Comments	Action on ischemic myocardium
Renin	None	None	None		No direct effect
Angiotensin I	Moderate positive effect	Moderate positive effect	Slight constriction		Deleterious
Angiotensin II	Large positive effect	Variable changes in heart rate	Large constriction	Can induce ischemia	Aggravates myocardial ischemia
Angiotensin III	Significant positive effect	Not studied	Large constriction		Aggravates myocardial ischemia

and II and appears to increase cardiac contractility to about the same extent as glucagon.

Trachte and Lefer (1979) also found angiotensin III to constrict isolated cat coronary vessels (Fig. 2). The constriction induced by angiotensin III was only slightly less than that observed in response to angiotensin II. Angiotensin III, therefore, constricts the coronary vasculature with a potency comparable to angiotensin II.

Angiotensin III induces inotropic and coronary constrictor actions closely related to those of angiotensin II. Angiotensin III produces undesirable effects in ischemic or failing cardiac states for the same reasons as angiotensin II. Converting enzyme inhibitors have been demonstrated to decrease angiotensin III production in addition to blocking angiotensin II formation (Freeman *et al.*, 1978). The beneficial actions of converting enzyme inhibitors in chronic heart failure, therefore, may involve elimination of angiotensin III in addition to angiotensin II.

V. Pituitary Hormones

A. Anterior Pituitary

Although the hormones of the anterior pituitary are well defined and have been known for many years, their cardiac effects are not clearly defined. This is even more surprising, since hypophysectomy has been shown to reduce the size of the heart (Whitehorn *et al.*, 1962) as well as to decrease cardiac output (Beznak, 1959, 1960). The tension developed by the heart in hypophysectomized rat was found to be unaltered in isolated ventricular muscle (Whitehorn *et al.*, 1962) but was impaired in the whole heart (Beznak, 1960). Moreover, there are six distinct adenohypophyseal hormones as well as one from the pars intermedia (i.e., melanocyte stimulating hormone, MSH). In addition, these peptide hormones have potent effects on a variety of target endocrine organs, stimulating the secretion of other hormones. Although these factors complicate the investigation of the cardiac actions of anterior pituitary hormones, significant progress on the cardiac effects of pituitary hormones has been made in recent years.

1. Adrenocorticotropin (ACTH)

In the early 1960s there was a burst of interest in the cardiac effects of ACTH. In 1961, Krayer and colleagues reported that ACTH stimulated the dog heart–lung preparation to increase heart rate. However, this positive chronotropic effect was somewhat erratic. In some preparations ACTH produced a large increase in heart rate, leading to an elevation in cardiac filling pressure (i.e., left atrial pressure) and decreased cardiac output. These effects are indicative of a negative inotropic effect. However, in other hearts no significant alterations in atrial pressure or cardiac output occurred despite a marked increase in heart rate. Moreover, the effects were obtained with relatively high concentration of ACTH (i.e., 100 μg/liter).

In 1963 Wollenberger and Halle extended these studies to embryonic chick hearts. These workers confirmed the finding that ACTH increased heart rate in a dose-dependent manner at concentrations of 2–200 ng/ml. They used the synthetic peptide, β^{1-24}-corticotropin in their studies similar to that of Krayer and co-workers (1961). However, Wollenberger and Halle (1963) also used A_1-corticotropin, consisting of 39 amino acids, and found this peptide also to increase heart rate to a similar extent as β-corticotropin.

Soon after these reports ACTH was shown to have chronotropic effects in the intact animal (i.e., the anesthetized rat). Juris and co-workers (1964) showed that at high doses ACTH increased heart rate in the rat, but at massive doses ACTH induced a significant bradycardia. No effect was observed at physiological concentrations. Thus the positive chronotropic effect of ACTH occurs in the intact animal but is a function of dose. In 1974 Lindner and Scholkins studied the chronotropic action of ACTH (α^{1-39}-corticotropin) in several mammalian species. In anesthetized dogs ACTH increased heart rate and dP/dt, suggesting a stimulation of mechanical activity of the heart. The effect was dose-dependent with an optimal dose of 8–32 μg/kg. The positive chronotropic effect was not altered by β-adrenergic blocking agents. However, only very small effects were seen in cats, and no effect was observed in rats and rabbits. These findings suggest that the chronotropic effect of ACTH may be more of a pharmacological curiosity in dogs and probably does not reflect an important physiological regulatory effect on the circulation. The increase in heart rate may be reflexly due to the decrease in blood pressure reported in cats and rabbits (Ueda *et al.*, 1970). Since the changes in heart rate described usually do not alter blood flow or myocardial performance and supraphysiological concentrations are necessary, the chronotropic effect of ACTH is not of major importance in the normal control of cardiac function, but may be significant in situations where ACTH secretion is enhanced.

2. Melanocyte-Stimulating Hormone (MSH)

MSH is a peptide closely related to ACTH. α-MSH is composed of 13 amino acid residues, 8 of which are identical and in the same sequence as amino acids occurring in corticoptropin. Aldinger *et al.* (1973) reported that α-MSH at 0.1–5.0 μg/kg increased heart rate moderately with slight increases in cardiac contractile force without altering blood pressure or cardiac rhythm. High doses of β-MSH induced cardiac arrhythmias symptomatic of myocardial ischemia. Since β-MSH exhibited vasopressinlike activity, it could have constricted the coronary vasculature inducing a relative myocardial ischemia (Aldinger *et al.*, 1973). However, β-MSH exhibited some antiarrhythmic activity (Lindner and Scholkens, 1974) in the dog heart–lung preparation, but as with ACTH, the effect was variable from one preparation to another. No antiarrhythmic effect of this peptide was observed.

MSH has not been extensively studied with respect to its cardiac effects. The few studies available on the subject indicate that there are actions on heart rate and cardiac rhythm, but these effects are of doubtful physiological significance and occur at concentrations probably above normal circulatory levels. It does not appear that MSH has extraordinary cardioactive properties that would confer special therapeutic value on this hormone. More probably, MSH has certain properties in common with ACTH, because of their similarity in amino acid sequence, and these effects are only of interest under supraphysiological secretion states.

3. Somatotropin (STH), Growth Hormone

STH is a relatively large protein hormone. Bovine STH contains 396 amino acid residues with a molecular weight of about 45,000 daltons, whereas human STH contains 245 amino acid residues. STH exerts important effects on protein, lipid, and carbohydrate metabolism, and it augments the action of other anterior pituitary tropic hormones. In contrast to most hormones, STH exerts its effects over periods of months and years. Nevertheless, there are several studies of the effects of growth hormone on the heart.

In 1960, Beznak reported that the decrease in heart weight observed in hypophysectomized rats could be reversed by treatment with LH, TSH, and STH or STH alone. Nevertheless, STH alone did not alter heart rate, or basal cardiac output. However, STH was able to stimulate the maximal cardiac output during volume loading, but not to the same extent as TSH. Growth hormone was able to influence the size of the heart alone, but TSH was important, perhaps in concert with STH for full restoration of cardiac performance.

Whitehorn and co-workers (1962) confirmed the findings of Beznak (1959) showing that hypophysectomized rats exhibited a small heart. However, they failed to obtain a reversal of heart size using STH at doses that restored normal body growth. Nevertheless, both groups concluded that there are no significant direct effects of STH on myocardial contractility and that alterations in cardiac performance in hypophysectomized rats are secondary to alterations in the peripheral vasculature (e.g., increased total peripheral resistance).

In 1966, Korecky, Beznak, and Korecka showed that STH was capable of influencing the performance of heart–lung preparations from hypophysectomized rats. STH given for 3–4 weeks to these rats partially restored stroke volume of the hypophysectomized rat heart–lung preparation toward normal without altering heart rate. Minelli and Korecky (1969) followed these effects in isolated rat papillary muscles obtained from hypophysectomized rats. These cardiac muscle preparations exhibited decreased myocardial contractility. This cardiac impairment was not restored by STH, but was by thyroxine. Thus STH does not appear to reverse directly the cardiac impairment of hypophysectomized rats. Thyroid hormone is a more vital factor in restoring this hypodynamic cardiac state. Moreover, STH may exert peripheral vascular effects that further complicate the interpretation of its cardiac effects. These studies in isolated cardiac tissue clearly show that STH does not restore cardiac performance to normal in hypodynamic states or increase cardiac performance above normal. Growth hormone, therefore, should not be considered as a cardioactive hormone.

None of the anterior pituitary hormones appear to be potentially useful agents in the treatment of myocardial ischemia (Table IV). ACTH, by increasing heart rate, would tend to increase myocardial oxygen demand and thus act to extend infarct size. MSH slightly increases heart rate and contractile force and would also increase myocardial oxygen demand. β-MSH may even act as a coronary vasoconstrictor, further compromising perfusion of cardiac tissue, and would aggravate myocardial ischemia. Growth hormone does not appear to exert any significant inotropic or chronotropic effect acutely, nor are any coronary vasoactive effects known. However, the well-known lipid-mobilizing effect of STH would tend to be an oxygen-wasting effect that also could induce arrhythmias and exert other potential deleterious actions in myocardial ischemia.

B. Neurohypophyseal Hormones

1. Vasopressin

Vasopressin (ADH) is an octapeptide that is known for its antidiuretic effect at low concentrations as well as a pressor effect at high concentrations. Nakano (1973) has reviewed the circulatory effects of vasopressin, particularly with regard to its vascular actions. Many of the early studies (i.e., prior to 1940) were made on crude pituitary extracts and on impure hormonal preparations and therefore cannot be cited here. Another problem in evaluating the inotropic effects of vasopressin in isolated perfused

TABLE IV

Cardiac Effects of Pituitary Hormones

Hormone	Inotropic effect	Chronotropic effect	Coronary vasodilation effect	Comments	Action on ischemic myocardium
ACTH	Little or no effect	Increases heart rate	None	May release corticosteroids	No benefit directly
MSH	Slight increase	Slight increase in heart rate	Constricts	High doses cause arrhythmias	Would be deleterious in ischemia
STH	None	None	None	Mobilizes lipids	No benefit, slightly deleterious due to lipolysis
Vasopressin	Negative inotropic effect Secondary to coronary constriction	Modest increase in heart rate	Large constrictor effect	Elevates S–T segment	Induces ischemia and may produce shock
Oxytocin	Little or no effect	Increases heart rate	Reduces flow slightly	Antiarrhythmic	No preservation of ischemia, may protect against arrhythmias

hearts is that vasopressin is a potent coronary vasoconstrictor (Drapanas *et al.*, 1961; Green *et al.*, 1942; Heeg and Meng, 1965; Hanson and Johnson, 1957; Nakano, 1967) and that this effect tends to result in a negative inotropic effect secondary to the reduced coronary flow. Also, high doses of vasopressin significantly increase peripheral resistance and thus evoke reflex adjustments in cardiac function. Finally, the cardiac effects of vasopressin are dose dependent. Thus low concentrations (i.e., less than about 25 mU/ml) exert little or no direct inotropic effect, whereas higher concentrations (i.e., greater than 200 mU/ml) depress myocardial contractility (Nakano and Shakford, 1965; Nolasko, 1976). Using left ventricular function curves, Nakano (1967) showed that infusion of low concentrations of vasopressin (10–20 mU/kg/min) resulted in a definite dose-dependent shift of the cardiac function curves downward and to the right, indicating a negative inotropic effect. This infusion rate is one that could be achieved *in vivo* by enhanced secretion of vasopressin. This cardiodepressant effect could be largely attributed to the coronary vasoconstrictor and vasopressor effects of the vasopressin. Thus when coronary blood flow was held constant, vasopressin did not alter myocardial contractile force. Furthermore, vasopressin exerts no negative inotropic effect in isolated cat papillary muscles and even exerts a very small positive inotropic effect at high concentrations (Heeg and Meng, 1965). However, in isolated guinea pig atria, vasopressin exerts a modest negative inotropic effect. Guinea pig and rabbit atria, however, are known to be very sensitive to hormones and can yield results that are consistent with *in vivo* effects.

Vasopressin also induces a modest positive chronotropic effect in the isolated cat heart (Nakano, 1973). However, in the guinea pig heart (Heeg and Meng, 1965) no such effect was found. In the intact circulatory system vasopressin produces a decrease in heart rate (Kullander and Wide, 1966; Lipton *et al.*, 1962; Longo *et al.*, 1964; Ribot *et al.*, 1961), presumably reflexly in response to the increased blood pressure. In this regard, vagotomy or atropine largely blocks the bradycardia (Baber *et al.*, 1960; Segel *et al.*, 1963). However, vasopressin may exert other effects on the sinoatrial node to reduce heart rate. The mechanism of these extravagal effects are not clear at the present time.

Vasopressin, by virtue of its coronary vasoconstrictor effect and its increase in total peripheral resistance, thereby reducing venous return, is clearly not an agent of choice in myocardial ischemia. Vasopressin, in fact, produces electrocardiographic alterations consistent with acute myocardial ischemia (e.g., S-T segment elevation, broadening of T-waves) (Black, 1960; Dearing *et al.*, 1944; Longo *et al.*, 1964). Furthermore, injection of vasopressin can induce myocardial infarction (Slotnik and Teigland, 1951) and even lead to the development of circulatory shock (Kanter and Klawans, 1948).

Octapressin (PLV-2) is a synthetic analogue of vasopressin that retains the vasopressor action but not the antidiuretic effect of vasopressin. Octapressin increases arterial blood pressure but profoundly decreases cardiac output in anesthetized dogs (Longo *et al.,* 1964). Heart rate does not change significantly. In hypotensive animals higher doses of octapressin are required to increase systemic blood pressure, but cardiac output is still not increased. Maxwell (1965) further studied octapressin and confirmed the results of Longo *et al.* (1964). Maxwell (1965) further studied octapressin at doses that increase blood pressure while reducing coronary blood flow by increasing coronary vascular resistance. Thus octapressin is not a particularly useful agent in myocardial ischemia and should be used with caution even in shock states (e.g., hemorrhagic or septic shock).

2. Oxytocin

Oxytocin exerts important well-known actions on uterine contractility, but its effects on cardiac vascular smooth muscle are less well defined. Some difficulty in interpretation of oxytocin results has occurred in early experiments because of use of pituitary extracts or mixtures of hormones and in more recent experiments because of the use of chlorbutanol as a preservative in some synthetic preparations of oxytocin (e.g., syntocinon).

Oxytocin generally has not been found to exert an inotropic effect in isolated cardiac preparations. Nakano and Fisher (1963) reported that oxytoxin does not alter contractile force in guinea pig atria or dog ventricular strips. This lack of inotropic effect occurred at concentrations that exerted well-developed uterine contractile effects (i.e., 20–40 mU/ml). At very high concentrations (i.e., 100–300 mU/ml) oxytocin depressed myocardial contractility in these preparations, although some of this negative inotropic effect may have been due to the effects of preservatives in the oxytocin preparation. Covino (1963) also reported that oxytocin at low concentrations did not influence the contractile force of isolated cat papillary muscles but that concentrations of 15–30 mU/ml exerted a moderate positive inotropic effect. This may reflect conditions of this particular experiment (e.g., rate of stimulation, resting tension, etc.)., since others have not found the cat heart to be particularly sensitive to oxytocin (Woodbury and Abreu, 1944). Moreover, Covino (1963) reported that spontaneously beating cat atria are slowed by similar concentrations of oxytocin.

Utilizing a variety of species, Priola and co-workers (1973) reported that oxytocin failed to augment the contractility of rat and monkey papillary muscles, nor did it augment contractility in the isovolumic dog heart. This lack of effect occurred at a variety of oxytocin concentrations. The failure of oxytocin in the isovolumic dog heart is particularly noteworthy, since no inotropic effect was obtained even with direct intracoronary administration of this hormone. This lack of effect of oxytocin in the dog heart confirmed the earlier work of Fortner *et al.* (1969), who measured myocardial contractile force in the intact animal using a strain gage arch sutured to the left ventricle. These workers could not observe an effect of oxytocin in myocardial contractile force even at high concentrations of oxytocin (e.g., 500 mU) that decreased coronary blood flow. In the intact rat, oxytocin at infusion rates of 90 mU/kg/min either did not modify cardiac output or only slightly increased cardiac output (i.e., by 10–20%). However, this effect may be the result of reflex adjustments in blood pressure and heart rate.

Oxytocin has usually been found to increase heart rate in man as well as in experimental animals. This tachycardia is generally thought to be a reflex response to the peripheral vascular effects of oxytocin in the intact animal. Thus Nakano (1964) showed that oxytocin exerted a vasoconstrictor effect in rats, guinea pigs, rabbits, and opossums. This was manifested as an increase in perfusion pressure under constant flow perfusion of the abdominal aorta. Nakano and Fisher (1963) found that catecholamine depletion with reserpine abolished this tachycardia, suggesting that it is not a direct effect of oxytocin on the sinoatrial node.

In human subjects oxytocin also reduces systemic blood pressure and reflexly increases heart rate (Anderson *et al.,* 1965). However, this tachycardia may not occur in anesthetized patients (Brotanek and Kazda, 1965), suggesting that certain anesthetics depress reflexes necessary for the changes in heart rate.

Oxytocin, when given in usual therapeutic oxytocic doses, does not usually alter the pattern of the electrocardiogram. However, oxytocin can depress the S-T segment and invert or broaden T-waves in women (Bergquist and Kaiser, 1959), as well as in men (Lipton *et al.,* 1962). This may be attributable to the reduced coronary blood flow or tachycardia induced by oxytocin (Fortner *et al.,* 1969; Brotanek and Kazda, 1965). Nevertheless, oxytocin has been reported to have significant antiarrhythmic effects. Melville and Varma (1961) first reported oxytocin to abolish S-T segment changes induced by hypoxia and to reverse ventricular fibrillation induced by picrotoxin. Others have also confirmed these antiarrhythmic effects of oxytocin (Bircher *et al.,* 1968; Brodeur and Beaulnes, 1963). Although the mechanism of this antiarrhythmic effect of oxytocin is not clearly understood, it appears to relate to the ability of oxytocin to lengthen the effective refractory period of the heart; some of this effect, however, may be due to the preservative (Beaulnes *et al.,* 1964).

Oxytocin does not appear to be a particularly useful agent in myocardial ischemia except perhaps to treat certain cardiac arrhythmias. Clearly, more studies are needed to determine whether oxytocin is effective against the arrhythmias occurring specifically during acute myocardial ishemia. However, since oxytocin decreases blood pressure and increases heart rate, it would tend to activate the sympathetic nervous system and thus increase myocardial oxygen demand. Moreover, oxytocin reduces coronary blood flow and may actually induce certain arrhythmias.

Table IV summarizes the cardiac effects of the pituitary hormones and evaluates their potential usefulness in the ischemic myocardium. Of the two major posterior pituitary hormones, oxytocin may have some antiarrhythmic potential but would not appear to preserve ischemic tissue based on its cardiodynamic profile. On the other hand, vasopressin would be detrimental to the ischemic heart largely on the basis of its potent coronary vasoconstrictor effect. In fact, vasopressin may actually contribute to or potentiate existing myocardial ischemia.

Acknowledgment

One of the authors (G.J.T.) is a Research Fellow of the Ischemia–Shock Research Institute of Thomas Jefferson University.

References

Ackerly, J. A., and Peach, M. J. (1975). *Pharmacologist* 17, 327.

Ahmed, S. S., Lee, C. H., Oldewurtel, H. A., and Regan, T. J. (1978). *J. Clin. Invest.* 61, 1123–1135.

Aldinger, E. E., Hawley, W. D., Schally, A. V., and Kastin, A. J. (1973). *J. Endocrinol.* 56, 613–614.

Anderson, T. W., De Padua, C. B., Stenger, V., and Prystowsky, H. (1965). *Clin. Pharmacol. Ther.* 6, 345–349.

Areskog, N. H. (1962). *Acta Soc. Med. Ups.* 67, 164–178.

Baber, J. J., Chafizadeh, M., Halligan, E. J., and Leevy, C. M. (1960). *Surg. Forum* 11, 354–355.

Ballard, K., Lefer, A., and Sayers, G. (1960). *Am. J. Physiol.* 199, 221–225.

Beardsley, A. C., Okuda, M., and Lefer, A. M. (1976a). *J. Surg. Res.* 20, 17–24.

Beardsley, A. C., Okuda, M., and Lefer, A. M. (1976b). *Proc. Soc. Exp. Biol. Med.* 151, 457–461.

Beaulnes, A., Panisset, J. C., Brodeur, J., Beltrami, E., and Gariepy, G. (1964). *Circ. Res., Suppl.* 2, 210–214.

Bergquist, J. R., and Kaiser, I. H. (1959). *Obstet. Gynecol.* 93, 547–552.

Beznak, M. (1959). *Circ. Res.* 7, 907–916.

Beznak, M. (1960). *J. Physiol. (London)* 150, 251–265.

Bircher, R. P., Tseng, D. T. C., and Wang, S. C. (1968). *Arch. Int. Pharmacodyn. Ther.* 172, 37–48.

Black, J. W. (1960). *J. Pharm. Pharmacol.* **12**, 87–94.

Blinks, J. R., and Koch-Weser, J. (1963). *Pharmacol. Rev.* **15**, 531–599.

Blumberg, A. L., Ackerly, J. A., and Peach, M. J. (1975). *Circ. Res.* **36**, 719–726.

Bonnardeaux, J. L., and Regoli. D. (1974). *Can. J. Physiol. Pharmacol.* **52**, 50–60.

Bonnardeaux, J. L., Park, W. K., and Regoli, D. (1977). *Arch. Int. Pharmacodyn. Ther.* **229**, 83–94.

Bottoms, G. D., Stitch, R. D., and Burger, R. O. (1969). *Proc. Soc. Exp. Biol. Med.* **132**, 1133.

Bouyard, P. (1965). *Ann. Anesthesiol. Fr.* **6**, 37–49.

Bouyard, P., and Klein, M. (1963). *C. R. Seances Soc. Biol. Ses. Fil.* **157**, 2252–2254.

Briggs, A. J., and Holland, W. C. (1959). *Am. J. Physiol.* **197**, 1161–1164.

Britton, S., and Di Salvo, J. (1973). *Am. J. Physiol.* **225**, 1226–1231.

Brodeur, J., and Beaulnes, A. (1963). *Rev. Can. Biol.* **22**, 275–285.

Bromer, W. W., Sinn, L. G., Staub, A., Behrens, O. K., Diller, E. R., and Bird, H. L. (1957). *J. Am. Chem. Soc.* **79**, 2807–2810.

Brotanek, V., and Kazka, S. (1965). *Am. J. Obstet. Gynecol.* **93**, 547–552.

Brunt, M. E., and McNeill, J. H. (1978). *Arch. Int. Pharmacodyn. Ther.* **233**, 42–52.

Busuttil, R. W., George, W. J., and Hewitt, R. L. (1975). *J. Thorac. Cardiovasc. Surg.* **70**, 955.

Busuttil, R. W., Paddock, R. J., Fisher, J. W., and George, W. J. (1976). *Circ. Res.* **38**, 162–167.

Cornman, I., and Gargus, J. L. (1957). *Am. J. Physiol.* **189**, 347–349.

Cornman, I., MacDonald, M., and Trams, E. (1957). *Am. J. Physiol.* **189**, 350–354.

Coutard, M., Osborne-Pellegrin, M. J., and Funder, J. W. (1978). *Endocrinology* **103**, 1144–1152.

Covino, B. G. (1963). *Am. Heart J.* **66**, 627–631.

Dalton, D. H., Hairston, P., and Lee, W. H. (1968). *Surg. Forum* **19**, 147–149.

Da Luz, P. L., Forrester, J. S., Wyatt, J. L., Diamond, G. A., Chag, M., and Swan, H. J. C. (1976). *Circulation* **53**, 847.

Dearing, W., Barnes, A. R., and Essex, H. E. (1944). *Am. Heart J.* **27**, 96–107.

Dempsey, D. J., McCallum, Z. T., Kent, K. M., and Cooper, T. (1971). *Am. J. Physiol.* **220**, 477–481.

Dhingra, R. C., Khan, A., Wu, D., Denes, P., Pouget, J. M., and Rosen, K. M. (1974). *Am. J. Cardiol.* **33**, 507–512.

Diamond, G., Forrester, J., Danzig, R., Parmley, W. W., and Swan, H. J. C. (1971). *Br. Heart J.* **33**, 290–295.

Downing, S. E., Lee, J. C., and Rieker, R. P. (1977). *Am. J. Obstet. Gynecol.* **127**, 649–656.

Drapanas, T., Crowe, C. P., Shim, W, K. T., and Worthington, G. S., Jr. (1961). *Surg., Gynecol. Obstet.* **113**, 484–489.

Ebaid, M., Caramelli, Z., Neto, S. M., Dos Santos, M. I. R., Tranchesi, J., Barbato, E., Oileggi, F., and Decourt, L. V. (1965). *Arch. Inst. Cardiol. Mex.* **35**, 3.

Eckstein, R. W. (1954). *Circ. Res.* **2**, 466.

Edelman, I. S., Bogoroch, R., and Porter, G. A. (1963). *Proc. Natl. Acad. Sci. U.S.A.* **50**, 1169–1177.

Emele, J. R., and Bonnycastle, D. D. (1956). *Am. J. Physiol.* **185**, 103–106.

Entman, M. L., Levey, G. S., and Epstein, S. E. (1969). *Circ. Res.* **25**, 429–438.

Farah, H., and Tuttle, R. (1960). *J. Pharmacol. Exp. Ther.* **129**, 49–55.

Farr, W. C., and Grupp, G. (1967). *J. Pharmacol. Exp. Ther.* **156**, 528–537.

Fortner, C. L., Manley, E. S., Jr., and Woodbury, R. A. (1969). *J. Pharmacol. Exp. Ther.* **165**, 258–266.

Freeman, R. H., Davis, J. O., and Khosla, M. C. (1978). *Am. J. Physiol.* **234**, F130–F134.

Funder, J. W., Duval, D., and Meyer, P. (1973). *Endocrinology* **93**, 1300–1308.

Gavras, H., Brown, J. J., Lever, A. F., Macadam, R. F., and Robertson, J. I. S. (1971). *Lancet* 2, 19–22.

Gavras, H., Faxon, D. P., Berkoben, J., Brunner, H. R., and Ryan, J. J. (1978a). *Circulation* 58, 770–776.

Gavras, H., Liang, C., and Brunner, H. R. (1978b). *Circ. Res.*, 43, I 59–I 62.

Gerlings, E. D., and Gilmore, J. P. (1973). *Basic Res. Cardiol.* 69, 222–227.

Glick, G., Parmley, W. W., Wechsler, A. S., and Sonnenblick, E. H. (1968). *Circ. Res.* 22, 789–799.

Gmeiner, R., Knapp, E., and Dienstl, F. (1974). *J. Mol. Cell. Cardiol.* 6, 201–206.

Gold, H. K., Prindle, K. H., Levey, G. S., and Epstein, S. E. (1970). *J. Clin. Invest.* 49, 999–1006.

Goldschlager, N., Rubin, E., Cowan, C. M., Leb, G., and Bing, R. J. (1969). *Circulation* 40, 829–837.

Goodner, C. J., Walike, B. C., Koerker, D. J., Ensinck, J. W., Brown, A. C., Chideckel, E. W., Palmer, J., and Kalnasy, L. (1977). *Science* 195, 177–179.

Green, H. D., Wegria, R., and Boyer, N. H. (1942). *J. Pharmacol. Exp. Ther.* 76, 378–391.

Gross, F. (1960). *Proc. Int. Congr. Edocrinol., 1st, 1960,* pp. 61–63.

Hajdu, S. (1957). *J. Pharmacol. Exp. Ther.* 120, 90–98.

Hajdu, S., and Szent-Györgyi, A. (1952). *Am. J. Physiol.* 168, 159–170.

Hanson, K. M., and Johnson, J. A. (1957). *Am. J. Physiol.* 190, 81–83.

Heeg, E., and Meng, K. (1965). *Naunyn-Schmiedebergs Arch. Exp. Pathol. Pharmacol.* 250, 35–41.

Hill, W. H. P., and Andrus, E. L. (1940). *Proc. Soc. Exp. Biol. Med.* 44, 213–214.

Hoffmann, G. (1954). *Naunyn-Schmiedebergs Arch. Exp. Pathol. Pharmacol.* 222, 224–226.

Hoffstein, S., Weissmann, G., and Fox, A. C. (1976). *Circulation* 53, 34.

Hollander, W., Kramsch, D. W., Chobanian, A. V., and Melby, J. C. (1966). *Circ. Res.* 18, Suppl. 1, 35–47.

Hurwitz, R. A. (1971). *Am. Heart J.* 81, 644–649.

Imai, S., Murase, H., Katori, M., Okada, M., and Shigei, T. (1965). *Jpn. J. Pharmacol.* 15, 62–71.

Jefferson, T., Glenn, T. M., and Lefer, A. M. (1971). *Proc. Soc. Exp. Biol. Med.* 136, 276–280.

Juris, S. M., Shovlin, M. B., and Watkins, S. M. H. (1964). *Nature (London)* 201, 474–475.

Kadowitz, P. J., and Yard, A. C. (1970). *Eur. J. Pharmacol.* 9, 311–318.

Kanter, A. E., and Klawans, A. H. (1948). *Am. J. Obstet. Gynecol.* 56, 366–369.

Koch-Weser, J. (1964). *Circ. Res.* 14, 337–344.

Koch-Weser, J. (1965). *Circ. Res.* 16, 230–237.

Kones, R. J. (1971). *South. Med. J.* 64, 459–461.

Korecky, B., Beznak, M., and Korecka, M. (1966). *Can. J. Physiol. Pharmacol.* 44, 13–20.

Krasney, J. A., Paudler, F. T., Smith, D. C., Davis, L. D., and Youmaus, W. G. (1965). *Am. J. Physiol.* 209, 539–544.

Krasney, J. A., Thompson, J. L., and Lowe, R. F. (1967). *Am. J. Physiol.* 213, 134–138.

Krayer, O., Astwood, E. B., Waud, D. R., and Alper, M. H. (1961). *Proc. Natl. Acad. Sci. U.S.A.* 47, 1227–1236.

Kullander, S., and Wide, E. (1966). *Acta Obstet. Gynecol. Scand.* 45, 102–110.

Lee, J. C., and Downing, S. E. (1976). *Am. J. Physiol.* 230, 1360–1365.

Lefer, A. M. (1967a). *In* "Factors Influencing Myocardial Contractility" (R. D. Tanz, ed.), pp. 611–631. Academic Press, New York.

Lefer, A. M. (1967b). *Proc. Soc. Exp. Biol. Med.* 125, 202–205.

Lefer, A. M. (1967c). *Am. Heart J.* 73, 674–680.

Lefer, A. M., and Spath, J. A., Jr. (1977). In "Cardiovascular Pharmacology" (M. Antonaccio, ed.), pp. 377–428. Raven, New York.

Lefer, A. M., Okuda, M., and Ogletree, M. L. (1977). J. Thorac. Cardiovasc. Surg. 74, 37–43.

Lesch, M., Teichholz, L. E., Soeldner, J. S., and Gorlin, R. (1974). Circulation 49, 1028–1037.

Levy, G. S., Prindle, K. H., and Epstein, S. E. (1970). J. Mol. Cell. Cardiol. 1, 403–410.

Levy, J. V., and Richards, V. (1962). Proc. Soc. Exp. Biol. Med. 3, 602–606.

Levy, J. V., and Richards, V. (1964). J. Pharmacol. Exp. Ther. 144, 104–109.

Libby, P., Maroko, P. R., Bloor, C. M., Sobel, B. E., and Braunwald, E. (1973). J. Clin. Invest. 52, 599.

Liedtke, A. J., Hughes, H. C., and Neely, J. R. (1976). Am. J. Cardiol. 38, 16–27.

Lindner, E., and Scholkens, B. (1974). Arch. Int. Pharmacodyn. Ther. 208, 19–23.

Lipski, J. I., Kaminsky, D., Donoso, E., and Friedberg, C. K. (1972). Am. J. Physiol. 222, 1107–1112.

Lipton, B., Hershey, S. G., and Baez, S. (1962). J. Am. Med. Assoc. 179, 410–416.

Longo, L. D., Morris, J. A., Smith, R. W., Beck, R., and Assali, N. S. (1964). Proc. Soc. Exp. Biol. Med. 115, 766–770.

Lorber, V. (1942). Am. Heart J. 23, 37–42.

Loubatières, A., and Sassine, A. (1963). C. R. Hebd. Seances Acad. Sci. 256, 781–782.

Loubatières, A., Bouyard, P., and Sassine, A. (1962). C. R. Hebd. Seances Acad. Sci. 255, 1147–1148.

Loubatières, A., Bouyard, P., and Klein, M. (1964). C. R. Seances Soc. Biol. Ses. Fil. 158, 1699–1701.

Loynes, J. S., and Gowdy, C. W. (1952). Can. J. Med. Sci. 30, 325–332.

Lucchesi, B. R. (1968). Circ. Res. 22, 777–787.

Lucchesi, B. R., Stutz, D. R., and Winfield, R. A. (1969). Circ. Res. 25, 183–190.

McCarl, R. L., Sjuhaj, B. F., and Houlihan, R. T. (1965). Science 150, 1611–1613.

Manchester, J. H., Parmley, W. W., Matloff, J. M., Liedtke, A. J., LaRaia, P. J., Herman, M. V., Sonnenblick, E. H., and Gorlin, R. (1970). Circulation 41, 579–588.

Marcus, M., Skelton, C. L., Prindle, K. H., and Epstein, S. E. (1971). J. Pharmacol. Exp. Ther. 179, 331–337.

Masters, T. N., Harbold, N. B., Jr., Hall, D. G., Jackson, R. D., Mullen, D. C., Daugherty, H. K., and Robicsek, R. (1976). Am. J. Cardiol. 32, 557.

Maxwell, G. M. (1965). Arch. Int. Pharmacodyn. Ther. 158, 17–23.

Mayer, S. E., Namm, D. H., and Rice, L. (1970). Circ. Res. 26, 225–233.

Melville, K. I., and Varma, D. R. (1961). Br. J. Pharmacol. Chemother. 17, 218–223.

Minelli, R., and Korecky, B. (1969). Can. J. Physiol. Pharmacol. 47, 545–552.

Moir, T. W., and Nayler, W. G. (1970). Circ. Res. 26, 29–34.

Morgan, H. E., Henderson, M. J., Regen, D. M., and Park, C. R. (1960). J. Biol. Chem. 236, 253–261.

Morrison, J., Maley, T., Reduto, L., Victa, C., Pyros, I., Brandon, J., and Gulotta, S. (1975). Crit. Care. Med. 3, 94.

Morrison, J., Reduto, L., Pizzarello, R., Geller, K., Maley, T., and Gulotta, S. (1976). Circulation 53, 200.

Morton, J. J., Semple, P. F., Ledingham, I. M., Stuart, B., Tehrani, M. A., Garcia, A. R., and McGarrity, G. (1977). Circ. Res. 41, 301–308.

Murthy, V. S., Waldron, T. L., Goldberg, M. E., and Vollmer, R. R. (1977). Eur. J. Pharmacol. 46, 207–212.

Nakano, J. (1964). Proc. Soc. Exp. Biol. Med. 115, 707–709.

Nakano, J. (1967). J. Pharmacol. Exp. Ther. 157, 19–31.

Nakano, J. (1973). *In* "The Handbook of Physiology" (R. O. Greep and E. B. Astwood, eds.), Sec. 7, Vol. 4, pp. 395–442. Am. Physiol. Soc., Washington, D.C.

Nakano, J., and Fisher, R. D. (1963). *J. Pharmacol. Exp. Ther.* **142**, 206–214.

Nakano, J., and Shakford, J. S. (1965). *Experientia* **21**, 474–475.

Nasmyth, P. L. (1957). *J. Physiol. (London)* **139**, 323–336.

Nayler, W. G. (1957). *Aust. J. Exp. Biol. Med. Sci.* **35**, 241–248.

Nayler, W. G. (1965). *J. Pharmacol. Exp. Ther.* **148**, 215–217.

Nayler, W. G., and Seabra-Gomes, R. (1976). *Cardiovasc. Res.* **10**, 349–358.

Nayler, W. G., McInnes, I., Chipperfield, D., Carcan, V., and Daile, P. (1970). *J. Pharmacol. Exp. Ther.* **171**, 265–275.

Nobel-Allen, N., Kirsch, M., and Lucchesi, B. R. (1973). *J. Pharmacol. Exp. Ther.* **187**, 475–481.

Nolasko, J. B. (1976). *Cardiology* **61**, 353–359.

Novak, E., Stubbs, S. S., Seckman, C. E., and Herron, M. S. (1970). *Clin. Pharmacol. Ther.* **11**, 711–717.

Nudel, D. B., Lee, J. C., and Downing, S. E. (1977). *Am. J. Physiol.* **233**, H665–H669.

Okuda, M., and Lefer, A. M. (1977). *J. Mol. Cell. Cardiol.* **9**, 989–1001.

Okuda, M., Young, K. R., Jr., and Lefer, A. M. (1976). *Circ. Res.* **39**, 640–646.

Osher, J., Lang, T., Meerbaum, S., Hashimoto, K., Farcot, J. C., and Corday, E. (1976). *Am. J.*

Okuda, M., Young, K. R., Jr., and Lefer, A. M. (1976). *Circ. Res.* **39**, 640–646.

Peach, M. J. (1971). *Circ. Res.* **28 & 29**, II 107–II 117.

Peach, M. J. (1977). *Physiol. Rev.* **57**, 313–370.

Priola, D. V., Vorherr, H., and Spurgeon, H. A. (1973). *Proc. West. Pharmacol. Soc.* **16**, 43–47.

Puri, P. S., and Bing, R. J. (1969). *Am. Heart J.* **78**, 660–668.

Regan, T. J., Frank, M. J., Lehan, P. H., and Hellems, H. K. (1963). *Am. J. Physiol.* **205**, 790–794.

Regan, T. J., Lehan, P. H., Henneman, D. H., Behar, A., and Hellems, H. K. (1964). *J. Lab. Clin. Med.* **63**, 638–647.

Regan, T. J., Ettinger, P. O., Khan, M. I., Terran, M. V., Lyons, M. M., Oldewurtel, H. A., and Weber, M. (1974). *Circ. Res.* **35**, 222–237.

Reid, I. A., Morris, B. J., and Ganong, F. W. (1978). *Annu. Rev. Physiol.* **40**, 377–410.

Ribot, S., Green, H., Small, M. J., and Abranowitz, S. (1961). *Am. J. Med. Sci.* **242**, 612–619.

Roberts, R., De Mello, V., and Sobel, B. E. (1976). *Circulation* **53**, 204.

Rogers, W. J., Stanley, A. W., Prenig, J. B., Prather, J. W., McDaniel, H. G., Moraski, R. E., Mantle, J. A., Russell, R. O., and Rackley, C. E. (1976). *Am. Heart J.* **92**, 441–454.

Rogers, W. J., Russell, R. O., McDaniel, H. G., and Rackley, C. E. (1977). *Am. J. Cardiol.* **40**, 421–428.

Sassine, A., Bourgeois, J. M., and Macabes, J. (1975). *Arch. Int. Pharmacodyn. Ther.* **219**, 196–201.

Sayers, G., and Solomon, N. (1960). *Endocrinology* **66**, 719–730.

Sayers, G., Lefer, A. M., and Nadzam, G. R. (1966). *Endocrinology* **78**, 211–213.

Segel, N., Bayley, T. J., Paton, A., Dykes, P. W., and Biship, J. M. (1963). *Clin. Sci.* **25**, 43–55.

Shatney, C. H., MacCarter, D. J., and Lillehei, R. C. (1976). *Surgery* **80**, 61.

Sherwin, R. S., Hendler, R., De Fronzo, Wahren, J., and Felig, P. (1977). *Proc. Natl. Acad. Sci. U.S.A.* **74**, 348–352.

Slotnik, I. L., and Teigland, J. D. (1951). *J. Am. Med. Assoc.* **146**, 1126.

Small, H. S., Weitzner, S. W., and Nahas, G. G. (1959). *Am. J. Physiol.* **196**, 1025–1028.

Snow, T. R. (1976). *Experientia* **32**, 1550–1551.

Solomon, N., Travis, R. H., and Sayers, G. (1959). *Endocrinology* **64**, 535–541.

Spath, J. A., Jr., and Lefer. A. M. (1975). *Am. Heart J.* **90**, 50–55.

Spath, J. A., Gorczynski, R. J., and Lefer, A. M. (1973). *Surg., Gynecol. Obstet.* **137**, 597.

Spath, J. A., Jr., Lane, D. L., and Lefer, A. M. (1974). *Circ. Res.* **25**, 44–51.

Steiner, C., Wit, A.L., and Damato, A. N. (1969). *Circ. Res.* **24**, 167–177.

Stirewolt, W. S., and Wool, I. G. (1966). *Science* **154**, 284–285.

Tanz, R. D. (1960). *J. Pharmacol. Exp. Ther.* **128**, 168–175.

Tanz, R. D., and Kerby, C. F. (1961). *J. Pharmacol. Exp. Ther.* **131**, 56–64.

Tanz, R. D., Clark, G. M., and Whitehead, R. W. (1956). *Proc. Soc. Exp. Biol. Med.* **92**, 167–169.

Tanz, R. D., Whitehead, R. W., and Weir, G. J. (1957). *Proc. Soc. Exp. Biol. Med.* **94**, 258–262.

Toyama, M., and Reis, R. L. (1975). *J. Thorac. Cardiovasc. Surg.* **70**, 458.

Trachte, G. J., and Lefer, A. M. (1979). *Recent Adv. Stud. Card. Struct. Metab.* **14**.

Travis, R. H., and Sayers, G. (1958). *Endocrinology* **62**, 816–821.

Turini, G. A., Brunner, H. R., Ferguson, R. K., Rivier, J. L., and Gavras, H. (1978). *Arch. Int. Pharmacodyn. Ther.* **233**, 166–176.

Ueda, M., Matsuda, S., Kawakami, M., and Takeda, H. (1970). *Jpn. J. Pharmacol.* **20**, 585–598.

Ullrick, W. C., and Hazelwood, R. L. (1963). *Am. J. Physiol.* **204**, 1001–1004.

Vinas, J. F., Fewel, J. G., Grover, F. L., Richardson, J. D., Arom, K. V., Webb, G. E., and Trinkle, J. K. (1977). *Surgery* **81**, 646–652.

Visscher, M. B., and Lee, Y. C. P. (1972). *Proc. Natl. Acad. Sci. U.S.A.* **69**, 463–465.

Visscher, M. B., and Muller, E. A. (1927). *J. Physiol. (London)* **621**, 341–348.

Vyden, J. K., Nagasawa, K., Rabinowitz, B., Parmley, W. W., Tomoda, H., Corday, E., and Swan, H. J. C. (1974). *Am. J. Cardiol.* **34**, 677.

Whitehorn, W. V., Grimm, A. F., and King, T. M. (1962). *Circ. Res.* **10**, 853–858.

Whitsitt, L. S., and Lucchesi, B. R. (1968). *Circ. Res.* **23**, 585–595.

Wildenthal, K. (1973). *Nature (London)* **243**, 226–227.

Winokur, S., Nobel-Allen, N. L., and Lucchesi, B. R. (1975). *Eur. J. Pharmacol.* **32**, 349–356.

Wollenberger, A., and Halle, W. (1963). *Byull. Eksp. Biol. Med.* **56**, T1215–T1218.

Woodbury, R. A., and Abreu, B. E. (1944). *Am. J. Physiol.* **142**, 114–120.

Young, K. R., Jr., Polansky, E. W., and Lefer, A. M. (1977). *Cardiology* **61**, 341–352.

2

Prostaglandins and the Heart

Åke Wennmalm

I. A Historical Outline

Prostaglandin (PG) research entered its most expansive phase in the early 1960s, but its origins lie in the beginning of the present century. The possibility that the male genital glands, apart from producing a nutritive transport solvent for the male gametes, also form biologically active agents attracted several investigators. The first observation that may be ascribed to the action of a prostaglandin or related compound was made by Camus and Gley in 1907. These authors injected the secretion from the internal prostate of the hedgehog intravenously into rabbits and found that the animals became severely dyspnoic and died. Götzl (1910) reported analogously that pressed juice from human prostate glands (autopsy material) on iv injection killed rabbits, apparently by inducing intravascular clotting. These early observations deserve attention since they suggest that products formed in the prostate gland may be related in some way to blood clotting, an idea that is of considerable current interest.

Experiments with extracts from fresh human prostate gland were carried out by Battez and Boulet (1913). The material was obtained from a 20-year-old man who had been executed. Injection of the extract intravenously in the dog led to a pronounced fall in blood pressure. This was probably the first observation to indicate the occurrence of a depressor substance in the male prostate gland. The first communication on a pharmacodynamic action of human seminal fluid originates from Kurzrok and Lieb (1931). They observed, after addition of seminal fluid to an isolated human uterine strip, an increase or a decrease in spontaneous movement or tone. The conclusion, apparently erroneous, was that the active agent in the seminal fluid was acetylcholine.

The occurrence of a depressor and smooth-muscle-stimulating substance in human seminal fluid was reported independently by Goldblatt (1933) and von Euler (1934). Initially the active principle was indistinctly separated from substance P, likewise a strong depressor agent. However, the chemical disparity between the new agent and substance P was rapidly elucidated, and the substance was given the name prostaglandin (von Euler, 1935a). Chemically it was defined as an acid soluble in ether and chloroform. It was clearly separated from other vasoactive substances (von Euler, 1935b). Later its entire blood-pressure-lowering action was shown to be due to a relaxing influence in the resistance vascular bed, the mammalian heart being completely unaffected by prostaglandin (von Euler, 1936). That prostaglandin is not a general vasodilator was pointed out; both qualitative and quantitative organ and species differences exist (von Euler, 1939).

The lack of suitable chemical methods at that time rendered further prostaglandin studies difficult. Not until the late 1940s was a second wave of research begun. It was then that the fruitful work of the Bergström group started, initiated by von Euler. This resulted in the important discovery that prostaglandin, rather than being a single compound, is a whole family of active agents. One of the first consequences of this discovery was the isolation of two prostaglandins in crystalline form (Bergström and Sjövall,

1957). Subsequently, research activity in the prostaglandin field has snow-balled.

Von Euler focused his interest at an early stage on the cardiovascular effects of prostaglandin. Today, 45 years later, prostaglandins appear as significant as ever before in connection with cardiac function in health and disease.

II. Chemistry and Biochemistry of Prostaglandins

A. Prostaglandin Nomenclature

Prostaglandins are fatty acid derivatives. In the PG nomenclature, prostanoic acid, a saturated C-20 fatty acid with cyclization between carbon atoms 8 and 12, is the theoretical mother substance and PGs are sub-grouped by the letters A–I, depending on their chemical structure (see Fig. 1). Prostaglandins of the A–H series all bear the basic prostanoic acid structure but differ in the type of active groups added to the molecule, as well as in the position of these groups. The PGs also differ regarding the degree of unsaturation in the molecule, the number of double bonds being indicated as a subscript (e.g., PGE_1, PGE_2). Thus PGs of the 1 series carry just a trans double bond in the 13,14 position, whereas PGs of the 2 series also have a 5,6-cis double bond. In addition to these bonds, PGs of the 3 series, which is sparse biologically, have a 17,18-cis double bond. The substituents of the cyclopentane ring in the prostanoic acid molecule are stereochemically indicated as α or β, α standing for a radical below the plane of the drawing and β standing for a radical rising out of the drawing. α-Configuration is usually indicated by a dotted or broken line and β-configuration by a wedge-formed or solid line. The two side chains in the prostanoic acid molecule are *trans* to each other, the enanthic acid attached to the cyclopentane ring in the C-8 position being in an α-direction and the octyl group binding to the C-12 being directed β. All biologically active prostaglandins have a C-15 hydroxy group in α-position (apart from PGG, which instead carries a hydroperoxy group).

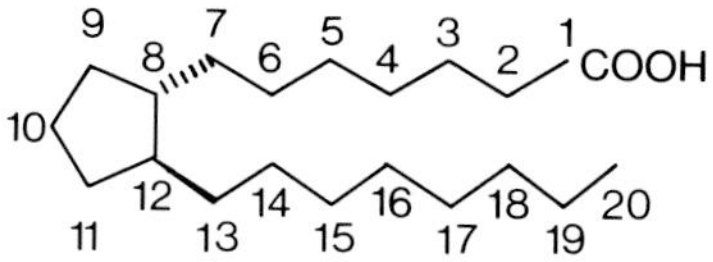

Fig. 1. Prostanoic acid, the theoretical mother substance in PG nomenclature.

The E prostaglandins [*E* standing for *e*ther, in which the PGs are more soluble than the F prostaglandins, which on partition between ether and phosphate (*f*osfat in Swedish) accumulate in the latter phase] are, in addition to the basic structure, characterized by an oxogroup in C-9 position and an α-directed hydroxy group at C-11 (Fig. 2). F prostaglandins have hydroxy groups at both C-9 and C-11. Depending on the direction of the C-9 radical, F PGs are designated α or β.

The A and B PGs are derived from the E series by treatment with *a*cid and *b*ase, respectively. PGA and PGB lack the C-11 hydroxy group of the E series and carry instead a trans double bond in 10,11 and 8,12 position, respectively. An unstable isomer to A is PGC, in which the double bond is located at 11,12. PGD is an isomer to PGE, carrying an α-hydroxy group at C-9 and a carbonyl group at C-11.

The G and H series are intermediates in the PG metabolism, characterized by an 9,11-endoperoxy bridge. PGH differs from PGG by having a hydroperoxy group at C-15 instead of the common hydroxy radical. In the I series, which is the most recent discovered group of PGs, an additional cyclization, a 6(9)-oxy bridge, is present. The only prostaglandin of the I series hitherto described is prostacyclin (PGI$_2$).

Although not true prostaglandins, the *thromboxanes* (Tx) are generally described in connection with the PGs, since they are intimately connected biochemically and physiologically. The thromboxanes (A and B) carry an oxane ring instead of the cyclopentane structure common to all PGs. The radicals at C-8 and C-12 are the same as in the PG series. TxA has a 9(11)-oxy bridge in the oxane ring, whereas TxB has a 9α,11β-dihydroxy structure.

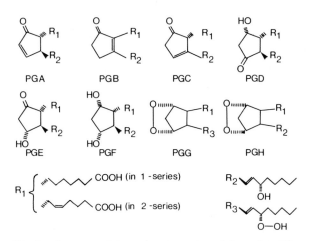

Fig. 2.   Structure of the cyclopentane ring of the various PGs.

B. Precursors in Prostaglandin Biosynthesis

Prostaglandins are formed in most tissues in the body. The immediate precursor to PGs of the 1 series (PGE_1, $PGF_{1\alpha}$, etc.) is dihomo-γ-linolenic acid ($C_{20:3}$), and the precursor to the 2 series (e.g., PGE_2, PGI_2) is arachidonic acid ($C_{20:4}$, AA) (Bergström *et al.*, 1964; van Dorp *et al.*, 1964). In the 3 series 5,8,11,14,17-eicosapentaenoic acid ($C_{20:5}$) is the precursor. γ-Linolenic acid and arachidonic acid occur in higher animals as well as in the lower flora and fauna. Although the immediate essential fatty acid (EFA) precursors to prostaglandins apparently are present in the diet, their quantitative importance is limited because the amounts ingested are so small. More interesting as a dietary PG precursor is linoleic acid ($C_{18:2}$), the intake of which by man is estimated at more than 10 g every 24 hr (van Dorp, 1975). It is well known that linoleic and linolenic acid are converted to dihomo-γ-linolenic acid and arachidonic acid in animal tissues and that this conversion probably occurs mainly in the liver mitochondria. The total daily excretion of PG metabolites is about 1 mg. Thus it is obvious that formation of PGs is a quantitatively unimportant byway in the overall metabolism of AA, this being completely dependent on a regular dietary supply of linoleic acid, as shown in studies where animals fed with a diet low on fatty acids decreased their production of PGs.

It has been known for a long time that polyunsaturated fatty acids occur mainly in the cell membranes in various organs, in contrast to saturated fatty acids, which are stored only in fat tissue. Polyunsaturated cell-membrane-bound EFA, apart from being candidates in PG formation, are important for the physical and biochemical properties they impart to the cell membrane. They are incorporated as phospholipid esters and are released by acyl hydrolases, possibly acting unspecifically as well as specifically (liberating PG precursors only). The mechanism controlling the liberation of $C_{20:3}$ and $C_{20:4}$ from the storage pools is of considerable interest, since it serves as the rate-limiting step in the formation of PGs.

C. Biosynthesis of Prostaglandins

Quantitatively the chief precursor in the bioformation of PGs is arachidonic acid (AA). This section accordingly deals only with the formation of the 2 series of PGs (having AA as precursor). The bioformation of the 1 and 3 series involves the same converting enzymes and is therefore analogous to that of the 2 series.

AA liberated into the cytoplasm can be transformed oxidatively via a variety of metabolic routes. So far eight pathways have been recognized, of which only four lead to formation of PGs or Tx. The first step in the conversion of AA to PG is the formation of a cyclic endoperoxide. The existence of such an intermediate in PG metabolism was proposed in 1965 by Samuelsson, but 8 years passed before the compound was isolated (Hamberg and Samuelsson, 1973; Nugteren and Hazelhof, 1973). Although the enzyme behind this conversion is usually denoted cyclooxygenase, its correct name is prostaglandin endoperoxide synthetase. This protein has been demonstrated to mediate not only the peroxidation at C-9–C-11 and the cyclization between C-8 and C-12 but also the introduction of a hydroperoxy group at C-15.

The compound achieved by the action of PG endoperoxide synthetase on AA is usually called PGG$_2$ (Fig. 3). PGG$_2$ is converted to another endoperoxide, PGH$_2$, by reduction of the C-15 hydroperoxy group to a hydroxy group by a specific enzyme (PGG–PGH reductase). These enzymatic steps, although proceeding at different rates in different tissues, are common to all organs capable of producing PGs or Tx. Biochemical studies have

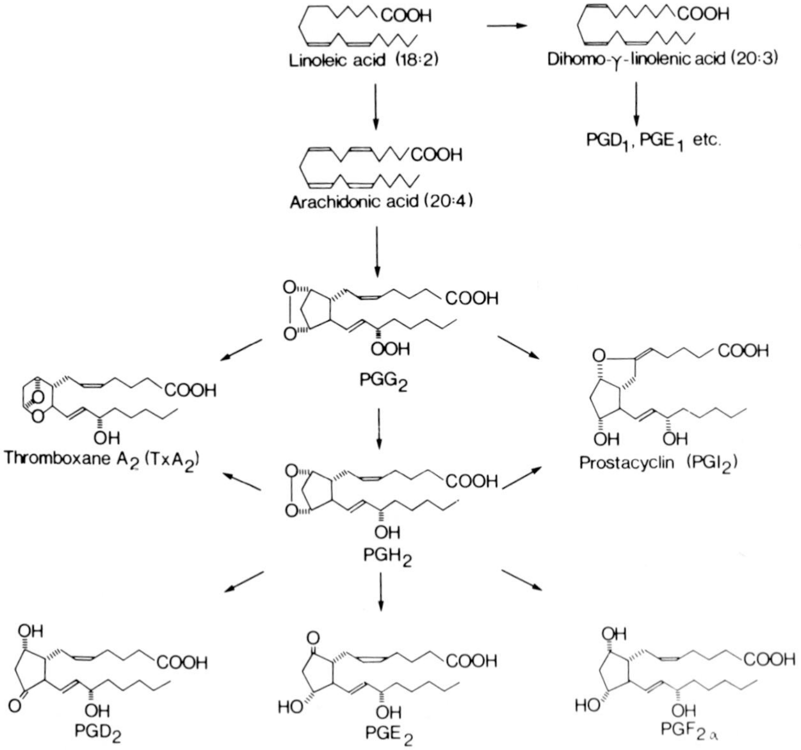

Linoleic acid (18:2)

Dihomo-γ-linolenic acid (20:3)

PGD$_1$, PGE$_1$ etc.

Arachidonic acid (20:4)

PGG$_2$

Thromboxane A$_2$ (TxA$_2$)

Prostacyclin (PGI$_2$)

PGH$_2$

PGD$_2$

PGE$_2$

PGF$_{2\alpha}$

Fig. 3.   Biosynthesis of PGs from precursor fatty acids.

revealed that the cyclooxygenase (PG endoperoxide synthetase) is particle bound, the highest activity being associated with a microsomal fraction obtained by high-speed centrifugation of homogenized tissue supernatant, after removal of other cell particles at lower speed.

The PG endoperoxides, although possessing biological activity of their own, are generally regarded as intermediates in PG bioformation. Their further conversion to PGs of the D, E, F, and I series, and to thromboxanes, requires access to specific terminal enzymes. The concentration of these enzymes varies from tissue to tissue, so that one tissue may produce an endoperoxide metabolite that is completely absent in another. The most common pattern is, however, for a certain tissue to produce a number of PG endoperoxide metabolites, of which one or two quantitatively exceed the others. This means that the PG production profile is to some extent specific for a particular tissue or organ. Clearly, such a profile of PGs may play a significant part in giving the tissue or organ specific biologic properties, distinguishing it from other tissues. Pathways that seem to be present in most tissues, although operating at different rates, are the isomerization of PG endoperoxides to PGD_2 and PGE_2 and the reduction to $PGF_{2\alpha}$. All these steps are brought about by specific enzymes (Granström et al., 1968; Hamberg and Samuelsson, 1973; Nugteren and Hazelhof, 1973). The thromboxane pathway, converting PGG_2 and PGH_2 into TxA_2 by a specific enzyme, thromboxane A_2 synthetase (Hamberg et al., 1975), is the most important pathway in platelets. TxA_2 formation has also been demonstrated in guinea pig lung, spleen, and brain as well as in rat lung, spleen, and brain, and it was completely absent in other tissues (e.g., myocardium, vascular tissue, and liver).

Prostacyclin (PGI_2) formation from PG endoperoxides is brought about by a specific cyclase, which occurs in vascular tissues from several species, including man. Prostacyclin is also found in other tissues (e.g., in dog renal cortex and in rat stomach).

D. Catabolism and Excretion of Prostaglandins

The metabolic inactivation of PG and Tx involves several steps. Spontaneous as well as enzymatic conversions occur. Two steps that seem to be common to most PGs are oxidation of the C-15 hydroxy group by means of 15-OH-PG-dehydrogenase and reduction of the 13,14 double bond by Δ^{13}-PG-reductase. The first of these steps, 15-OH-dehydrogenation, is especially important since it makes PGs biologically inactive. The respective 13,14-dihydro-15-keto derivatives of the various PGs undergo further degradation before being excreted via the urine. β- and ω-oxidations have been shown to occur, the main urinary PG metabolites in man being tetranor derivatives of prostanoic acid. In this connection it should be stressed that authentic PGs found in the urine are renal in origin and consequently do not reflect PG production or release in other tissues.

E. Analysis of Prostaglandins

It is beyond the scope of this chapter to present a thorough description of the problems involved in the analysis of PGs in organ effluents, plasma, or tissue extracts. The interested reader is referred to special literature on this issue (e.g., Frölich, 1978). This section will simply mention some of the methods commonly used and some of the many pitfalls involved.

Most authentic PGs, as well as TxA_2, are unstable in aqueous solutions. This means that plasma samples, effluents, or tissue extracts in which PG is to be analyzed should be extracted with organic solutions and stored dry at low temperature if immediate analysis is not feasible. Since all PGs and Tx are easily extracted from water solution to less polar solvents at slightly acidic reaction (pH 3–4.5), this prerequisite is readily fulfilled. The most unstable AA metabolites, like the PG endoperoxides, PGI_2, and TxA_2, require further, more rigorous precautions concerning extraction and storage. PGs extracted to organic solvents are concentrated by evaporation. After acidic lipid extraction special separation procedures have to be applied in most cases to separate PG, from other compounds, followed by a quantitative analysis.

The most common methods for separation of prostaglandins are silicic acid column chromatography and thin-layer chromatography (TLC). These methods are easy to handle and, when properly used, are valid and reproducible. A further advantage is that no expensive equipment is needed. Caldwell and co-workers (1972) have reported on a micro-method for separating groups of PGs. Originally it was used for the separation of prostaglandins into the A/B, E, and F subgroups, respectively, but by changing the polarity of the elution solvents, other subgroups may be separated as well. In our laboratory a modified version is used for routine purposes (Fig. 4). The modification involves, among other things, the use of disposable glass columns (Pasteur pipettes) and the replacement of the carcinogenic elution solvent benzene by toluene. Those planning to use column chromatography for separation of PGs should bear in mind two methodological points: (1) commercially available solvents usually require distillation before use, and (2) control of separation and recovery of compounds applied to the column are absolutely essential (best done using ^{3}H-labeled PGs); even when methodological instructions from a paper or another laboratory are followed exactly, the results may diverge considerably.

In the case of TLC a variety of systems have been devised for separating

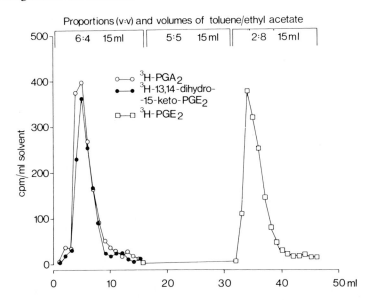

Fig. 4. Separation of PGE from less polar PGs using a microcolumn (5 × 45 mm) of silicic acid. Separation of [³H]PGE₂ from ³H-labeled PGA₂ and 13,14-dihydro-15-keto-PGE₂ is shown. The sample was applied to the column in solvent toluene/ethyl acetate 9 1, which was also used for preparation of the column. Increasing proportions of ethyl acetate in toluene elutes more polar compounds from the column. The technique is easily applied to other PGs.

groups and individual PGs, generally as their free acids. For routine purposes, commercially available TLC plates (e.g., Merck F 254) are sufficient. Some convenient solvent systems are listed in Table I. TLC has become increasingly popular with the development of sensitive equipment for radioscanning of thin-layer chromatograms of labeled PGs. Radio-scanning permits rapid evaluation of PG profiles obtained, for example, in effluent from isolated organs infused with ¹⁴C-labeled PG precursor (AA or PGG₂/PGH₂) or in incubates of homogenized organs with labeled precursor.

The quantitative analysis of PGs can be performed with a variety of methods, all of which are rather time-consuming, besides requiring extensive equipment and/or prolonged training of the laboratory staff. The most sophisticated of these methods is gas-liquid chromatography (GLC) in combination with electron capture detection (ECD) or mass spectrometry (MS). Both GLC-ECD and GLC-MS have the drawbacks indicated above, but in return they are completely specific and rather sensitive. In addition, GLC-MS is the most adequate too, for identification of unknown PGs or PG metabolites.

Radioimmunoassay (RIA) of PG, Tx, and their metabolites has been

TABLE I

Some Solvent Systems Suitable for Separation of Prostaglandins with Thin-Layer Chromatography (Silica Gel Plates)

Solvent system designation	Separation between prostaglandins	Composition of solvent system	Reference
AII	PGE_1, PGE_2, PGE_3, $PGF_{1\alpha}$, $PGF_{2\alpha}$, $PGF_{3\alpha}$	Ethyl acetate:acetic acid:methanol:2,2,4-trimethylpentane:water (110:30:35:10:100, organic phase)	Gréen and Samuelsson (1964)
AIX	$PGA_2/PGB_2/13,14$-dihydro-15-keto-PGE_2, PGD_2, PGE_2, $PGF_{2\alpha}$, 6-keto-$PGF_{1\alpha}$	Ethyl acetate:acetic acid:2,2,4-trimethylpentane:water (90:20:50:100, organic phase)	Hamberg and Samuelsson (1966)
BDA	$PGA_2/PGB_2/13,14$-dihydro-15-keto-PGE_2, TxB_2, PGD_2, PGE_2, $PGF_{2\alpha}/$6-keto-$PGF_{1\alpha}$	Benzene:dioxane:acetic acid (60:30:3)	Isakson et al. (1977)
C	$PGA_2/PGB_2/13,14$-dihydro-15-keto-PGE_2, TxB_2, PGD_2, $PGE_2/$6-keto-$PGF_{1\alpha}$, $PGF_{2\alpha}$	Chloroform:methanol:acetic acid:water (90:8:1:0.8)	Isakson et al. (1977)

frequently used in recent years. In analogy with other methods for quantitative analysis of PGs, RIA usually requires pretreatment of the samples (purification, concentration, and separation) to yield data of acceptable validity. Such pretreatment has not been a regular feature of the studies reported, and this has somewhat tarnished the method's reputation. A critical analysis of the requirements for RIA analysis of PGs has been presented recently (Granström, 1978).

Bioassay still plays an important role in the analysis of authentic PGs. This method is by far the most rapid, and, correctly handled, it is almost as sensitive and specific as GLC-MS. Its main disadvantages are that it requires certain experimental conditions (perfused organs, tissue incubates) and that the compound to be analyzed must be biologically active. Nevertheless, discoveries of the utmost significance may still be made using mainly bioassay, a case in point being the detection of prostacyclin and its unique effects (Gryglewski *et al.,* 1976; Moncada *et al.,* 1977); this was made solely with the aid of various isolated smooth muscle preparations as analytical instruments. Depending on the type of PG to be analyzed, as well as the medium containing the principle, different techniques have been used. For example, purified samples of PGEs may be assayed using a rat or hamster stomach strip (Vane, 1957; Ubatuba, 1973) in a small (5 ml) chamber, and the PG profile in circulating blood may be screened with a cascade of superfused organs (Vane, 1969). During the last few years it has been customary among some prostaglandinists to regard bioassay as a method of inferior scientific value. The discovery of prostacyclin has certainly created a basis for reassessing bioassay, a method that utilizes natural target organs for evaluation of biologic function.

III. Cardiac Biosynthesis of Prostaglandins

Although the formation and release of PGs in various organs have attracted considerable interest in laboratories for many years, it is only in the present decade that this has applied to their synthesis and liberation in cardiac tissue. The first indication of cardiac release of a prostaglandinlike substance (PLS) was made in isolated rabbit hearts, subjected to sustained sympathetic nerve stimulation (Wennmalm and Stjärne, 1971). Using TLC for separation and enzymatic degradation with 15-OH-PG-dehydrogenase for identification, this PLS was subsequently identified as PGE (Samuelsson and Wennmalm, 1971). Later, increased release of PLS from isolated hearts was also observed following infusion of the adenine nucleotides, adenosine diphosphate (ADP) and adenosine triphosphate (ATP) (Minkes *et al.,* 1973) or noradrenaline (Junstad and Wennmalm, 1973a). That the enzymatic basis for PG production was in fact present in the heart was demonstrated at the same time in a study where the microsomal fraction of homogenized canine left ventricular wall was found capable of forming PGE_2 from arachidonic acid (Limas and Cohn, 1973).

Evidence that cardiac tissue is capable of forming other PGs than those of the E series was not presented until some years ago, when the technique for incorporating [^{14}C]AA into the cardiac lipid stores (Isakson et al., 1976) was evolved. Using this technique, the Needleman group presented a series of observations indicating that the main AA metabolite in rabbit heart (Isakson et al., 1977) and in coronary arteries (Needleman et al., 1977a; Raz et al., 1977) is not PGE_2 but 6-keto-$PGF_{1\alpha}$. These authors also pointed out the pronounced coronary vasodilator properties of a hitherto unknown intermediate formed during the conversion of PGH_2 to 6-keto-$PGF_{1\alpha}$ (Raz et al., 1977). Independently and in parallel the Vane group descirbed the marked platelet antiaggregatory and vasodilating properties of a new PG formed by rabbit or pig aortic microsomes (Moncada et al., 1976a; Gryglewski et al., 1976). The new PGs detected by these groups proved to be a single entity, isolated shortly afterward and identified by its chemical structure (Johnson et al., 1976). The new compound (until then denoted PGX) was given the name prostacyclin (PGI_2) because of its content of a second cyclization (a 6,9,α-epoxy bridge). Prostacyclin is highly unstable and degrades in aqueous solution to 6-keto-$PGF_{1\alpha}$, the compound initially observed in the heart (cf. above).

Following these developments, the profile of PG formation in the hearts of various laboratory animals has been studied in more detail. Isakson et al. (1977) reported that [^{14}C]AA infused into isolated rabbit hearts (cf. Fig. 5) perfused at a constant flow was converted to labelled 6-keto-$PGF_{1\alpha}$, PGE_2, and $PGF_{2\alpha}$, in falling order of magnitude. Their data were mainly confirmed by DeDeckere et al. (1977). These authors used the GLC-ECD technique to estimate the outflow of PGs from isolated rabbit and rat hearts perfused at constant pressure and found that 6-keto-$PGF_{1\alpha}$ was the main PG released. In addition, they described a considerable increase in the outflow of authentic prostacyclin from the rabbit hearts (but not from rat hearts) after a period of anoxia. Schrör and co-workers (1978), infusing [^{14}C]AA into isolated guinea pig hearts perfused at a constant flow, likewise reported 6-keto-$PGF_{1\alpha}$ as the main cardiac prostaglandin, followed by PGE_2, PGD_2, and $PGF_{2\alpha}$. Conflicting somewhat with these data, repeated studies in our laboratory on [^{14}C]AA metabolism in isolated rabbit hearts perfused at a constant pressure consistently display PGE_2 or $PGF_{2\alpha}$ as the main metabolite, each of these constituting 25–35% of the total amounts of [^{14}C]PGs formed, followed by 6-keto-$PGF_{1\alpha}$ (20–25%) (Wennmalm, 1978b,c). Whether differences in techniques, species, or strains are responsible for

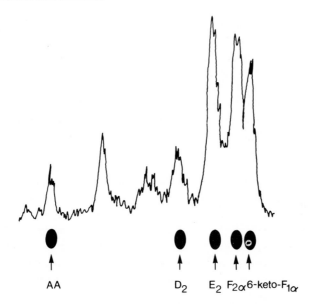

AA　　　　　　　　　　D_2　　E_2　$F_{2\alpha}$6-keto-$F_{1\alpha}$

Fig. 5. Rabbit perfused heart. This is a radioscan of a thin-layer chromatogram of the lipid extract from the cardiac effluent, collected during infusion of [^{14}C]arachidonic acid into the heart. As seen from the scan the ^{14}C-activity appears in peaks parallel to the unlabeled PG standards.

the moderate discrepancies observed is difficult to decide and may be considered of academic interest. Of major importance are the common features in these studies, namely, that isolated hearts from laboratory animals convert AA mainly into three types of prostaglandin—E_2, $F_{2\alpha}$, and I_2.

In the studies on the conversion of [^{14}C]AA in isolated bovine coronary arteries (Raz *et al.*, 1977), the profile of [^{14}C]PGs formed displayed surprisingly good agreement with the patterns of [^{14}C]PG appearing in the effluent from rabbit hearts infused with labeled precursor. This conformity led the authors to suggest that the biosynthesis of PG in the heart is largely restricted to the coronary vessels. Data supporting this hypothesis were obtained recently in our laboratory. Sustained (75–200 min) perfusion of isolated rabbit hearts with anoxic solution, leading to complete extinction of their mechanical activity, did not change the metabolism of [^{14}C]AA in the hearts. This suggests that the myocardium is not the main site of PG production in the heart and, consequently, highlights the alternative that cardiac PG mainly originates form the coronary vasculature (Wennmalm, 1979b).

Human cardiac PG formation is incompletely documented. Kulkarni *et al.* (1976) observed that AA relaxed isolated strips of human coronary artery and that such relaxation was counteracted by inhibition of PG synthesis. With present knowledge it appears reasonable to conclude that the coronary relaxation these authors observed was due to formation of prostacyclin. Some studies have also been performed on human cardiac PG formation *in vivo*. Berger and co-workers (1977) observed release of PGF into the coronary sinus blood in patients paced to angina, but were unable to detect release of PGA or PGE. At rest no PG release was observed. Neither prostacyclin nor 6-keto-PGF$_{1\alpha}$ was analyzed in that study. In a recent study in our laboratory, [^{14}C]AA was infused into the aortic root in male volunteers and the coronary sinus blood was analyzed for [^{14}C]PGs (Nowak *et al.*, 1980). Apart from [^{14}C]PG metabolites, labeled 6-keto-PGF$_{1\alpha}$ was found to constitute the largest radiopeak, indicating formation of prostacyclin in the human heart *in vivo*. Small peaks of labeled PGD$_2$, PGE$_2$, and PGF$_{2\alpha}$ were also observed. Interestingly, in a 54-year-old subject, 6-keto-PGF$_{1\alpha}$ constituted a greater proportion of [^{14}C]PG (60%) than in the other subjects. Whether that difference reflects a general effect of aging or indicates the presence in that subject of ischemic heart disease (cf. Section VI,B in this chapter) remains an open question.

IV. Physiological and Pharmacological Interference with Cardiac Biosynthesis

A. Stimulation of Cardiac Prostaglandin Formation

1. General Considerations

Various stimuli of PG bioformation have been described. Most of the data presented are based on experiments with isolated perfused organs. Under such experimental conditions there is often a moderate basal release of PG. An increasing amount of evidence indicates, however, that *in vivo*, basal release of PG from tissues, if present at all, is very low. One should therefore be very cautious about applying experimental results from isolated organs to the *in vivo* situation. Even if factors that stimulate PG formation in isolated organs may be capable of doing so *in vivo*, too, the effect of the PG released may be different in the two situations. The isolated organ perfusion involves a number of artificial factors, including the use of a low-oxygen perfusion medium without colloid pressure, an unregulated perfusion (constant pressure or constant flow), and lack of neuronal or hormonal regulation of vascular tone. This tends to put the organ in a distress that probably activates endogenous defense mechanisms. More physiological conditions are obtained if PG release is studied *in vivo*, but even then the anesthetic or analgesic used, as well as the operation or catheterization, may tend to disturb the data.

Normally, PG bioformation is controlled via the rate-limiting step, that is, the mobilization of AA from the physiological stores (cf. Section II,C in this chapter). Most agents that stimulate PG bioformation do so by activating phospholipase A, which in turn promotes hydrolysis of the AA-phospholipid esters and thereby increases the amount of precursor available for synthesis. The rate-limiting step in PG bioformation can be evaded by the exogenous administration of AA, to the organ to be studied, in the heart as well as in other organs (cf. Mentz and Förster, 1977). If AA is given to a tissue or organ, the precursor is transformed into the type(s) of PG that accords with the enzymatic set of that tissue. Whether AA, on the basis of such promotion of PG synthesis, should be regarded as a true stimulator of the bioformation of PG is questionable.

Agents that apparently initiate or accelerate PG formation by activating phospholipase A may be chemical, neuronal, or physical in nature. To the chemical stimulants belong some adenine nucleotides and certain peptides, as well as autonomic neurotransmitters (noradrenaline, acetylcholine). The neuronal stimuli of PG bioformation are sympathetic and parasympathetic nerve activity. The physical stimuli are hypoxia or ischemia and certain mechanical events (e.g., vibration). In the following sections these stimuli are discussed in more detail, with special reference to the heart. The possible physiological implications of an accelerated PG synthesis elicited by the various agents will be considered in Section VI of this chapter.

2. Adenine Nucleotides

Infusion of the adenine nucleotides, adenosine triphosphate (ATP) and adenosine diphosphate (ADP), at doses of 10^{-8} to 10^{-7} moles consistently released prostaglandinlike substances (PLS) from isolated perfused rabbit hearts (Minkes et al., 1973). PLS was analyzed with bioassay, which ruled out definite conclusions concerning the type of PG released. Later the same authors reported that ATP and ADP acted as PG releasers in a variety of perfused organs, and they were also able to strengthen the identity of the PLS by showing that the release was blocked by the PG synthesis inhibitor indomethacin (Needleman et al., 1974). In that study it was also reported that guanosine diphosphate, adenosine, and cyclic AMP were ineffective as PG releasers.

3. Peptides

Angiotensin II (AII) was demonstrated initially by McGiff and co-workers (1970a) to be a PG releasing agent in the canine kidney. These authors infused AII into the renal artery of anesthetized dogs and assayed PLS in the venous effluent with a cascade of blood-bathed assay organs. Their observation was confirmed by others, infusing AII into the saline-perfused cat spleen (Ferreira et al., 1973), the isolated perfused rabbit spleen (Douglas et al., 1973), splenic fat pad (Needleman et al., 1973a), and kidney (Needleman et al., 1973b).

The first attempt to stimulate cardiac PG formation by infusion of angiotensin was not equally successful. AI (50–200 ng) and AII (50–200 ng) proved inefficient in eliciting release of PLS from isolated rabbit hearts (Minkes et al., 1973). However, in a later report the same group reported that infusion of AII into isolated rabbit hearts, perfused for 1–2 hr, did in fact elicit a release of PLS that was abolished by indomethacin (Needleman et al., 1975a). In that study the dose required to stimulate PG bioformation was 1–2 μg, but in recent studies even lower doses have been reported efficient (cf. Fig. 8).

Bradykinin has also been reported to stimulate PG formation and release in various organs. Piper and Vane (1969) observed that infusion of bradykinin at a rate of 1–2.5 μg/ml into isolated perfused sensitized guinea pig lungs caused release of PLS into the effluent. Later it was shown that the release of PLS was short-lasting, even when the administration of bradykinin was continued (Palmer et al., 1973). Bradykinin is also capable of eliciting a transient PLS release from canine (McGiff et al., 1972) and rabbit (Needleman et al., 1973b) kidney. Bradykinin was reported initially to be incapable of stimulating cardiac release of PLS (Minkes et al., 1973), but efflux of PGE_2-like activity was detected later in the effluent from isolated rabbit hearts injected with bradykinin (50–200 ng) (Needleman et al., 1975b). This efflux was markedly enhanced by simultaneous infusion of a bradykininase inhibitor and was completely blocked by indomethacin. Even in the rabbit heart the efflux of PLS was transient; this was also true when bradykinin infusion was sustained (Needleman et al., 1975a, cf. Fig. 8).

Few studies have been performed on the effects of AII and bradykinin in the heart in situ. A comprehensive investigation was presented recently, however, on the effect of these peptides on coronary flow in anesthetized open-chest dogs before and after administration of PG synthesis inhibitors (Hintze and Kaley, 1977). It was found that the total increment to blood flow caused by bradykinin, or the reduction induced by AII, was not altered significantly by inhibition of cardiac PG formation. These data are not consistent with the hypothesis that AII and bradykinin elicit stimulation of cardiac PG formation, but rather emphasize the necessity of being extremely cautious about extrapolating data from experiments on isolated organs to the in vivo situation.

4. Nerve Stimulation and Neurotransmitters

The first indication of a release of PG from organs during activation of their autonomic nerve supply was obtained by Davies and co-workers (1967, 1968) using the sympathetically stimulated canine spleen. In the same tissue PG release was also evoked by injection of adrenaline (Gilmore *et al.,* 1968). In both these experiments the release of PG was abolished by pretreatment with α-adrenergic blocking agents, indicating that the mechanical response to either of these stimuli was necessary to evoke release of PG. Release of PG or PG-like material from cardiac tissue in response to sympathetic nerve stimulation has also been demonstrated (Wennmalm and Stjärne, 1971; Samuelsson and Wennmalm, 1971). In analogy with the observation in the dog spleen, the release in the rabbit heart could be evoked by other types of adrenoceptor activation, as shown in a study where noradrenaline was infused and found capable of releasing PLS (Junstad and Wennmalm, 1973a). The mechanism behind the release of PG from organs in response to adrenergic stimulation is still incompletely known. Blockade of α- and β-adrenergic receptors completely abolished the release of PLS from hearts infused with NA, indicating that activation of adrenergic receptors is crucial (Wennmalm, 1975). However, the picture is probably more complicated, since it has been demonstrated that neither administration of a pure α-adrenergic agonist (methoxamine) nor that of a β-adrenergic agonist (isoprenaline) is capable of evoking release of PLS from isolated rabbit hearts. In view of these data it has been suggested that cardiac release of PLS induced by noradrenaline is due to activation of a hitherto unobserved adrenoceptive mechanism, optimally stimulated by noradrenaline (Wennmalm and Brundin, 1978) (see Fig. 6).

Concerning the type of PG formed during nerve stimulation or infusion of noradrenaline, almost nothing is known. In most studies the activity released has been identified biologically. In one study, however, hearts prelabeled with [^{14}C]AA and subjected to sustained sympathetic nerve stimulation displayed a profile of [^{14}C]PG release (Wennmalm, 1978d) that did not differ from that obtained during infusion of [^{14}C]AA without simultaneous sympathetic stimulation. Consequently, there is no reason to assume that cardiac PG formation under adrenergic influence is directed from the normal pathway toward, for example, formation of just one type of PG.

Like sympathetic nerve stimulation, parasympathetic activity evokes release of PLS from isolated hearts. Bilateral vagal stimulation at 5 Hz, as well as infusion of acetylcholine, elicited outflow of PLS in isolated perfused rabbit hearts (Junstad and Wennmalm, 1974). The release was completely blocked by atropin, indicating that muscarinic receptors were involved.

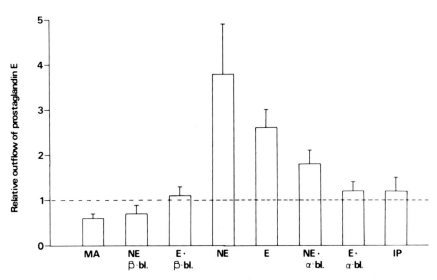

Fig. 6. Outflow of PGE from the isolated rabbit heart during infusion of sympathomimetic amines in the absence and in the presence of adrenolytic agents. The PGE outflow is expressed as the ratio between the outflow during the drug infusion period and the mean outflow during the preceding and the following period. Relative outflow figures under the broken horizontal line consequently indicate that no increase in PGE outflow was obtained during the drug infusion. The different sympathomimetic drugs are arranged from the left to the right in decreasing α-agonistic and increasing β-agonistic effect. MA, Methoxamine; NE, norepinephrine; E, epinephrine; IP, isoprenaline; α-bl, phentolamine; β-bl, propanolol. (Reproduced from Wennmalm and Brundin, 1978, with the permission of the publisher.)

Comparing the capacity of the two cardiac neurotransmitters, noradrenaline and acetylcholine, reveals that on a molar basis, noradrenaline is at least four times more efficient in liberating PLS than acetylcholine (Wennmalm, 1975). The same difference did not apply to stimulation of the sympathetic versus parasympathetic nerve supply to the heart, the former releasing 17–25 pg/impulse and the latter 11 pg/impulse (Junstad and Wennmalm, 1974). The basis for this discrepancy between the liberating ability of sympathetic or parasympathetic nerve activity, on the one hand, and infusion of the corresponding neurotransmitters, on the other, is not clear. The morphological relation between the two kinds of nerve terminals and the sites where PG production was stimulated may have differed, but data supporting such a hypothesis are not available.

5. Ischemia, Hypoxia, and Other Physical Interventions

Induction of unilateral renal ischemia in anesthetized dogs evokes release of PLS into the effluent of the ischemic kidney (McGiff *et al.,* 1970b). This very important observation may be regarded as the basis for all subsequent investigations that imply that endogenous PG plays a role in the vascular defense mechanism (reactive hyperemia) against tissue damage due to hypoxia. The fact that not only the ischemic but also the contralateral kidney was found to increase its formation of PLS initially complicated the interpretation of the data and some years passed before ischemia was tested as a stimulus of PG bioformation in extrarenal tissues. It was then demonstrated that periods of coronary occlusion in anesthetized dogs (Kraemer and Folts, 1973; Kraemer *et al.*, 1976) or in canine heart–lung preparations (Kent *et al.*, 1973; Alexander *et al.*, 1975) elicited a release of PGE into the cardiac effluent during the postocclusive period. Evidence for an accelerated formation of PG during ischemia has also been obtained in human myocardium. In patients with coronary artery disease, pacing to angina was followed by increased levels of PGF in coronary sinus blood, while at the same time the aortic PGF level remained constant. No release of PGA or PGE was observed (Berger *et al.*, 1974, 1977). From these data it may be concluded that ischemia is a stimulus for the myocardial bioformation of PG in various species. As to the type(s) of PG formed, however, our knowledge is still very incomplete. In this connection it is also necessary to stress that an increased myocardial synthesis of PG does not necessarily reflect an event of physiological significance. The possible physiological role of endogenous PG is discussed in Section VI in this chapter.

The mechanism behind the stimulatory effect of ischemia on tissue PG formation has not been studied very extensively. In isolated rabbit hearts, sustained (6–15 min) anoxia was followed by release of PLS (Block and Vane, 1973; Block *et al.*, 1974), and similar results were obtained in our laboratory when isolated rabbit hearts were perfused with a solution aerated by 5% O_2 and 5% CO_2 in N_2 (Wennmalm *et al.*, 1974). The latter study also demonstrated that hypotension and hypoglycemia were unable to increase the cardiac PG formation, suggesting that the factor that actually increases the synthesis of PG in an ischemic tissue or organ is the hypoxia induced. Results pointing in the same direction were obtained in isolated bovine coronary artery strips exposed to decreased oxygen tension. Thus lowering the P_{O_2} in the bath in which the strips were suspended, from about 500 to less than 100 mm Hg, induced a considerable release of PG (Kalsner, 1976). However, when the oxygen tension in the bath was further reduced to 9 mm Hg, the output of PG was sharply curtailed. On the basis of these data the author concluded that PG synthesis is accelerated by hypoxia unless the oxygen deprivation is so severe that it limits the supply of oxygen for synthesis (Kalsner, 1977).

Available data thus suggest that cardiac tissue—myocardial cells or coronary vessels unspecified—accelerates its synthesis of PG when exposed to ischemia and that the virtual stimulus connected with the ischemia is the lowered tissue oxygen tension. Furthermore, it appears that below a certain level of tissue oxygen tension, the hypoxia counteracts rather than stimulates PG bioformation. The possible physiological significance of hypoxia-induced stimulation of cardiac PG formation is discussed in Section VI of this chapter. Here it will simply be noted that tissue oxygen tension *in vivo* may well reach the level where, according to the data cited earlier, formation of PG is facilitated.

Other physical or mechanical stimuli of cardiac PG formation have also been tested. Block and Vane (1973), on perfusion of isolated rabbit hearts, observed that when the rhythmic spontaneous contractions of the organ were abolished by electrically induced fibrillation, there was a concomitant reduction in the output of PLS. The concentration of PLS rose again, however, when the heart was squeezed or when it regained its normal rhythm. The authors suggested that an active cardiac contraction is a prerequisite for PG release in the organ (Block *et al.,* 1974). This conception was not supported by a comprehensive study performed in our laboratory on the effect of various alterations to the internal environment on the release of PLS from isolated hearts (Wennmalm, 1975). It was found that an increase in the contractile force of the heart could be induced by hyperosmolarity, hypothermia, and hypotension without affecting the liberation of PLS. Furthermore, in the same study a decreased contractile force could be evoked by increased K^+, increased perfusion temperature, and decreased pH, again without alterations in the effluent content of PLS. The observations led us to conclude that the mechanical performance per se is not decisive for the liberation of PG from the heart. According to our experience, liberation of PLS from isolated rabbit hearts depends to a considerable degree on the handling of the animal and the organ during killing and dissection. Thus prolongation of the dissection time (e.g., because of free dissection of the autonomic nerve supply) elevates the initial basal release of PLS two to three times (Junstad and Wennmalm, 1974). Hearts displaying a high basal release of PLS during the first phase of a perfusion experiment usually show a lower liberation as perfusion continues (unpublished observation). Consequently, when studying release of PLS from an isolated heart *in situ* or *in vitro,* the animal and the organ must be treated very gently. Otherwise there is an obvious risk of jumping to unwarranted conclusions.

B. Inhibition of Cardiac Prostaglandin Formation

1. General Considerations

Sooner or later almost every scientist working in the PG field comes up against the problem of inhibiting PG bioformation. The reason for this is obvious: the easiest way to evaluate the role of an endogenous compound in the function of a tissue or organ is to study the effect of its withdrawal. This is especially true in PG research, since agents are still not available for blocking the actions of various PGs in tissues ("receptor blocking agents").

Inhibition of PG bioformation has, after the extremely important finding by Vane (1971), become almost synonymous with administration of nonsteroid antiinflammatory agents. That discovery unquestionably added a new dimension to PG research, not only through the wider insight it provided concerning the role of PG in the inflammatory process, but also because of the excellent tool it offered for studying the physiological effects of PGs in various tissues. Nevertheless, some other ways of interfering with PG bioformation, both *in vivo* and *in vitro,* do in fact exist and for certain experimental purposes they may provide a valuable alternative to the aspirinlike drugs.

2. Interference with Precursor Availability or Mobilization

An analysis of the current possibilities for interfering with PG bioformation reveals that several levels in the synthesis process may be attacked. Since PGs are formed from AA or dihomo-γ-linolenic acid, withdrawal of polyunsaturated fatty acids from the diet leads to precursor deficiency and consequently also to decreased synthesis of PG. Using this method has a certain advantage: No drug is needed and consequently no drug side effects have to be considered. The drawbacks are that proper food may be difficult to obtain, that a certain breeding time is needed, and that the diet may evoke other types of deficiency symptoms.

Apart from a decrease in dietary unsaturated fatty acids, PG bioformation can be inhibited either by interfering with the phospholipase-mediated mobilization of PG precursor from the membrane phospholipids or by inhibiting the enzymatic conversion of AA to various PGs.

Inhibition of lipolysis in rat adipose tissues occurs with a variety of hydrophobic antimalarial agents, such as quinacrine, cloroquine, and meparcine (Markus and Ball, 1969). The mechanism behind such inhibition is not known. Meparcine appears to be effective as an inhibitor of AA mobilization, and thereby also of PG bioformation. This was demonstrated in isolated perfused guinea pig lungs, in which the formation and subsequent release of RCS (rabbit aorta contracting substance, a mixture of TxA$_2$ and PG endoperoxides) induced by AA infusion was unaffected by mepacrine, while following injection of bradykinin (which requires activation of acylhydrolases) release of RCS was completely blocked (Vargaftig and DaoHai, 1972). No reports have appeared on inhibition of cardiac PG formation by drugs that block acylhydrolase activity, but there is reason to assume that tissue-to-tissue variations in the inactivation of phospholipase

A_2 should be small, and consequently that mepacrine and related drugs should be effective also in the heart. The principle of blocking mobilization of endogenous AA may be of great value when studying the conversion of exogenous AA to PG in an organ or tissue without interference from endogenous AA (mobilized, for example, during the manipulation of the tissue). A disadvantage with these drugs is that at higher concentrations they may interfere with cyclo-oxygenase activity.

Another group of drugs that interferes with AA mobilization is the antiinflammatory steroids. Release of PLS into the venous effluent from working dog's hindleg was demonstrated to be diminished by hydrocortisone by Herbaczynska-Cedro and Staszewska-Barczak (1974, 1977). Similar data were reported by Lewis and Piper (1975). The latter authors suggested that corticosteroids inhibit the release of PG by preventing their transport across the cell membrane. The validity of that hypothesis was questioned when release of PGE induced by noradrenaline, but not by AA, was abolished by various corticosteroids (Gryglewski *et al.*, 1975).

3. Inhibition of Arachidonic Acid Conversion to PG Endoperoxides

Agents that inhibit PG release by actually interfering with the conversion of precursor (AA) to PGs may be grouped into two unrelated classes: the first is substrate analogs, of which only one, 5,8,11,14-eicosatetraynoic acid (ETA) (Downing *et al.*, 1970), an acetylenic derivation of AA, has been used at all frequently in animal experiments, and the second is the aspirin-like drugs (Vane, 1971) (Fig. 7). ETA has been used to inhibit PG formation in isolated rabbit hearts (Samuelsson and Wennmalm, 1971; Junstad and Wennmalm, 1973b). In these experiments the ammonium salt of the compound, infused to produce a concentration in the perfusate of 10^{-6} to 4×10^{-5} M, was sufficient to produce an almost complete inhibition of PG formation. The use of ETA for inhibition of PG formation has certain disadvantages: Synthesis inhibition elicited by ETA is irreversible, the compound is very unstable and degrades spontaneously even in solid form, and is cardiotoxic (myocardial performance is impaired) at concentrations above 5×10^{-5} M.

The most common way of blocking the biosynthesis of PGs in tissues is to inhibit cyclooxygenase activity with nonsteroid antiinflammatory drugs. PG synthesis inhibition by aspirin and related agents was first demonstrated by Vane (1971), using cell-free homogenates of guinea pig lung. Subsequently, a large number of antiinflammatory drugs have been reported to counteract PG formation in various tissues. Aspirin and indomethacin are the two drugs that have attracted most interest as inhibitors of PG biosynthesis. Many investigators have reported on $(I)_{50}$ concentrations for aspirin and

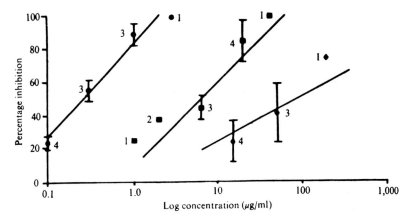

Fig. 7. Concentration (μg/ml) of indomethacin (●), aspirin (■), and salicylate (◆) plotted on a log scale against the percentage inhibition of PG synthesis (assayed as $PGF_{2\alpha}$ on rat colons). The lines are those calculated for best fit. Numbers by the points indicate number of experiments. Where three or more estimates were averaged, the standard error of the mean is shown. (Reproduced from Vane, 1971, with the permission of the publisher.)

indomethacin as PG synthesis inhibitors in a wide variety of animal tissues. In most tissues indomethacin is considerably (10–20,000 times) more effective—on a molar basis—than aspirin, the $(I)_{50}$ concentration varying between 0.1 and 10 M. In intact tissues or animals the dose required to inhibit PG biosynthesis has not been studied as carefully; i.e., the pharmacokinetics of indomethacine in the tissue or species to be investigated has generally not been taken into account. In the most usual cardiac preparation in our laboratory, the isolated perfused rabbit heart, an indomethacin concentration in the perfusion solution of 5×10^{-5} M is used routinely to block PG formation completely. Using indomethacin may cause problems to the investigator in certain situations, since the substance is insoluble in water. However, solutions can be prepared in 0.1 M phosphate buffer at slightly alkaline pH, but in such solutions the drug decomposes spontaneously. In our experience the most convenient way of handling the drug is to prepare a stock solution (10–50 mg/ml) in ethanol, from which dilutions in phosphate buffer (pH 7.4) may be prepared immediately prior to use.

4. Inhibition of PG Endoperoxide Conversion to Thromboxane and Prostacyclin

Cyclooxygenase is not the only enzyme involved in the bioformation of PGs that can be blocked by drugs. Inhibition of thromboxane synthetase and of prostacyclin synthetase has been reported with various agents. Although thromboxanes are not found in cardiac tissue, agents blocking the enzymes required for their synthesis may be of interest to those working in the cardiology field in view of their possible therapeutic value in the prevention of coronary thrombosis. Thromboxane synthetase has been reported to be inhibited by benzydamine [$(I)_{50}$ = 100 μg/ml, Moncada *et al.*, 1976b]. Unfortunately, this effect of the drug is not completely selective, since it can also inhibit cyclo-oxygenase [$(I)_{50}$ = 250 μg/ml]. More selective inhibition of TxA$_2$ formation in platelets appears to be achieved following administration of imidazole (Needleman *et al.*, 1977b) or the antiinflammatory agent 2-isopropyl-3-nicotinylindole (L 8027, Gryglewski *et al.*, 1977). The former of these compounds, imidazole, has also been shown to exert an antithrombotic action *in vivo* (Puig-Parellada and Planas, 1977).

Prostacyclin synthetase can also be inhibited selectively. Unlike the inhibition of thromboxane synthetase, blockade of the prostacyclin-forming enzyme appears to be of limited clinical value. Nevertheless, inhibitors of prostacyclin synthetase may be valuable in various experimental situations. Hitherto, only two inhibitors of prostacyclin formation have been reported: 15-hydroperoxyarachidonic acid (15-HPAA, Gryglewski *et al.*, 1976) and nicotine (Wennmalm 1978a,b). The $(I)_{50}$ for 15-HPAA is 0.5 μg/ml (2 μM) and for nicotine it is about 1 μM. The action of nicotine on the formation of prostacyclin raises the question of the extent to which the use of tobacco may induce a similar effect in smoking subjects. This issue will be considered later in this chapter (Section VI).

V. Effects of Prostaglandins on Cardiac Tissue

A. Effects of Prostaglandin Precursor

Arachidonic acid (AA) is the quantitatively most important precursor in PG biosynthesis (cf. Section II,B in this chapter). Since the enzymes required for conversion of AA to various PGs are immediately available in cytoplasmic particles, the rate of PG formation depends on the amount of precursor available. Consequently, addition of PG precursor to a tissue or organ stimulates biosynthesis of PGs. The types of PGs formed, as well as the quantitative relation between them, is of course determined by the enzymatic set of the tissue studied. This implies that the normal pattern of PGs produced in a tissue also applies after administration of AA. This in turn makes it easier to predict the pharmacological effects of PG precursor; since the precursor fatty acids generally lack biological effects of their own, the actions evoked by their administration are usually elicited by the PGs they are converted into.

Few studies have in fact been made on the effect of PG precursors on aspects of cardiac function. This is not surprising, since the results tend to be trivial. Nevertheless, under certain circumstances the findings have proved interesting. Thus it was observed that infusion of AA into the perfusate as it entered the perfused rabbit heart led to a concentration-dependent decrease in the coronary resistance and that, furthermore, indomethacin abolished this decrease (Needleman, 1976) (Fig. 8). No doubt this finding must have been puzzling, since in the same preparation PGE_2 was unable to affect coronary resistance. At that time it was not known that infusion of AA resulted in bioformation of vasodilating prostacyclin. Dilation of the coronary vascular bed following administration of AA has also been reported to develop in perfused guinea pig hearts (Schrör et al., 1978). In analogy with the rabbit heart experiment referred to earlier, the coronary vasodilatation was inhibited by treatment of the heart with indomethacin, indicating that the PG formed, and not the AA itself, was the active principle.

Similar effects of AA have been reported in experiments with isolated strips of bovine, canine, and human coronary arteries. AA (100 ng to 10 μg/ml) caused relaxation of all types of strips, and this relaxation was inhibited by pretreatment with the PG synthetase inhibitors, indomethacine, meclofenamate, and aspirin (Kulkarni et al., 1976; Needleman et al., 1977a).

Apart from its effects on coronary tone, the actions of AA or cardiac function are unknown. When predicting effects of AA on various aspects of cardiac performance, it should be born in mind that the distribution of PG synthetizing enzymes in various parts of the heart is still somewhat obscure. This implies that even if a certain PG is active in the heart in a certain respect, administration of AA will mimic this effect only if the specific PG-producing enzyme is present in that part of the heart in which this effect is elicited.

B. Effects on Cardiac Pacemaker Activity

1. Chronotropic Actions

The study of chronotropic effects of PGs provides drastic examples of the significance of technique and species differences, not to mention the variations between the chronotropic actions of different PGs. Since most authors agree that reflex tachycardia is a possible, if not probable, consequence of administration of vasodilator PGs (e.g., PGEs) to intact animals, it seems reasonable to concentrate on the effects of PGs in preparations where the possibility of extracardiac influence on the heart rate is excluded or at least diminished.

The early experiments by von Euler (1936) demonstrated that extracts of

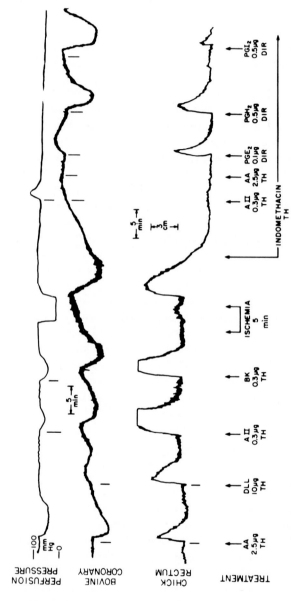

Fig. 8. Response of the isolated perfused rabbit heart and the superfused assay tissues to fatty acid or hormonal stimulation and to changes in oxygen tension. The following abbreviations were employed: AA, arachidonic acid; DLL, dihomo-γ-linolenic acid; A II, angiotensin II; BK, bradykinin. The numbers in the treatment section indicate nanograms of agonist employed. DIR denotes direct application of available standards to the assay tissue and TH denotes injection through the heart. Ischemia was produced by diverting the flow of media away from the heart (by means of a three-way stopcock) and directly across the assay tissues. 20 min was allowed to elapse after intracardiac indomethacin (300 ng/ml) treatment. The bioassay experiments were each repeated five times with the same results. An angiotensin antagonist (Sar[1], Ile[8]-AII) was continuously infused across the assay tissues to eliminate any direct effects of AII itself. (Reproduced from Needleman *et al.*, 1978, with the permission of the publisher.)

human seminal fluid were devoid of chronotropic activity when tested in isolated rabbit hearts. The spontaneous beating frequency did increase, however, in frog heart prepared according to Straub. Von Euler (1939) also demonstrated the lack of effect of a crude extract of sheep vesicular glands on the mechanical performance of the cat heart–lung preparation. Later studies have confirmed that E prostaglandins lack chronotropic effects in isolated rabbit and cat hearts (Berti *et al.*, 1965; Mantegazza, 1965), as well as in isolated chicken hearts (Horton and Main, 1967). The positive chronotropic effect observed by von Euler in frog hearts has likewise been confirmed and extended to isolated guinea pig hearts or atria (Berti *et al.*, 1965; Mantegazza, 1965; Courtney *et al.*, 1978). In some species isolated atria appear to behave differently from intact hearts when exposed to PGs of the E series. Thus PGE_1 was found to increase the beating frequency of isolated cat but not dog atria (Su *et al.*, 1973), while not changing the rate of isolated cat hearts (cf. earlier). Similarly, PGE_2 has been reported to increase the rate of spontaneously beating rat atria (Levy, 1973) while producing no chronotropic effect in isolated intact rat hearts (Vergroesen *et al.*, 1967).

The chronotropic effect of the prostaglandins of the A and F series has not been studied so frequently. Most investigations report a lack of effect in isolated hearts. Vergroesen *et al.* (1967) found that $PGF_{1\alpha}$ was unable to alter the rate of the isolated rat heart, and similar results were obtained by others, administering $PGF_{2\alpha}$ to rabbit or chicken hearts (Lee *et al.*, 1965; Horton and Main, 1967). In analogy with PGE_1, $PGF_{2\alpha}$ was found to increase the frequency of contraction of isolated cat but not dog atria (Su *et al.*, 1973). The overall picture of the effect of various PGs on pacemaker activity in isolated hearts is indeed complex, and no rational pattern has been discerned. Perhaps the most prominent feature is the lack of chronotropic effect of most PGs investigated in isolated hearts, apart from those of guinea pigs. The positive chronotropic effects that have in fact been observed in mammalian hearts were obtained under highly artificial experimental conditions, whose significance for the *in vivo* situation is unclear.

E and A prostaglandins have been shown in many studies to produce tachycardia and systemic hypotension in dogs (e.g., Steinberg *et al.*, 1964; Lee *et al.*, 1965; Bergström *et al.*, 1966; Nakano and McCurdy, 1967) (Fig. 9). Similar observations have been reported in cat (Koss *et al.*, 1973), calf (Anderson *et al.*, 1972; Lewis and Eyre, 1972), and man (Bergström *et al.*, 1959). The tachycardia induced is most probably due to reflex sympathetic activation. Already in 1939 von Euler had demonstrated that in cat or rabbit with denervated carotid sinus and heart, infusion of crude PG extracts produced marked hypotension without a simultaneous increase in heart rate. Further evidence has been presented to show that the tachycardia

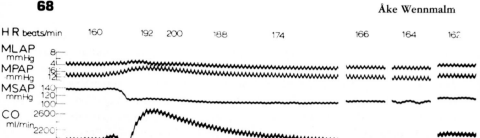

Fig. 9. Effects of the iv administration of 4.0 μg/kg of PGE₁ on heart rate (HR), mean left atrial pressure (MLAP), mean pulmonary arterial pressure (MPAP), mean systemic arterial pressure (MSAP), cardiac output (CO), and myocardial contractile force (MCF) in a dog. (Reproduced from Nakano and McCurdy, 1967, with the permission of the publisher.)

observed after systemic infusion of E prostaglandins is not due to a direct intrinsic effect on the cardiac pacemaker. PGA_1 did not produce any significant change in heart rate in conscious dogs, provided alterations in β-adrenergic activation and afterload were prevented (Higgins *et al.*, 1972), and direct infusion of PGE_1 into the sinus node artery did not produce any significant change in heart rate in anesthetized dogs (Chiba *et al.*, 1972). Hitherto, no data have been presented on the effect of prostacyclin on the cardiac pacemaker. Such data would be of considerable significance, since PGI_2 is the main PG formed in the heart in many species (cf. Section III in this chapter). Armstrong *et al.* (1977) reported that only variable changes in heart rate occurred in chloralose anesthetized dogs following iv infusion of PGI_2, despite a consistent decrease in systemic blood pressure.

A direct effect of PGs on the central control of heart rate has also been suggested. Infusion of PGE_1 increased the heart rate in dogs more powerfully when infused into the vertebral artery than when infused either intravenously or into the carotid artery, in all cases without affecting systemic blood pressure (Lavery *et al.*, 1970). Such an effect could not be evoked by infusion of PGA_1. All these data support the view that tachycardia that develops in conjunction with systemic hypotension during infusion of vasodilator PGs in intact animals is reflex in origin, possibly facilitated by a direct effect of the PG infused on the CNS.

2. Effects of Cardiac Arrhythmias

One should also consider the effect of E prostaglandins on cardiac arrhythmias. Zijlstra *et al.* (1972) demonstrated in dogs that infusion of PGE_1

effectively suppressed the bigeminy associated with thiobarbiturate anesthesia, as well as the ventricular tachycardia due to acute myocardial ischemia. An antiarrhythmic effect of $PGF_{2\alpha}$ on various models of experimental arrhythmias in rat, rabbit, and cat has also been reported (Förster et al., 1973) and of PGE_2 on catecholamine-induced arrhythmias in guinea pigs (Mest et al., 1977a). Recently, antiarrhythmic effects of the PG precursors AA and linoleic acid were demonstrated on various experimental arrhythmias in rabbit, cat, and guinea pig (Mest et al., 1977b). The effect was reduced by pretreatment of the animals with indomethacin, indicating that cardiac conversion of the infused precursor to PG preceded the antiarrhythmic action. The possible therapeutic value of PG in cardiac arrhythmias in man has also been studied (Mann, 1976). Infusion of $PGF_{2\alpha}$ resulted in a transitory regression of ventricular extrasystoles, the results being particularly evident in patients suffering from myocardial infarction. The mechanism behind the antiarrhythmic effect of PGs and their possible value in clinical routine work cannot be judged at present and require further investigation.

C. Effects on Myocardial Inotropy

Injections of human seminal fluid or corresponding amounts of purified solutions of PG produced a prolonged lowering of the blood pressure in rabbit, cat, and dog, without any definite influence on heart rate or blood pressure (von Euler, 1936). Addition of PG to fluid perfused through the rabbit's isolated heart (Langendorff preparation) did not elicit any clear effect on the amplitude of the contractions (von Euler, 1936). In contrast, frog's hearts prepared according to Straub displayed, on exposure to PG, a change in the type of contractions, characterized by a predominance of the systolic phase and an incomplete diastolic relaxation (von Euler, 1936). Later, the same author showed that crude PG extracts were devoid of inotropic actions in the cat heart–lung preparation (von Euler, 1939). These early observations are still valid and clearly suggest that PGs lack inotropic action in isolated mammalian heart.

PGE_1 has been shown to lack inotropic effect in isolated rabbit (Berti et al., 1965; Lee et al., 1965) and cat (Berti et al., 1965; Sunahara and Talesnik, 1974) heart. PGE_1 also appears to lack inotropic effect in isolated atria from humans (Levy and Killebrew, 1971), cats, and dogs (Su et al., 1973). Some studies, however, have elicited positive inotropic effects, both moderate and more pronounced. This was the case in isolated atria of rabbit (Tuttle and Skelly, 1968; Levy and Killebrew, 1971) and of normal and hypertensive rats (Levy, 1973), in the latter study after PGE_2 as well as PGE_1. The positive inotropic effect of PGE_1 in the frog's heart (cf. earlier) has also been confirmed (Berti *et al.*, 1965; Vergroesen and de Boer, 1968). In isolated guinea pig hearts an increased amplitude of contraction has likewise been reported following administration of PGE_1 (Berti *et al.*, 1965; Mantegazza, 1965; Sobel and Robison, 1969).

The F prostaglandins also display different inotropic effects in different species and preparations. $PGF_{1\alpha}$ or $F_{1\beta}$ produced positive inotropic effects in isolated rat hearts (Vergroesen *et al.*, 1967), and $PGF_{1\alpha}$ also increased the contractile force in the dog heart–lung preparation (Katori *et al.*, 1970). In guinea pig isolated hearts, however, $PGF_{1\alpha}$ was devoid of inotropic action (Sobel and Robison, 1969).

The inotropic effects of PGs in intact animals have been investigated by many authors. Bergström *et al.* (1959), infusing PGE_1 iv in two healthy males, reported a fall in systolic and diastolic pressure as well as a moderate decrease in cardiac output. In contrast, increased cardiac output following infusion of PGE_1 in healthy humans was observed by Carlson *et al.* (1969). These data have been confirmed recently in our laboratory. Infusion of PGE_1 (4–8 μg/min) in healthy males pretreated with indomethacin resulted in a drop in blood pressure and an increase in cardiac output from 6.1 to 8.7 liters/min (Nowak and Wennmalm, 1978). There is reason to assume that the increase in cardiac output observed in these studies is reflex in origin, i.e., due to baroreceptor activation and subsequent sympathetic stimulation of the heart resulting from the decrease in blood pressure. However, evidence has been presented of a direct effect of PGs on myocardial contractile force in intact animals. Intraarterial injection of PGE_1 into the anterior descending branch of the left coronary artery produced an increase in contractile force, even at doses that did not affect systemic blood pressure (Nakano and McCurdy, 1967). Similar data have been reported later by others (Hollenberg *et al.*, 1968; Nutter and Crumly, 1972). Katori *et al.* (1970), studying the dog heart–lung preparation, observed an increased myocardial contractility following administration of PGE_1 at a dose that did not affect heart rate or blood pressure. Prostacyclin, which in many respects resembles the E prostaglandins, has also been shown to increase myocardial performance. In chloralose anesthetized dogs, iv infusion of prostacyclin caused dose-dependent decreases in systemic blood pressure and total peripheral resistance and moderate increases in stroke volume and cardiac output (Armstrong *et al.*, 1977). However, in the same study direct injection of prostacyclin into the left circumflex coronary artery did not cause any change in systemic blood pressure or heart rate. This observation seems to exclude a direct positive inotropic effect of PGI_2 in this preparation. Similar data were reported by Fitzpatrick *et al.* (1978). They showed that PGI_2, unlike PGE_2, did not affect myocardial contractile force in anesthetized closed-chest dogs and that it elicited a slight decrease in contractile force in dogs with a left ventricular bypass preparation.

Taken together, the data obtained in isolated heart, atria, or papillary muscles and the results obtained in anesthetized or conscious animals or man indicate that PGs may have positive inotropic effects, but that considerable and unpredictable differences exist, both with respect to the animal investigated and the type of PG administered.

The mechanism by which PGs produce positive inotropic effects in certain species has been studied, too. Most results for intact and isolated hearts indicate that the PG effects are not mediated via adrenergic or cholinergic mechanisms, but rather reflect a direct action on the myocardium. Thus the positive inotropic effects of various PGs have been reported to persist after α-adrenergic blockade (Levy and Killebrew, 1971), β-adrenergic blockade (Berti *et al.*, 1965; Mantegazza, 1965; Nakano and McCurdy, 1967), and atropine (Levy and Killebrew, 1971). Furthermore, vagotomy (Nakano and McCurdy, 1968) or pretreatment with reserpine (Berti *et al.*, 1965; Mantegazza, 1965) did not change the inotropic effect of PG. A possible biochemical link between the administration of PG and the resulting increased contractile force would be activation of the adenylate cyclase-cyclic AMP system. In isolated guinea pig hearts the inotropic effects of PGE_1 and $PGF_{1\alpha}$ were linked to an increase in the cardiac activity of adenylate cyclase (Sobel and Robison, 1969), and in rat hearts increased intracellular cyclic AMP and activated phosphorylase were observed following addition of PGE_1 (Piccinini *et al.*, 1969; Curnow and Nuttal, 1971). In contrast, PGA_1, PGA_2, PGE_2, and $PGF_{2\alpha}$ did not affect accumulation of cyclic AMP in subcellular fractions of cat myocardial tissue. The connection between PG, inotropic effects, and the adenylate cyclase–cyclic AMP system consequently remains an open question.

D. Effect on Coronary Flow

The effect of various PGs on coronary vascular resistance has been investigated fairly frequently, using a wide range of techniques and preparations. Coronary strips, isolated hearts, and intact animals have been used, and the species investigated include man, cattle, pig, dog, cat, rabbit, rat, and others.

Isolated bovine, canine, and human coronary arteries exhibited dose-dependent contractions to the PGs E_2 and $F_{2\alpha}$. In contrast, PGE_1 caused a dose-dependent relaxation of bovine coronary arteries (Kulkarni *et al.*, 1976). Arachidonic acid was a relaxant of bovine, canine, and human coronary strips, in the absence of indomethacin (Kulkarni *et al.*, 1976), probably due to formation of prostacyclin in the strip.

In isolated perfused heart the actions of various PGs are mainly what one would expect from the experiments on isolated strips. Thus PGE_1 augmented coronary flow in isolated hearts from rat, cat, guinea pig, and rabbit (Mantegazza, 1965), and PGE_1, PGE_2, and PGA_1 increased coronary flow in the isolated rat heart (Vergroesen et al., 1967). PGE_2 and $PGF_{2\alpha}$ (up to 10^{-6} M) did not affect coronary flow in isolated rabbit hearts perfused at constant pressure (Hedqvist and Wennmalm, 1971) but caused a dose-dependent coronary dilatation in guinea pig hearts perfused at constant flow (Schrör et al., 1978). PGI_2 caused a sharp transient reduction in coronary perfusion pressure in rabbit hearts perfused at constant flow (Needleman et al., 1978) (Fig. 10) and the same effect was observed in similarly perfused guinea pig hearts (Schrör et al., 1978).

In anesthetized and conscious dogs, PGs of the A and E series increased coronary blood flow and decreased coronary vascular resistance without affecting heart rate or systemic blood pressure (Nakano and McCurdy, 1967, 1968; and others). The potency of PGE_1 as a coronary vasodilator has been shown to be greater than that of nitroglycerine (Nakano and McCurdy, 1968), and both PGE_1 and PGE_2 have been reported to be more powerful vasodilators than adenosine (Rowe and Afonso, 1974). F prostaglandins are probably not active in the coronary circulation. Thus in the anesthetized dog, intracoronary infusion of $PGF_{2\alpha}$ did not change the coronary blood flow (Nakano, 1968; Hollenberg et al., 1968) and similar results were obtained after iv infusion of $PGF_{2\alpha}$ in the dog (Bloor and Sobel, 1970). However, the effect of PGF in the coronary vasculature may be dose-dependent, since high doses of $PGF_{1\alpha}$ increased coronary flow in the isolated dog heart–lung preparation (Katori et al., 1970).

Hitherto, the effect of prostacyclin on coronary flow in intact animals has been studied only by Armstrong et al. (1977). These authors found that iv infusion of prostacyclin increased peak phasic coronary flow only at a high infusion rate and that mean coronary flow did not change significantly even though coronary vascular resistance was substantially reduced. However, direct injection of prostacyclin into the left circumflex artery increased both phasic and mean coronary flow and decreased coronary vascular resistance without any change in systemic blood pressure or heart rate. These data on the effect of prostacyclin on coronary flow are of special interest, since PGI_2 is the main cardiac PG formed, at least in some species (cf. Section III in this chapter). The discovery of prostacyclin as the principal cardiac PG formed, together with its coronary dilator effect, has stimulated various proposals concerning the role of PGs in the regulation of coronary vasculature. This problem will be discussed in detail in Section VI,B of this chapter.

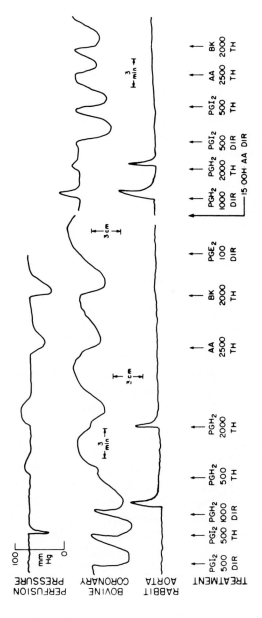

Fig. 10. Comparison of the effect of PGI_2 and PGH_2 on the isolated perfused rabbit heart. The PGI_2 was stored in an ethanol stock. The ethanol was evaporated in a stream of N_2 and was diluted as a 50 mM Tris buffer pH 9 solution just before use. The PGH_2 was stored as an acetone stock solution. The organic solvent was removed in a stream of N_2 and redissolved in a 50 mM phosphate buffer (pH 7.4) just before use. The number below each agonist indicates the amount in nanograms injected. DIR denotes direct application of standards to the assay tissues, and TH denotes injections through the heart. The 15-hydroperoxyarachidonic acid (15-OOH-AA) was dissolved in 0.1 M Tris pH 7.4 buffer and was infused over the assay tissues at a final concentration of 1 μg/ml for 15 min before testing. (Reproduced from Needleman *et al.*, 1978, with the permission of the publisher.)

E. Effect on Autonomic Neurotransmission in the Heart

1. Adrenergic Transmission

More than 10 years ago Hedqvist and Brundin (1969) observed that PGE_1 occasionally reduced the overflow of norepinephrine (NE), which sympathetic nerve stimulation elicited, into the effluent of the perfused cat spleen. Using PGE_2, the inhibitory effect on sympathetic transmitter release in this preparation was demonstrated regularly (Hedqvist, 1970a). This effect of exogenously applied PGs on sympathetic transmitter release appears to be almost ubiquitous in animal tissues. The basic mechanisms of prostaglandin action on autonomic neurotransmission have recently been reviewed (Hedqvist, 1977).

An inhibitory effect on NE release has also been demonstrated in the heart (Hedqvist *et al.,* 1970). In experiments with isolated perfused rabbit hearts (Langendorff preparation) with intact sympathetic nerve supply (Hukovic and Muscholl, 1962) it was demonstrated that the effluent content of NE, appearing in response to stimulation of the sympathetic supply to the heart (1–10 Hz, 30 sec), was markedly and reversibly reduced by PGE_2. This was followed by a more thorough investigation on the effects of various concentrations of PGs E_1, E_2, and $F_{2\alpha}$ on the sympathetically stimulated rabbit heart (Hedqvist and Wennmalm, 1971). A linear or semilinear relationship was found between the log concentration of PGs E_1 or E_2 in the medium perfusing the heart and the inhibition of the NE release elicited by nerve stimulation. As a result of the decreased transmitter release, the chronotropic and inotropic responses to stimulation were reduced, mainly in parallel to the reduction in NE liberation. When PG was omitted from the perfusion solution, the overflow of NE in response to nerve stimulation, as well as the chronotropic and inotropic responses, was completely restored (Fig. 11). PGE_1 appeared to be more efficient than PGE_2 as an inhibitor of NE release, but the difference was not marked. $PGF_{2\alpha}$ was completely devoid of inhibitory activity. The effect of prostacyclin on sympathetic neurotransmission has been studied recently (Wennmalm, 1978a). PGI_2 was about 700 times less active as an inhibitor compared to PGE_2. Although these experiments were not performed in the heart, there is reason—in view of earlier observations on the similarity of the effect of various PGs on different sympathetically innervated organs—to believe that prostacyclin is also a weak inhibitor of cardiac sympathetic neurotransmission.

The inhibitory effect of the E prostaglandins on NE release appears to be related to the depolarization frequency in the adrenergic neurons. Thus, at 10 Hz, PGE_1 (2×10^{-8} M) inhibited transmitter liberation only to about

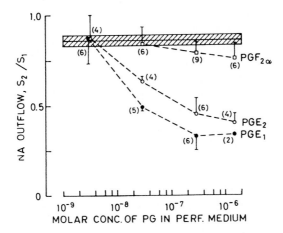

Fig. 11. Perfused rabbit heart. Effect of PGE_1, PGE_2, and $PGF_{2\alpha}$ on outflow of NA in response to sympathetic nerve stimulation (10 per second, 30 sec). All values presented as ratio between second and first stimulation. Hatched area: Control experiments in which PGs were omitted. Vertical bars: Means ± SE. Figures within brackets are the numbers of experiments. (Reproduced from Hedqvist and Wennmalm, 1971, with the permission of the publisher.)

50% of control, compared with 30% of control at 5 Hz and 20% at 2 Hz (Wennmalm, 1978e). Such a frequency dependence of transmitter release is probably the basis for the more efficient reduction of the chronotropic response to sympathetic stimulation elicited by PGE_2 (5×10^{-7} M) at 2 Hz (43% of control) compared with 10 Hz (87% of control) observed in this preparation (Junstad and Wennmalm, 1973b). A similar frequency-response relation was observed by Park *et al.* (1973), studying PGE_2 effects on autonomic neurotransmission in spontaneously beating rabbit sinoatrial nodes. They reported that PGE_2 (8×10^{-7} M) almost completely blocked positive chronotropic responses induced by stimulation of intranodal sympathetic fibers at low frequencies (2–5 Hz) but had no effect at high stimulation frequencies. Data have been presented that indicate that not only the depolarization frequency but also the total number of pulses delivered are decisive for the inhibitory effect of PG. Thus in guinea pig atria field-stimulated at 10 Hz, PGE_1 (3×10^{-8} M) was found to inhibit the inotropic response more powerfully after 10 than after 40 strokes (Illés *et al.*, 1973).

The mechanism behind the inhibitory effect of PG on transmitter liberation is not known in detail. Various studies have excluded the possibility that PGs interfere with the propagation of impulses in the sympathetic nerve trunk or with the spread of excitation throughout the terminal adrenergic network. Furthermore PG does not appear to interfere with the metabolic degradation or reuptake of NE released. It seems rather that the basis for PG action on NE release is to be found in the stimulus-secretion coupling in the terminal arborization. Data supporting such a view have been presented. Thus increased Ca^{2+} concentration in the perfusing medium counteracts the inhibitory effect of PGE_2 on NE release in isolated cat spleen (Hedqvist, 1970c) and guinea pig vas deferens (Stjärne, 1973a). Although the latter studies were not performed in hearts, there is, as mentioned earlier, good reason to assume that the results are valid in this organ too. There are no indications that PGs affect the postsynaptic part of the sympathetic neurotransmission in the heart (i.e., the cardiac adrenergic receptors). Hedqvist and Wennmalm (1971) found that neither PGE_1, PGE_2, nor $PGF_{2\alpha}$, in concentrations ranging from 3×10^{-9} M to 1.5×10^{-6} M, altered the chronotropic or inotropic responses to added NE. The data available consequently indicate that the inhibitory effects of E prostaglandins on cardiac sympathetic neurotransmission are prejunctional only (i.e., localized to the depolarization-induced liberation of NE from the adrenergic nerve terminals).

2. Cholinergic Transmission

The effects of PGs on cardiac parasympathetic neurotransmission have not been studied very extensively. There are several reasons for this. For one thing, the two branches of the vagal nerves to the heart, although easy to prepare, are very fragile and often cease to function for no obvious reason shortly after dissection is complete. For another, it is difficult to assess the outflow of acetylcholine (Ach) into the cardiac effluent because the concentrations of transmitter are small and there is a lack of suitable methods for analyzing them. Finally, the study of pharmacological effects of PGs on cholinergic nerves is rendered less attractive by doubts as to whether there is in fact an endogenous PG-mediated feedback of the cholinergic transmitter release, analogous with that on the sympathetic side (cf. Section VI,C in this chapter).

The first indication that E prostaglandins may interfere with cholinergic neurotransmission was obtained in isolated rabbit hearts in which the bilateral vagal supply was prepared and stimulated (Wennmalm and Hedqvist, 1971) (Fig. 12). It was observed that the bradycardia induced by a 10-sec stimulation of the nerves at 1–8 Hz was counteracted by PGE_1 ($5–8 \times 10^{-7}$ M), the negative chronotropic response being reduced to about 60% of control. The same study demonstrated that the response to infusion of acetylcholine was unaffected by simultaneous administration of PGE_1 in the dose range mentioned, indicating that the effect of PGE_1 was prejunctional, i.e., that PGE_1 interfered at some point in the chain of events propagation-depolarization-transmitter release in the cholinergic network in the heart.

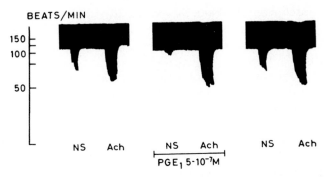

Fig. 12. Perfused rabbit heart. Chronotropic response to three consecutive vagal nerve stimulations (1 per second for 10 sec) and acetylcholine infusions. Second stimulation and infusion performed during infusion of PGE_1. (Reproduced from Wennmalm and Hedqvist, 1971, with the permission of the publisher.)

Interference by PGE_1 with the vagal negative chronotropic response has also been observed in hearts from guinea pig (Hall *et al.*, 1975) and mouse (Feniuk and Large, 1975). The mechanism may, however, be species dependent, since it has been reported that in guinea pig atria, PGE_1 block chronotropic responses to both vagal nerve stimulation and administration of Ach (Hadhazy *et al.*, 1973). In other studies, moreover, no effect of E prostaglandins was observed. Thus in isolated rabbit spontaneously beating nodes, Park *et al.* (1973) found that field stimulation in the presence of propranolol (given to block adrenergic responses in the tissue) resulted in a negative chronotropic response that was not affected by PGE_2 (8×10^{-7} M). Whether the use by these authors of PGE_2 (instead of PGE_1 by others studying cholinergic responses) is the sole explanation for the divergent results cannot be decided at present.

VI. Physiological Significance of Cardiac Prostaglandins

A. General Considerations

The discovery of the hypotensive actions of certain PGs (von Euler, 1936, 1939; Bergström *et al.*, 1959) stimulated many investigators in the early 1960s to further detailed studies on their actions in various parts of the cardiovascular system. Although no indications were found of their bioformation or occurrence in the heart or in vascular tissue, it was often assumed that PGs are involved in the regulation of cardiovascular function. It was suggested, for instance, that PGs were hypotensive hormones—

possibly released from the kidney—and this hypothesis was supported by the observation that A prostaglandins were not inactivated in the pulmonary circulation (McGiff *et al.,* 1969), as were the PGs of the E series (Ferreira and Vane, 1967).

Later the existence of A prostaglandins in biological tissues was questioned. In addition, it was emphasized that the concentrations of PGE in blood are probably very small, considerably lower than reported earlier (Samuelsson, 1973). All this revived the question of the PGs physiological role in cardiovascular function. After the discovery of prostacyclin (Gryglewski *et al.,* 1976), new credit was given cardiovascular PGs, especially PGI_2. The platelet antiaggregatory action and powerful vasodilator properties of PGI_2, together with its passage through the lungs without inactivation (Armstrong *et al.,* 1977), certainly makes this PG most interesting in relation to cardiovascular function in health and disease.

This section briefly reviews some of the hypotheses about the physiological significance of cardiovascular prostaglandins. PG research is a very dynamic field and one can only hope that at least some of these hypotheses will still be relevant by the time this volume has been published.

B. Regulation of Coronary Flow

It has long been known that coronary flow is autoregulated within a wide range of perfusion pressures and that this autoregulation is of considerable significance for myocardial metabolism and hence also for the mechanical performance of the heart. Experiments with isolated, and thereby denervated, hearts have indicated that this autoregulation is chemically mediated to a large extent and various vasoactive agents have been proposed in this connection. The active principle that has attracted most attention as a physiological regulator of coronary tone is no doubt adenosine (cf. Rubio and Berne, 1975). This substance, a breakdown product of adenine nucleotides, is a powerful vasodilator and is produced continuously by the normal heart in amounts sufficient to play a role in coronary flow regulation (Rubio and Berne, 1969).

Data obtained in various laboratories during the last few years have indicated that PGs formed in the coronary vasculature also may play a role in the regulation of coronary resistance, at least under certain conditions. As mentioned in Section IV,A,5 in this chapter, it has been shown that cardiac hypoxia or ischemia is a powerful stimulus for PG formation and release (Kent *et al.,* 1973; Kramer and Folts, 1973; Block *et al.,* 1974; Wennmalm *et al.,* 1974; Alexander *et al.,* 1975; Needleman *et al.,* 1975c). In some of these studies the type of PG released was not identified, whereas in others liberation of PGE (Kent *et al.,* 1973; Alexander *et al.,* 1975) or of both

PGA and PGE (Kraemer and Folts, 1973; Kraemer *et al.*, 1976) was indicated. More recent data have demonstrated that also prostacyclin is liberated from hearts after anoxia (DeDeckere *et al.*, 1977) or during hypoxia (Wennmalm, 1979a). Experiments have also been performed in man. In patients with multivessel coronary artery disease, Berger *et al.* (1977) induced angina by atrial pacing and observed a release of PGF in most cases.

In most of the studies mentioned, an increased coronary flow paralleled the hypoxia or anoxia (Block *et al.*, 1974; Needleman *et al.*, 1975a) or developed after the release of coronary artery occlusion (Kent *et al.*, 1973; Kraemer and Folts, 1973; Alexander *et al.*, 1975; Kraemer *et al.*, 1976). The crucial question then arises: Was the increased liberation of PGs from these anoxic, hypoxic, or ischemic hearts indicative of a stimulated cardiac PG bioformation that necessarily preceded the coronary vasodilatation, or was it merely a secondary phenomenon, resulting, for example, from a more efficient washout of PG in the dilated coronary vasculature. Divergent results have been reported, and at present there is no definite answer on this point. Kent *et al.* (1973) observed in open-chest dogs that both indomethacin and mechlofenamate, well-known inhibitors of PG bioformation, caused a marked reduction in the vasodilator response to arterial occlusion or to hypoxia. Similar results were reported by Afonso *et al.* (1974), who observed that in intact dogs indomethacin considerably blunted the increase in coronary blood flow caused by the inhalation of a gas mixture containing a lower concentration of oxygen. Experiments with isolated coronary arteries or perfused hearts also yielded results that support a role for endogenous PGs in the regulation of the coronary vascular response to hypoxia. In isolated bovine coronary artery strips, decreased oxygen tension in the organ bath surrounding the strip induced a relaxation and an increased release of PG, and both phenomena were counteracted by indomethacin (Kalsner, 1976). In the same preparation it was observed that extreme hypoxia sharply curtailed the output of PG into the bath, besides reversing the relaxation of the strip that was elicited by moderate hypoxia (Kalsner, 1977). In isolated rabbit hearts the increased coronary flow and the liberation of prostacyclin caused by perfusion of the heart with a hypoxic solution were both effectively inhibited by indomethacin (Wennmalm, 1979a).

However, contradictory results have also been presented. In perfused rabbit hearts the anoxia-induced vasodilatation was not impaired by indomethacin (Block *et al.*, 1974), and in the same preparation similar results were obtained for vasodilatation induced by ischemia, hypoxia, or anoxia (Needleman *et al.*, 1975c). In open-chest dogs the hyperemic responses to brief occlusions of the left coronary artery were unaffected in terms of the percentage repayment and peak increase as well as of the duration of the hyperemia response (Giles and Wilcken, 1977). Similar data were reported by Hintze and Kaley (1977), who found that although indomethacin or meclofenamate certainly decreased the peak dilatation and volume of reactive hyperemia induced by brief coronary artery occlusions in open-chest dogs, they did not change the percentage flow debt repaid. Furthermore, the drugs did not significantly modify the total increment to coronary flow from hypoxia-induced vasodilatation (Fig. 13).

It is still to early to draw any conclusions concerning the role of coronary PGs in the regulation of myocardial blood flow. The preceding studies have yielded divergent data, to some extent under very similar experimental conditions. Consequently, there are no clear grounds for explaining the conflicting results in terms of differences in technique or species used. It was recently demonstrated in our laboratory that in human skeletal muscle vasodiltation induced by muscle work was unaffected by indomethacin,

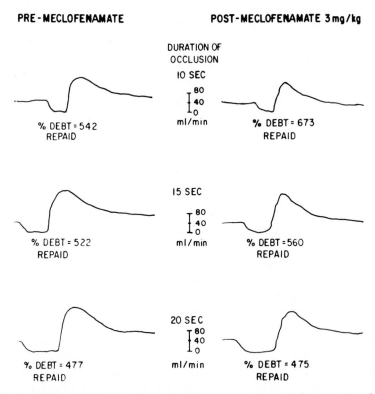

Fig. 13. Effects of inhibition of prostaglandin synthesis with meclofenamate (3 mg/kg) on the reactive hyperemias resulting from 10, 15, and 20 sec occlusions of the circumflex coronary artery in a single dog. (Reproduced from Hintze and Kaley, 1977, with the permission of the American Heart Association, Inc.)

whereas in the same tissue this drug considerably diminished reactive (post-occlusive) hyperemia (Nowak and Wennmalm, 1979). Perhaps these data are valid in the coronary vasculature too. If so, coronary PGs would be of minor importance for the normal regulation of tone in coronary vessels, while possibly playing a significant role for the relaxation of these vessels under conditions of more severe tissue hypoxia.

C. Regulation of Autonomic Transmitter Release

As mentioned in Section V,E in this chapter, PGs of the E series have been shown to inhibit the release of sympathetic neurotransmitter induced by depolarization in adrenergic nerves. Such an effect of PGEs has been shown in various species and tissues (cf. Hedqvist, 1970b). On the basis of this observation, together with earlier reports on release of endogenous prostaglandinlike substances from adrenergically stimulated canine spleen (Davies *et al.,* 1967), it was suggested (Hedqvist, 1970b) that the increased formation of PGs evoked by sympathetic nerve activity in a tissue gives rise, in the vicinity of adrenergic nerve endings, to PG concentrations that are sufficient to inhibit ("brake") further release of transmitter. It was also suggested that the increased formation of PG occurred in the effector organ stimulated by the liberated transmitter, i.e., a negative feedback control of transmitter release. Such a negative feedback control implies that transmit-ter released from the adrenergic nerve endings activates the adrenergic receptor *and* stimulates PG formation in the effector organ, that the PG formed is released from the effector organ, from which it crosses the synap-tic cleft back to the adrenergic nerves, and finally that the PG elicits an inhibitory effect on the further release of transmitter. The first evidence supporting this hypothesis was obtained in our laboratory in experiments on sympathetically stimulated rabbit hearts (Samuelsson and Wennmalm, 1971). It was observed that the PG synthesis inhibitor ETA (cf. Section IV,B in this chapter) decreased the outflow of PG from the heart that is induced by nerve stimulation and simultaneously increased the outflow of NE in response to nerve stimulation.

Using ETA for PG synthesis inhibition, this observation was confirmed shortly afterward in feline spleen (Hedqvist *et al.,* 1971). The common occurrence of such an endogenous control of sympathetic transmitter re-lease has subsequently been confirmed in studies where aspirinlike drugs were used to block PG bioformation (Chanh *et al.,* 1972; Stjärne, 1973b; Stjärne and Gripe, 1973; Fredholm and Hedqvist, 1973; Frame and Hedqvist, 1975). However, data questioning the universal validity of such an endogenous control of transmitter release have also been presented (Hoszowska and Panczenko, 1974; Dubocovich and Langer, 1975).

There is good reason to assume that regulation of sympathetic transmitter release by endogenous PGs occurs not only in isolated organs but also in intact animals. Thus indomethacin was reported to increase the excretion of NE into the urine in rats, cold stressed (Stjärne, 1972) or kept at room temperature (Junstad and Wennmalm, 1972) (Fig. 14). Furthermore, oral administration of indomethacin increased the NE turnover rate in a variety of tissues in the rat, such as heart, spleen, submandibular gland, and adipose tissue (Fredholm and Hedqvist, 1975). Most of the evidence obtained *in vitro* and *in vivo* consequently supports the hypothesis that inhibition of PG bioformation does in fact increase the amount of NE released per nerve impulse. This implies that a PG-mediated regulation of NE release does exist even in the intact animal. However, no evidence has yet been presented to justify the term "feedback" for such a regulation. "Feedback" would require that the transmitter substance accelerate PG bioformation in the target structure, and no such data have been presented. On the contrary, a recent study in our laboratory demonstrated that in the heart, PG bioformation and sympathetic transmitter release are not strictly related morphologically (Wennmalm, 1979b). Apparently, further studies are

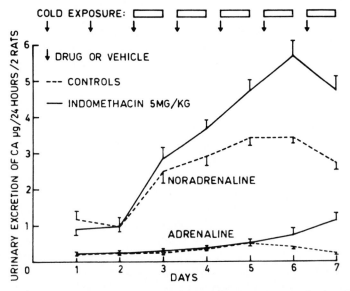

Fig. 14. Effect of indomethacin 5 mg/kg·day on the urinary excretion of NA and A in rats kept at room temperature for 2 days and subsequently exposed to +2°–to +4°C for 15 hr each 24 hr period. Comparisons to controls receiving vehicle. Drug group 18 rats, control group 18 rats. Two rats were kept in each cage. Mean ± SE. (Reproduced from Stjärne, 1972, with the permission of the publisher.)

necessary before the concept of a PG-mediated negative "feedback" regulation of sympathetic transmitter release can be established as physiologically significant.

The possibility that a regulation of cholinergic transmitter release exists, in analogy with that occurring on the adrenergic side, has also been discussed. It has been reported that PGE_1 inhibits the negative chronotropic response to vagal nerve stimulation, while not affecting the corresponding response induced by injection of Ach. Based on these data, it was suggested that PGE_1 depressed the depolarization-induced release of transmitter from the cholinergic nerve terminals (Wennmalm and Hedqvist, 1971). Later findings that vagal nerve stimulation, as well as injection Ach, increased the outflow of PLS from isolated hearts (Junstad and Wennmalm, 1974) appeared to support the concept that an endogenous regulation of cholinergic transmitter release analoguous to the regulation of the liberation of sympathetic transmitter was operating and that the mediator was cardiac prostaglandins. Fairly extensive investigations in our laboratory have, however, failed to deliver further evidence in support of this concept. Inhibition of cardiac PG formation with ETA or indomethacin did not affect the negative chronotropic response to vagal nerve stimulation, and the overflow of acetylcholinelike activity into the effluent from the heart during vagal stimulation was mainly the same before and after indomethacin (Å. Wennmalm, unpublished). In other cholinergically innervated tissues, endogenous PGs, rather than inhibiting the release of Ach, seem to facilitate this (cf. Hedqvist, 1977).

D. Platelet Aggregation and Coronary Prostacyclin Formation

As mentioned earlier in this chapter, the main AA derivative formed in platelets is thromboxane A_2. TxA_2 is a strong vasoconstrictor and has powerful platelet antiaggregatory properties. Platelets supplied with AA or PG endoperoxide immediately aggregate and, in addition, liberate TxA_2 into the surrounding medium. It has been suggested that TxA_2 is involved in the physiological regulation of platelet aggregation (Samuelsson, 1976). Prostacyclin is both a powerful vasodilator and a potent inhibitor of platelet aggregation (Gryglewski et al., 1976), being in the latter respect the most active endogenous substance so far described. Recent results indicate that prostacyclin is continuously released from the lungs, thereby controlling platelet aggregation in vivo (Moncada et al., 1978; Gryglewski et al., 1978). An interaction between platelets and vessel walls has also been suggested, implying that PG endoperoxide released by platelets tending to adhere to an intact vascular intima is retained by the endothelium and converted to

antiaggregatory prostacyclin (Gryglewski *et al.*, 1976). The PGI₂ thus
formed would actively prevent further aggregation and subsequent thrombus formation and thereby protect an intact vessel against thrombotization.
Furthermore, in vessels with damaged endothelium, in which no prostacyclin formation may occur, the antiaggregatory effect would not be present.
This hypothesis implies that normally, the pro-aggregatory effect of TxA₂
found in the platelets is efficiently counteracted by the antiaggregatory
PGI₂ formed in the vascular endothelium and that persistent platelet aggregation and thrombus formation must be preceded by a destruction of the
prostacyclin-producing part of the vessel wall. This hypothesis offers an
explanation for the striking ability of healthy vascular endothelium to prevent adhesion of platelets, besides shedding new light on the relation between atherosclerotic vascular disease and thrombus formation (see Fig.
15). It has been shown that vascular prostacyclin production *in vitro* is
inhibited by a lipid peroxide (Moncada *et al.*, 1976c). Since atherosclerosis
is characterized by an increased lipid peroxidation in the vessel walls, the
increased risk of thrombosis associated with this disease may be due to
inhibition of prostacyclin formation in the atherosclerotic endothelium
(Moncada *et al.*, 1977). Clearly this hypothesis is also of considerable interest in connection with the coronary circulation in health and disease; prostacyclin is one of the major coronary PG formed (Isakson *et al.*, 1977;

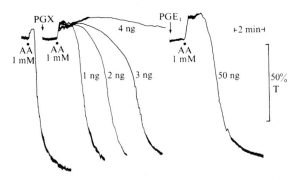

Fig. 15. The tracings show changes in light transmission through platelet-rich human
plasma in a Born aggregometer. Comparison of antiaggregatory potencies of PGX (early
designation of PGI₂) and PGE₁. PGX was obtained by incubation of 100 ng PGH₂ with 500 μg
of aortic microsomes in 100 μl 0.05 M Tris buffer (pH 7.5) for 2 min at 22°C and then stored
on ice. PGX and PGE₁ (10 μl) were added to plasma rich in human platelets 1 min before
arachidonic acid (AA 1 mM). In this experiment PGX was at least 25 times more potent as an
antiaggregatory agent than PGE₁. Doses of PGX (1–4 ng) or PGE₁ (50 ng) are shown at the
sides of the tracings. (Reproduced from Moncada *et al.*, 1976a, with the permission of the
publisher.)

DeDeckere *et al.*, 1977) and may therefore be of great value, according to this hypothesis, in protecting the coronary vessels against thrombosis.

VII. Cigarette Smoking, Nicotine, and Cardiac Prostaglandins

In epidemiological studies a definite relation has been established between cigarette smoking and cardiovascular diseases (cf. e.g., Doyle *et al.*, 1962). However, the biochemical or pathophysiological link between the inhalation of tobacco smoke and the development of aggravation of cardiovascular disease remains obscure. It has been suggested that a discrepancy between the myocardial oxygen demand and oxygen supply develops during administration of nicotine or cigarette smoking (Bellet *et al.*, 1962), possibly as a consequence of the nicotine-induced increase in cardiac activity (Forte *et al.*, 1960; Leb *et al.*, 1970) or the increased consumption of free fatty acids (Mjös and Ilebekk, 1973). Alternative mechanisms should, however, be considered.

Recent data obtained in our laboratory indicate that nicotine interferes with PG bioformation in various tissues, including the heart. On the basis of the proposed physiological or pathophysiological actions of cardiac PG, such an effect by nicotine is of interest in relation to ischemic heart disease. A brief review of the relation between nicotine and PG bioformation and its possible implications for the relation between cigarette smoking and cardiovascular function therefore seems justified.

In isolated rabbit hearts it was observed that the addition of nicotine at a concentration of 5×10^{-5} M elicited an almost seven-fold increase in the outflow of PGE-like activity from the organ (Wennmalm and Junstad, 1976). This outflow was probably not an indirect effect of the concomitant release of NA induced by nicotine; it appeared instead to be a direct action of the drug administered. The increased release of PLS was abolished by pretreatment of the heart with indomethacin (Wennmalm, 1977). In hearts perfused with $[^{14}C]AA$ the cardiac effluent content of 6-keto-$[^{14}C]PGF_{1\alpha}$ was decreased by nicotine (Wennmalm, 1978b). This observation, indicating an inhibitory effect of nicotine on cardiac PG bioformation, seemed at first to conflict with the earlier finding of an enhanced efflux of PGE-like activity. A detailed analysis of the effect of nicotine on the overall cardiac conversion of $[^{14}C]AA$ to $[^{14}C]PGs$ provided an explanation. Increasing concentrations of nicotine counteract the proportion of 6-keto-$[^{14}C]PGF_{1\alpha}$ formed, at the same time facilitating the formation of $[^{14}C]PGE_2$ (Wennmalm, 1978c). It thus appears that nicotine redistributes cardiac PG formation away from prostacyclin to PGE_2. Whether the increased formation of PGE_2 is the result of an active facilitation of the PGH_2–PGE_2 pathway or merely a consequence of the inhibition of prostacyclin synthetase remains an open question.

In addition to its apparent effect on prostacyclin synthetase, nicotine seems to inhibit cyclooxygenase. In rabbit kidney microsomes, nicotine dose-relatedly inhibited the formation of primary PGs from AA, the $(I)_{50}$ concentrations ranging from $7 \times 10^{-6} M$ to $10^{-5} M$ (Alster and Wennmalm, 1980a). In the same preparation the conversion of PGH_2 to primary PGs was almost unaffected by nicotine, indicating that the drug acted on the conversion of AA to PGH_2. The effect of nicotine on the efflux of prostacyclin-like activity (PCLA) has also been studied in superfused human and rabbit vascular tissue, as well as in perfused rabbit hearts. The amount of PCLA formed by these tissues was dose-dependently decreased by nicotine in comparison to controls (Sonnenfeld and Wennmalm, 1980), as was the efflux of PCLA in rabbit hearts in which the PG formation was facilitated by hypoxia or by infusion of AA (Wennmalm, 1980). The inhibitory action by nicotine on cardiac and vascular formation of PCLA does, however, not reflect a uniform action by the alkaloid on cyclooxygenase. In contrast, AA-induced aggregation and formation of thromboxane in human platelets was completely unaffected by nicotine (Alster and Wennmalm, 1980b). This implies a selective action by nicotine-inhibiting vascular PGI_2, but not by platelet TxA_2 formation. Such a selective action might change platelet aggregability (see Section VI,D in this chapter) and favor thrombus formation.

Some indications have also been found that tobacco smoking directly interferes with vascular prostacyclin formation. In healthy volunteers the forearm reactive hyperemia that develops in response to arterial occlusion was reduced by about 30% by cigarette smoking (Fig. 16). Pretreatment with indomethacin reduced the hyperemia further; with indomethacin, however, cigarette smoking prior to the arterial occlusion did not add further to the reduction in postocclusion flow increase (Wennmalm, 1979c). The data imply that smoking counteracts reactive hyperemia by interfering with the same mechanism as indomethacin, i.e., with the vascular formation of PG.

It seems these data may be of significance for the connection between smoking and cardiovascular disease. Reactive hyperemia is probably an important vascular defense mechanism against tissue hypoxia, and an impairment of this mechanism in the coronary vasculature may result in an insufficient myocardial oxygen supply and possibly also myocardial tissue damage. In addition, a selective inhibition of coronary prostacyclin formation may result in an imbalance between the formation of proaggregatory TxA_2 in the platelets and antiaggregatory prostacyclin in the coronary vessels. This would promote platelet aggregation and thrombus formation. The hazardous effect of nicotine would consequently be dual: reducing the possibility

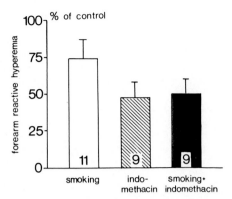

Fig. 16. Effect of cigarette smoking and of indomethacin, separate or in combination, on the reactive hyperemia in the forearm induced by 5 min of arterial occlusion. The data are presented as percentage (mean ± SE of 9–11 experiments) of the reactive hyperemia in control experiments, performed without preceding smoking or drug administration. As shown, smoking alone induced a considerable reduction of the hyperemia. After pretreatment with indomethacin the hyperemia was even more decreased, but smoking did not add further to this reduction.

of developing reactive hyperemia and promoting platelet aggregation. It is hoped that future experiments will reveal to what extent these mechanisms are in fact significant in relation to cardiovascular function in health and disease.

References

Afonso, S., Bandow, G. T., and Rowe, G. G. (1974). *J. Physiol. (London)* **241**, 299–308.

Alexander, R. W., Kent, K. M., Pisano, J. J., Keiser, H. R., and Cooper, T. (1975). *J. Clin. Invest.* **55**, 1174–1181.

Alster, P., and Wennmalm, Å. (1980a). To be published.

Alster, P., and Wennmalm, Å. (1980b). To be published.

Anderson, F. L., Kralios, A. C., Tsagaris, T. J., and Kuida, H. (1972). *Proc. Soc. Exp. Biol. Med.* **140**, 1049–1053.

Armstrong, J. M., Chapple, D., Dusting, G. J., Hughes, R., Moncada, S., and Vane, J. R. (1977). *Br. J. Pharmacol.* **61**, 136P.

Battez, G., and Boulet, L. (1913). *C.R. Seances Soc. Biol. Ses. Fil.* **74**, 8–9.

Bellet, S., West, J. W., Müller, O. F., and Manzoli, U. C. (1962). *Circ. Res.* **10**, 27–34.

Berger, H. J., Zaret, B. L., Speroff, L., Cohen, L. S., and Wolfson, S. (1974). *Circ. Res., Suppl.* **3**, 122.

Berger, H. J., Zaret, B. L., Speroff, L., Cohen, L. S., and Wolfson, S. (1977). *Am. J. Cardiol.* **39**, 481–487.

Bergström, S., and Sjövall, J. (1957). *Acta Chem. Scand.* **11**, 1086.

Bergström, S., Dunér, H., von Euler, U.S., Pernow, B., and Sjövall, J. (1959). *Acta Physiol. Scand.* **45**, 145–151.

Bergström, S., Danielsson, H., and Samuelsson, B. (1964). *Biochim. Biophys. Acta* **90**, 207–210.

Bergström, S., Carlson, L. A., and Orö, L. (1966). *Acta Physiol. Scand.* **67**, 185–193.

Berti, F., Lentati, R., and Usardi, M. M. (1965). *Med. Pharmacol. Exp.* **13**, 233–240.

Block, A. J., and Vane, J. R. (1973). *Naunyn-Schmiedeberg's Arch. Pharmacol.* **279**, R19.

Block, A. J., Poole, S., and Vane, J. R. (1974).*Prostaglandins* **7**, 473–486.

Bloor, C. M., and Sobel, B. E. (1970). *Circulation* **42**, Suppl. III, 123.

Caldwell, B. V., Brock, W. A., Gordon, W. J., and Speroff, L. (1972). In "Prostaglandins in Fertility Control" (S. Bergström, K. Gréen, and B. Samuelsson, eds.), Vol. 2, pp. 83–91.

Camus, L., and Gley, E. (1907). *C. R. Seances Soc. Biol. Ses. Fil.* **63**, 204–208.

Carlson, L. A., Ekelund, L. G., and Orö, L. (1969). *Acta Physiol. Scand.* **75**, 161–169.

Chanh, Pham-Huu-, Junstad, M., and Wennmalm, Å. (1972). *Acta Physiol. Scand.* **86**, 563–567.

Chiba, S., Nakajima, T., and Nakano, J. (1972). *Jpn. J. Pharmacol.* **22**, 734–736.

Courtney, K. R., Colwell, W. T., and Jensen, R. A. (1978). *Prostaglandins* **16**, 451–459.

Curnow, R. T., and Nuttall, F. Q. (1971). *Fed. Proc., Fed. Am. Soc. Exp. Biol.* **30**, 625.

Davies, B. N., Horton, E. W., and Withrington, P. G. (1967). *J. Physiol. (London)* **188**, 38P–39P.

Davies, B. N., Horton, E. W., and Withrington, P. G. (1968). *Br. J. Pharmacol. Chemother.* **32**, 127–135.

DeDeckere, E. A. M., Nugteren, D. H., and TenHoor, F. (1977). *Nature (London)* **268**, 160–163.

Douglas, J. R., Jr., Johnson, E. M., Jr., Marshall, G. R., Jaffe, B. M., and Needleman, P. (1973). *Prostaglandins* **3**, 67–74.

Downing, D. T., Ahern, D. G., and Bachta, M. (1970). *Biochem. Biophys. Res. Commun.* **40**, 218–223.

Doyle, J. T., Dawber, T. R., Kannel, W. B., Heslin, A. S., and Kahn, H. A. (1962) *N. Engl. J. Med.* **266**, 796–801.

Dubocovich, M. L., and Langer, S. Z. (1975). *J. Physiol. (London)* **251**, 737–762.

Feniuk, W., and Large, B. J. (1975). *Br. J. Pharmacol.* **55**, 47–49.

Ferreira, S. H., and Vane, J. R. (1967). *Nature (London)* **216**, 868–873.

Ferreira, S. H., Moncada, S., and Vane, J. R. (1973). *Br. J. Pharmacol.* **47**, 48–58.

Fitzpatrick, T. M., Alter, I., Corey, E. J., Ramwell, P. W., Rose, J. C., and Kot, P. A. (1978). *Circ. Res.* **42**, 192–194.

Förster, W., Mest, H.-J., and Mentz, P. (1973). *Prostaglandins* **3**, 895–904.

Forte, I. E., Williams, A. J., Potgieter, L., Schmitthenner, J. E., Hafkenschiel, J. H., and Rigel, C. (1960). *Ann. N.Y. Acad. Sci.* **90**, 174–185.

Frame, M. H., and Hedqvist, P. (1975). *Br. J. Pharmacol.* **54**, 189–196.

Fredholm, B. B., and Hedqvist, P. (1973). *Acta Physiol. Scand.* **87**, 570–572.

Fredholm, B. B., and Hedqvist, P. (1975). *Br. J. Pharmacol.* **54**, 295–300.

Frölich, J. C. (1978). In "Methods in Prostaglandin Research" (B. Samuelsson and R. Paoletti, eds.), Vol. 5. Raven Press, New York.

Giles, R. W., and Wilcken, D. E. L. (1977). *Cardiovasc. Res.* **11**, 113–121.

Gilmore, N., Vane, J. R., and Wyllie, J. H. (1968). *Nature (London)* **218**, 1135–1140.

Goldblatt, M. W. (1933). *Chem. Ind. (London)* **52**, 1056–1057.

Götzl, A. (1910). *Z. Urol.* **4**, 743–748.

Granström, E. (1978). *Prostaglandins* **15**, 3–17.

Granström, E., Lands, W. E. M., and Samuelsson, B. (1968). *J. Biol. Chem.* **243**, 4104–4108.

Gréen, K., and Samuelsson, B. (1964). *J. Lipid Res.* **5**, 117–120.

Gryglewski, R. J., Panczenko, B., Korbut, R., Grodzińska, L., and Ocetkiewicz, A. (1975). *Prostaglandins* **10**, 343–355.

Gryglewski, R. J., Bunting, S., Moncada, S., Flower, R. J., and Vane, J. R. (1976). *Prostaglandins* 12, 685–713.

Gryglewski, R. J., Zmuda, A., Korbut, R., Krecioch, E., and Bieron, K. (1977). *Nature (London)* 267, 627–628.

Gryglewski, R. J., Korbut, R., and Ocetkiewicz, A. (1978). *Nature* 273, 765–767.

Hadházy, P., Illés, P., and Knoll, J. (1973). *Eur. J. Pharmacol.* 23, 251–255.

Hall, W. J., O'Neill, P., and Sheehan, J. D. (1975). *Eur. J. Pharmacol.* 34, 39–47.

Hamberg, M., and Samuelsson, B. (1966). *J. Biol. Chem.* 241, 257–263.

Hamberg, M., and Samuelsson, B. (1973). *Proc. Natl. Acad. Sci. U.S.A.* 70, 899–903.

Hamberg, M., Svensson, J., and Samuelsson, B. (1975). *Proc. Natl. Acad. Sci. U.S.A.* 72, 2994–2998.

Hedqvist, P. (1970a). *Life Sci.* 9, 269–278.

Hedqvist, P. (1970b). *Acta Physiol. Scand.* 79, Suppl. 345, 1–40.

Hedqvist, P. (1970c). *Acta Physiol. Scand.* 80, 269–275.

Hedqvist, P. (1977). *Annu. Rev. Pharmacol.* 17, 259–279.

Hedqvist, P., and Brundin, J. (1969). *Life Sci.* 8, 389–395.

Hedqvist, P., and Wennmalm, Å. (1971). *Acta Physiol. Scand.* 83, 156–162.

Hedqvist, P., Stjärne, L., and Wennmalm, Å. (1970). *Acta Physiol. Scand.* 79, 139–141.

Hedqvist, P., Stjärne, L., and Wennmalm, Å. (1971). Acta Physiol. Scand. 83, 430–432.

Herbaczyńska-Cedro, K., and Staszewska-Barczak, J. (1974). *Abstr. Congr. Hung. Pharmacol. Soc., 2nd, 1974* p. 19.

Herbaczyńska-Cedro, K., and Staszewska-Barczak, J. (1977). *Prostaglandins* 13, 517–531.

Higgins, C. B., Vatner, S. F., Franklin, D., and Braunwald, E. (1972). *Am. J. Physiol.* 222, 1534–1538.

Hintze, T. H., and Kaley, G. (1977). *Circ. Res.* 40, 313–320.

Hollenberg, M., Walker, R. S., and McCormick, D. P. (1968). *Arch. Int. Pharmacodyn. Ther.* 174, 66–73.

Horton, E. W., and Main, I. H. M. (1967). *Br. J. Pharmacol. Chemother.* 30, 568–581.

Hoszowska, A., and Panczenko, B. (1974). *Pol. J. Pharmacol. Pharm.* 26, 137–142.

Huković, S., and Muscholl, E. (1962). *Naunyn-Schmiedebergs Arch. Exp. Pathol. Pharmakol.* 244, 81–96.

Illés, P., Hadházy, P., Torma, Z., Vizi, E. S., and Knoll, J. (1973). *Eur. J. Pharmacol.* 24, 29–36.

Isakson, P. C., Raz, A., and Needleman, P. (1976). *Prostaglandins* 12, 739–748.

Isakson, P. C., Raz, A., Denny, S. E., Pure, E., and Needleman, P. (1977). *Proc. Natl. Acad. Sci. U.S.A.* 74, 101–105.

Johnson, R. A., Morton, D. R., Kinner, J. H., Gorman, R. R., McGuire, J. C., and Sun, F. F. (1976). *Prostaglandins* 12, 915–928.

Junstad, M., and Wennmalm, Å. (1972). *Acta Physiol. Scand.* 85, 573–576.

Junstad, M., and Wennmalm, Å. (1973a). *Acta Physiol. Scand.* 87, 573–574.

Junstad, M., and Wennmalm, Å. (1973b). *Acta Physiol. Scand.* 89, 544–549.

Junstad, M., and Wennmalm, Å. (1974). *Br. J. Pharmacol.* 52, 375–379.

Kalsner, S. (1976). *Blood Vessels* 13, 155–166.

Kalsner, S. (1977). *Can. J. Physiol. Pharmacol.* 55, 882–887.

Katori, M., Takeda, K., and Imai, S. (1970). *Tohoku J. Exp. Med.* 101, 67–75.

Kent, K. M., Alexander, R. W., Pisano, J. J., Keiser, H. R., and Cooper, T. (1973). *Physiologist* 16, 361.

Koss, M. C., Gray, J. W., Davison, M., and Nakano, J. (1973). *Eur. J. Pharmacol.* 24, 151–157.

Kraemer, R. J., and Folts, J. D. (1973). *Fed. Proc., Fed. Am. Soc. Exp. Biol.* 32, 454.

Kraemer, R. J., Phernetton, T. M., and Folts, J. D. (1976). *J. Pharmacol. Exp. Ther.* **199**, 611–619.

Kulkarni, P. S., Roberts, R., and Needleman, P. (1976). *Prostaglandins* **12**, 337–353.

Kurzrok, R., and Lieb, C. C. (1931). *Proc. Soc. Exp. Biol. Med.* **28**, 268–272.

Lavery, H. A., Lowe, R. D., and Scroop, G. C. (1970). *Br. J. Pharmacol.* **39**, 511–519.

Leb, G., Derntl, F., Robin, E., and Bing, R. J. (1970). *J. Pharmacol. Exp. Ther.* **173**, 138–144.

Lee, J. B., Covino, B. G., Takman, B. H., and Smith, E. R. (1965). *Circ. Res.* **17**, 57–77.

Levy, J. (1973). *Prostaglandins* **4**, 731–736.

Levy, J. V., and Killebrew, E. (1971). *Proc. Soc. Exp. Biol. Med.* **136**, 1227–1231.

Lewis, A. J., and Eyre, P. (1972). *Prostaglandins* **2**, 55 64.

Lewis, G. P., and Piper, P. J. (1975). *Nature (London)* **254**, 308–311.

Limas, C. J., and Cohn, J. N. (1973). *Cardiovasc. Res.* **7**, 623–628.

McGiff, J. C., Terragno, N. A., Strand, J. C., Lee, J. B., and Lonigro, A. J. (1969). *Nature (London)* **223**, 742–745.

McGiff, J. C., Crowshaw, K., Terragno, N. A., and Lonigro, A. J. (1970a). *Circ. Res.* **26**, Suppl. I, I-121–I-130.

McGiff, J. C., Crowshaw, K., Terragno, N. A., Lonigro, A. J., Strand, J. C., Williamson, M. A., Lee, J. B., and Ng, K. K. F. (1970b). *Circ. Res.* **27**, 765–782.

McGiff, J. C., Terragno, N. A., Malik, K. U., and Lonigro, A. J. (1972). *Circ. Res.* **31**, 36–43.

Mann, D. (1976). *Acta Biol. Med. Ger.* **35**, 1113–1117.

Mantegazza, P. (1965). *Atti Accad. Med. Lomb.* **20**, 66–72.

Markus, H. B., and Ball, E. G. (1969). *Biochim. Biophys. Acta* **187**, 486–491.

Mentz, P., and Förster, W. (1977). *Prostaglandins* **14**, 173–179.

Mest, H.-J., Winkler, J., and Förster, W. (1977a). *Acta Biol. Med. Ger.* **36**, 1193–1196.

Mest, H.-J., Blass, K. E., and Förster, W. (1977b). *Prostaglandins* **14**, 163–172.

Minkes, M. S., Douglas, J. R., and Needleman, P. (1973). *Prostaglandins* **3**, 439–445.

Mjös, O. D., and Ilebekk, A. (1973). *Scand. J. Clin. Lab. Invest.* **32**, 75–80.

Moncada, S., Gryglewski, R., Bunting, S., and Vane, J. R. (1976a). *Nature (London)* **263**, 663–665.

Moncada, S., Needleman, P., Bunting, S., and Vane, J. R. (1976b). *Prostaglandins* **12**, 323–335.

Moncada, S., Gryglewski, R. J., Bunting, S., and Vane, J. R. (1976c). *Prostaglandins* **12**, 715–737.

Moncada, S., Higgs, E. A., and Vane, J. R. (1977). *Lancet* **1**, 18–20.

Moncada, S., Korbut, R., Bunting, S., and Vane, J. R. (1978). *Nature (London)* **273**, 767–768.

Nakano, J. (1968). *Proc. Soc. Exp. Biol. Med.* **127**, 1160–1163.

Nakano, J., and McCurdy, J. R. (1967). *J. Pharmacol. Exp. Ther.* **156**, 538–547.

Nakano, J., and McCurdy, J. R. (1968). *Proc. Soc. Exp. Biol. Med.* **128**, 39–42.

Needleman, P. (1976). *Fed. Proc., Fed. Am. Soc. Exp. Biol.* **35**, 2376–2381.

Needleman, P., Marshall, G. R., and Douglas, J. R. (1973a). *Eur. J. Pharmacol.* **66**, 316–319.

Needleman, P., Kauffman, A. H., Douglas, J. R., Jr., Johnson, E. M., Jr., and Marshall, G. R. (1973b). *Am. J. Physiol.* **224**, 1415–1419.

Needleman, P., Minkes, M. S., and Douglas, J. R., Jr. (1974). *Circ. Res.* **34**, 455–460.

Needleman, P., Marshall, G. R., and Sobel, B. E. (1975a). *Circ. Res.* **37**, 802–808.

Needleman, P., Key, S. L., Denny, S. E., Isakson, P. C., and Marshall, G. R. (1975b). *Proc. Natl. Acad. Sci. U.S.A.* **72**, 2060–2063.

Needleman, P., Key, S. L., Isakson, P. C., and Kulkarni, P. S. (1975c). *Prostaglandins* **9**, 123–134.

Needleman, P., Kulkarni, P. S., and Raz, A. (1977a). *Science* **195**, 409–412.

Needleman, P., Raz, A., Ferrendelli, J. A., and Minkes, M. (1977b). *Proc. Natl. Acad. Sci. U.S.A.* **74**, 1716–1720.

Needleman, P., Bronson, S. E. D., Wyche, A., Sivakoff, M., and Nicolaou, K. C. (1978). *J. Clin. Invest.* **61**, 839–849.

Nowak, J., and Wennmalm, Å. (1978). *Acta Physiol. Scand.* **102**, 484–491.

Nowak, J., and Wennmalm, Å. (1979). *Acta Physiol. Scand.* **106**, 365–369.

Nowak, J., Kaijser, L., and Wennmalm, Å. (1980). *Prostaglandins Med.* **4**, 205–214.

Nugteren, D. H., and Hazelhof, E. (1973). *Biochem. Biophys. Acta* **326**, 448–461.

Nutter, D. O., and Crumly, H. J. (1972). *Cardiovasc. Res.* **6**, 217–225.

Palmer, M. A., Piper, P. J., and Vane, J. R. (1973). *Br. J. Pharmacol.* **49**, 226–242.

Park, M. K., Dyer, D. C., and Vincenzi, F. F. (1973). *Prostaglandins* **4**, 717–730.

Piccinini, F., Pomarelli, P., and Chiarra, A. (1969). *Pharmacol. Res. Commun.* **1**, 381–389.

Piper, P. J., and Vane, J. R. (1969). *Nature (London)* **223**, 29–35.

Puig-Parellada, P., and Planas, J. M. (1977). *Lancet* **2**, 40.

Raz, A., Isakson, P. C., Minkes, M. S., and Needleman, P. (1977). *J. Biol. Chem.* **252**, 1123–1126.

Rowe, G. G., and Afonso, S. (1974). *Am. Heart J.* **88**, 51–60.

Rubio, R., and Berne, R. M. (1969). *Circ. Res.* **25**, 407–415.

Rubio, R., and Berne, R. M. (1975). *Cardiovasc. Dis.* **18**, 105–122.

Samuelsson, B. (1965). *J. Am. Chem. Soc.* **87**, 3011–3013.

Samuelsson, B. (1973). *Adv. Biosci.* **9**, 7–14.

Samuelsson, B. (1976). *Adv. Prostaglandin Thromboxane Res.* **1**, 1–6.

Samuelsson, B., and Wennmalm, Å. (1971). *Acta Physiol. Scand.* **83**, 163–168.

Schrör, K., Moncada, S., Ubatuba, F. B., and Vane, J. R. (1978). *Eur. J. Pharmacol.* **47**, 103–114.

Sobel, B. E., and Robison, A. K. (1969). *Circulation* **40**, Suppl. III, 189.

Sonnenfeld, T., and Wennmalm, Å. (1980). *Br. J. Pharmacol.* (in press).

Steinberg, D., Vaughan, M., Nestel, P. J., Strand, O., and Bergström, S. (1964). *J. Clin. Invest.* **43**, 1533–1540.

Stjärne, L. (1972). *Acta Physiol. Scand.* **86**, 388–397.

Stjärne, L. (1973a). *Prostaglandins* **3**, 105–109.

Stjärne, L. (1973b). *Eur. J. Pharmacol.* **22**, 233–238.

Stjärne, L., and Gripe, K. (1973). *Naunyn-Schmiedebergs Arch. Pharmacol.* **280**, 441–466.

Su, J. Y., Higgins, C. B., and Friedman, W. F. (1973). *Proc. Soc. Exp. Biol. Med.* **143**, 1227–1230.

Sunahara, F. A., and Talesnik, J. (1974). *J. Pharmacol. Exp. Ther.* **188**, 135–147.

Tuttle, R. S., and Skelly, M. M. (1968). *In* "Prostaglandin Symposium of the Worcester Foundation for Experimental Biology" (P. W. Ramwell and J. E. Shaw, eds.), pp. 309–320. Wiley (Interscience), New York.

Ubatuba, F. B. (1973). *Br. J. Pharmacol.* **49**, 662–666.

van Dorp, D. A. (1975). *Proc. Nutr. Soc.* **34**, 279–286.

van Dorp, D. A., Beerthuis, R. K., Nugteren, D. H., and Vonkeman, H. (1964). *Biochim. Biophys. Acta* **90**, 204–207.

Vane, J. R. (1957). *Br. J. Pharmacol. Chemother.* **12**, 344–349.

Vane, J. R. (1969). *Br. J. Pharmacol.* **35**, 209–242.

Vane, J. R. (1971). *Nature (London), New Biol.* **231**, 232–235.

Vargaftig, B. B., and DaoHai, N. (1972). *J. Pharm. Pharmacol.* **24**, 159–161.

Vergroesen, A. J., and de Boer, J. (1968). *Eur. J. Pharmacol.* **3**, 171–176.

Vergroesen, A. J., de Boer, J., and Gottenbos, J. J. (1967). *In* "Prostaglandins" (S. Bergström and B. Samuelsson, eds.), pp. 211–218.

von Euler, U. S. (1934). *Naunyn Schmiedebergs Arch. Exp. Pathol. Pharmacol.* 175, 78–84.
von Euler, U. S. (1935a). *Klin: Wochenschr.* 14, 1182–1183.
von Euler, U. S. (1935b). *Proc. Physiol. Soc. (London)* 84, 21P–22P.
von Euler, U. S. (1936). *J. Physiol. (London)* 88, 213–234.
von Euler, U. S. (1939). *Skand. Arch. Physiol.* 81, 65–80.
Wennmalm, Å. (1975). *Acta Physiol. Scand.* 93, 15–24.
Wennmalm, Å. (1977). *Br. J. Pharmacol.* 59, 95–100.
Wennmalm, Å. (1978a). *Acta Physiol. Scand.* 102, 199–204.
Wennmalm, Å. (1978b). *Acta Physiol. Scand.* 103, 107–109.
Wennmalm, Å. (1978c). *Br. J. Pharmacol.* 63, 559–563.
Wennmalm, Å. (1978d). *Prostaglandins* 15, 113–121.
Wennmalm, Å. (1978e). *Prostaglandins & Medicine* 1, 49–54.
Wennmalm, Å. (1979a). *Acta Physiol. Scand.* 106, 47–52.
Wennmalm, Å. (1979b). *Acta Physiol. Scand.* 105, 254–256.
Wennmalm, Å. (1979c). *Prostaglandins Med.* 3, 321–326.
Wennmalm, Å. (1980). *Br. J. Pharmacol.* (in press).
Wennmalm, Å., and Brundin, T. (1978). *Acta Physiol. Scand.* 102, 374–381.
Wennmalm, Å., and Hedqvist, P. (1971). *Life Sci.* 10, 465–470.
Wennmalm, Å., and Junstad, M. (1976). *Acta Physiol. Scand.* 96, 281–282.
Wennmalm, Å., and Stjärne, L. (1971). *Life Sci.* 10, 471–479.
Wennmalm, Å., Pham-Huu-Chanh, and Junstad, M. (1974). *Acta Physiol. Scand.* 91, 133–135.
Ziljstra, W. G., Brunsting, J. R., TenHoor, F., and Vergroesen, A. J. (1972). *Eur. J. Pharmacol.* 18, 392–395.

3

Thyroid Hormone Effects on the Heart

Robert C. Smallridge*

*The opinions and assertions contained herein are the private views of the author and are not to be construed as official or reflecting the views of the Department of the Army or the Department of Defense.

I. Thyroid Hormone Synthesis, Metabolism, and Mechanisms of Action

Thyroid hormone synthesis occurs within the follicles of the thyroid gland and proceeds through a series of steps: (1) inorganic iodide is transported into the gland, (2) intrathyroidal iodide is oxidized to iodine under the influence of H_2O_2 and peroxidase, (3) iodine is bound in thyroglobulin to tyrosine, forming monoiodotyrosine (MIT) and diiodotyrosine (DIT), (4) the iodotyrosines are enzymatically coupled to form thyroxine (T4) and triiodothyronine (T3), (5) the iodothyronines, T4 and T3, are stored in thyroglobulin until released into the circulation, and (6) the unused iodotyrosines are deiodinated and the iodide recycled. Thyroid hormone secretion is regulated by the central nervous system. In this negative feedback system thyrotropin releasing hormone (TRH), secreted by the hypothalamus, travels via the pituitary portal blood system to thyrotrophs in the pituitary where it stimulates the release of thyrotropin (TSH). TSH in turn travels in the bloodstream to the thyroid gland. Acutely TSH stimulates iodide binding by increasing H_2O_2 formation, whereas chronically it enhances thyroidal peroxidase content and iodide trapping. The intrathyroidal enzymatic control of these pathways has been reviewed recently (Degroot and Niepomniszcze, 1977).

Once thyroid hormone is released from the gland, it travels to virtually every tissue in the body. All the T4 produced must necessarily be derived from intrathyroidal synthesis, whereas only a third of circulating T3 emanates from the gland. The rest is produced by peripheral monodeiodination of T4. Since T3 is felt to be the major active iodothyronine, factors that affect its production are extremely important, and there has been considerable interest in the pathways of peripheral monodeiodination. It has been established that T4 deiodinates enzymatically to both T3 and reverse T3 (Chopra, 1977; Cavalieri et al., 1977). These hormones may be further deiodinated to several diiodothyronines (Burman et al., 1977; Chopra et al., 1978; Pangaro et al., 1979) and 3'-monoiodothyronine (Smallridge et al., 1978c, 1979a,b) (Fig. 1). Although deiodination occurs primarily in the liver and kidney, T4 to T3 conversion has been demonstrated in the isolated perfused rat heart (Rabinowitz and Hercker, 1971) and T3 degradation has been reported in cultured chick embryo heart cells (Dickstein et al., 1978). The thyroid state has a profound influence on these metabolic pathways. Hyperthyroidism induces a rise in serum levels and production rates of T4 and T3 (Nicoloff et al., 1972), reverse T3 (Smallridge et al., 1978b), and 3', 5'-T2 (Burman et al., 1978; Smallridge et al., 1979c), whereas hypothyroidism produces the opposite effect. Alterations in circulating

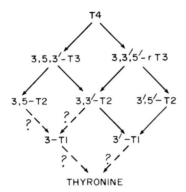

THYROXINE (T4)

Fig. 1.   Pathways of deiodinative metabolism of thyroxine. Solid arrows indicate known, and interrupted arrows presumed, pathways of monodeiodination.

levels of the iodothyronines, particularly T3, may influence the function of many target organs.

With the recent discovery of specific tissue binding sites for T3, an intense effort has been made to determine the mechanism of action of thyroid hormone at the cellular level. There is evidence that T3 may act at several locations within the cell. Segal *et al.* (1977) have demonstrated that T3 acutely stimulates 2-deoxyglucose uptake in cultured chick embryo heart cells, suggesting an effect on the cell membrane. T3 may bind to the inner mitochondrial membrane of many tissues, including rat myocardium, where binding is promptly followed by an increase in oxidative phosphorylation (Sterling *et al.*, 1977, 1978). The physiological importance of these actions is not resolved because of the nonphysiological concentrations of T3 required to effect a response. High-affinity T3 binding to a nonhistone nuclear protein has also been identified in many tissues, including rat heart (Oppenheimer *et al.*, 1974; Tsai and Chen, 1976), and various responses occur with physiological T3 concentrations. Several recent reviews have summarized the current knowledge on T3 receptors (Latham *et al.*, 1978;

Oppenheimer and Dillmann, 1978a,b; Oppenheimer, 1979; Sterling, 1979).

If thyroid hormone action is mediated through T3 receptors, then it is possible that pathological serum T3 concentrations might regulate either the number or affinity of the receptors. In rat liver it has been claimed that neither T3 administration (Degroot *et al.*, 1976; Bernal *et al.*, 1978) nor hypothyroidism (Spindler *et al.*, 1975; Oppenheimer *et al.*, 1975) influences the receptor. However, there is evidence that thyroidectomy in the neonatal rat increases liver T3 receptor number (Valcana and Timiras, 1977), and that nuclear T3 receptors in cultured pituitary tumor cells are depleted by T3 (Samuels *et al.*, 1976). There are minimal data on the effects of thyroid disorders on myocardial nuclear T3 receptors. Latham *et al.* (1979) have observed a reduction in T3 and T4 receptor numbers in both hypothyroid and hyperthyroid rat myocardium. Further studies will be necessary to determine whether or not the dramatic changes in cardiac structure and function in states of altered thyroid economy as described in the following sections are regulated in any measure by thyroid hormone receptors.

II. Thyroid Hormone Excess: Its Effects on the Heart

A. Protein Synthesis and Cardiac Hypertrophy

Thyroid hormone, by inducing protein synthesis, may produce cardiac hypertrophy. Michels *et al.* (1963) treated rats with 100 μg L-T4 for 2–3 days and demonstrated an increased incorporation of L-[1-^{14}C]leucine into heart protein. Bressler and Wittels (1966) found that 50 μg T4 administered for 10 days to guinea pigs increased both myocardial protein and the RNA/DNA ratio, whereas uridine kinase activity increased after T4 to provide the uracil nucleotides necessary for RNA synthesis (Gertz and Haugaard, 1979). An initial increase in protein synthesis and ^{32}P uptake into RNA after 2 weeks of thyroid therapy has also been described in rabbits (Golber and Kandror, 1969). However, at 4 weeks the left ventricular protein and RNA concentrations were less than in the control animals. The relative contributions of increased synthesis as compared with decreased degradation of protein in the development of cardiac hypertrophy by T4 have been studied in isolated perfused rat hearts (Sanford *et al.*, 1978). The increased rate of synthesis, estimated by [^{3}H]phenylalanine incorporation, was most marked after 3 days of thyroxine, returning to normal by 2 weeks (Fig. 2). Protein degradation was mildly delayed initially, but by a week had returned to normal. Four days after discontinuation of T4, the rate of pro-

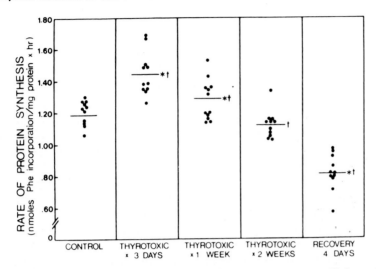

Fig. 2. Influence of progressive thyrotoxicosis and recovery on the rate of left ventricular protein synthesis. Each point represents one rat and the bar represents the mean. * = $p < 0.05$ compared to control; † = $p < 0.05$ compared to preceding group. (Reprinted by permission of the American Heart Association, Inc., from Sanford *et al.*, 1978.)

tein synthesis was markedly decreased and degradation was mildly delayed as well. Carter and Faas (1978) have also noted a decreased breakdown of both sarcoplasmic and myofibrillar proteins. The effect of T3 (20 μg/100 g × 3–14 days) on myocardial chromatin in rats has been reported by Limas and Chan-Stier (1978). Both an enhanced chromatin template activity (pmol [^{3}H]UMP/mg per min) and an increased number of transcription initiation sites were noted; chromatin dissociation and reconstitution experiments further localized the augmented RNA synthesis to the nonhistone chromatin proteins (NHPs). Interestingly, the NHPs were neither increased in number nor altered in their electrophoretic pattern. The effect on RNA synthesis was maximal at 7 days, and then regressed toward normal. These studies indicate that thyroid hormone increases RNA and protein synthesis. The augmented synthetic rates are temporary, however, returning toward control values after 2 weeks. T3 is also capable of stimulating myocardial DNA α-polymerase activity in rats, but only during neonatal life (Limas, 1979). The consequences of these alterations may be reflected in both the structural and functional modifications known to occur in cardiac muscle after treatment with thyroid hormone.

Increased protein synthesis, ultimately producing cardiac hypertrophy, has been appreciated for many years (Gemmill, 1958; Sandler and Wilson, 1959). The change in cardiac size, defined as an increase in the heart weight to body weight (HW/BW) ratio, occurs in many species, including rats (Sandler, 1959; Whitehorn *et al.*, 1959; Cairoli and Crout, 1967; Frazer and Hess, 1969; Sanford *et al.*, 1978), mice (Gemmill, 1958; Cohen *et al.*, 1966), guinea pigs (Bressler and Wittels, 1966; Murayama and Goodkind, 1968), cats (Strauer and Scherpe, 1975), and rabbits (Banerjee *et al.*, 1976). This change, which has been observed as early as 3–5 days after initiation of large doses of T4 (Brus and Hess, 1973; Frazer *et al.*, 1969; Newcomb *et al.*, 1978; Sanford *et al.*, 1978) usually is of the order of 30–50% greater than seen in control hearts. Thyroid hormone stimulates a true myocardial hypertrophy as there is no change in the water content and the changes are reversible even though thyroid is administered for as long as 8 weeks (Gemmill, 1958; Sandler and Wilson, 1959). Likewise, there is no increase in the collagenous portion of the heart (Bartošová *et al.*, 1969; Limas and Chan-Stier, 1978). In humans, a reversible cardiac hypertrophy has been described by Nixon *et al.* (1979), who measured, by echocardiography, a mean 27% reduction in left ventricular mass after successful therapy for thyrotoxicosis. Electrocardiographic evidence of left ventricular hypertrophy is also reversible (Wong *et al.*, 1979).

What is unresolved is whether the effects of the hormone are uniform. Although right ventricular hypertrophy disproportionate to left ventricular hypertrophy has been reported (Van Liere *et al.*, 1969; Mowery and Lindsay, 1973), this observation is not universally accepted (Bartošová *et al.*, 1969). The reason for these differences is not certain but may be related to the duration of hormone administration, the particular hormone used, or other factors. The former authors used T3 for only 2 weeks, whereas the latter study used T4 for 4 weeks. The stimulatory effect of thyroid hormone on atria is also unsettled, since hyperthyroid animals have been described to have either increased (Cairoli and Crout, 1967) or normal (Murayama and Goodkind, 1968) atrial weights when compared to euthyroid animals. Further investigations are warranted to resolve this issue. Thus it may be concluded that thyroid hormone produces cardiac hypertrophy. The changes in cardiac size seem to follow temporally the increases in protein synthesis (Sanford *et al.*, 1978), with the HW/BW ratio increasing during the first few days to 2 weeks and then reaching a plateau (Fig. 3).

B. Hemodynamic Effects

1. Animal Studies

The hyperdynamic circulatory manifestations of hyperthyroidism naturally led to studies on the effects of thyroid hormone on measurements of blood flow and resistance. *In vivo* and *in vitro* experiments have demon-

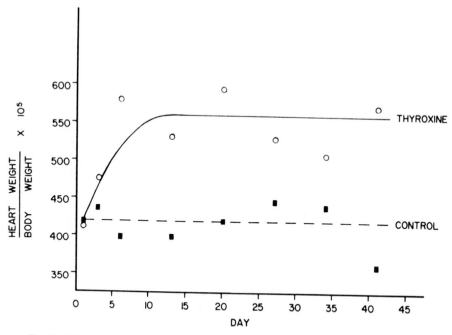

Fig. 3. Wet heart weight: body weight ratios as a function of time in control mice and in mice fed synthetic L-thyroxine for approximately 6 weeks. Each point represents a mean value for five animals, with a standard error of less than 10% of the mean value in each case. (Reprinted by permission of the American Heart Association, Inc., from Cohen et al., 1966.)

strated the profound influence of this hormone on the circulation (Table I). The isolated rat auricle, deprived of neural control, has an increased rate of contraction after 3 days of T3 or T4 (Hirvonen and Lybeck, 1956a). Subsequent studies in rats have shown that oxygen consumption (Q_{O_2})(Peacock and Moran, 1963; van der Schoot and Moran, 1965; Van Liere et al., 1969) and cardiac index (C.I.) increase (Beznák, 1962; Frazer et al., 1969), and peripheral resistance falls while systolic blood pressure rises (Beznák, 1962), and mean arterial pressure rises (Frazer et al., 1969).

Buccino et al. (1967) observed an increase of 71% and 93% in cardiac index and oxygen consumption, respectively, in cats. Skelton et al. (1970) noted that basal Q_{O_2} was elevated 28% in papillary muscle from hyperthyroid cats, whereas it rose 87% above euthyroid levels during isometric contraction. Although Q_{O_2} increased markedly during exercise, the developed tension also rose significantly. In situ measurements were performed in cats after 2 weeks of T4 (Strauer and Scherpe, 1975). These animals had an increased heart rate, cardiac index, mean arterial pressure,

TABLE I

Effect of Hyperthyroidism on Hemodynamic Indices in Experimental Animals[a]

Species and Reference	Heart rate	Cardiac index	Q_{O_2}	Peripheral Resistance	Coronary blood flow	MAP	Systolic BP	Mean PA pressure	LVEDP	RVEDP
Rat										
Hirvonen and Lybeck (1956a)	↑									
Beznák (1962)	↑	↑70%	↑100%	↓50%			↑58%			
Peacock and Moran (1963)	↑35%		↑54%							
van der Schoot and Moran (1965)			↑91%							
Van Liere et al. (1969)			↑40%							
Frazer et al. (1969)	↑35%	↑53%				↑29%				
Cat										
Buccino et al. (1967)	N.C.	↑71%	↑93%							
Skelton et al. (1970)		↑83%	↑28%							
Strauer and Scherpe (1975)	↑48%					↑24%	↑		N.C.	
Dog										
Brewster et al. (1956)	↑29%	↑53%	↑55%							
van der Schoot and Moran (1965)	↑92%		↑50%			↑53%	N.C.			
Piatnek-Leunissen and Olson (1967)										
Without CHF	↑38%	↑74%	↑24%		↑20%	↓12%		↑20%	N.C.	↑35%
With CHF	↑88%	↑34%	↑89%		↑98%	↑8%		↑53%	N.C.	↑97%
Rabbit										
Golber et al. (1967)	↑42%	↑66%		↓12%			↑31%			

[a] Q_{O_2} = oxygen consumption; MAP = mean arterial pressure; systolic BP = systolic blood pressure; mean PA pressure = mean pulmonary artery pressure; LVEDP and RVEDP = left ventricular and right ventricular end diastolic pressures, respectively; N.C. = no change.

systolic blood pressure, and systolic left ventricular pressure. Mean right atrial pressure, left ventricular end-diastolic pressure (LVEDP), and vena cava pressures were unchanged.

Brewster *et al.* (1956) induced a tachycardia and an elevated cardiac index and Q_{O_2} in dogs fed thyroid hormone 1–3 weeks. Thyroxine for 3 weeks doubled the heart rate and increased Q_{O_2} and mean arterial pressure by 50% in both open chest and hind limb perfused dogs (van der Schoot and Moran, 1965). Piatnek-Leunissen and Olson (1967) induced congestive heart failure in 13 of 30 dogs treated with thyroid hormone. In the group without heart failure, heart rate and Q_{O_2} rose moderately in comparison to cardiac index. In the group with heart failure, although the cardiac index was above the euthyroid value, it was considerably less than in uncomplicated hyperthyroidism, and heart rate and Q_{O_2} were both markedly increased. Other parameters that were elevated during the hyperthyroid state, and increased even further in the animals with heart failure, were coronary blood flow, mean pulmonary artery (PA) pressure, and right ventricular end-diastolic pressure (RVEDP). LVEDP was unaffected.

In rabbits, there was a rise in heart rate after 2 weeks of thyroid hormone with no further change at 4 weeks. Cardiac index was maximally elevated by 2 weeks, with a slight fall at 4 weeks and no changes in stroke volume at either interval. In contrast the arteriovenous (A-V) O_2 difference was unchanged early, but was significantly increased by 4 weeks. There was an initial decrease in peripheral resistance with return to normal at 4 weeks, and venous pressures were normal throughout the study (Golber *et al.*, 1967).

2. Human Studies

Blumgart *et al.* (1930a,b) observed that hyperthyroid individuals had tachycardia and a shortened circulation time, both of which improved with administration of Lugol's iodine. Since that time, many of the hemodynamic parameters noted in experimental hyperthyroidism have also been studied in humans with thyrotoxicosis, and Table II summarizes the major changes observed. The hemodynamic changes consistently seen in hyperthyroidism include elevations in heart rate, cardiac index, coronary blood flow, oxygen consumption, and right and left ventricular work; these parameters return to normal in treated patients (Rowe *et al.*, 1956). Mean systemic arterial and pulmonary artery pressures are either increased or normal, and peripheral resistance is generally decreased.

The reason for the increased cardiac output has been questioned for years, and several studies have indicated that peripheral vasodilatation with decreased peripheral resistance are at least partly responsible. Kontos *et al.* (1965) found an increase of 320% in forearm and hand blood flow and noted

TABLE II

Effect of Hyperthyroidism on Hemodynamic Indices in Humans[a]

Reference	Heart rate	Cardiac index	Q_{O_2}	Peripheral resistance	Stroke volume	MAP	$\overline{RA}$ pressure	PA pressure	RV work	LVWI	A–V Q_{O_2} Diff.
Bishop et al. (1955)	↑	↑	↑		↑	↑	N		↑		
Rowe et al. (1956)	↑ 39%	↑ 58%	↑ 44%			N	↑ 33%		↑ 78%	↑ 38%	N
Graettinger et al. (1959)											
IA	↑ 43% (↑)[b]	↑ 100% (↑)	↑ 59% (↑)	↓ 56%	44% (↑)					↑ 91%	
IB	↑ 29% (↑)	↑ 48% (↑)	↑ 46% (↑)	↓ 24%	18% (↑)					↑ 84%	
IIA	↑ 39% (↑)	↑ 12% (↑)	↑ 48% (↑)	↓ 3%	18% (→)					↑ 20%	
IIB	↑ 59% (↑)	↑ 200% (↓)	↑ 65% (↑)	↓ 69%	87% (↓)					↑ 335%	
Kontos et al. (1965)	↑ 63%	↑ 215%	↑ 55%	↓ 53%	33%	N					
Ueda et al. (1965)	↑ 27%	↑ 255%			201%		↑ 59%				
Theilen and Wilson (1967)	↑ 55%	↑ 52%		N.C.	N.C.	N.C.	N.C.				
Amidi et al. (1968)	↑ 78%	↑ 211%	↑ 52%		N	↑ 11%	N				↓ 30%
Grossman et al. (1971)	↑	↑	↑			↑					
Pietras et al. (1972)	↑									↑	
Ikram (1977)											
No CHF	↑	↑ 57%				N	N				
CHF		N				N	↑				

[a] Q_{O_2} = oxygen consumption; MAP = mean arterial pressure; $\overline{RA}$ pressure = mean right atrial pressure; PA pressure = pulmonary artery; LVWI = left ventricular work index; N = normal; N.C. = no change; CHF = congestive heart failure.

[b] ( ) indicates increase or decrease in parameter after exercise.

also that the circulation to the forearm skin was under cholinergic control. Theilen and Wilson (1967) proposed that the vasodilation was secondary to increased heat production from excessive metabolic activity within the tissues. In order to test this, they infused phenylephrine (1–2 μg/kg · min) into hyperthyroid and euthyroid subjects to produce vasoconstriction, at the same time keeping heart rate constant by atropine pretreatment. There was a significant reduction in cardiac index (from 4.8 to 3.3 liters/min·m²), indicating that the high cardiac output of thyrotoxicosis is at least partially due to peripheral vasodilatation. Cardiac output (C.O.) is a function of both heart rate and stroke volume. Virtually all reports, both in experimental animals and in humans, document an elevated heart rate: Although no change in stroke volume has been reported (Theilen and Wilson, 1967), many studies have described an increase in either stroke volume or stroke volume index (Bishop *et al.*, 1955; Kontos *et al.*, 1965; Ueda *et al.*, 1965; Massey *et al.*, 1967).

The data in Table II generally refer to patients studied at rest. Bishop *et al.* (1955) observed a high cardiac output response after exercise, manifest by an increased heart rate and an even greater stroke volume. Mean PA pressures were also higher than in normals after exercise. Graettinger *et al.* (1959) divided his patients into two groups. Group I had no evidence of congestive heart failure at any time during their hyperthyroidism. Group IA patients had normal hearts, whereas those in IB had underlying organic heart disease. Group II patients had congestive heart failure (CHF) during their thyroid illness; IIA had normal cardiac outputs at rest, whereas IIB subjects had unusually high outputs. Table II depicts the hemodynamic measurements in the patients before and after exercise, compared to a group of normal individuals. Some patients with organic heart disease (IB) tolerated the additional strain of thyrotoxicosis, although their C.I./Q_{O_2} ratios were not as high as those of patients in group IA. Of those who developed CHF, most who had underlying heart disease had normal resting cardiac outputs. They had "relative" low output failure, with a low C.O./Q_{O_2} ratio and widened (A-V) O_2 difference; moreover, there was no change in cardiac output during exercise. This was due primarily to an inability of the myocardium to increase its stroke volume, as heart rate rose. Of special interest were the few patients in group IIB who had much higher cardiac outputs and C.O./Q_{O_2} ratios at rest than did IA patients. However, exercise elicited a decrease in stroke volume index and cardiac index with a rise in oxygen consumption. Hemodynamic studies in patients with and without CHF were also conducted by Ikram (1977). Patients with uncomplicated hyperthyroidism had high resting cardiac indices and normal mean right atrial pressures, whereas the patients with CHF had high right atrial pressures and a mean cardiac index that was in the midnormal range for euthyroid individuals.

In summary, many hemodynamic alterations resulting from excess thyroid hormone have been documented both in experimental animals and in humans. Although these stresses on cardiac function may be well tolerated, some patients (particularly those with underlying heart disease) may be unable to meet the increased metabolic demands. Although they maintain an absolute cardiac output in the normal range for euthyroidism, this is insufficient during hyperthyroidism and leads to a relative "low-output" heart failure. On the other hand, some patients may indeed develop congestive heart failure despite extraordinarily high cardiac outputs, a true "high-output" failure.

C. Contractility Effects

1. Animal Studies

Thyroid hormone exerts a major influence on myocardial contractility. Most animal experiments, performed *in vitro,* have measured either isometric or isotonic contractions. The parameters measured during isometric contractions include the rate of tension development (dP/dt), the time to peak tension (msec), and total tension, whereas isotonic studies measure the maximal velocity of muscle shortening (V_{max}). Another method for assessing myocardial mechanics has been to determine left ventricular isovolumic tension or pressure *in vivo* after aortic occlusion.

Early studies using rat auricles or ventricle strips indicated that muscle from hyperthyroid animals produced less contractile force and maximum tension (Hirvonen and Lybeck, 1956b; Whitehorn *et al.,* 1959), whereas T4-treated rats *in vivo* had greater than normal maximum work per gram of left ventricle with an increased reserve after an acute stress on the heart (Beznák, 1962). Anton and Gravenstein (1970) also reported an increased contractile force in isolated hyperthyroid rabbit ventricle strips.

Buccino *et al.* (1967, 1968), using cat papillary muscles, found significant differences in the development of isometric tension in various thyroid states (Fig. 4). Most striking was the more rapid rate of tension development with less time required to reach peak tension in the muscles from hyperthyroid animals. The total tension achieved did not exceed that seen in the euthyroid state, although it was significantly higher than in hypothyroid cats. Several variables, including temperature and frequency of contractions, also affected contractility.

Other authors have reported similar results. Murayama and Goodkind (1968) found a triphasic frequency–force curve in guinea pig atria. They

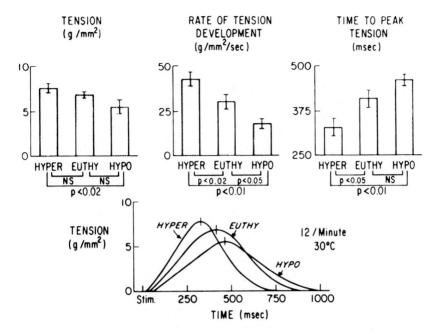

Fig. 4. Isometric tension examined in relation to time and analyzed in terms of its component factors as a function of level of thyroid state. Tension represents maximum active tension, measured at the peak of the length–active tension curve. Rate of tension development was measured as the maximum slope of the tension curve, and time to peak tension was measured from the stimulus. Tension curves in the lower panel represent average data, as presented in columns of the upper panel, for muscles from 11 hyperthyroid, 8 euthyroid, and 13 hypothyroid cats. NS = $P > 0.05$. (Reprinted by permission from Buccino *et al.*, 1967.)

also noted that tension development was greater at contraction frequencies less than 100/min, with no difference at rates above 100/min. If the studies were conducted at a low calcium concentration (0.625 mM), the tension was greater at all frequencies in the hyperthyroid animals. This calcium dependency suggested that thyroid hormone may augment calcium uptake and hence contractility. Parmley *et al.* (1968) found a 32% decrease in time to peak tension and a 27% increase in maximum isometric tension in papillary muscles from hyperthyroid cats. Using the same animal model, Taylor (1970) found that at 12 contractions per minute, time to peak tension was shorter, and the rate and developed tension were greater in hyperthyroidism, but at a frequency of 60/min the developed tension and rate of tension rise were similar to the euthyroid state. It was proposed that the increased oxygen consumption at the faster rate produced a hypoxic depressant effect on the myocardium.

Skelton *et al.* (1970), also using cat papillary muscles, showed a 27% decrease in time to peak tension, a 68% increase in rate of tension development, and a 34% increase in total tension. These changes were associated with a 52% increase in myocardial Q_{O_2}. In a subsequent experiment total tension was less in the hyperthyroid animals (Skelton *et al.*, 1971). In the latter study the authors examined energy utilization by removing the energy formation processes. They were able to do this by inhibiting glycolysis with iodoacetic acid and by inhibiting oxidative phosphorylation by bathing the muscles in a solution equilibrated with 95% N_2–5% CO_2. Their results suggested that hyperthyroid cardiac muscle had an altered conversion of chemical energy to mechanical work and that the process was an inefficient utilization of energy. Palacios *et al.* (1979) confirmed that the augmented contractility of hyperthyroid cat papillary muscles could be abolished in a hypoxic environment (95% N_2, 5% CO_2). Skelton *et al.* (1973) also examined the time course of the effect of thyroid hormone on contractility. In cardiac muscle from euthyroid cats and guinea pigs, incubation with T4 or T3 for 8 hr failed to enhance contractility, whereas if cats were pretreated for 3 days with T4, there was a faster rate of tension development and shorter time to peak tension. Contractility was also unaffected in intact euthyroid dogs whose hearts were perfused acutely with T4 or T3. Although these studies indicated that thyroid hormone required a lag period before enhancing the inotropic response, Tsai (1975) observed an increase in contractility by T3 within 20 min in a newborn rat myocardial cell culture system.

Isotonic contraction studies have been conducted to assess the maximum velocity of shortening (V_{max}) in various thyroid states. Buccino *et al.* (1967) demonstrated a greater V_{max} at every load studied (Fig. 5) in hyperthyroid animals. Similar results have been reported (Parmley *et al.*, 1968; Taylor, 1970; Skelton *et al.*, 1970; Strauer and Scherpe, 1975), with the V_{max} being 60–85% greater in the hyperthyroid state. Parmley *et al.* (1968) also noted that since the series elastic compliance was unchanged, the altered V_{max} was due to a change in the contractile element.

In vivo studies have generally corroborated the *in vitro* results. Goodkind (1968) determined the maximal left ventricular pressure response to aortic constriction in guinea pigs as a measure of contractility and found that both the maximum rate of rise of systolic pressure and the maximum left ventricular systolic pressure were greater in hyperthyroid animals. Taylor *et al.* (1969) observed an increased velocity and a slightly higher total tension when isovolumic contractions were measured after sudden balloon occlusion of the aorta. Strauer and Scherpe (1975) found an increase in the isovolumetric rate of ventricular pressure development in hyperthyroid cats *in vivo*. Golber *et al.* (1967) and Golber and Kandror (1969) found in rabbits

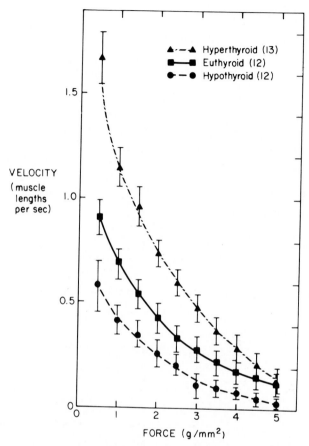

Fig. 5. The average force–velocity relationship for papillary muscles from hyperthyroid, euthyroid, and hypothyroid cats. Initial velocity of shortening is normalized in terms of muscle lengths per second, and load, corrected for cross-sectional area of individual muscles, is expressed in g/mm^2. Brackets represent $\pm$ SEM. (Reprinted by permission from Buccino *et al.*, 1967.)

that maximum left ventricular pressure increased by 50% after 2 weeks of thyroid hormone therapy, with no further increase after 4 weeks. After ligating the aorta, maximal pressure was decreased after 4 weeks. The authors felt that these animals had an impaired functional reserve (as opposed to the increased reserve noted by Beznák, 1962) and that it correlated with the reduction in left ventricular protein after 4 weeks of thyroid treatment. The results obtained by Golber may be explained by the more prolonged study period, as most experiments have given T4 for 14 days or less.

2. Human Studies

Direct measurements of contractility are lacking in humans with thyrotoxicosis because of the necessity of performing invasive procedures. Howitt *et al.* (1968) did, however, report indirect indices of contractility by means of aortic catheterization and pressure recordings. The shorter ejection time and increased mean systolic ejection rate suggested that ejection velocity was enhanced. A number of studies have examined contractility noninvasively by recording systolic time intervals. Figure 6 illustrates the parameters measured: QS$_2$ is the total duration of electromechanical systole. It is composed of the preejection period (PEP) and the left ventricular ejection time (LVET). The PEP is in turn subdivided into the QS$_1$ and the isovolumic contraction period (ICP). The latter is the time needed for the ventricle to generate enough pressure to open the aortic valve and should reflect the velocity of shortening and time to peak tension.

Using these parameters as a reflection of myocardial performance, Amidi *et al.* (1968) noted a shortening of the isovolumic contraction time, PEP, and the ejection time in untreated hyperthyroid patients. In the past several years a number of similar studies have been conducted (Parisi *et al.,* 1974;

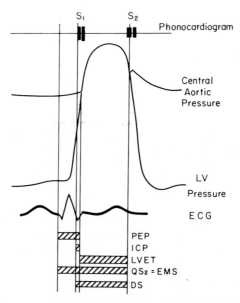

Fig. 6. Schematic representation of the events of a cardiac cycle and definitions of systolic time intervals: preejection period (PEP), isovolumic contraction period (ICP), left ventricular ejection time (LVET), electromechanical systole (EMS), and duration of systole (DS). S$_1$ = first heart sound; S$_2$ = second heart sound. (Reprinted by permission from Grossman *et al.,* 1971.)

Hillis *et al.*, 1975; Burckhardt *et al.*, 1978; Chakravarty *et al.*, 1978; Rubler *et al.*, 1977). The results have been quite consistent, demonstrating a short QS_2, short PEP (primarily the ICP), and normal LVET. There is a significant negative correlation between serum T4 and the PEP, and normalization of the former is associated temporally with return to normal of the PEP (Chakravarty *et al.*, 1978). At least one study evaluating diastolic time intervals has reported a short, rapid filling time in hyperthyroidism that becomes normal after treatment (Rubler *et al.*, 1977). Serial M-mode echocardiograms have also been used to document increased velocity of myocardial fiber shortening (Friedman *et al.*, 1979), stroke volume, and cardiac output, which are effectively reduced after successful therapy (Nixon *et al.*, 1979).

In summary, thyroid hormone has a direct effect on contractility. Animal studies have shown the major effect to be enhancement of the velocity of shortening or time to peak tension, whereas the total tension achieved is affected to a much smaller degree. A number of factors may alter the response, including frequency of contraction, temperature, and ionic calcium concentration. Although most studies have been conducted after 2 weeks or less of thyroid hormone, some evidence suggests that more prolonged therapy may lead to a reduced myocardial reserve. Human studies have been performed indirectly and have confirmed that the velocity of contraction is enhanced by thyroid hormone.

D. Catecholamine Interactions with Thyroid Hormone

1. Circulatory Effects

a. ANIMAL STUDIES

Many of the symptoms and signs of hyperthyroidism resemble those of sympathetic stimulation, suggesting that the enhanced hemodynamics of hyperthyroidism may be due to hypersensitivity of the autonomic nervous system. Brewster *et al.* (1956) provided such evidence by showing that the increases in heart rate and cardiac index following infusion of epinephrine and norepinephrine were greater in thyrotoxic than in euthyroid dogs, and that both responses were completely abolished by an epidural preganglionic block. Stimulation of stroke work after catecholamines was also greater in the thyroid-fed animals. Mendelsohn *et al.* (1961) found that treatment of rats with reserpine prevented the increased heart rate of isolated atria, suggesting to the authors that the main reason for thyroxine-induced tachycardia was an enhanced sensitivity to catecholamines. A similar result was obtained in dogs whose ectopic ventricular pacemakers induced by T3 myocardial implants were inhibited by reserpine (Folkman and Edmunds, 1962).

Barker and Makiuchi (1965) reported that guanethidine pretreatment of rats did not prevent the subsequent heart rate response to T4, and that bretylium only partially blocked this chronotropic effect. They concluded that the peripheral effects of T4 could be diminished but not abolished by sympathetic blockade. A number of experiments testing dose–response relationships for catecholamines provided strong evidence that the sensitivity of the cardiovascular system to catecholamines is not altered by thyroid hormone. Graded doses of norepinephrine and epinephrine produced similar increases in heart rate and contractile force (Figs. 7 and 8) in control and thyroxine-treated dogs (van der Schoot and Moran, 1965). The same results for chronotropic responses to catecholamines were also observed in rats (van der Schoot and Moran, 1965; Cravey and Gravenstein, 1965), dogs (Margolius and Gaffney, 1965), guinea pigs (Goodkind, 1969), and rabbits (Anton and Gravenstein, 1970). Inhibition of heart rate by β-blockers has usually produced only a partial reduction in the heart rate of thyrotoxic animals (Cairoli and Crout, 1967; Goodkind, 1968; Thompson, 1973), although complete inhibition has also been reported (Hirvonen and Paavilainen, 1967). Evidence for an augmentation of norepinephrine-stimulated heart rate by T3 has been reported by Wildenthal (1972) in fetal mouse heart organ cultures. However, these results were obtained only with very large doses of T3 (5×10^{-6} M) and only in atria.

Numerous studies have also evaluated the possibility of a catecholamine–thyroid hormone interaction on inotropic responses. Van der Schoot and Moran (1965) found that the increase in isometric contraction after catecholamines was actually less in hyperthyroid than in control dogs. Similar results have been reported in cat papillary muscles (Buccino *et al.,* 1967; Levey *et al.,* 1969b). In addition, Buccino observed that norepinephrine depletion by reserpine had no effect on the V_{max} of isotonic shortening. In hyperthyroid guinea pigs it has been found that catecholamines do not augment the developed tension *in vitro* (Murayama and Goodkind, 1968) or the maximum left ventricular systolic pressure response to aortic constriction (Goodkind, 1969) and that the pressure response is not affected by propranolol (Goodkind, 1968). The details of the chronotropic dose responses to catecholamines are summarized by Levey (1971).

b. Human Studies

Numerous investigations have demonstrated that the sympathetic nervous system is at least partially responsible for the chronotropic effects observed in hyperthyroidism. Reserpine, which causes myocardial depletion of catecholamines, decreases tachycardia and improves clinical symptoms (Canary *et al.,* 1957; deGroot *et al.,* 1960, 1961; Amidi *et al.,* 1968),

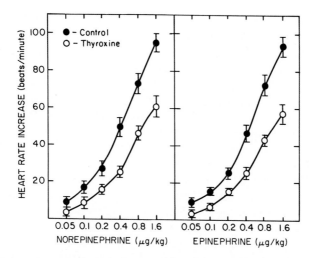

Fig. 7. Influence of graded doses of norepinephrine and epinephrine on heart rate of 17 normal dogs and 17 dogs pretreated with thyroxine (1 mg/kg·day) for 3 weeks. Pentobarbital-barbital anesthesia. Mean control heart rates were 122 and 170 beats/min, respectively, for normal and thyroxine-treated dogs. (Reprinted by permission from van der Schoot and Moran, 1965.)

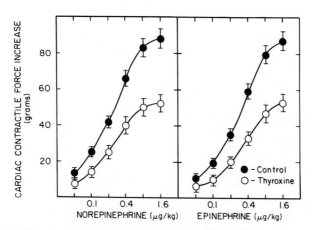

Fig. 8. Influence of graded doses of norepinephrine and epinephrine on cardiac contractile force of 17 normal dogs and 17 dogs pretreated with thyroxine (1 mg/kg·day) for 3 weeks. Pentobarbital-barbital anesthesia. Mean control contractile forces were 77 and 79 gs, respectively. (Reprinted by permission from van der Schoot and Moran, 1965.)

although cardiac output and oxygen consumption are usually unaffected. Guanethidine also reduces both heart rate and cardiac output, but not to normal (Goldstein and Killip, 1965). In studies of β-blockade, Wilson *et al.* (1964) reported that whereas nethalide abolished the isoproterenol induced increase in heart rate, it had no effect on basal heart rate in hyperthyroid subjects. Similar results by Wilson *et al.* (1966) were reported using propranolol in euthyroid subjects given exogenous triiodothyronine. A reduction in heart rate has generally been shown by other reports of β-blockers, including sotalol (Grossman *et al.*, 1971) and propranolol (McDevitt *et al.*, 1968; Wiener *et al.*, 1969; Pietras *et al.*, 1972; Howitt *et al.*, 1968; Toft *et al.*, 1976; Zwillich *et al.*, 1978). The heart rate, though reduced, has not necessarily become normal, suggesting both a thyroid hormone and sympathetic nervous system effect. An interesting report by Ikram (1977) showed that heart rate and cardiac output were significantly reduced in thyrotoxic patients who had congestive heart failure, but not in patients without heart failure. It was felt that the sympathetics played a greater role in the patients with heart failure.

The data on the effect of β-blockade on inotropic responses in hyperthyroidism in general indicate that the sympathetic nervous system plays little role. Although Wiener *et al.* (1969) found an inhibitory effect of propranolol on some inotropic responses, left ventricular efficiency was actually increased. β-Blockade has been reported to have no effect on the preejection period, isovolumic contraction time, or ejection time (Amidi *et al.*, 1968; Grossman *et al.*, 1971), although some authors (Howitt *et al.*, 1968; Pietras *et al.*, 1972) found some effect on ejection rate. It should be noted, however, that Pietras' patients had preexisting cardiovascular disease. DeGroot et al. (1961) found that neither guanethidine nor reserpine normalized the ICT or duration of ventricular ejection.

2. Metabolic Effects

Since catecholamine effects are mediated through the adenyl cyclase–cyclic AMP pathway, any synergism between thyroxine and the adrenergic nervous system might be reflected in increased cAMP levels in heart. The consensus is, however, that pretreatment of animals with thyroid hormone does not enhance catecholamine stimulation of adenyl cyclase activity (Section II,G,1). On the other hand, there is evidence that myocardial glycogenolysis is augmented by interaction of these hormones. Glycogenolysis requires the presence of phosphorylase *a,* and T3 is known to enhance the activity of this enzyme in response to catecholamines (Section II,G,2). Wilson *et al.* (1967) investigated the effects of isoproterenol and propranolol on free fatty acids and glucose in euthyroid and T3-treated subjects. Although isoproterenol increased plasma free fatty acid levels and the response was inhibited by propranolol, the changes were the same in both treated and control subjects. Isoproterenol infusions had no effect on blood glucose concentrations in either study group.

3. Catecholamine Concentrations

Although hyperthyroidism does not appear to alter the sensitivity to catecholamines, there is ample evidence that activity of the adrenergic system contributes to the hyperdynamic peripheral circulation. The results of studies measuring catecholamine tissue concentrations and metabolism have been variable and do not afford a unifying explanation. Goodkind *et al.* (1961) reported that the myocardial content of norepinephrine in guinea pig auricles was increased when the animals were pretreated with large doses of T3. Kurland *et al.* (1963), on the other hand, found that norepinephrine and epinephrine concentrations in rabbit whole heart or ventricles were unaffected by thyroxine, whereas the atrial contents of both hormones were decreased. Normal ventricular norepinephrine content has been reported in cats (Buccino *et al.,* 1967), rats (Barker and Makiuchi, 1965), and dogs (Conway *et al.,* 1976), although decreased concentrations were found in rabbit ventricles (Anton and Gravenstein, 1970). A normal catecholamine content has been reported in animals receiving myocardial T3 implants (Folkman and Edmunds, 1962). Serum and urine catecholamine concentrations and their turnover rates in hyperthyroidism have been reviewed by Landsberg (1977). The studies showed either no change or a decrease in serum and urine concentrations and turnover rates of norepinephrine with no change in epinephrine metabolism.

4. Catecholamine Receptors

Catecholamines produce their effects by binding to receptors, and recent methodological developments have permitted the direct measurement of cardiac membrane adrenoreceptors. If thyroid hormone interplays with the adrenergic nervous system, it might do so by affecting the adrenergic receptors. β-Receptor number and affinity may be determined by labeling the receptor with the β-antagonist [^{3}H]dihydroalprenolol. Similar results for the α-receptor may be obtained using [^{3}H]dihydroergokryptine. Williams *et al.* (1977) found a twofold increase in the number of β-receptors with no change in binding affinity after 3 days of T3 (Fig. 9). Acute exposure to T4 during incubation of membranes from euthyroid animals failed to increase receptor number, suggesting that the effect in hyperthyroidism may be secondary to new protein and receptor synthesis. A T3-induced increase in β-receptors may be seen in cultured myocardial cells incubated for 24 hr, however (Tsai and Chen, 1978). Banerjee and Kung (1977) demonstrated an increase in the number of β-adrenergic binding sites when thyroidec-

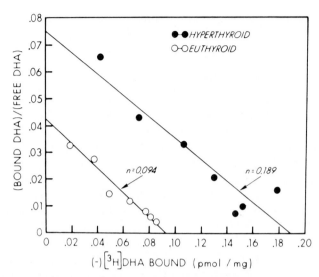

Fig. 9. Scatchard plot of (−) [³H]dihydroalprenolol (DHA) binding to cardiac membranes from control (euthyroid) and hyperthyroid rats. Hyperthyroidism was induced by injection of triiodothyronine. Cardiac membranes were incubated with a series of concentrations of (−) [³H]dihydroalprenolol and specific binding was determined. The lines for euthyroid ($r = 0.97$) and hyperthyroid ($r = 0.93$) membranes were determined by linear regression analysis. The intercept with the abscissa indicates the number of binding sites (n). Each point represents the mean of duplicate determinations. (Reprinted by permission from Williams *et al.*, 1977.)

tomized rats were given T3, although there was no increase in euthyroid rats treated with T3. The effect on α-receptors was a reduction in the number of sites and no change in the affinity when the animals received T3 (Sharma and Banerjee, 1978a). Ciaraldi and Marinetti (1977), on the other hand, have demonstrated in hyperthyroid rats a marked increase in numbers of β-receptors with no change in the affinity and a decrease in both number and affinity of α-receptors.

It is apparent that the thyroid state affects myocardial adrenergic receptor numbers. Whether this is achieved through T3 induction of receptor synthesis, a direct effect of T3, or serum concentrations of catecholamines is not clear. An important unresolved question is why, if β-receptors are increased by thyroid hormone, there is not a clearly definable synergism between these hormones and the inotropic and chronotropic responses (Section II,D,1). Further studies directed at assessing receptor occupancy and the possibility of postreceptor insensitivity may help resolve this issue. The recent development of an antiserum to a purified propranolol binding site from solubilized cardiac membranes should also aid in understanding these unresolved problems (Wrenn and Haber, 1979).

E. Cholinergic Interaction with Thyroid Hormone

The tachycardia of hyperthyroidism has attracted the interest of investigators for many years. The evidence indicates that although the adrenergic nervous system is functional in this condition, it is not supersensitive. It appears that the chronotropic effects are due to both catecholamine stimulation and the direct action of thyroid hormone on the heart (Section II,D,1). There is yet another means by which the tachycardia could be at least partially explained, and that is via an alteration in the parasympathetic nervous system. This system decreases heart rate, as demonstrated by vagal nerve stimulation or acetylcholine (ACh) infusions. Early work by Hoffmann et al. (1947) supported the proposition that thyroid hormone might influence cholinergic activity. *In situ* studies showed that hyperthyroid cats, rats, and rabbits all had less of a bradycardia response to vagal stimulation than did control animals, and isolated cat and guinea pig hearts yielded similar results after ACh injection. Vagal nerve stimulation *in vitro* produced a shorter duration of cardiac arrest in hyperthyroid cat hearts (Hoffmann et al., 1953).

Subsequent experiments have given variable results. Some authors have found less of a reduction in heart rate after vagal stimulation in thyroxine-treated rats (Cairoli and Crout, 1967; Frazer and Hess, 1969). The latter authors also reported no differences in (1) myocardial cholinesterase activity or (2) response to ACh injections in the thyrotoxic animals. In contrast, Zaimis et al. (1969) reported no difference in the cholinergic sensitivity of T4-treated guinea pigs and an increased sensitivity in cats. Leveque (1956) found an increased sensitivity to acetylcholine in dogs and Anton and Gravenstein (1970) observed no alteration in cholinergic receptor sensitivity to mecholyl and atropine in hyperthyroid rabbits. Attempting to examine the role of the parasympathetic nervous system without any sympathetic activity, Bilder and Hess (1973) prepared their rats with bretylium and adrenal demedullation. The hyperthyroid animals had a smaller chronotropic response than did the euthyroid ones. These authors reported that atrial choline acetyltransferase activity was unchanged in the experimental group, but choline infusions normalized the chronotropic response to vagal stimulation. They speculated that either a decreased extracellular choline content or an impaired uptake by the hyperthyroid myocardium could explain these results. Recently White and Zimmerman (1976) evaluated both the effect of atropine (with propranolol adrenergic blockade) and sinus node artery perfusion with acetylcholine. In the basal state cholinergic activity was impaired in the hyperthyroid dogs. This defect was not due to an efferent disturbance as both vagal stimulation and ACh perfusion produced slowing of heart rate similar to their controls (differing from previous data, *vide supra*).

Comparable data in humans are scarce, but Heimbach and Crout (1972) did demonstrate that graded doses of atropine induced a smaller heart rate increase in hyperthyroid than in euthyroid subjects. Although the data are not unanimous, the consensus is that the tachycardia of hyperthyroidism may be in part a reflection of impaired parasympathetic stimulation. The differences observed in these studies may reflect species differences, variation in dose or duration of thyroid therapy, or other unknown factors.

F. Electrophysiological Changes Due to Thyroid Hormone

Although cardiac rhythm disturbances in patients with thyroid disease have been appreciated for many years, recent advances in cardiac electrophysiology have permitted a better understanding of their genesis. In experimental hyperthyroidism in several species, alterations in electrical conduction have been demonstrated. Freedberg *et al.* (1970), using isolated atria from rabbits, showed that whereas the resting potential and the heights of action potentials did not differ, the duration of action potential repolarization was shortened in animals who received T4 for 6 weeks. Arnsdorf and Childers (1970) found a shortened effective refractory period (as did Frolov *et al.*, 1967) and a lowered diastolic threshold for atrial responses in isolated perfused hearts of rabbits treated for 7 days with T4 (250 μg/kg). A delay in the atrial response was evident, however, since acute perfusion of control hearts with T4 had no effect on spontaneous heart rate or intraatrial conduction time. Atrial and ventricular electrograms from denervated hearts of open chest anesthetized dogs who received thyroid powder for 4–6 weeks were studied by Goel *et al.* (1972). The A-V functional refractory period and conduction time were both significantly shortened in these animals. Infusion of epinephrine and/or norepinephrine (Arnsdorf and Childers, 1970; Goel *et al.*, 1972) or atropine (Arnsdorf and Childers, 1970) showed that catecholamines and acetylcholine did not enhance the effect of T4 on conduction time or refractory period. El-Shahawy (1974) attempted to localize the conduction disturbance by performing His bundle recordings in dogs after an acute injection of T3. T3 induced a significant shortening of the atrial to His bundle (A-H) interval, whereas atrial pacing prolonged this interval. Neither pacing nor T3 affected the His bundle to ventricle (H-V) time, and propranolol (in a dose sufficient to block acutely an isoproterenol increase in heart rate) did not affect the A-H or the H-V times. Although unable to determine transmembrane potentials in humans, Cotoi *et al.* (1972) were able to record intracardiac monophasic action potentials (MAPs) using suction electrodes in two hyperthyroid individuals. These patients showed a shorter duration of the MAP and a faster rate of rise of the action potential than did a group of seven hypothyroid patients.

From these investigations it can be concluded that hyperthyroidism enhances the conduction velocity and shortens the refractory period in atria of both animals and humans. The effects are presumably the result of a direct action of thyroid hormone on the myocardium, as catecholamines and atropine did not augment the responses to T4. Limited data (El-Shahawy, 1974) suggest that the enhanced conductivity is limited to the A-H interval, with H-V conduction being normal. Though the reason for enhanced electrical activity is unclear, the ultrastructural changes described (Section II,I) may alter membrane ion transport. The result may lead to what has been known for years, an increased propensity for arrhythmias.

G. Thyroid Hormone Effect on Myocardial Enzymes

1. Adenyl Cyclase–Cyclic AMP

Catecholamines, which induce positive inotropic and chronotropic responses in the heart, also activate adenyl cyclase (Sutherland and Robison, 1966). It was proposed by Levey and Epstein (1968) that thyroxine might also produce inotropic and chronotropic effects through adenyl cyclase. These authors demonstrated a rise in cardiac adenyl cyclase when thyroxine ($5 \times 10^{-7} M$) was added *in vitro* to a particulate fraction of cat left ventricle. Furthermore, they suggested the existence of two adenyl cyclase systems when they found that propranolol inhibited the catecholamine but not the T4-induced activation of adenyl cyclase (Levey and Epstein, 1969; Fig. 10). They noted, however, that this *in vitro* phenomenon might not be physiologically relevant because (1) acutely T4 did not alter contractility; (2) D-thyroxine, a much less potent analogue, was equally as effective as L-thyroxine in stimulating adenyl cyclase; and (3) reverse T3 also stimulated this activity. Subsequent studies of *in vivo* T4 administration have generally substantiated their concern that the *in vitro* activation of adenyl cyclase by T4 might not be applicable to the whole animal. If T4 did indeed augment the adenyl cyclase–cyclic AMP system, then the cardiac catecholamine effects might be enhanced, since they are thought to be cyclic AMP mediated. Administration of thyroid hormone to either cats (Levey *et al.*, 1969b; Sobel *et al.*, 1969) or rats (Brus and Hess, 1973) had no effect on basal or norepinephrine-stimulated levels of adenyl cyclase (Fig. 11).

Catecholamines may also act via the adenyl cyclase–cyclic AMP–phosphorylase *b* kinase system to increase phosphorylase *a* activity (Frazer

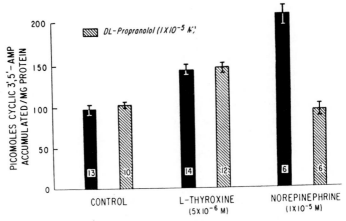

Fig. 10. Effect of DL-propranolol on L-thyroxine and L-norepinephrine activation of adenyl cyclase. Each bar represents the mean ± SE; the number of determinations is shown at the base of each bar. (Reprinted by permission from Levey and Epstein, 1969.)

et al., 1969). Similarly, T3 treatment *in vivo* will increase phosphorylase *a*. This effect by T3, unlike the response to catecholamines, is not related to enhanced adenyl cyclase activity or cyclic AMP levels in the heart (Frazer *et al.*, 1969; McNeill *et al.*, 1969; Young and McNeill, 1974). Recently Limas (1978a) reported that cyclic AMP-dependent phosphorylation of cardiac sarcoplasmic reticulum was enhanced in rats treated with T4 for 2 weeks. Since cardiac contractility may depend on Ca^{2+} transport by the sarcoplasmic reticulum, these data suggest a role for cyclic AMP in myocardial performance although the finding of normal myocardial adenylate cyclase and phosphodiesterase activities in these hyperthyroid animals is not supportive.

2. Phosphorylase and Protein Kinase

Glycogen metabolism is dependent on conversion of the inactive enzyme phosphorylase *b* to its active form, phosphorylase *a*. Catalysis of this reaction may involve both phosphorylase kinase and a cyclic AMP-dependent protein kinase (Walsh *et al.*, 1971). Since hyperthyroidism is a state of augmented energy consumption, a number of studies have investigated the effect of thyroid hormone on cardiac phosphorylase *a*. Hornbrook and Brody (1963) described an elevated level of phosphorylase *a* activity in hearts from rats pretreated with thyroid. Wollenberger *et al.* (1964) felt that the baseline elevations may have been due to tissue anoxia, since the rapid rise in activity in hyperthyroid dog hearts was abolished if tissue was frozen *in situ*. However, McNeill and Brody (1968) demonstrated an increased

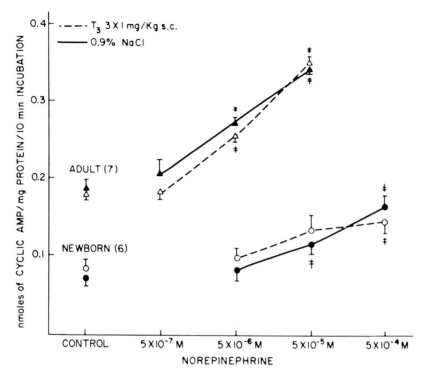

Fig. 11. Effect of norepinephrine on adenyl cyclase activity in hearts from euthyroid and hyperthyroid adult and newborn rats. Each point is the mean of 6–7 experiments with standard error of the mean. ≠ indicates significant difference from corresponding control. (Reprinted by permission from Brus and Hess, 1973.)

basal level of phosphorylase *a* in hyperthyroid heart tissue frozen immediately on removal, and they felt anoxia had no effect on these changes.

Of interest has been the possible interaction of thyroid hormone and catecholamines on phosphorylase *a* activity. Wollenberger *et al.* (1964) showed that the β-adrenergic blocking agent nethalide could reduce the formation of phosphorylase *a* after anoxia. Likewise, pretreatment with propranolol, reserpine, or MJ-1999 (a β-blocker) decreased the basal and catecholamine-stimulated phosphorylase *a* levels in hyperthyoid rats (McNeill and Brody, 1968; Frazer *et al.*, 1969). The mechanism for the catecholamine effect involves cyclic AMP stimulation, which in turn activates phosphorylase *b* kinase, the enzyme that converts phosphorylase *b* to phosphorylase *a*. However, the cyclic AMP–phosphorylase *b* kinase–phosphorylase *b* (and *a*) system may not be necessary for the T4-induced rise in phosphorylase *a*, as adenylate cyclase activity, cAMP, and phosphorylase *b* kinase levels are normal (Frazer *et al.,* 1969; McNeill *et al.,* 1969; Young and McNeill, 1974). Calcium may also enhance phosphorylase *a* activity, though the finding of similar dose-dependent increases after $CaCl_2$ in euthyroid and hyperthyroid rats indicates no supersensitivity to the phosphorylase-activating effect of calcium (McNeill, 1978). Although cAMP levels are normal, McNeill (1977, 1978) has reported that dibutyryl-cAMP enhances phosphorylase *a* activity in hearts of hyperthyroid rats, and he suggested that this may occur at the level of protein kinase. Protein kinase, however, like phosphorylase kinase, is also cAMP dependent (Keely *et al.,* 1978) and its activation is temporally associated with the transformation of phosphorylase kinase to a form capable of catalyzing conversion of phosphorylase *b* to *a* (Dobson, 1978). In hyperthyroid rats the levels of protein kinase in myocardial cytosol have been found to be either normal (Katz *et al.,* 1977) or elevated (Newcomb *et al.,* 1978).

It is clear from these studies that hyperthyroidism induces a rise in phosphorylase *a* activity both basally and in response to catecholamines and that these changes are prevented by pretreatment with β-blockers. The rise in phosphorylase may be augmented by dibutyryl-cAMP. Nevertheless, the documentation of normal myocardial adenyl cyclase, cAMP, and phosphorylase *b* kinase levels and the conflicting data on protein kinase activity in hyperthyroidism leave unsettled the issue of whether cyclic AMP is operative in the T4-induced glycogenolytic pathway.

3. Myocardial ATPases

a. DIVALENT CATION ATPASES

The effect of thyroid hormone on contractility may be through myosin calcium-activated ATPase (Ca^{2+}-ATPase). Thyrum *et al.* (1970) showed that hyperthyroid guinea pigs had not only an increased myosin ATPase activity, but also a high helical content and altered amino acid composition in myosin. Suko (1971) demonstrated a rise in Ca^{2+}-ATPase and calcium uptake in rabbits treated for 3–4 weeks with T4; he suggested that myocardial contraction may be regulated in part by thyroid hormone influencing cardiac sarcoplasmic reticulum function. Goodkind *et al.* (1974) found that Ca^{2+}-ATPase and papillary muscle time-to-peak tension were both altered after 8 days of T4, whereas other measures of contractility (developed tension and maximum rate of tension rise) were changed as early as 1 day after T4. They concluded that only the late effects on contractility were due to increased myosin ATPase activity. Subsequent studies have demonstrated that unlike euthyroid animals, the cardiac myosin ATPase from hyperthyroid rabbits failed to stimulate after sulfhydryl modification by

N-ethylmaleimide. Furthermore, there was no change in the myosin amino acid composition (unlike Thyrum's results) or the electrophoretic pattern of the light chains, suggesting that thyroid hormone may act by producing a conformational change in the molecule near the SH_1 thiols (Banerjee *et al.*, 1976). Yazaki and Raben (1975) reported species differences in Ca^{2+}-ATPase activity. Rabbits had increased activity after 3 days of T4, whereas rats (with high activity levels in the euthyroid state) had no augmentation. This may explain why Rovetto *et al.* (1972) saw no increase in activity in rats after large doses of T4. Noting some differences both in the light-chain amino acid composition and in the enzymatic properties of myosin, they concluded that T4 stimulates new myosin synthesis with altered enzymatic properties. The reason for the different species responses between the rabbit and rat is unclear. The subunit composition and thiol group content of cardiac tropomyosin, although known to vary among species, appear to be the same in these small animals (Leger *et al.*, 1976). Nevertheless, these authors demonstrated differences in myosin Ca^{2+}-ATPase activity among the rat, rabbit, and guinea pig. Similar species differences (including humans) have been noted for cardiac atrial myosin Ca^{2+}-ATPase activity (Yazaki *et al.*, 1979).

Recent studies have provided further evidence that thyroid hormone induces changes in ATPase activity and that structural alterations may be involved. Flink and Morkin (1977) showed that cyanogen bromide digests of hyperthyroid rabbit myosin had different electrophoretic patterns. In addition, there was a difference in the distribution of radiolabeled cysteine peptides, and they felt that a new myosin species was present. The enhanced Ca^{2+}-ATPase activity in myosin of hyperthyroid rabbits has been shown to reside in the heavy meromyosin subfragment (Banerjee *et al.*, 1977). Thyroxine affects not only the ATPase activity stimulated by calcium, but the Mg^{2+}- and actin-activated ATPase activities as well (Morkin *et al.*, 1977; Banerjee *et al.*, 1977). It has been suggested that these thyroxine-induced changes in divalent cation–stimulated ATPase are responsible for the contractile responses seen in hyperthyroidism (Morkin, 1979).

Another possible effect of thyroxine on calcium transport involves the formation of a phosphoprotein intermediate. Suko and Hasselbach (1976) have suggested that a calcium–phosphoprotein complex involving ATPase forms on the outer membrane of the sarcoplasmic reticulum before calcium transport can occur. The role of T4 in this process was nicely demonstrated by Limas (1978a,b). He found, as had been previously reported, that Ca^{2+} uptake and Ca^{2+}-ATPase activity were increased in hyperthyroid animals (Fig. 12). The rise in ATPase activity, however, was preceded temporally by phosphoprotein formation in both hyperthyroid and euthyroid animals, with the greatest increase being in the former group (Fig. 13). Chronic

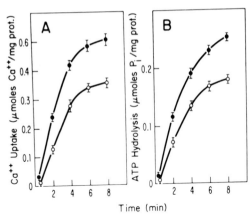

Fig. 12. Ca^{2+} uptake (A) and Ca^{2+}-ATPase activity (B) of cardiac microsomes from control (O) and hyperthyroid (●) animals. (Reprinted by permission from Limas, 1978b.)

thyroid hormone administration to dogs, however, may elevate Ca^{2+}-activated ATPase, yet be associated with reduced Ca^{2+} uptake (Conway *et al.*, 1976).

In general, the results of these studies support the theory that the thyroid hormone effects of enhancing speed of contractility are due to an increased calcium transport in the sarcoplasmic reticulum. The change in calcium uptake, presumably through the action of Ca^{2+}-ATPase, is preceded by formation of a phosphoprotein complex. There appear to be changes not only in the enzymatic properties of the ATPase enzyme, but in its structure as well. Mg^{2+}- and actin-activated ATPases are also enhanced.

b. MONOVALENT CATION ATPASES

Several studies have indicated that K^+-ATPase is not altered by the administration of thyroid hormone (Yazaki and Raben, 1975; Katagiri *et al.*, 1975; Conway *et al.*, 1976), but these results may not reflect the overall effect of thyroxine on monovalent cation transport. It is known that T4 stimulates protein synthesis (Michels *et al.*, 1963) and that actinomycin D and puromycin (inhibitors of RNA and protein synthesis) will inhibit calorigenesis (Tata, 1963). Ismail-Beigi and Edelman (1971) have proposed that the mechanism for the calorigenic response to thyroid hormone involves stimulation of Na^+, K^+-ATPase activity. It is therefore possible that part of the increased myocardial oxygen consumption in hyperthyroidism is due to enhanced Na^+, K^+-ATPase activity. Curfman *et al.* (1977) observed in T3-treated guinea pigs that this enzymatic activity was significantly increased in both atrial and ventricular homogenates. Based on ouabain binding

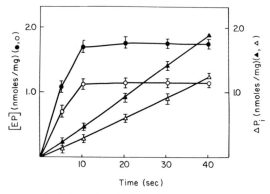

Fig. 13. Time course of EP formation (●, ○) and P_i liberation (▲, △) by cardiac sarcoplasmic reticulum from hyperthyroid (●, ▲) and euthyroid (○, △) rats. Results are given as means ± SE for seven experiments. (Reprinted by permission from Limas, 1978b.)

studies, they suggested that the activity was due to an increased number of Na, K-ATPase enzyme units. Philipson and Edelman (1977) have reported an increase in Na, K-ATPase 24 hr after T3 was given to hypothyroid rats. The enzyme effect was not secondary to a prior alteration in ion concentrations, as the rise in intracellular $[K^+]$ also occurred at 24 hr and there was no change in $[Na^+]$. Kinetic studies showed that T3 had no effect on the affinity but increased the maximum velocity of the enzyme, indicating that T3 enhanced synthesis of additional Na, K-ATPase without altering its characteristics. Banerjee and Sharma (1979) have claimed that the T3-induced increase in cardiac Na, K-ATPase is not responsible for the thermogenic action of thyroid hormone, since the increase in enzyme activity is primarily located in nonthermogenic sympathetic nerve endings.

4. Dehydrogenases and Cathepsin D

Glycerol-phosphate dehydrogenase participates in the glycerophosphate shuttle, a cycle that serves to transport electrons into the mitochondria and increase oxygen consumption. Those tissues that respond to T4 by increasing their metabolic rate are able to form more of this enzyme, and in heart the cytochrome-linked glycerol-phosphate dehydrogenase in mitochondria was increased in hyperthyroid rats (Lee and Lardy, 1965; Isaacs *et al.*, 1969). Numerous other dehydrogenases, in contrast, were unaltered (Lee and Lardy, 1965). During regression of thyroxine-induced cardiac hypertrophy in rats the level of myocardial cathepsin D, a proteolytic enzyme, increases 40% while lysosomal glucosaminidase and acid phosphatase are unchanged (Wildenthal and Mueller, 1974).

H. Energy Metabolism

1. Carbohydrates

Glucose, on entering the cell, may be stored as glycogen or be metabolized to pyruvic acid through the process of glycolysis. The pyruvic acid then combines with acetoacetic acid to form acetyl-CoA, which enters the mitochondria for generation of high-energy phosphate stores. After 20–40 hr, T3 (10^{-8} M) can increase the rate of glucose metabolism in cultured rat myocardial cells (Tsai and Chen, 1976). A series of experiments by Segal et al. (1977; Segal and Gordon, 1977a,b) examined the process of sugar uptake in chick embryo heart cells. They found that free T3 concentrations of 8.7×10^{-10} M produced half maximal stimulation of [1-^{3}H]deoxyglucose (DOG), a nonmetabolizable sugar that enters the cell by facilitated diffusion. During the first 6 hr of stimulation by T3, DOG uptake rose linearly. From 6–24 hr, uptake was inhibited by actinomycin D, puromycin, and cycloheximide (Fig. 14) but not by hydroxyurea. The results indicated a biphasic response to T3. The initial response, independent of protein synthesis, may be a direct effect of T3. The latter stimulation appeared to be dependent on RNA and protein, but not DNA synthesis. Kinetic studies revealed that T3 increased the V_{max} but not the K_m for sugar uptake. Bressler and Wittels (1966) found that myocardium from hyperthyroid guinea pigs had (1) decreased rates of conversion of glucose to lactate and CO_2, (2) increased conversion of glucose to glycogen and of pyruvate to CO_2, and (3) increased rates of hexosemonophosphate formation. Overall, the rate of glucose oxidation was depressed. Altschuld et al. (1969) showed that during anoxia less lactic acid was produced from glucose or glucose 6-phosphate in rat heart homogenates. Their data suggested that anaerobic inhibition of glycolysis occurred through a decrease in phosphofructokinase activity, and it was associated with diminished left ventricular function.

Piatnek-Leunissen and Olson (1967) induced hyperthyroidism in dogs, some of whom developed congestive heart failure. Those animals in failure had a decreased ability of the myocardium to extract glucose and pyruvate, which suggested to the authors a relative hypoxia. Zaimis et al. (1969) documented by histochemical techniques a decrease in glycogen content in the hearts of T4-treated cats and guinea pigs. Isaacs et al. (1969) also found a markedly depressed cardiac glycogen concentration in hyperthyroid rats, which they attributed to the greater demand for carbohydrate.

2. Lipids

Free fatty acids (FFA) are transported enzymatically into mitochondria. Once inside, the fatty acids are oxidized with progressive release of

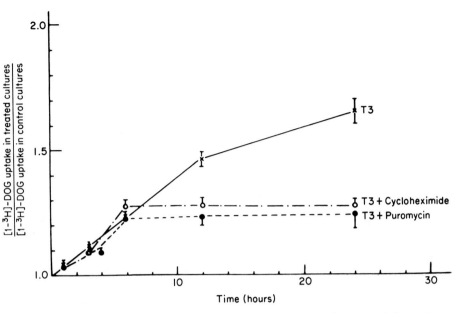

Fig. 14. The effect of puromycin (2 μg/ml) or cycloheximide (0.1 μg/ml) on 2-deoxy-D-[1-³H]glucose uptake in 10^{-8} M T3-treated cultured chick embryo heart cells. Four-day-old cultures were treated for different periods either with T3, puromycin, or cycloheximide alone and with either a combination of T3 and puromycin or with T3 and cycloheximide. At the end of the specified periods, the uptake of 2-deoxy-D-[1-³H]glucose was determined under each treatment. The ratio of the uptakes of the following treatments is depicted in this figure: (x), the ratio of T3-treated to nontreated cultures; (O), the ratio of T3 + cycloheximide-treated to cycloheximide-treated cultures, and (●), the ratio of T3 + puromycin-treated to puromycin-treated cultures. There were at least four plates in each treatment group at each point in time. The bars represent one standard deviation of the mean. (Reprinted by permission from Segal and Gordon, 1977a.)

2-carbon acetyl-CoAs. The acetyl-CoAs then enter the tricarboxylic acid (TCA) cycle, leading to ATP production. Thyroid hormone mobilizes lipids and increases both the plasma levels and turnover of free fatty acids (Eaton *et al.*, 1965). Bressler and Wittels (1966) have shown that myocardium from thyroxine-treated guinea pigs had increased concentrations of FFA and triglycerides, and higher rates of fatty acid oxidation. Bound and free carnitines were elevated, as was the activity of palmityl-CoA-carnitine acyltransferase. These changes are beneficial since carnitine helps form long-chain fatty acylcarnitines which can permeate the mitochondria. Similar results have been obtained in hyperthyroid dogs with increased plasma FFA concentrations in whom myocardial delivery and uptake of FFAs and free fatty acid oxidation were enhanced (Gold *et al.*, 1967). The authors were uncertain whether the observed changes were due to a direct myocardial effect of T4 or were secondary to the elevated plasma FFA levels. The importance of elevated plasma levels and myocardial extraction of FFAs in hyperthyroidism was also demonstrated in dogs by Piatnek-Leunissen and Olson (1967). When their animals developed heart failure, both the plasma levels and tissue extraction of FFAs were depressed.

Recent investigations have demonstrated that certain cellular fractions have altered lipid compositions. Steffen and Platner (1976) found that T4-treated rats had a decrease in the percent of unsaturated fatty acids in heart mitochondria and microsomes. Both cell fractions had increased levels of stearate and palmitate, with decreased concentrations of linoleate and arachidonate. The reduced levels may be due to their enhanced β-oxidation. This study documented that structural changes occurred, and the authors suggested that these lipid changes might allow increased membrane permeability or they might regulate enzyme activity. Limas (1978b) described an increase in total lipids, phospholipids, and phosphatidylcholine in sarcoplasmic reticulum of T4-treated rats, with the same individual fatty acid changes noted earlier by Steffen and Platner (1976). These membrane phospholipid alterations may have contributed to the augmentation of Ca^{2+}-ATPase activity in these animals.

3. Oxidative Phosphorylation

Pyruvate, fatty acids, and amino acids are converted to acetyl-CoA, and then enter the TCA cycle. Through a series of enzymatic processes CO_2 and hydrogen atoms are formed and ATP is generated. The electron equivalents of the hydrogen atoms enter the respiratory chain, where a series of electron carriers transport these electrons to molecular oxygen. During this process, known as oxidative phosphorylation, phosphorylation of ADP yields considerable amounts of energy stored as ATP, which is then available for cellular metabolism. Since hyperthyroidism increases the energy requirements of the cell, it is possible that energy production could be affected. The integrity of the respiratory chain can be assessed by measuring the P/O ratio, that is, the moles of inorganic phosphate recovered in organic form per atom of oxygen taken up.

Wiswell and Braverman (1957) added large doses of thyroxine (1.6 × 10^{-5} M) to rat heart homogenates and observed both a marked increase in O_2 utilization and a decrease to zero in the P/O ratio, indicating uncoupling of oxidative phosphorylation. Challoner (1968) also presented evidence for uncoupling in hyperthyroid rats who were in congestive heart failure after massive doses of T3 (100 μg/day for 3 weeks). Numerous studies have challenged the claim that thyroid hormone (at least in concentrations that might be observed in hyperthyroidism) uncouples oxidative phosphoryla-tion. Piatnek-Leunissen and Olson (1967) found that the P/O ratio was normal in sarcosomes from hyperthyroid dogs with and without heart fail-ure. Normal amounts of high-energy phosphate stores were determined in these dogs, as they have been in hyperthyroid cats (Buccino *et al.*, 1967). In guinea pigs chronic T4 administration augmented both basal (state 4) and ADP-stimulated (state 3) O_2 consumption of ventricular myocardium (Zaimis *et al.*, 1969). The respiratory control index and ADP/O ratio were unchanged, and the degree of uncoupling induced by dinitrophenol was the same as in euthyroid animals. In the same study, hyperthyroid cats had some evidence for uncoupling. The overall increase in respiratory activity might have been due to the observed increase in mitochondrial mass.

Tarjan (1971) examined the various substrates involved in energy forma-tion. Following a single dose of T4 in rabbits, pyruvate decarboxylation was inhibited whereas oxidation of fatty acids and activities of several TCA cycle enzymes were unaltered. Thus substrates other than pyruvate that fed into the respiratory chain were not affected. Further studies from the same laboratory (Kimata and Tarjan, 1971; Tarjan and Kimata, 1971) next tested the degree of coupling of oxidative phosphorylation in rabbit ventricle mitochondria after 1–31 days of T4. Using the results of respiratory control ratios, ADP/O ratio, and reversal of electron transport, they found no evi-dence for "loose coupling" or uncoupling. Additional evidence supporting tight coupling of oxidative phosphorylation was recently presented by Nishiki *et al.* (1978). Mitochondrial respiration in hearts of rats receiving T4 for 10–15 days was tested using malate and glutamate as substrates. There was an equal increase in state 3 and state 4 respiration, with ADP/O ratios equal to euthyroid rats. Both the mitochondrial mass and cytochrome content were increased by T4. It is obviously impossible to determine, in man, the effect of thyroid hormone on myocardial oxidative phosphoryla-tion. Stocker *et al.* (1968), however, studied mitochondria obtained from skeletal muscle biopsies of hyperthyroid patients. When compared to euthyroid subjects, they found normal P/O ratios, respiratory control ratios, and ATPase activity after dinitrophenol.

One can conclude that although in very large doses *in vivo* or *in vitro* T4 might uncouple oxidative phosphorylation, most studies indicate that there is tight coupling. This does not mean, however, that myocardial metabolism is unimpaired in hyperthyroidism. Altschuld *et al.* (1969) have shown that anaerobic glycolysis is impaired. Skelton *et al.* (1971) inhibited both glycolysis and oxidative phosphorylation by exposing heart muscle to iodoacetic acid and a nitrogen atmosphere. When both these mechanisms for energy generation were removed, they observed an inefficiency in the conversion of chemical energy to mechanical work.

I. Histopathology

The changes produced by thyroxine, although definite, are not particularly characteristic when assessed by light microscopy. By 6 days, thyroxine-fed mice developed an increased fiber size without any edema (Cohen *et al.*, 1966), whereas treatment of rats for 8 weeks produced a prominent intercellular infiltration of plasma cells and lymphocytes (Sandler and Wilson, 1959). The effect of thyroid hormone on myocardial cellular architecture is considerably more apparent when examined by electron microscopy. Myofibrillar edema and mitochondrial disturbances (disintegrated cristae, granulation, and edema) may occur in rabbits treated for 28 days (Frolov *et al.*, 1967). Increases in myocardial mitochondrial volume were observed by Zaimis *et al.* (1969), with these changes being due to hypertrophy in guinea pigs and to hypertrophy and hyperplasia in cats. The mitochondrial changes included infoldings, lengthening (involving the cristae), and sometimes swelling with loss of cristae. The formation of contraction bands and myelin figures were also observed in some cases, indicating nonspecific cellular injury.

Reith and Fuchs (1973) determined by morphometric techniques that in euthyroid rats, myocardial fibers comprise 87% of the myocardium. The major components of the fibers were myofibrils (42%) and mitochondria (37%). When these animals received T3 (25 μg/100g BW daily for 5 days) there was a decrease in myofiber bulk and an increase in the intracellular space. Although the fraction of the fibers composed of mitochondria was unchanged, there were alterations in both mitochondrial shape and internal structure. This included an increase in the cristae membrane concentrations and more mitochondrial invaginations and tiplike processes. Page and McCallister (1973) also performed quantitative electron microscopic studies of rat myocardial fibers and reported an almost identical cellular composition of mitochondria and myofibrils. The membrane areas were predominantly those of the cristae (the sites of oxidative phosphorylation). When hypothyroid rats were given T4 (180 μg/kg BW for 24 days) there was an increase in cell volume, the amount of myofibrils and mitochondria, and the percent of the cell occupied by mitochondria (but not myofibrils). Both total cristal membrane area and the percentage of mitochondrial volume composed of cristae were also increased by T4. These changes were confirmed by microchemical assays of Mg^{2+} (to assess myofibrils) and copper (to assess cytochrome content). This type of tissue growth in response to thyroid hormone differed from that which is seen in ventricular hypertrophy in which myofibrillar content increases while mitochondrial content decreases.

J. Thyroid Analogues

Thyroxine and T3 have profound and widespread effects on the heart whereas other analogues are generally less potent. Hirvonen and Lybeck (1956a) found that DL-thyroxine was as effective as L-T4 and L-T3 in increasing the rate of isolated rat auricles while the arsenophenyl and sulfophenyl-T3 azo derivatives were much less potent. The adenyl cyclase response to D-T4 was equal to that of L-T4, whereas DL reverse T3 and 3,3'-diiodothyronine were 60% as effective (Levey and Epstein, 1969; Epstein et al., 1970; Levey, 1971). Other analogues, including 3,5-diiodothyronine, thyronine, diiodotyrosine, monoiodotyrosine, and tyrosine, were ineffective. D-T4 was also active in terms of contractility and energy metabolism. In papillary muscles of cats receiving D-T4 for up to 14 days, there was an increase in cardiac index, isometric and isotonic contractions, and myocardial oxygen consumption with no evidence for uncoupling of oxidative phosphorylation (Gunning et al., 1974). Triiodothyroacetic acid, when injected chronically into rats, produced cardiac hypertrophy and an increased number of mitochondria (Symons et al., 1975). The measurement of 2-deoxyglucose uptake by cultured chick embryo heart cells revealed that compared to L-T3, the molar potencies were 20% for L-T4, 17% for D-T3, less than 1% for rT3 (reverse T3), 3,5-diiodothyronine and thyronine, but 500% for 3'-isopropyl- 3,5-diiodothyronine (Segal et al., 1977).

K. Clinical Cardiovascular Complications of Hyperthyroidism

Having reviewed the biochemical and physiological changes attributed to thyroid hormone, this section will summarize the cardiac complications associated with hyperthyroidism. Some of these disturbances are adduced directly to the effects of thyroid hormone on a normal heart, whereas others arise due to the additional stress of the hyperkinetic state on an already diseased heart. In either situation, it can be fairly claimed that the hyperthyroidism is responsible for the clinical result.

1. Arrhythmias

Animal studies have demonstrated that thyroid hormone predisposes to cardiac rhythm disturbances. Leveque (1956) reported that thyroid-fed dogs were more susceptible to acetylcholine-induced atrial fibrillation than were control animals, and rabbits given thyroid hormone had a shorter refractory period and more readily developed heart block and ventricular fibrillation (Frolov *et al.,* 1967). *In vitro,* after a lag time of 4–6 days, T3 $(10^{-7}–10^{-5}\ M)$ induced atrial and ventricular tachycardia and irregular rhythms in fetal mouse hearts maintained in organ culture (Wildenthal, 1971).

The influence of thyroid hormone on arrhythmias in humans has fascinated investigators for many years. Ernstene (1938) found that atrial fibrillation occurred in 207 of 1000 thyrotoxic patients, 94 of whom had no evidence of organic heart disease. In about half the patients this disorder was present preoperatively, and in the other half it presented itself postoperatively; in both situations reversion to sinus rhythm usually occurred. Atrial fibrillation was more common in older patients ($\simeq 75\%$ were over 45 years old) with adenomatous goiters who had had thyrotoxicosis for more than 3 years. Likoff and Levine (1943), reporting on 409 cases, found atrial fibrillation in 29 of 78 patients with known organic heart disease. Of the 331 individuals with no antecedent heart disease, 30 had atrial fibrillation. The patients who developed congestive heart failure more commonly had atrial fibrillation and a longer duration of their hyperthyroidism. Atrial fibrillation was reported in 15 of 123 patients by Hoffman and Lowrey (1960) and in 18 of 200 patients by Summers and Surtees (1961). In the latter series, the eventual reversion to sinus rhythm was considerably higher in subjects with no underlying organic heart disease. Atrial fibrillation may also be the presenting feature in patients that are not clinically suspected of having hyperthyroidism. Forfar *et al.* (1979), measuring serum T4, T3, and the TSH response to TRH, made the diagnosis of thyrotoxicosis in 10 of 75 patients having atrial fibrillation. Despite the frequency with which this arrhythmia is seen in adults, it is rare in children (Perry and Hung, 1971). Other types of arrhythmias have been noted much less frequently. In the 1000 patients reported by Ernstene (1938), paroxysmal atrial tachycardia was observed in only five, atrial flutter in two, and paroxysmal ventricular tachycardia in two. The rarity of ventricular arrhythmias is such that only recently Lyngborg and Jacobsen (1972) reported a thyrotoxic patient who had multiple atrial and ventricular arrhythmias, ultimately progressing to ventricular tachycardia and death.

It is not surprising that atrial arrhythmias might be prevalent, given the electrophysiological alterations seen in thyrotoxicosis (Section II,F). What is less well appreciated is that various types of conduction delays also may occur. Although Sandler (1959) found no differences in the P-R interval of thyrotoxic individuals, a prolonged P-R interval was observed in five of 76 patients (four returned to normal when euthyroid) by Blizzard and Rupp (1960) and in 11 of 123 patients by Hoffman and Lowrey (1960). More advanced degrees of conduction disturbances including second- and third-degree heart block have been reported in individual cases (Stern *et al.,*

1970; Campus *et al.*, 1975; Eraker *et al.*, 1978). Other electrocardiographic abnormalities described by Hoffman and Lowrey (1960) included ST–T-wave changes (noted particularly in young adults) and shortening of the Q-Tc interval, but these changes were not seen by Sandler (1959). Both studies did find notching of the P waves. Although sinus tachycardia and atrial fibrillation are the arrhythmias usually associated with thyrotoxicosis, a variety of additional disturbances have been reported, and therefore hyperthyroidism must be considered in the differential diagnosis of their etiology.

2. Organic Heart Disease and Hyperthyroidism

a. ATHEROSCLEROTIC HEART DISEASE

Myocardial infarction (M.I.) occurring in a patient with active hyper-thyroidism has been stated to be rare, possibly because of the lipid-lowering effect of hyperthyroidism (Littman *et al.*, 1957). However, because of the increased cardiac output and myocardial oxygen consumption, one might expect instead an exacerbation of angina or precipitation of myocardial infarction in hyperthyroid patients. Several recent reports have described young patients who have developed angina and infarction while hyper-thyroid, and who have been found to have normal coronary arteries by arteriography (Kotler *et al.*, 1973; Proskey *et al.*, 1977). Resnekov and Falicov (1977) performed ventricular pacing and phenylephrine infusions in three such patients and determined that all had myocardial lactate produc-tion rather than lactate extraction. Wei *et al.* (1979) have also reported a patient with normal coronaries who had angina, coronary ischemia and spasm, and ventricular arrhythmia, all of which subsided with return to the euthyroid state. The studies suggest that although myocardial infarction is claimed to be uncommon in hyperthyroidism, it clearly does occur. More-over, a striking number of these patients are young, have normal coronary arteries, and may suffer adverse consequences due to increased myocardial oxygen demands or coronary arterial spasm.

The effect in euthyroid individuals of acute myocardial infarction on thyroid function is of potential importance and has received some attention. Harland *et al.* (1972) determined that the thyroxine secretion rate was normal after an acute M.I. Serum concentrations of total T4 and T3, free T4 and T3, and basal and TRH-stimulated TSH were normal within the first 24 hours and 14 days after an acute M.I. (Thomson *et al.*, 1979). The sampling time may be crucial, though, as McLarty *et al.* (1975) have shown that serum T3 decreases markedly during the first 7 days post-M.I. Kaplan *et al.* (1977) observed in 16 patients that serum T3 and T4 concentrations fell 29% and 21%, respectively, whereas serum reverse T3 rose 56% during the first 5 days after an infarct, and all values returned toward normal by 1–2 weeks. Similar alterations in T3 and rT3 were recently described by Faber *et al.* (1979b). In addition, their patients had normal serum 3',5'-T2 but low 3,3'-T2 levels, indicating a disturbance of the integrity of several enzymatic pathways of monodeiodination. The change in serum T3, presumably caused by impaired T4 to T3 conversion, is apparently not related to alterations in endogenous cortisol levels (Ljunggren *et al.*, 1979). A low serum T3, however, may be a prognosticator of outcome, as one patient whose T3 level failed to rise ultimately died (McLarty *et al.*, 1975). Whether these alterations in thyroid hormone metabolism are significant, either causally or in regard to recovery, deserves further study.

b. CARDIOMEGALY AND CONGESTIVE HEART FAILURE

Summers and Surtees (1961) observed cardiomegaly in 18 of 200 thyrotoxic patients who had no other cause for the cardiac enlargement, and Likoff and Levine (1943) diagnosed congestive heart failure in 21 of 331 hyperthyroid subjects with no known history of organic heart disease. However, reversible mitral regurgitation and CHF have been reported only rarely in children (Reynolds and Woody, 1971) and in infants (Section II,K,3). Cardiomegaly in children has also been demonstrated recently by echocardiography (George *et al.*, 1978). In this study there was an increase in chamber size without ventricular hypertrophy.

3. Neonatal Thyrotoxicosis

Hyperthyroidism, although having a multitude of effects on the cardiovascular system, usually does not produce significant cardiac complications except in older patients with coexistent organic heart disease. The question as to whether thyroid hormone, through a direct effect on the myocardium, can induce cardiac failure has interested physicians for years. Several studies in animals and adults have provided evidence that congestive failure occurs (Piatnek-Leunissen and Olson, 1967; Graettinger *et al.*, 1959) in otherwise healthy hearts. An impressive human model for confirming the detrimental effects of thyroxine on normal myocardium can be seen in infants born with neonatal thyrotoxicosis. This uncommon disorder was first reported in a child with a pulse of greater than 200 beats/min and who ultimately died (White, 1912). These infants are frequently born with cardiomegaly and/or congestive heart failure, requiring treatment with digitalis and diuretics in addition to antithyroid drugs (Elsas *et al.*, 1967; Smith and Howard, 1973; Ørbeck, 1973; Mujtaba and Burrow, 1975; Leszynsky *et al.*, 1971). Electrocardiographic abnormalities have included right atrial and ventricular hypertrophy and strain, sinus arrest, and A-V dissociation (Rosenberg *et al.*, 1963; Mahoney *et al.*, 1964; Shapiro *et al.*, 1975). The etiology of this illness is due not to maternal hyperthyroidism per se, since affected infants have been born of euthyroid mothers with a prior history of Graves' disease, but rather to the transplacental passage of thyroid-stimulating immunoglobulins such as LATS (long-acting thyroid stimulator) (Sunshine *et al.,* 1965; Maisey and Stimmler, 1972) or LATS-protector (Dirmikis and Munro, 1975; Smallridge *et al.,* 1978a). LATS has a half-life of approximately a week in these babies, and resolution regularly occurs within weeks to a few months.

4. Pharmacological Agents

a. CARDIAC GLYCOSIDES

Experimental studies in animals have questioned whether or not hyperthyroidism alters the chronotropic or inotropic responses to glycosides. Peacock and Moran (1963) found that the percent increase in contractility of hyperthyroid rat ventricle strips after ouabain was unaltered, and Rosen and Moran (1963) reported a smaller increase *in vivo* in hyperthyroid dogs. The latter authors also noted that ouabain-induced arrhythmias appeared later in T4-treated than in euthyroid animals. Similar results were obtained in euthyroid dogs with pacemaker-induced tachycardia, suggesting enhanced clearance because of the increased heart rate. Buccino *et al.* (1967) observed a smaller than normal increase in contractility after acetylstrophanthidin in hyperthyroid cats, although maximum tension developed was not depressed. Additional evidence of species differences was shown in a study in which hyperthyroid rabbits, but not guinea pigs, were more likely to develop arrhythmias after ouabain (Thompson, 1973). The reason hyperthyroid guinea pigs might not be more susceptible is unclear, as they have been reported to have more cardiac ouabain binding sites (Curfman *et al.,* 1977).

Early claims of cardiac glycoside effect in states of altered thyroid function in humans were variable, so Frye and Braunwald (1961) attempted to determine whether or not thyroid hormone influenced the dose requirements for digitalis to control ventricular rate in patients with atrial fibrillation. When their patients were made hyperthyroid by ingesting 100–250 μg T3 per day, their digoxin requirements to control the chronotropic response increased fourfold. Doherty and Perkins (1966) analyzed the pharmacokinetic behavior of the glycosides to see what was responsible for the increased dose requirements in hyperthyroidism. Using [^{3}H]digoxin, they found low serum concentrations. With no significant change in serum half-life ($t_{\frac{1}{2}}$), they postulated an increased tissue distribution. Although they were unable to demonstrate increased stores in most tissues of hyperthyroid dogs, the hearts did have elevated digoxin levels. Several studies have confirmed low serum digoxin levels, but they have also demonstrated a short $t_{\frac{1}{2}}$, apparently due to an enhanced renal digoxin and creatinine clearance (Croxson and Ibbertson, 1975; Bonelli *et al.*, 1978). Increased bilary excretion has also been observed (Huffman *et al.*, 1977). With improvement in thyroid function, the plasma digoxin level normalizes (Fig. 15). Nielsen *et al.* (1974) found that even in euthyroid patients there was a significant negative correlation between serum T3 and digoxin concentrations. At variance with these studies, Lawrence *et al.* (1977) found no change in serum digoxin and no overall increase in renal clearance of the drug. They did describe an increase in digoxin concentration in the deep tissue compartment.

In general, it does not appear that cardiac muscle from hyperthyroid animals has impaired or increased contractility after cardiac glycosides. Presumably hyperthyroid patients may need additional digoxin to control ventricular rate not because of altered sensitivity but for reasons related to lower serum digoxin levels. Although the data are not uniform, the low

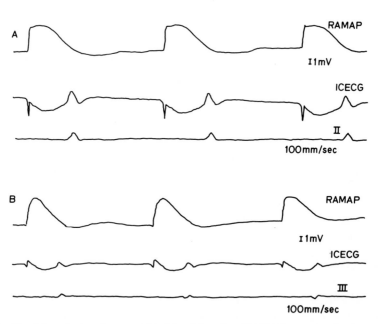

Fig. 15. Monophasic action potential of the right atrium (RAMAP) recorded simultaneously with an intracavitary electrocardiogram (ICECG) and one standard ECG lead. (A) Before treatment. The mean duration of monophasic action potential measured at 90% of the amplitude is 330 msec. (B) After 2 weeks of treatment with thyroid hormone. The mean duration of the monophasic action potential shortened to 240 msec. (Reprinted by permission from Cotoi *et al.*, 1972.)

serum levels are probably due to a combination of factors including enhanced renal and biliary clearance and a larger distribution space.

b. β-ADRENERGIC BLOCKING AGENTS

The effect of the β-adrenergic blocking drugs has been previously examined (Section II,D,1), with dramatic improvement in the peripheral manifestations of thyrotoxicosis being noted. These findings naturally led to the proposition that propranolol might be adequate for the surgical management of hyperthyroid patients. An early review by Riddle and Schwartz (1970) advised against the routine use of sympatholytic agents alone but agreed that they were helpful in selected cases. However, Pinstone and Joffe (1970) used propranolol and Lugol's iodine successfully in over 100 patients operated on for thyrotoxicosis. Numerous studies have confirmed the feasibility of using β-blockers preoperatively (Lee et al., 1973; Michie et al., 1974; Bewsher et al., 1974; Starling and Thomas, 1977; Toft et al., 1978; Zonszein et al., 1979). The dose of propranolol has varied widely, being individualized to maintain a pulse of less than 90/min. Using propranolol alone, morbidity has been very low, but one must remember to continue the drug for up to a week postoperatively while the peripheral pool of stored hormone is metabolized.

Caution must be taken when β-adrenergic blockers are employed, since they alleviate the sympathetic symptoms without altering the dysfunction in the thyroid. Propranolol in conventional doses may not provide complete β-adrenergic blockade, as thyroid storm has been reported in two patients receiving 160 mg of propranolol a day (Eriksson et al., 1977). Adequacy of this dose has been challenged by subsequent studies in which plasma propranolol levels were measured. Hellman et al. (1977) noted that in 8 of 11 thyrotoxic patients this dose of propranolol was insufficient to maintain plasma levels above 50 ng/ml, and similar data were reported in 4 of 12 patients by Rubenfeld et al. (1979).

Although β-blockers have been known for years to assuage the symptoms and signs of hyperthyroidism, an additional biochemical effect has recently been documented. Propranolol does not alter thyroid iodine release or thyroxine turnover (Wartofsky et al., 1975). However, although serum T4 levels are unaffected, serum T3 levels decrease from 18 to 33% (Nauman et al., 1974; Wiersinga and Touber, 1977; Lotti et al., 1977), and there is also an associated rise in serum reverse T3 (Verhoeven et al., 1977; Theilade et al., 1977; Faber et al., 1979a). The mechanism of action of propranolol, evaluated by kinetic analysis in humans utilizing radiolabeled isotopes, was proven to be due to impaired T4 to T3 conversion (Lumholtz et al., 1978). An in vitro study using rat liver parenchymal cells has also demonstrated that propranolol inhibits T4 to T3 conversion (van Noorden et al., 1979).

It may be concluded that β-adrenergic blocking drugs deserve a prominent place in the therapeutic armamentarium. Not only do they act rapidly to control many of the peripheral side effects of thyrotoxicosis, but they provide some biochemical relief as well. One must be aware, however, that in certain circumstances their use may be contraindicated. Ikram (1977) found that although propranolol had no adverse effect in uncomplicated thyrotoxicosis, it produced a significant reduction in heart rate and cardiac index and rise in mean right atrial pressure in patients with congestive heart failure and hyperthyroidism. The data suggested that in the latter situation cardiac function was being sustained by the sympathetic nervous system.

III. Thyroid Hormone Deficiency: Its Effects on the Heart

A. Cardiac Size

Hypothyroidism produces a decrease in the HW/BW ratio within 6–8 weeks, which may be corrected by a return to the euthyroid state (Rovetto *et al.*, 1972; Benforado and Wiggins, 1965; Lifschitz and Kayne, 1966; Strauer and Schulze, 1976). In those animals having undergone hypophysectomy, growth hormone replacement will increase heart and body weights, but not their ratio; only T4 is permissive in normalizing this parameter (Lifschitz and Kayne, 1966; Rovetto *et al.*, 1972; Minelli and Korecky, 1969).

B. Hemodynamic Effects (Table III)

1. Animal Studies

In the rat, hypothyroidism induces a 55% reduction in heart rate (Hirvonen and Paavilainen, 1967), which may be reversed with 3 days of thyroid hormone (Hirvonen and Lybeck, 1956b). A decrease in oxygen consumption has been described (Minelli and Korecky, 1969), although the Q_{O_2} may normalize after the initial decrease (Peacock and Moran, 1963). Beznák (1964) studied the hemodynamic effects of both thyroid hormone and growth hormone in hypophysectomized rats. There was an $\approx$60% reduction in heart rate, cardiac index, and oxygen consumption. The low cardiac output was not absolute, however, as intracardiac infusions of poly (vinylpyrrolidone) elicited a two- to fourfold increase in cardiac output. These basal parameters were all reversible by thyroid alone, and were not corrected by growth hormone. However, maximum cardiac output and

TABLE III

Hemodynamic Effects of Hypothyroidism[a]

Species	Heart rate	Cardiac index	Q_{O_2}	Stroke volume	Peripheral resistance	(A–V) O_2 difference	LV work
Human							
Blumgart et al. (1930b)	↓						
Stewart et al. (1938)		↓ 47%	↓ 37%			↑ in 4/5	
Scheinberg et al. (1950)		↓ 44%	↓		↑	↑ but N.S.	
Ellis et al. (1952)		↓ 36%	↓ 31%		↑	↑ in 3/5	
Graettinger et al. (1958)		↓ 31%	↓ 34%	↓ 27%	↑ 65%		
Amidi et al. (1968)	N.S.			↓ 38%			
Burack et al. (1971)	N.C.						
Paine et al. (1977)		↓ 45%	↓ 30%			↑ in 3/6	
Rats							
Hirvonen and Lybeck (1956b)	↓ 43%						
Peacock and Moran (1963)			↓ 15% (day 25) N.C. (day 58)				
Beznák (1964)	↓ 55%	↓ 65%	↓ 65%				
Hirvonen and Paavilainen (1967)	↓ 55%						
Minelli and Korecky (1969)			↓ 43%				
Cats							
Buccino et al. (1967)	↓ 25%	↓ 9%	↓ 21%	N.C.			
Strauer and Schulze (1976)	↓ 15%	↓ 12.5%		N.C.			
Dogs							
Scott et al. (1961)	↓ 19%	↓ 27%	↓ 26%				
Scott et al. (1962)		↓	↓	N.C.			
Gold et al. (1967)	N.C.	↓ 65%	↓ 38%				↓ 70%

[a] Q_{O_2} = oxygen consumption; LV work = left ventricular work; N.S. = nonsignificant; N.C. = no change.

work, as well as the development of cardiac hypertrophy after aortic constriction, required both hormones.

Buccino *et al.* (1967) observed that in cats, hypothyroidism had considerably less of an effect on cardiac function than did hyperthyroidism. Although the mean values for cardiac index and Q_{O_2} decreased, the only significant alteration was a bradycardia. Strauer and Schulze (1976), on the other hand, found a decrease in both heart rate and cardiac index. Neither study reported a significant change in stroke volume or SV index.

In hypothyroid dogs Scott *et al.* (1961, 1962) noted a reduced heart rate, cardiac index, and left ventricular oxygen consumption. To assess whether these changes were appropriate for their metabolic state, the animals were then made hypoxemic. The normal response to hypoxemia in euthyroidism is an increase in heart rate, cardiac index, left ventricular work, and coronary blood flow, and a decrease in coronary vascular resistance. The hypothyroid dogs had no change in cardiac output during hypoxemia, and the other responses were diminished approximately 50%, suggesting that the hypothyroid heart does not function normally. Gold *et al.* (1967) have reported a significant reduction in cardiac index, myocardial Q_{O_2}, and left ventricular work. Myocardial efficiency (derived by comparing left ventricular work to myocardial Q_{O_2}) was diminished 52%.

2. Human Studies

Blumgart *et al.* (1930b) studied the velocity of blood flow in seven patients with myxedema. These patients had a mild bradycardia, and their prolonged arm to heart and pulmonary circulation times became normal after therapy. Stewart *et al.* (1938) made similar observations in five patients, and also described an increased arteriovenous oxygen difference which improved with therapy. The cardiac index and oxygen consumption were both significantly below normal in seven hypothyroid patients reported by Scheinberg *et al.* (1950). Although the increase in (A-V) O_2 difference was nonsignificant as compared with their controls, it did narrow in both patients examined before and after treatment. Ellis *et al.* (1952) noted in 5 hypothyroid individuals that all had a low cardiac index and Q_{O_2} and an increased peripheral resistance, with three of five having an increased (A-V) O_2 difference. In three of the patients the low cardiac output paralleled the low Q_{O_2} and their myocardial efficiency was normal whereas the other two had a depressed C.O./Q_{O_2}. One of the latter patients was only 21 years old and her hemodynamic alterations and heart size normalized with thyroid therapy, suggesting a true "myxedema heart." A low oxygen consumption was confirmed by Asper *et al.* (1953), who reported that pulse rate and Q_{O_2} were increased within a day following parenteral T3 administration.

Graettinger *et al.* (1958) evaluated 12 hypothyroid patients before and after exercise to determine whether they might have an impaired myocardial reserve. At rest the cardiac index, Q_{O_2}, and stroke volume index were all depressed, and peripheral resistance was increased. The C.I./Q_{O_2} ratio, however, did not differ from that seen in euthyroid controls. Exercise induced a rise in cardiac output (although in two patients it was minimal) and the response was much greater than that observed in a group of patients with chronic congestive failure. Although no hypothyroid patients developed congestive heart failure, the C.O./Q_{O_2} ratio after exercise fell considerably in many patients. There was also a greater (A-V) O_2 difference during exercise in the hypothyroid than in the euthyroid patients. Parameters which did not differ from normal included mean right atrial, mean pulmonary artery and mean brachial artery pressures and total pulmonary resistance, although several patients did have elevated atrial pressures, mild pulmonary hypertension, and pulmonary resistance. Burack et al. (1971) evaluated the effect of exercise on cardiac output and oxygen uptake before and after thyroid replacement therapy. Exercise produced a rise in the C.O. and oxygen uptake which were similar in both treatment periods. However, the rise in C.O. in the hypothyroid patients was due chiefly to a faster heart rate, with little increase in stroke volume. Although there was considerable variability, the average increment in oxygen utilization with exercise was also greater in the hypothyroid group. Amidi et al. (1968) and Paine et al. (1977) confirmed previous findings of a low cardiac index and Q_{O_2}. The former authors also demonstrated a 38% fall in stroke volume index, while the latter noted an increase in the (A-V) O_2 difference in three of their six patients.

Hypothyroidism thus has a considerable effect on blood flow and oxygen consumption. Although the cardiac index is virtually always low, in animals this is frequently due to a slower heart rate and in humans to a decreased stroke volume index. Oxygen consumption is also depressed, whereas both peripheral resistance and the (A-V) O_2 difference are often increased. Although the C.I./Q_{O_2} ratio is often unchanged, indicating an appropriate functional capacity of the heart, it has been observed both experimentally and in humans that mycocardial efficiency may on occasion be impaired in the absence of known underlying heart disease.

C. Contractility Effects

1. Animal Studies

Hypothyroidism has a definite influence on contractility, with the results being opposite to those observed in hyperthyroidism (Section II,C). Hirvonen and Lybeck (1956b) found a lower than normal contraction force in hypothyroid rat auricles. Benforado and Wiggins (1965), on the other hand, observed in rat ventricle strips that the total tension developed was equal to euthyroid animals, and they concluded that short-term hypothyroidism did not produce cardiac muscle weakness. Several studies in cat papillary muscles have also shown no significant depression of maximum isometric tension (Buccino *et al.*, 1967, 1968; Strauer and Schulze, 1976). Most other studies of isometric contractions in either cat (Levey *et al.*, 1969a; Skelton *et al.*, 1971) or rat (Minelli and Korecky, 1969) hypothyroid papillary muscles have demonstrated a reduction in maximum tension, a decrease in the rate of tension development, and a prolonged time to peak tension. Minelli and Korecky (1969) felt that the decrease in maximum tension was due to a marked impairment in the rate of tension developed, with only partial compensation by the longer time to peak tension. Using a hypophysectomized rat model, they found that T4 but not growth hormone corrected the abnormalities. When isotonic contractions were analyzed, the maximum velocity of shortening was decreased by $\approx 35\%$ (Buccino *et al.*, 1967; Strauer and Schulze, 1976). Similarly, *in vivo* isovolumic contraction studies have demonstrated an impaired rate of tension development in cats (Strauer and Schulze, 1976) and dogs (Taylor *et al.*, 1969), with the latter also finding a decrease in maximum tension.

2. Human Studies

Systolic time intervals (Section II,C,2) have illustrated that hypothyroidism has a clear-cut effect on contractility. Amidi *et al.* (1968) observed that these patients may have a long preejection period, isovolumic contraction time, and ejection time. A number of other studies have confirmed that there is a long electromechanical systole (QS_2). This was due primarily to a long PEP, as the LVET was normal or short (Hillis *et al.* 1975; Burckhardt *et al.*, 1978; Chakravarty *et al.*, 1978; Bough *et al.*, 1978; Plotnick *et al.*, 1979). The ΔPEP and PEP/LVET correlated with serum TSH and were reversible with thyroxine therapy. Both the dose of T4 and duration of therapy appeared to have an effect on cardiac function (Fig. 16). Another noninvasive technique for estimating contractility and pulse wave velocity involves measuring the time interval from the QRS complex to pulse arrival at the brachial artery (the QK interval). Hypothyroidism prolongs this interval, and thyroid hormone restores it to normal (Young *et al.*, 1976).

D. Catecholamines and Hypothyroidism

1. Circulatory Effects

The relationship between catecholamines and hypothyroidism has been less extensively studied than it has been in hyperthyroidism, but most

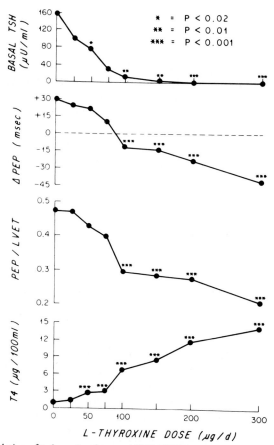

Fig. 16.   Relation of L-thyroxine dose to △PEP, PEP/LVET, serum total thyroxine (T4), and serum thyrotropin (TSH) concentration. Asterisks indicate statistical significance of differences from baseline measurements. Note that the △PEP, PEP/LVET, serum T4, and serum TSH have returned to normal with an L-thyroxine dose of 150 μg per day. (Reprinted by permission from Crowley *et al.*, 1977.)

studies are in agreement. There is some evidence that hypothyroidism decreases the sensitivity of rat atria to epinephrine (Cravey and Gravenstein, 1965). Their results, however, are at variance with a number of other reports. Benforado and Wiggins (1965) reported that although the spontaneous atrial rate was significantly faster in euthyroid rats, the maximum rate achieved during exposure to norepinephrine was no higher than that in the hypothyroid group. Margolius and Gaffney (1965) found almost identical chronotropic responses to graded doses of norepinephrine in dogs, though the arterial pressor effect was somewhat diminished in the hypothyroid animals. The isometric tension response of hypothyroid cat papillary muscles to varying doses of norepinephrine (10^{-10}–$10^{-6}M$) was assessed by Buccino *et al.* (1967). As was the case in their hyperthyroid animals, there was an inverse relationship between the initial tension and the increment observed. Hypothyroid animals, with the lowest basal tension, had the greatest increase during exposure to norepinephrine. The maximum tension was thus no different from that seen in the euthyroid and hyperthyroid animals. Howitt *et al.* (1968) demonstrated in hypothyroid humans that the low heart rate could be reduced further with propranolol, suggesting that insensitivity to sympathetic stimulation was not responsible for the bradycardia.

2. Catecholamine Concentrations

The myocardial content of norepinephrine in hypothyroidism varies depending on which tissue is examined. Atria have a decreased norepinephrine level (Goodkind *et al.*, 1961; Kurland *et al*, 1963), whereas the latter authors reported increased concentrations in whole heart and ventricle. There were no changes in epinephrine levels. Buccino *et al.* (1967) observed no difference in right ventricular norepinephrine concentrations. Landsberg and Axelrod (1968) showed not only an increase in the myocardial content of norepinephrine but also a shortened half-life and increased rate of synthesis in hypothyroidism. Landsberg (1977), in reviewing the serum levels, reported that urine norepinephrine was either normal or increased, serum levels were increased, and the epinephrine levels in both urine and serum were unchanged.

3. Catecholamine Receptors

An early study by Kunos *et al.* (1974) demonstrated that altering the thyroid state could affect adrenergic receptor binding. The maximum inotropic response was normal in isolated atria from thyroidectomized rats, but the heart changed its sensitivity to selected amines. The inotropic response was less sensitive to the β-agonists norepinephrine and isoproterenol, and propranolol was less potent in inhibiting contraction. Conversely, the atria were more sensitive to the α-agonist phenylephrine, and phenoxybenzamine was a more potent antagonist in the hypothyroid than in the euthyroid animals. These findings suggested that hypothyroidism either altered the response of two independent receptors or, as the authors felt, produced a change in the characteristics of a single receptor. Kunos (1977) subsequently found that the chronotropic response in thyroidectomized animals was reduced by isoprenaline and increased by phenylephrine.

Banerjee and Kung (1977) found that the number of β-adrenergic binding sites decreased by 33% in heart microsomes from hypothyroid rats, while the receptor affinity was unchanged. Similar results were observed in skeletal muscle, except that the affinity was also increased (Sharma and Banerjee, 1978b). The studies on α-adrenergic receptors, using [^{3}H]dihydroergokryptine, have given conflicting results. Ciaraldi and Marinetti (1977) described a marked decrease in α-receptor number and an increase in their affinity in PTU-treated animals. β-Receptors were also slightly decreased and affinity was increased. Sharma and Banerjee (1978a) reported an increase in α-receptor binding in thyroidectomized animals as compared to hypothyroid animals given T3. The affinity was the same in both groups. These studies indicate that hypothyroidism influences cardiac α- and β-receptor numbers and that they may vary reciprocally. The effect on binding affinity is less clear and will require further investigation.

E. Hypothyroidism and the Cholinergic Nervous System

The possible relationship between thyroid hormone deficiency and parasympathetic control of heart rate has been virtually unexplored. Hoffmann *et al.* (1947, 1953) indicated both *in situ* and *in vitro* that vagal stimulation and acetylcholine infusion evoked a greater chronotropic depressant effect in the hypothyroid animals, but more recent studies (Section II,E) have examined the cholinergic system only in hyperthyroidism.

F. Electrophysiological Alterations in Hypothyroidism

Electrophysiological studies have contributed to the understanding of cardiac conduction in response to low levels of thyroid hormone. Experimental hypothyroidism produced a prolonged duration of repolarization and slowed conduction velocity (Freedberg *et al.*, 1970; Goel *et al.*, 1972) and, in humans, hypothyroidism was associated with a long right atrial monophasic action potential (MAP) duration (Cotoi *et al.*, 1972; Gavrilescu *et al.*, 1976). Two to 4 weeks of T4 corrected both the prolonged duration of repolarization and MAP in the latter reports (Fig. 17). Gavrilescu *et al.* (1976) performed His bundle recordings in six hypothyroid patients. Three were normal, one had a SupraHisian A-V block, and two had H-V interval prolongation. From these studies it appears that hypothyroidism prolongs intracardiac conduction and that it may be reversible. The prolonged refractory period presumably is responsible for the infrequency of arrhythmias as compared with hyperthyroidism.

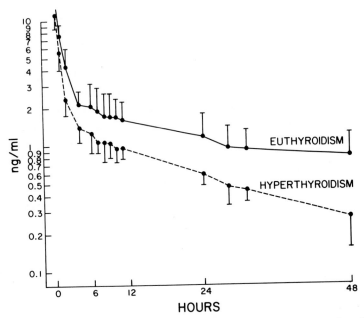

Fig. 17. Mean plasma digoxin concentration (ng/ml) ± S after i.v. administration of 1 mg digoxin in nine patients with manifest hyperthyroidism and after thyrostatic therapy. (Reprinted by permission from Bonelli *et al.*, 1978.)

G. Effect of Hypothyroidism on Myocardial Enzymes

1. Adenyl Cyclase–Cyclic AMP

There is ample evidence that hyperthyroidism does not alter the basal levels of myocardial adenyl cyclase activity or cyclic AMP (Section II,G,1). Although less extensively studied, it appears that hypothyroidism has an effect on cyclic AMP. Levey *et al.* (1969a) have shown that although basal adenyl cyclase activity measured in heart homogenates was no different in euthyroid and hypothyroid cats, the maximum response to graded doses of norepinephrine was less in the latter group. The net accumulation of cyclic 3′,5′-AMP was also less (Fig. 18), and the phosphodiesterase activity was unaltered. Since isolated papillary muscles from the hypothyroid cats responded normally to norepinephrine, the authors felt that only a portion of the cyclic AMP produced by catecholamines was necessary for the inotropic response. Bode and Meara (1978) have reported preliminary data showing that glucagon-stimulated myocardial adenylate cyclase activity is depressed in hypothyroid but normal in hyperthyroid rats, and that T4 corrected this response.

2. Myocardial ATPases

Lifschitz and Kayne (1966) demonstrated a significant reduction in myofibrillar ATPase activity in both thyroidectomized and hypophysectomized rats. This activity was normalized by thyroxine, but not growth hormone. Hjalmarson *et al.* (1970) noted that myosin Ca^{2+}-activated ATPase was reduced 30–45% in hypophysectomized rats, that peak ventricular pressure and maximum rate of tension development were reduced, and that T4 for 7 days but not growth hormone corrected the abnormality. K^+ and NH_4^+-ATPase activities were unaltered. Diminished Ca^{2+}-ATPase was associated with a reduced rate of Ca^{2+} uptake by sarcoplasmic reticulum in rabbits (Suko, 1971).

Several studies have indicated that hypothyroidism may alter the ATPase structure. Jacobson *et al.* (1972), using skeletal muscle, found an increased helical content of myosin with some differences in amino acid composition. Electrophoretic patterns showed the myosin from hypothyroid and euthyroid animals to have similar size and shape. Rovetto *et al.* (1972) subsequently showed that myosin Ca^{2+}-ATPase from the hearts of hypophysectomized rats was low, that contractility was impaired, and that

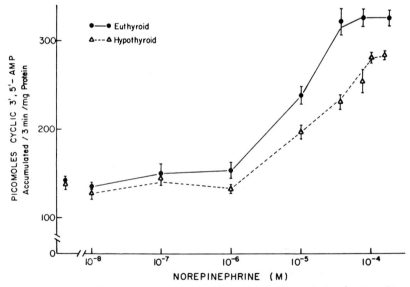

Fig. 18.   Norepinephrine concentration–response curves in the particulate fraction of heart homogenates from euthyroid and hypothyroid cats. The values represent the mean ± SE of 10–15 samples from six cats. The differences are significant at 1×10^{-5} mole/liter ($P < 0.05$); 5×10^{-5} mole/liter ($P < 0.02$); 8×10^{-5} mole/liter ($P < 0.02$); 1–2×10^{-4} mole-liter ($P < 0.05$). (Reprinted by permission from Levey *et al.,* 1969a.)

both parameters were corrected by T4 but not by growth hormone. The failure of N-ethylmaleimide to stimulate Ca^{2+}-ATPase in either normal or hypothyroid rats suggested that the differences seen were not due to a modification of sulfhydryl groups. K^+ and NH_4^+-ATPases were unaffected. Yazaki and Raben (1975) found that hypothyroid rat myosin had low Ca^{2+}-ATPase activity which was activated by N-ethylmaleimide, whereas myosin from hypothyroid rabbits had normal Ca^{2+}-ATPase which was not activated by N-ethylmaleimide. Both species had normal K^+-ATPase. Thyroidectomy produced some change in the amino acid composition of rat myosin subunits, and the enzyme was more sensitive to temperature and alkaline pH. The ATPase activity was enhanced by T4 administration.

These data provide evidence that the Ca^{2+}-activated ATPase in hypothyroidism may have altered enzyme properties, and T4 corrects the abnormalities. These changes are associated with reduced calcium uptake in the sarcoplasmic reticulum and impaired contractility and suggest that the altered contractility of hypothyroidism may at least in part be under the control of ATPase.

H. Biochemical Effects of Thyroid Hormone Deficiency

1. Carbohydrates and Lipids

Cardiac glycogen stores have been shown by Bray and Goodman (1967) to be increased in thyroidectomized rats, which may be related to reduced phosphorylase a levels. Fasting increased the glycogen content in normal but not in hypothyroid animals.

Unlike the changes in lipid metabolism observed in thyroxine-treated animals, experimental hypothyroidism has little effect on lipid composition. Plasma FFAs were normal in thyroidectomized rats (Bray and Goodman, 1967), and in dogs it has been shown that plasma FFAs, their delivery to, uptake, and oxidation by the myocardium were all normal (Gold *et al.,* 1967). The total body turnover of plasma FFAs was, however, decreased. Steffen and Platner (1976) observed that propylthiouracil-induced hypothyroidism in rats had no influence on either the percent of unsaturated fatty acids or the specific lipids when the animals were warm, although mitochondrial stearate levels were diminished in cold-acclimatized rats.

2. Oxidative Phosphorylation

Buccino *et al.* (1967), in examining the contractile properties of hypothyroid cat papillary muscles, found no significant change in total high-energy phosphate stores (ATP plus creatine phosphate) as compared to euthyroid animals. Skelton *et al.* (1971) confirmed that high-energy phosphate stores were not significantly altered in hypothyroid cat papillary muscles. Moreover, these muscles used only 64% as much energy while performing 81% as much work as euthyroid muscles, suggesting that energy metabolism was not impaired by thyroid hormone deficiency. Recent work by Nishiki *et al.* (1978) has furnished additional information. In rats studied 10–20 days after thyroidectomy the Q_{O_2} was decreased, and this was associated with a greater depression in state 4 than in state 3 respiration. Thus the respiratory control ratio was actually increased and there was no change in the ADP/O ratio. Although the myocardial cytochrome content was lowered by 30%, 6 days of T4 normalized this deficiency.

I. Histopathology

Hypothyroidism produces rather characteristic pathological changes in the myocardium. Goldberg (1927) noted dilated, pale, flabby hearts with normal valves in thyroidectomized sheep. Histologically, the muscle cross striations were frequently absent, and the Purkinje tissue was swollen and vacuolated. Brewer (1951) described the presence of a weakly acid mucoprotein infiltration that was periodic acid Schiff (PAS) stain positive but did not stain metachromatically. He claimed that the numerous areas of basophilic degeneration were characteristic. Douglass and Jacobson (1957) examined the hearts of 10 hypothyroid patients and found swollen myocardial fibers staining PAS-positive for intracellular vacuoles. These vacuoles, along with interstitial edema, were also observed by Dainauskas *et al.* (1974). At an ultrastructural level, thyroidectomized rats had a smaller volume of myocardial cells and fewer myofibrils and mitochondria than thyroxine-treated animals, although the percent of the cell volume comprised of these organelles was unchanged. Mitchondrial cristae were also reduced. The alterations in myofibrils and cristae were both confirmed by microchemical assays (Page and McCallister, 1973).

J. Clinical Cardiovascular Complications of Hypothyroidism

1. Electrocardiographic Disturbances

The effect of hypothyroidism on cardiac electrophysiology is to delay conduction and prolong the refractory period (Section III,F), presumably accounting for the infrequency of arrhythmias. ECG abnormalities have included low voltage, sinus bradycardia, flat P waves, and flattened or inverted T waves (Zondek, 1964). DeSwiet (1971), however, described an unusual hypothyroid patient who had inverted U waves, a long Q-T interval, and a sinus tachycardia of 120 beats/min which improved with thyroid hormone. Urschel and Gates (1953) described serial ECGs in a patient who became repeatedly hypothyroid and euthyroid. The T vector changed during hypothyroidism, indicating delayed repolarization. The rapidity with which the ECG abnormalities were reversible has been described by Zondek (1964). Thyroid hormone improved voltage and T waves within a day. However, the response was variable, as some patients had a delay of many weeks. A-V conduction disturbances may also occur. In three cases reported by Singh et al. (1973), patients had complete A-V block which resolved with T3 replacement. The authors speculated that this response might be due to a direct effect of thyroid hormone on nodal and conduction tissue, a view given support by the finding of thyroid hormone localization in the bundle of His (Tommaselli et al., 1965).

2. Organic Heart Disease and Hypothyroidism

a. ATHEROSCLEROTIC HEART DISEASE

The possible association between hypothyroidism and atherosclerotic heart disease (ASHD) has been the topic of debate for many years, yet no relationship has been proven. Smyth (1938) speculated over 40 years ago that there was a high incidence of ASHD in myxedema, and that this might be due to hypercholesterolemia. This concept was challenged by Blumgart et al. (1953), whose patients, following prophylactic thyroidectomies for heart failure, had an elevation of serum cholesterol but no progression of atherosclerosis. This study failed to exclude the possibility of hypothyroidism facilitating ASHD for several reasons: There was no control group, many of the patients were young with only mild hypercholesterolemia, and the mean duration of follow-up was only 7.4 years.

The incidence of angina pectoris was 6–8% in two large series of hypothyroid patients (Keating et al., 1960; Watanakunakorn et al., 1965) and hypercholesterolemia was present in over 80% of patients. Other investigators have reported groups of patients with myocardial infarction and antecedent lymphocytic thyroiditis, with there being evidence of hypercholesterolemia before the development of thyroid failure or coronary disease (Fowler and Swale, 1967; Bastenie et al., 1967). Steinberg (1968) reviewed the autopsy records of 38 women with thyroid atrophy and found that, when compared to an age- and sex-matched control group, there was an increased incidence of coronary artery disease in the hypertensive (but not the normotensive) patients. This study had the problem of being retrospective and, since it included only autopsied cases, may not be representative of the population at large of hypothyroid individuals. Nevertheless, the results of this study, as well as the previously cited observations, at least suggest that coronary artery disease may be aggravated by hypothyroidism. Whether the reversal of hypercholesterolemia from thyroid replacement (Miettinen, 1968) will reverse this tendency is unknown. It is interesting, however, that not only L-T4 and L-T3 but D-T4, 3,5-diiodothyronine, and the formic, acetic, and propionic acid analogues of T3 and T4 have varying effects on lipid metabolism (Sachs, 1961). Although D-thyroxine has been used for management of hyperlipidemia, caution must be exercised since the dextroisomer is calorigenic and suppresses TSH (Gorman et al., 1979).

What has been better understood is the special problem involved in managing hypothyroidism in the patient with symptomatic heart disease. Smyth (1938) pointed out that injudicious thyroid hormone replacement may aggravate angina pectoris. Keating et al. (1960), examining the effect of thyroid hormone in a large group of patients, found that chest pain improved or disappeared in 21 of 55 patients with preexisting angina. Twenty-five other patients had no change in symptoms, and 9 became worse. Of 35 patients who first developed angina after initiating thyroid therapy, it occurred within a month in 6, within a year in 6, and more than a year later in 23. Although many patients have benefited from thyroid replacement, there are occasional patients who cannot tolerate even suboptimal therapy without worsening of their angina. The combination of small doses of T3 and propranolol has been suggested for these patients (Steinberg and Schrader, 1971), but the benefit derived from using propranolol is unproven. Two recent reports have provided an alternative in the hypothyroid patient severely incapacitated by angina, and that is coronary artery saphenous vein bypass surgery (Nelson et al., 1974; Paine et al., 1977). A total of nine patients were evaluated and all tolerated arteriography without thyroid therapy. The patients who were not given thyroid until the peri- or postoperative period generally did well and often returned to fully active lines. Surprisingly, two patients who were cautiously treated with thyroid hormone for several weeks preoperatively both suffered myocardial infarctions and died before bypass surgery. One must therefore be extremely careful when attempting to even partially correct the metabolic defect in someone with severe ischemic heart disease, since any increase in cardiac output and oxygen consumption may lead to disastrous consequences.

b. Myxedema Heart Disease

Cardiac enlargement, with or without congestive heart failure, has been observed as a complication of hypothyroidism for many years, although it may be due to coexistent hypertension or coronary artery disease (Aber and Thompson, 1963). Heart failure, while occurring in 42 of 400 hypothyroid patients (Watanakunakorn et al., 1965), may have been secondary to hypertension in some instances. An enlarged cardiac silhouette could be due to cardiac hypertrophy, dilatation, or pericardial effusion. Several individual cases have demonstrated cardiomegaly and dilatation by angiography (Monroe and Fearrington, 1966; Dainauskas *et al.*, 1974), and Santos *et al.* (1978) recently found echocardiographic evidence of asymmetric thickening of the ventricular septum in 14 subjects. The extent of thickening was greater with long-standing hypothyroidism, and the changes were reversible with thyroid hormone.

Pericardial effusions have been responsible for extreme widening of the cardiac silhouette (Kern *et al.*, 1949; Kittredge *et al.*, 1963; Gupta *et al.*, 1971), and echocardiography has been invaluable in assessing the incidence of effusions in hypothyroidism. Kerber and Sherman (1975) noted effusions in 10 of 33 subjects, and Crowley *et al.* (1977) observed them in 9 of 14 patients. While the effusions disappeared with thyroid hormone replacement, a few patients had residual cardiomegaly. Since these effusions accumulate slowly, cardiac tamponade is not usually a problem, although it may occur (Martin and Spathis, 1965; Davis and Jacobson, 1967; Smolar *et al.*, 1976).

3. Cardiac Glycosides

Peacock and Moran (1963) found less of a contractility response in hypothyroid than in euthyroid rats, although this may have been due to a high basal value. Buccino *et al.* (1967), in contrast, demonstrated enhanced contractile tension after strophanthidin. Pharmacokinetic studies in humans have shown either increased serum digoxin levels with a normal half-life (Doherty and Perkins, 1966), increased serum levels and a prolonged half-life (Croxson and Ibbertson, 1975), or else both were normal (Lawrence *et al.*, 1977). Huffman *et al.* (1977), while finding normal serum digoxin levels in hypothyroid rats, found that biliary excretion of this drug was low. The significant correlation between creatinine and digoxin clearances both in hypo- and hyperthyroidism indicates that proper management of digitalis therapy may require monitoring of serum digoxin concentrations and renal function in patients with thyroid disease (Croxson and Ibbertson, 1975).

IV. Summary

Considerable knowledge has been accumulated concerning the effect of thyroid hormone on myocardial structure and function. These studies have examined the hormonal effect on cellular ultrastructure, enzymes, electrophysiologic events, hemodynamics, and contractility. The information obtained has provided insight into the molecular and cellular alterations that occur, and has greatly aided in understanding the clinical cardiac symptomatology of hyperthyroidism and hypothyroidism.

Recent investigations of T3 binding to hepatic nuclear receptors have shown that T3-induced changes in specific messenger RNAs lead to the synthesis of particular proteins that mediate the response to thyroid hormone (Baxter and Funder, 1979). It is likely that over the next several years, studies of the interaction of T3 with myocardial receptors and the postreceptor events initiated after receptor binding will clarify the mechanism of the action of thyroid hormone at the cardiac molecular level and its associated clinical manifestations.

References

Aber, C. P., and Thompson, G. S. (1963). *Br. Heart J.* **25**, 421–424.

Altschuld, R. A., Weiss, A., Kruger, F. A., and Weissler, A. M. (1969). *J. Clin. Invest.* **48**, 1905–1913.

Amidi, M., Leon, D. F., deGroot, W. J., Kroetz, F. W., and Leonard, J. J. (1968). *Circulation* **38**, 229–239.

Anton, A. H., and Gravenstein, J. S. (1970). *Eur. J. Pharmacol.* **10**, 311–318.

Arnsdorf, M. F., and Childers, R. W. (1970). *Circ. Res.* **26**, 575–581.

Asper, S. P., Jr., Selenkow, H. A., and Plamondon, C. A. (1953). *Bull. Johns Hopkins Hosp.* **93**, 164–198.

Banerjee, S. P., and Kung, L. S. (1977). *Eur. J. Pharmacol.* **43**, 207–208.

Banerjee, S. P., and Sharma, V. K. (1979). *Brit. J. Pharmacol.* **65**, 615–621.

Banerjee, S. K., Flink, I. L., and Morkin, E. (1976). *Circ. Res.* **39**, 319–326.

Banerjee, S. K., Kabbas, E. G., and Morkin, E. (1977). *J. Biol. Chem.* **252**, 6925–6929.

Barker, S. B., and Makiuchi, M. (1965). *J. Pharmacol. Exp. Ther.* **148**, 71–74.

Bartošová, D, Chvapil, M., Poupa, O., Rakušan, K., Turek, Z., and Vízek, M. (1969). *J. Physiol. (London)* **200**, 285–295.

Bastenie, P. A., Vanhaelst, L., and Neve, P. (1967). *Lancet* **2**, 1221–1222.

Baxter, J. D., and Funder, J. W. (1979). *N. Engl. J. Med.* **301**, 1149–1161.

Benforado, J. M., and Wiggins, L. L. (1965). *J. Pharmacol. Exp. Ther.* **147**, 70–75.

Bernal, J., Coleoni, A. H., and Degroot, L. J. (1978). *Endocrinology* **103**, 403–413.

Bewsher, P. D., Pegg, C. A. S., Stewart, D. J., Lister, D. A., and Michie, W. (1974). *Ann. Surg.* **180**, 787–790.

Beznák, M. (1962). *Can. J. Biochem. Physiol.* **40**, 1647–1654.

Beznák, M. (1964). *Circ. Res.* **15**, Suppl. II, 141–152.

Bilder, G. E., and Hess, M. E. (1973). *J. Pharmacol. Exp. Ther.* **185**, 468–478.

Bishop, J. M., Donald, K. W., and Wade, O. L. (1955). *Clin. Sci.* **14**, 329–360.

Blizzard, J. J., and Rupp, J. J. (1960). *J. Am. Med. Assoc.* **173**, 1845.

Blumgart, H. L., Gargill, S. L., and Gilligan, D. R. (1930a). *J. Clin. Invest.* **9**, 69–89.

Blumgart, H. L., Gargill, S. L., and Gilligan, D. R. (1930b). *J. Clin. Invest.* **9**, 91–106.

Blumgart, H. L., Freedberg, A. S., and Kurland, G. S. (1953). *Am. J. Med.* **14**, 665–673.

Bode, H. H., and Meara, P. A. (1978). *Program, 60th Annu. Meet. Endocrine Soc.* p. 427.

Bonelli, J., Haydl, H., Hruby, K., and Kaik, G. (1978). *Int. J. Clin. Pharmacol.* **16**, 302–306.

Bough, E. W., Crowley, W. F., Ridgway, E. C., Walker, H., Maloof, F., Myers, G. S., and Daniels, G. H. (1978). *Arch. Intern. Med.* **138**, 1476–1480.

Bray, G. A., and Goodman, H. M. (1967). *Proc. Soc. Exp. Biol. Med.* **125**, 1310–1313.

Bressler, R., and Wittels, B. (1966). *J. Clin. Invest.* **45**, 1326–1333.

Brewer, D. B. (1951). *J. Pathol. Bacteriol.* **63**, 503–512.

Brewster, W. R., Jr., Isaacs, J. P., Osgood, P. F., and King, T. L. (1956). *Circulation* **13**, 1–20.

Brus, R., and Hess, M. E. (1973). *Endocrinology* **93**, 982–985.

Buccino, R. A., Spann, J. F., Jr., Pool, P. E., Sonnenblick, E. H., and Braunwald, E. (1967). *J. Clin. Invest.* **46**, 1669–1682.

Buccino, R. A., Spann, J. F., Jr., Sonnenblick, E. H., and Braunwald, E. (1968). *Endocrinology* **82**, 191–192.

Burack, R., Edwards, R. H. T., Green, M., and Jones, N. L. (1971). *J. Pharmacol. Exp. Ther.* **176**, 212–219.

Burckhardt, D., Staub, J.-J., Kraenzlin, M., Raeder, E., Engel, U., and Cloppenburg, P. (1978). *Am. Heart J.* **95**, 187–196.

Burman, K. D., Strum, D., Dimond, R. C., Djuh, Y.-Y., Wright, F. D., Earll, J. M., and Wartofsky, L. (1977). *J. Clin. Endocrinol. Metab.* **45**, 339–352.

Burman, K. D., Wright, F. D., Smallridge, R. C., Green, B. J., Georges, L. P., and Wartofsky, L. (1978). *J. Clin. Endocrinol. Metab.* **47**, 1059–1064.

Cairoli, V. J., and Crout, J. R. (1967). *J. Pharmacol. Exp. Ther.* **158**, 55–65.

Campus, S., Rappelli, A., Malavasi, A., and Satta, A. (1975). *Arch. Intern. Med.* **135**, 1091–1095.

Canary, J. J., Schaaf, M., Duffy, B. J., Jr., and Kyle, L. H. (1957). *N. Engl. J. Med.* **257**, 435–442.

Carter, W. J., and Faas, F. H. (1978). *Proc. 60th Annu. Meet. Endocrine Soc.* p. 125 (abstr.).

Cavalieri, R. R., Gavin, L. A., Bui, F., McMahon, F., and Hammond, M. (1977). *Biochem. Biophys. Res. Commun.* **79**, 897–902.

Chakravarty, J., Guansing, A. R., Chakravarty, S., and Hughes, C. V. (1978). *Acta Endocrinol. (Copenhagen)* **87**, 507–515.

Challoner, D. R. (1968). *Am. J. Physiol.* **214**, 365–369.

Chopra, I. J. (1977). *Endocrinology* **101**, 453–463.

Chopra, I. J., Wu, S.-Y., Nakamura, Y., and Solomon, D. H. (1978). *Endocrinology* **102**, 1099–1106.

Ciaraldi, T., and Marinetti, G. V. (1977). *Biochem. Biophys. Res. Commun.* **74**, 984–991.

Cohen, J., Aroesty, J. M., and Rosenfeld, M. G. (1966). *Circ. Res.* **18**, 388–397.

Conway, G., Heazlitt, R. A., Fowler, N. O., Gabel, M., and Green, S. (1976). *J. Mol. Cell. Cardiol.* **8**, 39–51.

Cotoi, S., Constantinescu, L., and Gavrilescu, S. (1972). *Experientia* **28**, 797–798.

Cravey, G. M., and Gravenstein, J. S. (1965). *J. Pharmacol. Exp. Ther.* **148**, 75–79.

Crowley, W. F., Jr., Ridgway, E. C., Bough, E. W., Francis, G. S., Daniels, G. H., Kourides, I. A., Myers, G. S., and Maloof, F. (1977). *N. Engl. J. Med.* **296**, 1–6.

Croxson, M. S., and Ibbertson, H. K. (1975). *Br. Med. J.* **3**, 566–568.

Curfman, G. D., Crowley, T. J., and Smith, T. W. (1977). *J. Clin. Invest.* **59**, 586–590.

Dainauskas, J. R., Susmano, A., and Bogdonoff, M. L. (1974). *Am. Heart J.* **88**, 229–239.

Davis, P. J., and Jacobson, S. (1967). *Arch. Intern. Med.* **120**, 615–619.

Degroot, L. J., and Niepomniszcze, H. (1977). *Metab., Clin. Exp.* **26**, 665–718.

Degroot, L. J., Torresani, J., Carrayon, P., and Tirard, A. (1976). *Acta Endocrinol. (Copenhagen)* **83**, 293–304.

deGroot, W. J., Leonard, J. J., Paley, H. W., and Warren, J. V. (1960). *J. Lab. Clin. Med.* **56**, 1960.

deGroot, W. J., Leonard, J. J., Paley, H. W., Johnson, J. E., and Warren, J. V. (1961). *J. Clin. Invest.* **40**, 1033.

DeSwiet, J. (1971). *Postgrad. Med. J.* **47**, 626–627.

Dickstein, Y., Schwarts, H., Gordon, A., and Gross, J. (1978). *Program 54th Annu. Meet. Am. Thyroid Assoc.* T-21.

Dirmikis, S. M., and Munro, D. S. (1975). *Br. Med. J.* **2**, 665–666.

Dobson, J. G., Jr. (1978). *Am. J. Physiol.* **234**, H638-H645.

Doherty, J. E., and Perkins, W. H. (1966). *Ann. Intern. Med.* **64**, 489–507.

Douglass, R. C., and Jacobson, S. D. (1957). *J. Clin. Endocrinol. Metab.* **17**, 1354–1362.

Eaton, R. P., Steinberg, D., and Thompson, R. H. (1965). *J. Clin. Invest.* **44**, 247–260.

Ellis, L. B., Mebane, J. G., Maresh, G., Hultgren, H. N., and Bloomfield, R. A. (1952). *Am. Heart J.* **43**, 341–356.

Elsas, L. J., Whittemore, R., and Burrow, G. N. (1967). *J. Am. Med. Assoc.* **200**, 250–252.

El-Shahawy, M. (1974). *Circulation* **50**, Suppl. III, 171.

Epstein, S. E., Skelton, C. L., Levey, G. S., and Entman, M. (1970). *Ann. Intern. Med.* **72**, 561–578.

Eraker, S. A., Wickamasekaran, R., and Goldman, S. (1978). *J. Am. Med. Assoc.* **239**, 1644–1646.

Eriksson, M., Rubenfeld, S., Garber, A. J., and Kohler, P. O. (1977). *N. Engl. J. Med.* **296**, 263–264.

Ernstene, A. C. (1938). *Am. J. Med. Sci.* **195**, 248–256.

Faber, J., Friis, T., Kirkegaard, C., Lumholtz, I. B., Hansen, J. M., Siersbaek-Nielsen, K., Skovsted, L., and Theilade, P. (1979a). *Horm. Metab. Res.* **11**, 34–36.

Faber, J., Kirkegaard, C., Lumholtz, I. B., Siersbaek-Nielsen, K., and Friis, T. (1979b). *J. Clin. Endocrinol. Metab.* **48**, 611–617.

Flink, I. L., and Morkin, E. (1977). *FEBS Lett.* **81**, 391–394.

Folkman, J., and Edmunds, L. H., Jr. (1962). *Circ. Res.* **10**, 632–641.

Forfar, J. C., Miller, H. C., and Toft, A. D. (1979). *Am. J. Cardiol.* **44**, 9–12.

Fowler, P. B. S., and Swale, J. (1967). *Lancet* **1**, 1077–1079.

Frazer, A., and Hess, M. E. (1969). *J. Pharmacol. Exp. Ther.* **170**, 1–9.

Frazer, A., Hess, M. E., and Shanfeld, J. (1969). *J. Pharmacol. Exp. Ther.* **170**, 10–16.

Freedberg, A. S., Papp, J. G., and Williams, E. M. V. (1970). *J. Physiol. (London)* **207**, 357–369.

Friedman, M. J., Okada, R. D., Hellman, D., Sahn, D. J., and Ewy, G. A. (1979). *Clin. Res.* **27**, 3A.

Frolov, V. A., Abinder, A. A., Kryukova, I. V., Mitin, K. S., Dvurechenskii, Y. I., and Kandror, V. I. (1967). *Cor Vasa* **9**, 288–296.

Frye, R. L., and Braunwald, E. (1961). *Circulation* **23**, 376–382.

Gavrilescu, S., Luca, C., Streian, C., Lungu, G., and Deutsch, G. (1976). *Br. Heart J.* **38**, 1350–1354.

Gemmill, C. L. (1958). *Am. J. Physiol.* **195**, 385–390.

George, L., Connors, M., Riemenschneider, T. A., Mathewson, J. W., DeMaria, A. N., and Mason, D. T. (1978). *Clin. Res.* **26**, 169A.

Gertz, B. J., and Haugaard, E. S. (1979). *Fed Proc. Fed. Am. Soc. Exp. Biol.* **38**, 427 (abstr.).

Goel, B. G., Hanson, C. S., and Han, J. (1972). *Am. Heart J.* **83**, 504–511.

Golber, L. M., and Kandror, V. I. (1969). *Cor Vasa* **11**, 35–47.

Golber, L. M., Kandror, V. I., and Ester, K. M. (1967). *Cor Vasa* **9**, 210–218.

Gold, M., Scott, J. C., and Spitzer, J. J. (1967). *Am. J. Physiol.* **213**, 239–244.

Goldberg, S. A. (1927). *Quart. J. Exp. Physiol.* **17**, 15–30.

Goldstein, S., and Killip, T., III (1965). *Circulation* **31**, 219–227.

Goodkind, M. J. (1968). *Circ. Res.* **22**, 605–614.
Goodkind, M. J. (1969). *Circ. Res.* **25**, 237–244.
Goodkind, M. J., Fram, D. H., and Roberts, M. (1961). *Am. J. Physiol.* **201**, 1049–1052.
Goodkind, M. J., Dambach, G. E., Thyrum, P. T., and Luchi, R. J. (1974). *Am. J. Physiol.* **226**, 66–72.
Gorman, C. A., Jiang, N-S., Ellefson, R. D., and Elveback, L. R. (1979). *J. Clin. Endocrinol. Metab.,* **49**, 1–7.
Graettinger, J. S., Muenster, J. J., Checchia, C. S., Grissom, R. L., and Campbell, J. A. (1958). *J. Clin. Invest.* **37**, 502–510.
Graettinger, J. S., Muenster, J. J., Selverstone, L. A., and Campbell, J. A. (1959). *J. Clin. Invest.* **38**, 1316–1327.
Grossman, W., Robin, N. I., Johnson, L. W., Brooks, H. L., Selenkow, H. A., and Dexter, L. (1971). *Ann. Intern. Med.* **74**, 869–874.
Gunning, J. F., Harrison, C. E., Jr., and Coleman, H. N., III (1974). *Am. J. Physiol.* **226**, 1166–1171.
Gupta, M. P., Kim, S., Kang, J., Sherman, L., Kolodny, H. D., and Hamby, R. I. (1971). *J. Am. Med. Assoc.* **217**, 205–207.
Harland, W. A., Orr, J. S., Dunnigan, M. G., and Sequeira, R. F. C. (1972). *Br. Heart J.* **34**, 1072–1074.
Heimbach, D. M., and Crout, J. R. (1972). *Arch. Intern. Med.* **129**, 430–432.
Hellman, R., Kelly, K. L., and Mason, W. D. (1977). *N. Engl. J. Med.* **297**, 671–672.
Hillis, W. S., Bremner, W. F., Lawrie, T. D. V., and Thomson, J. A. (1975). *Clin. Endocrinol. (N.Y.)* **4**, 617–624.
Hirvonen, L., and Lybeck, H. (1956a). *Acta Physiol. Scand.* **36**, 23–28.
Hirvonen, L., and Lybeck, H. (1956b). *Acta Physiol. Scand.* **36**, 29–37.
Hirvonen, L., and Paavilainen, T. O. A. (1967). *Acta Physiol. Scand.* **69**, 284–294.
Hjalmarson, A. C., Whitfield, C. F., and Morgan, H. E. (1970). *Biochem. Biophys. Res. Comm.* **41**, 1584–1589.
Hoffman, I., and Lowrey, R. D. (1960). *Am. J. Cardiol.* **6**, 893–904.
Hoffmann, F., Hoffmann, E. J., and Talesnik, J. (1947). *Am. J. Physiol.* **148**, 689–699.
Hoffmann, F., Middleton, S., Molina, A., and Talesnik, J. (1953). *Acta Physiol. Lat. Am.* **3**, 118–124.
Hornbrook, K. R., and Brody, T. M. (1963). *J. Pharmacol. Exp. Ther.* **140**, 295–307.
Howitt, G., Rowlands, D. J., Leung, D. Y. T., and Logan, W. F. W. E. (1968). *Clin. Sci.* **34**, 485–495.
Huffman, D. H., Klaassen, C. D., and Hartman, C. R. (1977). *Clin. Pharmacol. Ther.* **22**, 533–538.
Ikram, H. (1977). *Br. Med. J.* **1**, 1505–1507.
Isaacs, G. H., Sacktor, B., and Murphy, T. A. (1969). *Biochim. Biophys. Acta* **177**, 196–203.
Ismail-Beigi, F., and Edelman, I. S. (1971). *J. Gen. Physiol.* **57**, 710–722.
Jacobson, A. L., Humphrey, B., and Grey, V. (1972). *Int. J. Biochem.* **3**, 518–524.
Kaplan, M. M., Schimmel, M., and Utiger, R. D. (1977). *J. Clin. Endocrinol. Metab.* **45**, 447–456.
Katagiri, T., Freedberg, A. S., and Morkin, E. (1975). *Life Sci.* **16**, 1079–1087.
Katz, S., Hamilton, D., Tenner, T., and McNeill, J. H. (1977). *Res. Commun. Chem. Pathol. Pharmacol.* **18**, 777–780.
Keating, F. R., Jr., Parkin, T. W., Selby, J. B., and Dickinson, L. S. (1960). *Prog. Cardiovasc. Dis.* **3**, 364–381.
Keely, S. L., Jr., Lincoln, T. M., and Corbin, J. D. (1978). *Am. J. Physiol.* **234**, H432–H438.
Kerber, R. E., and Sherman, B. (1975). *Circulation* **52**, 823–827.

Kern, R. A., Soloff, L. A., Snape, W. J., and Bello, C. T. (1949). *Am. J. Med. Sci.* 217, 609–618.

Kimata, S.-I., and Tarjan, E. M. (1971). *Endocrinology* 89, 378–384.

Kittredge, R. D., Arida, E. J., and Finby, N. (1963). *Radiology* 80, 430–433.

Kontos, H. A., Shapiro, W., Mauck, H. P., Jr., Richardson, D. W., Patterson, J. L., Jr., and Sharpe, A. R., Jr. (1965). *J. Clin. Invest.* 44, 947–956.

Kotler, M. N., Michaelides, K. M., Bouchard, R. J., and Warbasse, J. R. (1973). *Arch. Intern. Med.* 132, 723–728.

Kunos, G. (1977). *Br. J. Pharmacol.* 59, 177–189.

Kunos, G., Vermes-Kunos, I., and Nickerson, M. (1974). *Nature (London)* 250, 779–781.

Kurland, G. S., Hammond, R. P., and Freedberg, A. S. (1963). *Am. J. Physiol.* 205, 1270–1274.

Landsberg, L. (1977). *Clin. Endocrinol. Metab.* 6, 697–718.

Landsberg, L., and Axelrod, J. (1968). *Circ. Res.* 22, 559–571.

Latham, K. R., MacLeod, K. M., Papavasiliou, S. S., Martial, J. A., Seeburg, P. H., Goodman, H. M., and Baxter, J. D. (1978). *Recept. Horm. Action* 3, 75–100.

Latham, K. R., Smallridge, R. C., Tseng, Y. L., Burman, K. D., and Wartofsky, L. (1979). *Clin. Res.* 27, 255A.

Lawrence, J. R., Sumner, D. J., Kalk, W. J., Ratcliffe, W. A., Whiting, B., Gray, K., and Lindsay, M. (1977). *Clin. Pharmacol. Ther.* 22, 7–13.

Lee, T. C., Coffey, R. J., Mackin, J., Cobb, M., Routon, J., and Canary, J. J. (1973). *Ann. Surg.* 177, 643–647.

Lee, Y.-P., and Lardy, H. A. (1965). *J. Biol. Chem.* 240, 1427–1436.

Leger, J., Bouveret, P., Schwartz, K., and Swynghedauw, B. (1976). *Pfluegers Arch.* 362, 271–277.

Leszynsky, H. E., Gross-Kieselstein, E., and Abrahamov, A. (1971). *Pediatrics* 47, 1069–1073.

Leveque, P. E. (1956). *Circ. Res.* 4, 108–111.

Levey, G. S. (1971). *Am. J. Med.* 50, 413–420.

Levey, G. S., and Epstein, S. E. (1968). *Biochem. Biophys. Res. Commun.* 33, 990–995.

Levey, G. S., and Epstein, S. E. (1969). *J. Clin. Invest.* 48, 1663–1669.

Levey, G. S., Skelton, C. L., and Epstein, S. E. (1969a). *J. Clin. Invest.* 48, 2244–2250.

Levey, G. S., Skelton, C. L., and Epstein, S. E. (1969b). *Endocrinology* 85, 1004–1009.

Lifschitz, M. D., and Kayne, H. L. (1966). *Biochem. Pharmacol.* 15, 405–407.

Likoff, W. B., and Levine, S. A. (1943). *Am. J. Med. Sci.* 206, 425–434.

Limas, C. J. (1978a). *Am. J. Physiol.* 234, H426–H431.

Limas, C. J. (1978b). *Am. J. Physiol.* 235, H745–H751.

Limas, C. J. (1979). *Biochem. J.* 180, 59–67.

Limas, C. J., and Chan-Stier, C. (1978). *Circ. Res.* 42, 311–316.

Littman, D. S., Jeffers, W. A., and Rose, E. (1957). *Am. J. Med. Sci.* 233, 10–15.

Ljunggren, J-G., Falkenberg, C., and Savidge, G. (1979). *Acta. Med. Scand.* 205, 267–269.

Lotti, G., Delitala, G., Devilla, L., Alagna, S., and Masala, A. (1977). *Clin. Endocr.* 6, 405–410.

Lumholtz, I. B., Siersbaek-Nielsen, K., Faber, J., Kirkegaard, C., and Friis, T. (1978). *J. Clin. Endocrinol. Metab.* 47, 587–589.

Lyngborg, K., and Jacobsen, J. G. (1972). *Acta Med. Scand.* 192, 427–431.

McDevitt, D. G., Shanks, R. G., Hadden, D. R., Montgomery, D. A. D., and Weaver, J. A. (1968). *Lancet* 1, 998–1000.

McLarty, D. G., Ratcliffe, W. A., McColl, K., Stone, D., and Ratcliffe, J. G. (1975). *Lancet* 2, 275–276.

McNeill, J. H. (1977). *Res. Commun. Chem. Pathol. Pharmacol.* 16, 735–743.

McNeill, J. H. (1978). *Recent Adv. Stud. Card. Struct. Metab.* 11, 413–418.

McNeill, J. H., and Brody, T. M. (1968). *J. Pharmacol. Exp. Ther.* 161, 40–46.

McNeill, J. H., Muschek, L. D., and Brody, T. M. (1969). *Can. J. Physiol. Pharmacol.* **47**, 913–916.

Mahoney, C. P., Pyne, G. E., Stamm, S. J., and Bakke, J. L. (1964). *Am. J. Dis. Child.* **107**, 516–522.

Maisey, M. N., and Stimmler, L. (1972). *Clin. Endocrinol.* **1**, 81–90.

Margolius, H. S., and Gaffney, T. E. (1965). *J. Pharmacol. Exp. Ther.* **149**, 329–335.

Martin, L., and Spathis, G. S. (1965). *Br. Med. J.* **2**, 83–85.

Massey, D. G., Becklake, M. R., McKenzie, J. M., and Bates, D. V. (1967). *N. Engl. J. Med.* **276**, 1104–1112.

Mendelsohn, I. E., Bassett, A., Kelly, J. J., Jr., and Hoffman, B. F. (1961). *Am. J. Cardiol.* **7**, 694–696.

Michels, R., Cason, J., and Sokoloff, L. (1963). *Science* **140**, 1417–1418.

Michie, W., Hamer-Hodges, D. W., Pegg, C. A. S., Orr, F. G. G., and Bewsher, P. D. (1974). *Lancet* **1**, 1009–1011.

Miettinen, T. A. (1968). *J. Lab. Clin. Med.* **71**, 537–547.

Minelli, R., and Korecky, B. (1969). *Can. J. Physiol. Pharmacol.* **47**, 545–552.

Monroe, E. W., and Fearrington, E. L. (1966). *Am. Heart J.* **72**, 94–101.

Morkin, E. (1979). *Circ. Res.* **44**, 1–7.

Morkin, E., Banerjee, S. K., and Stern, L. Z. (1977). *FEBS Lett.* **79**, 357–360.

Mowery, M. B., and Lindsay, H. A. (1973). *Proc. Soc. Exp. Biol. Med.* **143**, 138–140.

Mujtaba, Q., and Burrow, G. N. (1975). *Obstet. Gynecol.* **46**, 282–286.

Murayama, M., and Goodkind, M. J. (1968). *Circ. Res.* **23**, 743–751.

Nauman, J., Nauman, A., and Roszkowska, K. (1974). *Mater. Med. Pol. (Engl. Ed.)* **6**, 178–182.

Nelson, J. C., Palmer, F. J., and Bowyer, A. F. (1974). *Med. Arts Sci.* **28**, 15–22.

Newcomb, M., Gibson, K., and Harris, P. (1978). *Biochem. Biophys. Res. Commun.* **81**, 596–601.

Nicoloff, J. T., Low, J. C., Dussault, J. H., and Fisher, D. A. (1972). *J. Clin. Invest.* **51**, 473–483.

Nielsen, T. P., Bodfish, R. E., and Kabok, A. (1974). *Ann. Intern. Med.* **81**, 126–127.

Nishiki, K., Erecińska, M., Wilson, D. F., and Cooper, S. (1978). *Am. J. Physiol.* **235**, C212–C219.

Nixon, J. V., Anderson, R. J., and Cohen, M. L. (1979). *Am. J. Med.* **67**, 268–276.

Oppenheimer, J. H. (1979). *Science* **203**, 971–979.

Oppenheimer, J. H., and Dillmann, W. H. (1978a). *Clin. Endocrinol. Metab.* **7**, 145–165.

Oppenheimer, J. H., and Dillmann, W. H. (1978b). *Recept. Horm. Action* **3**, 1–33.

Oppenheimer, J. H., Schwartz, H. L., and Surks, M. I. (1974). *Endocrinology* **95**, 897–903.

Oppenheimer, J. H., Schwartz, H. L., and Surks, M. I. (1975). *Endocr. Res. Commun.* **2**, 309–325.

Ørbeck, H. (1973). *Acta Paediatr. Scand.* **62**, 313–316.

Page, E., and McCallister, L. P. (1973). *Am. J. Cardiol.* **31**, 172–181.

Paine, T. D., Rogers, W. J., Baxley, W. A., and Russell, R. O., Jr. (1977). *Am. J. Cardiol.* **40**, 226–231.

Palacios, I., Sagar, K., and Powell, W. J. Jr. (1979). *Am. J. Physiol.* **237**, H293–H298.

Pangaro, L., Smallridge, R. C., Cahnmann, H. J., Wright, F. D., and Burman, K. D. (1979). *Program 61st Annu. Meet. Endocrine Soc.* Abstract 75.

Parisi, A. F., Hamilton, B. P., Thomas, C. N., and Mazzaferri, E. L. (1974). *Circulation* **49**, 900–904.

Parmley, W. W., Spann, J. F., Jr., Taylor, R. R., and Sonnenblick, E. H. (1968). *Proc. Soc. Exp. Biol. Med.* **127**, 606–609.

Peacock, W. F., III, and Moran, N. C. (1963). *Proc. Soc. Exp. Biol. Med.* **113**, 526–530.

Perry, L. W., and Hung, W. (1971). *J. Pediatr.* **79**, 668–671.
Philipson, K. D., and Edelman, I. S. (1977). *Am. J. Physiol.* **232**, C202–C206.
Piatnek-Leunissen, D., and Olson, R. E. (1967). *Circ. Res.* **20**, 242–252.
Pietras, R. J., Real, M. A., Poticha, G. S., Bronsky, D., and Waldstein, S. S. (1972). *Arch. Intern. Med.* **129**, 426–429.
Pimstone, B., and Joffe, B. (1970). *S. Afr. Med. J.* **44**, 1059–1061.
Plotnick, G. D., Vassar, D. L., Parisi, A. F., Hamilton, B. P., Carliner, N. H., and Fisher, M. L. (1979). *Am. J. Med. Sci.* **277**, 263–268.
Proskey, A. J., Saksena, F., and Towne, W. D. (1977). *Chest* **72**, 109–111.
Rabinowitz, J. L., and Hercker, E. S. (1971). *Science* **173**, 1242–1243.
Reith, A., and Fuchs, S. (1973). *Lab. Invest.* **29**, 229–235.
Resnekov, L., and Falicov, R. E. (1977). *Br. Heart J.* **39**, 1051–1057.
Reynolds, J. L., and Woody, H. B. (1971). *Am. J. Dis. Child* **122**, 544–548.
Riddle, M. C., and Schwartz, T. B. (1970). *Ann. Intern. Med.* **72**, 749–750.
Rosen, A., and Moran, N. C. (1963). *Circ. Res.* **12**, 479–486.
Rosenberg, D., Grand, M. J. H., and Silbert, D. (1963). *N. Engl. J. Med.* **268**, 292–296.
Rovetto, M. J., Hjalmarson, Ä. C., Morgan, H. E., Barrett, M. J., and Goldstein, R. A. (1972). *Circ. Res.* **31**, 397–409.
Rowe, G. G., Huston, J. H., Weinstein, A. B., Tuchman, H., Brown, J. F., and Crumpton, C. W. (1956). *J. Clin. Invest.* **35**, 272–276.
Rubenfeld, S., Silverman, V. E., Welch, K. M. A., Mallette, L. E., and Kohler, P. O. (1979). *N. Engl. J. Med.* **300**, 353–354.
Rubler, S., Arvan, S. B., Rafii, F., Shah, N., and Olowe, O. (1977). *Angiology* **28**, 702–711.
Sachs, M. L. (1961). *J. Chronic Dis.* **14**, 515–536.
Samuels, H. H., Stanley, F., and Shapiro, L. E. (1976). *Proc. Natl. Acad. Sci. U.S.A.* **73**, 3877–3881.
Sandler, G. (1959). *Br. Heart J.* **21**, 111–116.
Sandler, G., and Wilson, G. M. (1959). *Q. J. Exp. Physiol. Cogn. Med. Sci.* **44**, 282–289.
Sanford, C. F., Griffin, E. E., and Wildenthal, K. (1978). *Circ. Res.* **43**, 688–694.
Santos, A. D., Miller, R. P., Wallace, W. A., Mathew, P. K., and Hinojosa, L. (1978). *Clin. Res.* **26**, 268A.
Scheinberg, P., Stead, E. A., Jr., Brannon, E. S., and Warren, J. V. (1950). *J. Clin. Invest.* **29**, 1139–1146.
Scott, J. C., Balourdas, T. A., and Croll, M. N. (1961). *Am. J. Cardiol.* **7**, 690–693.
Scott, J. C., Finkelstein, L. J., and Croll, M. N. (1962). *Am. J. Cardiol.* **10**, 840–845.
Segal, J., and Gordon, A. (1977a). *Endocrinology* **101**, 150–156.
Segal, J., and Gordon, A. (1977b). *Endocrinology* **101**, 1468–1474.
Segal, J., Schwartz, H., and Gordon, A. (1977). *Endocrinology* **101**, 143–149.
Shapiro, S., Steier, M., and Dimich, I. (1975). *Clin. Pediatr. (Philadelphia)* **14**, 1155–1156.
Sharma, V. K., and Banerjee, S. P. (1978a). *J. Biol. Chem.* **253**, 5277–5279.
Sharma, V. K., and Banerjee, S. P. (1978b). *Biochim. Biophys. Acta* **539**, 538–542.
Singh, J. B., Starobin, O. E., Guerrant, R. L., and Manders, E. K. (1973). *Chest* **63**, 582–585.
Skelton, C. L., Coleman, H. N., Wildenthal, K., and Braunwald, E. (1970). *Circ. Res.* **27**, 301–309.
Skelton, C. L., Pool, P. E., Seagren, S. C., and Braunwald, E. (1971). *J. Clin. Invest.* **50**, 463–473.
Skelton, C. L., Karch, F. E., and Wildenthal, K. (1973). *Am. J. Physiol.* **224**, 957–962.
Smallridge, R. C., Wartofsky, L., Chopra, I. J., Marinelli, P. V., Broughton, R. E., Dimond, R. C., and Burman, K. D. (1978a). *J. Pediatr.* **93**, 118–120.

Smallridge, R. C., Wartofsky, L., Desjardins, R. E., and Burman, K. D. (1978b). *J. Clin. Endocrinol. Metab.* **47**, 345–349.

Smallridge, R. C., Latham, K. R., Ward, K. E., Dimond, R. C., Wartofsky, L., and Burman, K. D. (1978c). *Program 54th Annu. Meet. Am. Thyroid Assoc.* T-7.

Smallridge, R. C., Wartofsky, L., Green, B. J., Miller, F. C., and Burman, K. D. (1979a). *J. Clin. Endocrinol. Metab.* **48**, 32–36.

Smallridge, R. C., Latham, K. R., Ward, K. E., Wartofsky, L., and Burman, K. D. (1979b). *Clin. Res.* **27**, 260A.

Smallridge, R. C., Smith, C. E., Wright, F. D., and Wartofsky, L. (1979c). *Program 61st Annu. Meet. Endocrine Soc.* Abstract 74.

Smith, C. S., and Howard, N. J. (1973). *J. Pediatr.* **83**, 1046–1048.

Smolar, E. N., Rubin, J. E., Avramides, A., and Carter, A. C. (1976). *Am. J. Med. Sci.* **272**, 345–352.

Smyth, C. J. (1938). *Am. Heart J.* **15**, 652–660.

Sobel, B. E., Dempsey, P. J., and Cooper, T. (1969). *Proc. Soc. Exp. Biol. Med.* **132**, 6–9.

Spindler, B. J., MacLeod, K. M., Ring, J., and Baxter, J. D. (1975). *J. Biol. Chem.* **250**, 4113–4119.

Starling, J. R., and Thomas, C. G., Jr. (1977). *World J. Surg.* **1**, 251–257.

Steffen, D. G., and Platner, W. S. (1976). *Am. J. Physiol.* **231**, 650–654.

Steinberg, A. D. (1968). *Ann. Intern. Med.* **68**, 338–344.

Steinberg, A. D., and Schrader, Z. R. (1971). *Lancet* **2**, 213.

Sterling, K. (1979). *N. Engl. J. Med.* **300**, 117–123, 173–177.

Sterling, K., Milch, P. O., Brenner, M. A., and Lazarus, J. H. (1977). *Science* **197**, 996–999.

Sterling, K., Lazarus, J. H., Milch, P. O., Sakurada, T., and Brenner, M. A. (1978). *Science* **201**, 1126–1129.

Stern, M. P., Jacobs, R. L., and Duncan, G. W. (1970). *J. Am. Med. Assoc.* **212**, 2117–2119.

Stewart, H. J., Deitrick, J. E., and Crane, N. F. (1938). *J. Clin. Invest.* **17**, 237–248.

Stocker, W. W., Samaha, F. J., and Degroot, L. J. (1968). *Am. J. Med.* **44**, 900–909.

Strauer, B. E., and Scherpe, A. (1975). *Basic Res. Cardiol.* **70**, 115–129.

Strauer, B. E., and Schulze, W. (1976). *Basic Res. Cardiol.* **71**, 624–644.

Suko, J. (1971). *Biochim. Biophys. Acta* **252**, 324–327.

Suko, J., and Hasselbach, W. (1976). *Eur. J. Biochem.* **64**, 123–130.

Summers, V. K., and Surtees, S. J. (1961). *Acta Med. Scand.* **169**, 661–671.

Sunshine, P., Kusumoto, H., and Kriss, J. P. (1965). *Pediatrics* **36**, 869–876.

Sutherland, E. W., and Robison, G. A. (1966). *Pharmacol. Rev.* **18**, 145–161.

Symons, C., Olsen, E. G. J., and Hawkey, C. M. (1975). *J. Endocrinol.* **65**, 341–346.

Tarjan, E. M. (1971). *Endocrinology* **88**, 833–844.

Tarjan, E. M., and Kimata, S-I. (1971). *Endocrinology* **89**, 385–396.

Tata, J. R. (1963). *Nature (London)* **197**, 1167–1168.

Taylor, R. R. (1970). *Circ. Res.* **27**, 539–549.

Taylor, R. R., Covell, J. W., and Ross, J., Jr. (1969). *J. Clin. Invest.* **48**, 775–784.

Theilade, P., Hansen, J. M., Skovsted, L., Faber, J., Kirkegård, C., Friis, T., and Siersbaek-Nielsen, K. (1977). *Lancet* **2**, 363.

Theilen, E. O., and Wilson, W. R. (1967). *J. Appl. Physiol.* **22**, 207–210.

Thompson, E. B. (1973). *J. Pharm. Sci.* **62**, 1638–1643.

Thomson, J. E., Baird, S. G., and Thomson, J. A. (1979). *Am. Heart J.* **97**, 406–407.

Thyrum, P. T., Kritcher, E. M., and Luchi, R. J. (1970). *Biochim. Biophys. Acta* **197**, 335–336.

Toft, A. D., Irvine, W. J., and Campbell, R. W. F. (1976). *Clin. Endocrinol. (Oxford)* **5**, 195–198.

Toft, A. D., Irvine, W. J., Sinclair, I., McIntosh, D., Seth, J., and Cameron, E. H. D. (1978). *N. Engl. J. Med.* **298**, 643–647.

Tommaselli, A., Gravina, E., and Roche, J. (1965). *In* "Current Topics in Thyroid Research" (C. Cassano and M. Andreoli, eds.), pp. 382–393. Academic Press, New York.

Tsai, J.-S. (1975). *Clin. Res.* **23**, 243A.

Tsai, J.-S., and Chen, A. (1976). *Science* **194**, 202–204.

Tsai, J.-S., and Chen, A. (1978). *Nature* **275**, 138–140.

Ueda, H., Sugishita, Y., Nakanishi, A., Ito, I., Yasuda, H., Sugiura, M., Takabatake, Y., Ueda, K., Koide, T., and Ozeki, K. (1965). *Jpn. Heart J.* **6**, 396–406.

Urschel, D. L., and Gates, G. E. (1953). *Am. Heart J.* **45**, 611–622.

Valcana, T., and Timiras, P. S. (1977). *Proc. Intern. Congr. Endocrinol., 5th 1976* 579A.

van der Schoot, J. B., and Moran, N. C. (1965). *J. Pharmacol. Exp. Ther.* **149**, 336–345.

Van Liere, E. J., Sizemore, D. A., and Hunnell, J. (1969). *Proc. Soc. Exp. Biol. Med.* **132**, 663–665.

van Noorden, C. J. F., Wiersinga, W. M., and Touber, J. L. (1979). *Horm. Metab. Res.* **11**, 366–370.

Verhoeven, R. P., Visser, T. J., Docter, R., Hennemann, G., and Schalekamp, M. A. D. H. (1977). *J. Clin. Endocrinol. Metab.* **44**, 1002–1005.

Walsh, D. A., Perkins, J. P., Broström, C. O., Ho, E. S., and Krebs, E. G. (1971). *J. Biol. Chem.* **246**, 1968–1976.

Wartofsky, L., Dimond, R. C., Noel, G. L., Frantz, A. G., and Earll, J. M. (1975). *J. Clin. Endocrinol. Metab.* **41**, 485–490.

Watanakunakorn, C., Hodges, R. E., and Evans, T. C. (1965). *Arch. Intern. Med.* **116**, 183–190.

Wei, J. Y., Genecin, A., Greene, H. L., and Achuff, S. C. (1979). *Am. J. Cardiol.* **43**, 335–339.

White, C. (1912). *J. Obstet. Gynaecol. Br. Emp.* **21**, 231–233.

White, C. W., and Zimmerman, T. J. (1976). *Circulation* **54**, 890–895.

Whitehorn, W. V., Ullrick, W. C., and Andersen, B. R. (1959). *Circ. Res.* **7**, 250–255.

Wiener, L., Stout, B. D., and Cox, J. W. (1969). *Am. J. Med.* **46**, 227–233.

Wiersinga, W. M., and Touber, J. L. (1977). *J. Clin. Endocrinol. Metab.* **45**, 293–298.

Wildenthal, K. (1971). *Am. J. Physiol.* **221**, 238–241.

Wildenthal, K. (1972). *J. Clin. Invest.* **51**, 2702–2709.

Wildenthal, K., and Mueller, E. A. (1974). *Nature (London)* **249**, 478–479.

Williams, L. T., Lefkowitz, R. J., Watanabe, A. M., Hathaway, D. R., and Besch, H. R., Jr. (1977). *J. Biol. Chem.* **252**, 2787–2789.

Wilson, W. R., Theilen, E. O., and Fletcher, F. W. (1964). *J. Clin. Invest.* **43**, 1697–1703.

Wilson, W. R., Theilen, E. O., Hege, J. H., and Valenca, M. R. (1966). *J. Clin. Invest.* **45**, 1159–1169.

Wilson, W. R., Theilen, E. O., and Connor, W. E. (1967). *Proc. Soc. Exp. Biol. Med.* **124**, 298–303.

Wiswell, J. G., and Braverman, M. G. (1957). *Endocrinology* **61**, 153–159.

Wollenberger, A., Krause, E.-G., and Macho, L. (1964). *Nature (London)* **201**, 789–791.

Wong, T. C. Y., Barzilai, D. C., Smith, R. E., and McConahey, W. M. (1979). *Mayo Clin. Proc.* **54**, 763–768.

Wrenn, S., and Haber, E. (1979). *J. Biol. Chem.* **254**, 6577–6582.

Yazaki, Y., and Raben, M. S. (1975). *Circ. Res.* **36**, 208–215.

Yazaki, Y., Ueda, S., Nagai, R., and Shimada, K. (1979). *Circ. Res.* **45**, 522–527.

Young, B. A., and McNeill, J. H. (1974). *Can. J. Physiol. Pharmacol.* **52**, 375–383.

Young, R. T., Van Herle, A. J., and Rodbard, D. (1976). *J. Clin. Endocrinol. Metab.* **42**, 330–340.

Zaimis, E., Papadaki, L., Ash, A. S. F., Larbi, E., Kakari, S., Matthew, M., and Paradelis, A. (1969). *Cardiovasc. Res.* **3**, 118–133.

Zondek, H. (1964). *Br. Heart J.* **26**, 227–232.

Zonszein, J., Santangelo, R. P., Mackin, J. F., Lee, T. C., Coffey, R. J., and Canary, J. J. (1979). *Am. J. Med.* **66**, 411–416.

Zwillich, C. W., Matthay, M., Potts, D. E., Adler, R., Hofeldt, F., and Weil, J. V. (1978). *J. Clin. Endocrinol. Metab.* **46**, 491–500.

4

Catecholamines and the Heart

William M. Manger

I. Historical Background

In 1921 Otto Loewi made the important discovery that stimulation of the cardiac sympathetic nerves of the isolated perfused turtle heart resulted in an increase in the heart's rate and force of contraction. He further demonstrated that following stimulation of these nerves, the fluid perfusing the heart was capable of enhancing the rate and contraction of another isolated heart. His brilliant experiments firmly established that stimulation of cardiac sympathetic nerves resulted in the liberation of a chemical substance that could account for the chronotropic and inotropic effects on the heart. This then laid the foundation for the current concept of the mechanism of sympathetic nerve transmission.

About 12 years later Cannon and Rosenbluth (1933) demonstrated that the substance released by stimulating cardioaccelerator nerves entered the circulation and could cause a response in other organs (e.g., contraction of the nictitating membrane in the cat sensitized to cocaine). Since extracts of the heart produced biologic effects that resembled those caused by epinephrine, Cannon and Lissak (1939) concluded that sympathetic nerves contained epinephrine. A few years later Simeone and Sarnoff (1947) found that contraction of the nictitating membrane following cardioaccelerator nerve stimulation could be prevented by administering the adrenergic blocking agent, dibenamine. During the same period Hoffmann and coworkers observed that adding acetylcholine to an isolated mammalian heart preparation resulted in liberation of an epinephrinelike substance from the heart (Hoffmann *et al.,* 1945). However, it was von Euler who, in 1946, established the fact that the sympathetic neurotransmitter (i.e., the sympathomimetic substance liberated during sympathetic nerve stimulation) was norepinephrine. A few years later Goodall (1950) quantitated the content of norepinephrine and epinephrine in cattle heart and Raab and Gigee (1955) reported studies on the concentrations of these biogenic amines in normal and diseased human hearts.

From an evolutionary viewpoint it is interesting that epinephrine and norepinephrine are present in high concentrations in chromaffin cells lining the heart cavities of cyclostomes and the Pacific hagfish, primitive vertebrates (Bloom *et al.,* 1961; Chapman *et al.,* 1963). As stated by Braunwald and associates, this finding provides strong morphological evidence that even the hearts of organisms on a relatively low phylogenetic scale contain cells capable of secreting epinephrine and norepinephrine (Braunwald *et al.,* 1964).

In the mammalian heart the neurotransmitter, norepinephrine, is located in storage vesicles in the sympathetic nerves and not in the myocardial cells. Observations by Outschoorn and Vogt (1952) and Siegel and associates

(1961) revealed that stimulation of the cardioaccelerator nerves resulted in a marked elevation of the concentration of norepinephrine in coronary sinus blood and even some increase of the concentration in arterial blood. Then in 1962 and 1963 several investigators found that release of significant amounts of norepinephrine from the heart could be induced by a number of vasoactive agents (e.g., tyramine, quanethidine, reserpine, bretylium); furthermore, the amount released was enough to cause sympathomimetic responses (Chidsey *et al.,* 1962a; Gaffney *et al.,* 1962a,b; Harrison *et al.,* 1963).

Braunwald and co-workers made additional observations that indicated that the norepinephrine released by electrical stimulation of the sympathetic nerves to the dog heart could elevate arterial blood pressure by a peripheral effect. They pointed out that

the overflow of norepinephrine into the venous blood is of greater magnitude in the coronary vascular bed than in other vascular beds for three reasons: First, there is a relatively large total quantity of norepinephrine in the heart. Secondly, the basal perfusion rate of the heart per unit weight of tissue exceeds that of the spleen, liver and limbs, organs which contain smaller although still substantial quantities of norepinephrine. This relatively high perfusion rate facilitates the delivery of norepinephrine released from sympathetic nerve endings into the coronary venous blood prior to its return to the nerve endings or its enzymatic degradation. Finally, the vasodilatation in the coronary bed consequent to sympathetic nerve stimulation also aids passage of the neurohormone into the coronary venous blood, whereas the vasoconstrictor response to sympathetic stimulation in other vascular beds impedes the overflow of norepinephrine into the venous blood [Braunwald *et al.,* 1964].

In light of the facts cited in the foregoing historical review plus evidence that the isolated mammalian heart is capable of biosynthesis and storage of norepinephrine (Chidsey *et al.,* 1963b; Spector *et al.,* 1963), Braunwald and co-workers (1964) suggested the intriguing concept that the heart can function as a neuroendocrine organ.

During the past two decades there has been an explosion of information regarding catecholamine biosynthesis, storage, secretion, inactivation, receptors, and pharmacology. Considerable light has been shed on the important role catecholamines may play in a variety of diseases. In this chapter an attempt is made to present some of the current concepts of catecholamines and their effects on the mammalian heart. A potentially successful human cardiac transplantation (i.e., an extrinsically denervated heart that does not become reinervated) has caused some to deny the importance of neural regulation of the heart under normal physiological conditions. However, evidence has accumulated that now indicates that the autonomic nerves to the heart not only influence heart rate, contractile force, and atrial, ventricular, and systemic blood pressures, but also influence velocities and patterns of conduction, electrophysiological properties of different portions of the heart, rhythmicity of contraction, and coronary blood flow. Furthermore, it seems likely that local metabolic reactions, membrane ionic mechanisms, and intracardiac reflexes may be modulated by either or both of the sympathetic and parasympathetic cardiac nerves (Randall, 1977, p. 8).

II. Catecholamine Metabolism: Biosynthesis, Storage, Release, and Inactivation

A. General Remarks

Nomenclature, Occurrence, and Metabolism

Basic to an understanding of the function and pathophysiology of the catecholamines is a knowledge of the biosynthesis and inactivation of these biogenic amines. The term "catecholamine" refers to any compound composed of a catechol nucleus (a benzene ring with two adjacent hydroxyl groups) and an amine-containing side chain; these substances are of low molecular weight. The catecholamines known to occur in man are dopamine, norepinephrine, and epinephrine. They are importantly involved in neural and endocrine function.

Dopamine appears to serve as a neurotransmitter in the central nervous system and to a minor extent in some sympathetic ganglia. As will be mentioned later, there is accumulating evidence that dopaminergic nerves and receptors exert unique functions in the brain and elsewhere (Goldberg, 1974; Moskowitz and Wurtman, 1975a,b); however, this amine functions as a precursor for norepinephrine. Epinephrine and norepinephrine are of major importance in affecting metabolism and cardiovascular physiology. Biosynthesis of these amines occurs in the sympathetic neurons (mainly the nerve endings), brain, and chromaffin tissue. Both norepinephrine and epinephrine are synthesized in some chromaffin cells and parts of the brain, whereas only norepinephrine is synthesized in the postganglionic sympathetic nerves, where it serves the important function of the neurotransmitter (mediator of nerve activity) at most postganglionic sympathetic endings in the autonomic nervous system. All the enzymes necessary for conversion of the amino acid L-tyrosine to norepinephrine are present in the nerve ending, where the bulk of norepinephrine is synthesized and stored. Neurons that liberate catecholamines are called "sympathetic" or "adrenergic neurons." In the fetus the adrenal (Hökfelt, 1951; West *et al.*, 1951) and organ of Zuckerkandl (collections of chromaffin cells located anterior to the abdominal aorta just above its bifurcation and extending to the origin of the inferior mesenteric artery) (West *et al.*, 1951, 1953) contain only norepinephrine; however, epinephrine also appears in these organs within one year following birth (West *et al.,* 1953). The sites of norepinephrine storage in tissue are indicated in Table I.

Although norepinephrine and epinephrine are secreted into the blood, where they can be demonstrated in minute concentrations in the free (unconjugated) form, the presence of free dopamine in the blood of normal subjects was not quantitatively reported until 1973 (Christensen, 1973). More recently, with the use of a very sensitive assay, dopamine has been detected, although only sporadically, in a few normotensive and hypertensive subjects, and it has been suggested that the plasma concentration of this amine is independent of sympathetic activity (de Champlain *et al.,* 1976). In peripheral blood about 80% of norepinephrine and epinephrine and almost 100% of dopamine are conjugated (Buu and Kuchel, 1977; Kuchel *et al.,* 1977). All three catecholamines are, however, present in urine in both the free and conjugated form.

Figure 1 reveals the pathways of biosynthesis and metabolism of catecholamines and indicates the enzymes catalyzing the various reactions. The biosynthesis, storage, release, and inactivation of the catecholamines in sympathetic nerves and chromaffin cells will now be considered.

B. Sympathetic Nerves

1. Biosynthesis, Storage, and Release of Norepinephrine

Figure 2 reveals a schematic representation of the biosynthesis, storage, and secretion of norepinephrine in a sympathetic nerve ending. Each sympathetic nerve may contain as many as 25,000 varicosities (or "buttons"), which simply represent thickenings or bulges, at the nerve ending and along the course of the fibers, where norepinephrine is synthesized and stored in granulated vesicles. In addition to the norepinephrine contained in these latter organelles (i.e., synaptic vesicles) an intracellular pool of "free" norepinephrine is also assumed to exist (Moskowitz and Wurtman, 1975a,b). Most of the varicosities, which contain high concentrations of norepinephrine, lie in close proximity to effector (target) cells and represent synaptic regions of the sympathetic nerve terminals (Hillarp, 1959).

L-Tyrosine from the blood is thought to be transported across the membrane of the sympathetic nerves by a special concentrating mechanism. It is then converted by the enzyme tyrosine hydroxylase, which is found only within catecholamine-producing cells, to L-dihydroxyphenylalanine (dopa). This reaction, which requires tetrahydropteridine as a cofactor, proceeds slowly *in vivo* and is considered the rate-limiting step in the biosynthesis of the catecholamines (Kaufman and Friedman, 1965; Levitt *et al.,* 1965). Tyrosine hydroxylase is inhibited by catecholamines, and this inhibition

TABLE I

Sites of Norepinephrine Storage in Tissue[a,b]

Organ	Cell	Relative amount	Present in granulated vesicle
Brain and spinal cord	Adrenergic neuron Cell body Nerve ending	Moderate Very large	No Partly
Sympathetic ganglia	Adrenergic neuron Cell body	Small	No
Organs with sympathetic innervation (i.e., heart, spleen, liver, kidney, muscle, salivary gland)	Adrenergic neuron Sympathetic nerve ending Extraneural pool (in parenchymal cells)	Very large (most of the norepinephrine in the body) Small	Yes (adrenergic vesicle) No
Adrenal medulla (and extramedullary chromaffin cells)	Chromaffin cell	Very large	Yes (chromaffin granule)
Uterus	Parenchyma (?)	Moderate	No

[a] From Wurtman (1966, p. 17), reprinted by permission.

[b] The concentrations of norepinephrine in the adrenergic cell body and nerve ending have been estimated to be 10–100 and 10,000 $\mu g/g$, respectively.

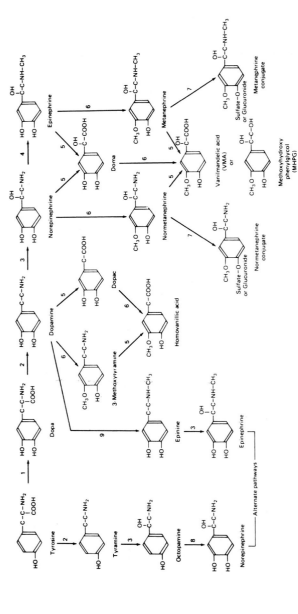

Fig. 1. Pathways of synthesis and metabolism of catecholamines with enzymes catalyzing various reactions. (1) Tyrosine hydroxylase; (2) aromatic amino acid decarboxylase; (3) phenylamine β-hydroxylase; (4) phenylethanol-amine N-methyltransferase; (5) monoamine oxidase plus aldehyde dehydrogenase; (6) catechol O-methyltransferase; (7) conjugating enzymes; (8) rabbit liver enzyme; (9) rabbit lung enzyme. (From Manger and Gifford, 1977, reprinted by permission.)

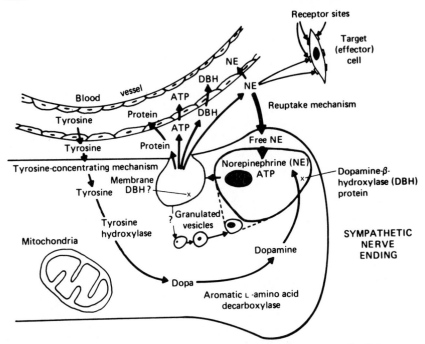

Fig. 2. Intracellular movements of substrates in the biosynthesis of norepinephrine; secretion via exocytosis of storage granules, and theoretical "recycling" of granule. (From Manger and Gifford, 1977, reprinted by permission.)

appears important in controlling the rate of biosynthesis of norepinephrine in the sympathetic nerves (Nagatsu *et al.*, 1964). Dopa, in turn, is rapidly decarboxylated to L-dihydroxyphenylethylamine (dopamine) by aromatic L-amino acid decarboxylase in the cytoplasm of the neurons. This second step proceeds rapidly and requires pyridoxal phosphate as a cofactor. Dopa decarboxylase is widely distributed even in tissues that do not normally synthesize catecholamines, and its high activity in kidney may explain the large amounts of dopamine found in urine.

Dopamine then enters minute granulated vesicles (400–600 Å) in the sympathetic nerve terminals, where it is then finally hydroxylated by dopamine-β-hydroxylase (DβH) to *l*-norepinephrine. DβH is found only in cells that produce norepinephrine. This third enzymatic reaction requires O_2 and ascorbic and fumaric acids as cofactors. Norepinephrine, the neurotransmitter, remains inactive and protected in these storage vesicles until released by activation of the sympathetic nerves. A small amount of norepinephrine leaks from these granules into the surrounding cytoplasm, but these vesicles also have the capacity to take up and bind norepinephrine from the cytoplasm. It is believed that excitation of the sympathetic nerves results in a process of exocytosis (emiocytosis, or "cell vomiting") whereby storage granules move, perhaps via microtubules, to the surface of the sympathetic nerve membrane, where they expel their contents into the extracellular fluid and circulation (Weinshilboum *et al.*, 1971). The contents of these vesicles consist of norepinephrine and adenosine triphosphate (ATP) in perhaps a 4:1 molar ratio, plus soluble DβH, and a small amount of protein (other than DβH) which is called chromogranin. It is possible that the empty vesicles are then reutilized (recycled) for the synthesis and storage of norepinephrine.

Primarily because of an efficient reuptake mechanism, a relatively small fraction of physiologically active neurotransmitter reaches receptors on the target (effector) cells and thereby activates these cells (e.g., vascular smooth muscle, myocardium, adipocyte, myometrium, or hepatocyte; receptors also exist at presynaptic neural sites). Even intense activation of the sympathetic nervous system may cause no appreciable increase in the plasma concentration of norepinephrine (Manger *et al.*, 1975). This finding is probably explained by the efficient reuptake mechanism and enzymatic degradation, which prevent norepinephrine from overflowing into the circulation in significant amounts. It is assumed that the relatively small amount of norepinephrine that reaches the circulation does so by a process of diffusion; however, there are no experimental studies that either validate or refute this concept.

The physiological response of target cells to injected or secreted catecholamines depends on (1) the fraction of catecholamine delivered to the target cell (this can vary with the state of the circulation); (2) the ability of the cell to inactivate the delivered catecholamines; and (3) the sensitivity of the target cell (Wurtman, 1966, p. 33).

Release of norepinephrine and DβH is enhanced by calcium ions and by some α-adrenergic blocking agents (e.g., phenoxybenzamine and phentolamine). This enhanced release can be inhibited by prostaglandin E$_2$, perhaps due to prostaglandin's interference with availability of Ca^{2+} (Axelrod, 1973).

During the past few years evidence has accumulated for the existence of a presynaptic regulation of norepinephrine release from adrenergic nerves (Langer, 1974). It has been postulated that norepinephrine released by nerve stimulation (once it reaches a threshold concentration in the synaptic gap) activates presynaptic α-receptors, triggering a negative feedback mechanism that inhibits further release of the neurotransmitter. Compatible with this hypothesis is the fact that α-receptor agonists inhibit, whereas α-receptors antagonists enhance, norepinephrine release by nerve stimulation. It now appears that, in addition to α-receptors in adrenergic nerve endings, there are dopaminergic and muscarinic receptors that are inhibitory to neurotransmitter release, and there are also nicotinic receptors that elicit norepinephrine release (Langer, 1974). The existence of a presynaptic β-adrenergic receptor seems to be an equally plausible concept: stimulation of a presynaptic β-receptor would enhance the norepinephrine release during adrenergic stimulation and thus constitute a positive feedback control of neurotransmitter secretion. Recently Stjärne and Brundin (1975) have demonstrated a dual adrenoceptor-mediated control of norepinephrine secretion from human vasoconstrictor nerves, i.e., a facilitation by β-receptors and an inhibition by α-receptors in the presynaptic region. From their elegant experimental observations it was suggested that low sensitivity for α-adrenoceptors can only be triggered by high concentrations of norepinephrine occurring in the synaptic cleft. On the other hand, the extremely high sensitivity of β-adrenoceptors should enable them to detect physiological concentrations of circulating catecholamines. These latter receptors may thus subserve the function of enhancing secretion of norepinephrine from synaptic nerves during conditions of increased secretion of epinephrine from the adrenal medulla. However, high epinephrine concentrations may depress norepinephrine secretion from synaptic nerves by stimulating the less sensitive α-adrenergic-mediated control mechanism.

It also appears that other presynaptic receptor systems exist that can modify catecholaminergic transmission: angiotensin II has been shown to increase the release of norepinephrine evoked by electrical stimulation of noradrenergic neurons, whereas some prostaglandins (PGE_1 and PGE_2) and some narcotic analgesics decrease release of the neurotransmitter (Starke et al., 1977).

2. Inactivation of Norepinephrine

a. CATABOLISM

Inactivation of norephrine occurs in several ways. The norepinephrine that is free in the cytoplasm of sympathetic nerves may be deaminated by monoamine oxidase (MAO) plus aldehyde dehydrogenase in mitochondria to form an unstable aldehyde, which can then be oxidized to an acid, 3,4-dihydroxymandelic acid (DHMA or DOMA); or norepinephrine may be reduced to an alcohol, dihydroxyphenylglycol (DHPG). The reduction product predominates in the rat, whereas the oxidation product predominates in man (Axelrod et al., 1959).

MAO, which is widely distributed and is particularly abundant in the brain, liver, and kidney, was once considered to play a key role in terminating the physiological action of the catecholamines. This enzyme is now thought to be primarily concerned with disposing of excess stores of catecholamines (Kopin, 1964). On the other hand, the norepinephrine that is released into the circulation is largely converted by meta-O-methylation to normetanephrine by the action of catechol O-methyltransferase (COMT) (Axelrod *et al.,* 1958; LaBrosse *et al.,* 1958). COMT, first identified by Axelrod (1957), is present in almost all tissues and particularly concentrated in liver and kidney. Although COMT has been considered to be located in extraneuronal sites, there is recent evidence of an intraneuronal location in some tissues (Goldberg and Marsden, 1975); it does not, however, appear to be present in very significant amounts in sympathetic nerves. COMT requires S-adenosylmethionine as the methyl donor. The biosynthesis, storage, secretion, and catabolism of norepinephrine in the sympathetic nerve is diagrammatically illustrated in Fig. 3.

Further degradation of normetanephrine and metanephrine by MAO and of 3,4-dihydroxymandelic acid by COMT in cells elsewhere in the body results in the formation of 3-methoxy-4-hydroxymandelic acid (VMA). A small amount of methoxyhydroxyphenylglycol (MHPG) is generated by the

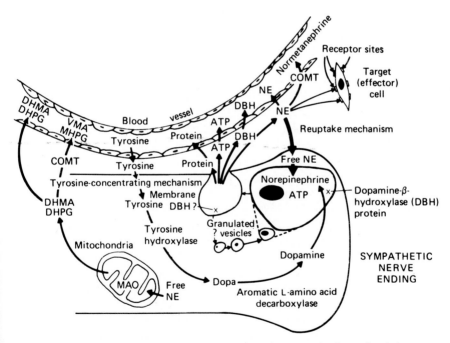

Fig. 3. Intracellular movements of substrates in the biosynthesis of norepinephrine; secretion via exocytosis of storage granules, and theoretical "recycling" of granule, and catabolism. COMT, Catechol O-methyltransferase (in cells); MAO, monoamine oxidase (in mitochondria); DHMA, dihydroxymandelic acid; DHPG, dihydroxyphenylglycol; VMA, vanillylmandelic acid; MHPG, methoxyhydroxyphenylglycol. (From Manger and Gifford, 1977, reprinted by permission.)

enzymatic reaction of MAO with metanephrine and normetanephrine, and by the reaction of COMT with dihydroxyphenylglycol. Some free norepinephrine and normetanephrine are converted to glucuronide and/or sulfate conjugates (Buu and Kuchel, 1977), which are biologically inert, as are the metabolites formed by the action of MAO and COMT (Evarts *et al.*, 1958; LaBrosse *et al.*, 1958).

b. Uptake and Binding

The inactivation of catecholamines entering the blood is extremely rapid. For example, radioactive norepinephrine and epinephrine, when injected into animals in physiological concentrations, have an initial half-life of 10–30 sec (Weil-Malherbe *et al.*, 1959; Whitby *et al.*, 1961; Wurtman, 1966). Vendsalu reported the half-life in plasma of norepinephrine infused into humans to be 2.3 min (Vendsalu, 1960).

The fate of the catecholamines in the circulation depends largely on the organs to which they are delivered (Wurtman, 1966, p. 27). Organs richly innervated with sympathetic nerves (e.g., heart and spleen) take up circulating catecholamines and bind most of them in a physiologically inactive form in the storage vesicles of sympathetic nerve endings. On the other hand, organs containing relatively high concentrations of COMT and MAO (e.g., liver and kidney) convert the catecholamines to their metabolites (i.e., normetanephrine, metanephrine, VMA, or MHPG). Because of the blood–brain barrier, only the hypothalamus takes up detectable amounts of catecholamines (Weil-Malherbe *et al.*, 1959).

Manger and co-workers (1959) and LaBrosse and Hertting (1964) demonstrated the remarkable ability of the liver to clear 85% or more of the catecholamines from the circulation. The heart extracts 70 or 80% of these amines from the circulation during a single passage (Wurtman *et al.*, 1963).

Rapid removal and physiological disposition of catecholamines from the circulation cannot be entirely accounted for by sympathetic nerve uptake (Vane, 1969). Avakian and Gillespie (1967, 1968) found that norepinephrine is taken up *in vitro*, not only by adrenergic nerves but also by smooth muscle, collagen, and elastic tissue, and they suggested that smooth muscle cells have a transport mechanism for intracellular norepinephrine uptake. Kaumann (1972) obtained results consistent with a saturable extraneuronal mechanism with high affinity for norepinephrine. Even catecholamine entry into blood cells has been demonstrated (Manger and Gifford, 1977, pp. 15, 16).

Thus there are "specific" (neuronal) and "nonspecific" (extraneuronal) catecholamine storage sites. The uptake of catecholamines by sympathetic nerves (uptake$_1$) and extraneuronal uptake of catecholamines (uptake$_2$) have been reviewed and studied by Iverson (1975a); however, the mechanisms and importance of extraneuronal catecholamine uptake are complex and have not been adequately investigated. The most important mechanisms for removing and inactivating circulating catecholamines are uptake into sympathetic nerves and metabolic degradation by the enzyme COMT (Axelrod, 1963).

c. REUPTAKE MECHANISM

Of major importance in terminating the physiological action of norepinephrine released at the sympathetic nerve terminals is the neuronal reuptake process. This high-affinity neuronal uptake is stereoselective and requires sodium; it can be utilized by other amines structurally similar to norepinephrine (e.g., epinephrine, dopamine, tyramine, α-methylnorepinephrine, metaraminol, and amphetamine) (Axelrod, 1973). These structurally related amines can also be taken up by the storage vesicles and displace norepinephrine. Potter and Axelrod (1963) demonstrated that organs having extensive sympathetic nerve innervation take up and store circulating catecholamines in a chemically unchanged form in granulated vesicles of sympathetic nerve terminals. Moskowitz and Wurtman (1957a) have imaginatively likened the release and reuptake of the neurotransmitter to the behavior of a sponge: "the wave of depolarization squeezes the metaphoric sponge, causing catecholamine molecules to drip out into synapses; with repolarization the sponge snaps back into shape, sopping up the catecholamines in the synaptic cleft."

Perhaps as much as 80% of norepinephrine liberated from synaptic nerves into the extracellular fluid is taken up into adjacent synaptic nerve terminals by an active transport mechanism (Fölkow, 1971). Such a reuptake mechanism is of great value to the economy and efficient function of the sympathetic nervous system. To emphasize the importance of the reuptake process in terminating the action of norepinephrine, it should be appreciated that the biologic activity of the catecholamines is promptly terminated even if catabolic degradation is pharmacologically blocked. Hypersensitivity of sympathetically denervated structures to catecholamines may partly be explained by degeneration of sympathetic nerves and disappearance of storage vesicles following nerve section. As a consequence, vesicles are not available to take up the catecholamines, and therefore an excess of these amines is available to stimulate the adrenergic receptors of the denervated structure.

C. Chromaffin Cells

Biosynthesis, Storage, Release, and Inactivation

The biosynthesis, release, and metabolism of norepinephrine in chromaffin cells is essentially the same as that in the sympathetic nerves; however, some chromaffin cells (e.g., certain cells in the adrenal medulla) have the capacity to convert *l*-norepinephrine to *l*-epinephrine. This reaction is brought about by the enzyme phenylethanolamine-*N*-methyltransferase (PNMT), which transfers a methyl group from *S*-adenosylmethionine to the nitrogen position of norepinephrine. In mammalian tissues only the heart, adrenal medulla, brain (Axelrod, 1962), and brainstem (Saavedra *et al.,* 1976) have measurable amounts of this epinephrine-synthesizing enzyme (PNMT). Since PNMT, when present, is located in the cytoplasm of chromaffin cells, norepinephrine must migrate from the chromaffin granule to the cytoplasm for methylation and then return to the granule for storage.

It is noteworthy that enzymes (tyrosine hydroxylase, DβH, and PNMT) controlling catecholamine biosynthesis in the adrenal medulla are under hormonal control (Axelrod, 1973). Furthermore, some recent evidence suggests that glucocorticoids modulate transsynaptic induction of tyrosine hydroxylase in sympathetic ganglia as well as in the adrenal medulla (Otten and Theonen, 1975).

Of the catecholamine content of the adult human adrenal medulla, 80–85% is epinephrine and 15–20% is norepinephrine. Plasma and urinary levels of norepinephrine correlate reasonably well with sympathetic nerve activity, since norepinephrine enters the circulation mainly as an "overflow" from the adrenergic nerves. Catecholamines released from the adrenal glands are inactivated mainly by COMT and MAO in the liver.

Bilateral adrenalectomy markedly reduces the concentration of epinephrine in the urine of man, whereas the norepinephrine concentration is not significantly altered (von Euler *et al.,* 1954; Goldenberg and Rapport, 1951). Any remaining epinephrine (perhaps one-fifth of that normally excreted in the urine) is presumed to come from chromaffin cells present elsewhere in the body (von Euler, 1956, p. 287). It should be pointed out that the adrenal medulla can be viewed as a sympathetic ganglion that is innervated by preganglionic cholinergic fibers. These fibers release acetylcholine, which causes secretion of catecholamines by a process of exocytosis from the chromaffin cells of the adrenal medulla. The control of secretion from other chromaffin cells has not been adequately elucidated.

Secretion of catecholamines by a process of exocytosis was first studied in the adrenal medulla, where it appears to be responsible for the release of catecholamines from these chromaffin cells (Douglas, 1968; Viveros *et al.,* 1968). It was further demonstrated that the presence of calcium was not only essential but was itself sufficient for the secretion of catecholamines in response to acetylcholine; other ions (potassium, sodium, chloride, and magnesium) were not necessary (Douglas, 1968). Secretion of adrenal catecholamines caused by other substances (e.g., histamine, serotonin, angiotensin, and bradykinin) appears to depend on depolarization of the chromaffin cells and the entry of calcium, the latter being a critical event in stimulus–secretion coupling of chromaffin cells (Douglas, 1968).

A similarly important role for calcium in stimulus–secretion coupling that involves exocytosis has been demonstrated in cholinergic and adrenergic nerves, where the respective neurotransmitters, acetylcholine and norepinephrine, are contained in membrane-limited structures (synaptic vesicles).

III. Adrenergic Receptors and Responses

Receptors can be viewed as target or binding sites on a cell that when activated by an agonist (i.e., a substance that interacts with a receptor and evokes a biologic response) can cause a series of events that lead to a response in that cell. Receptor sites have never been seen and identified as anatomic structures; rather, their existence has been postulated on the basis of biologic responses. Catecholamines are capable of activating receptor sites of a wide variety of cells. For example, catecholamines can cause lipolysis in adipose cells, glycogenolysis in liver and skeletal muscle, aggregation of platelets, chronotropic and inotropic effects on the myocardium, smooth muscle contraction or relaxation, and glandular secretion; they can even alter blood cell activity. The catecholamine receptors have been designated alpha (α) and beta (β) adrenergic receptors, depending on the type of response caused by the catecholamines. Some typical adrenergic responses are listed in Table II. α- and β-Responses can also be distinguished by specific antagonists that block specific responses, as schematically depicted in Fig. 4.

β-Adrenergic receptors can be further subdivided into β_1 (e.g., those that when stimulated cause a positive inotropic effect on the myocardium, lipolysis of fat cells, and inhibition of intestinal motility) and β_2-receptors (e.g., those which when stimulated cause bronchodilatation, glycogenolysis, and myometrial and smooth muscle relaxation). Epinephrine and norepinephrine are approximately equipotent in eliciting a β_1-response, whereas epinephrine is much more potent than norepinephrine in eliciting a β_2-response. Certain antagonists (i.e., substances that interact with α- or β-receptors and alter or occupy the receptors and thereby block biologic responses) have a greater potency in blocking β_1- than β_2-receptors; however, there are no known antagonists that specifically block only β_1- or β_2-receptors (Williams and Lefkowitz, 1978). Demonstration that the stereoisomers of epinephrine and norepinephrine with the levo ($-$) configuration are considerably more potent than those with the dextro ($+$) configuration indicates that a specific three-dimensional configuration is required for stimulation of the receptor site to cause a maximal response. β- ($-$) adrenergic agonists are more stereospecific than α- ($-$) agonists; β- ($-$) stereoisomers of the catecholamines are two to three orders of magnitude

TABLE II

Some Typical Adrenergic Responses[a]

Tissue	α-Response	β-Response
Smooth muscle		
Uterus (rabbit)	Contraction	Relaxation
Pyloric sphincter	Contraction	Relaxation
Bronchial		Relaxation
Bladder (detrusor)		Relaxation
Bladder (trigone and sphincter)	Contraction	
Iris (radial muscle)	Contraction	
Ciliary muscle (lens)		Relaxation
Intestine	Decreased motility	Decreased motility
Arterial	Contraction	Relaxation
Adipose tissue		Lipolysis
Salivary glands	$K^+ + H_2O$ secretion	Amylase secretion
Lymphocytes		Inhibition of cytolysis
Cardiac muscle		
Contractility	Increased	Increased
Heart rate		Increased
Functional refractory period	Increased	Decreased
Platelets	Aggregation	Inhibition of aggregation

[a] From Williams and Lefkowitz (1978, p. 11), reprinted by permission.

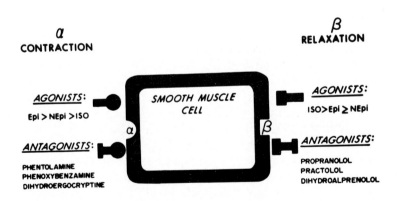

Fig. 4. The pharmacological differentiation of α- and β-adrenergic responses. A schematic diagram of a typical smooth muscle cell is shown. (Note: The response to α-receptor stimulation by an α-agonist appears to result from a change in ion permeability whereas the response to β-receptor stimulation by a β-agonist appears to involve accumulation of a cyclic nucleotide.) (From Williams and Lefkowitz, 1978, p. 8, reprinted by permission.)

more potent than the corresponding (+) stereoisomers, whereas the α- (−) stereoisomers are about one order of magnitude greater than their corresponding (+) stereoisomers (Williams and Lefkowitz, 1978). Representative α- and β-adrenergic compounds are listed in Table III.

TABLE III

Some Representative α- and β-Adrenergic Compounds[a]

α-Adrenergic agonists	α-Adrenergic antagonists
Catecholamines	Imidazolines
Epinephrine	Phentolamine
Norepinephrine	Tolazoline
Isoproterenol	Haloalkylamines
Dopamine	Dibenamine
Nordefrin	Phenoxybenzamine
Other phenylethylamines	Ergot Alkaloids
Phenylephrine	Ergotamine
Metaraminol	Ergocryptine
Hydroxyamphetamine	Ergocrystine
Methoxamine	Ergocornine
Ephedrine	Dihydroergotamine
Mephentermine	Dihydroergocryptine
Ergot alkaloids	Dihydroergocrystine
Ergonovine	Dihydroergocornine
Methysergide	Others
Ergotamine	Yohimbine
Others	Dibozane
Clonidine	Phenothiazines, e.g., chlorpromazine
	Butyrophenones, e.g., haloperidol
β-Adrenergic agonists	**β-Adrenergic antagonists**
Hydroxybenzylisoproterenol	Aryloxyethanolamines
Isoproterenol	Alprenolol
Epinephrine	Oxprenolol
Norepinephrine	Propranolol
Protokylol	Practolol
Salbutamol	Hydroxybenzylpindolol
Cobefrin	Dihydroalprenolol
Soterenol	Phenylethanolamines
Metaproterenol	Isoxuprine
Isoetharine	Nylidrin
Phenylephrine	Ritodrine
	Butoxamine
	Dichlorisoproterenol

[a] From Williams and Lefkowitz (1978, p. 7), reprinted by permission.

In addition to α- and β-adrenergic receptors that respond to epinephrine and norepinephrine (Table IV), a third type of adrenergic response caused by dopamine has been defined. Specific dopaminergic receptors have been identified in the brain and in renal, mesenteric, and cerebral vascular beds, where dopamine causes vasodilatation (Goldberg, 1972; Goldberg et al., 1978a,b; Iverson, 1975a). Some evidence indicates that coronary vessels contain dopaminergic receptors that when stimulated can cause vasodilatation (Schuelke et al., 1971; Vatner et al., 1973). Goldberg and co-workers (1978a,b) have also shown that dopamine acts on β_1- and α-receptors and possibly on β_2- and serotonin receptors.

A high degree of binding specificity and a strong affinity for catecholamines characterize the receptor–catecholamine interaction. The interaction is rapid and reversible. Several thousand receptors have been demonstrated in a single cell. These receptors are macromolecules that appear to be protein and that are located in the plasma membrane (Lefkowitz, 1976). Stimulation of adrenergic receptors results in a sequence of biochemical events that produce a biologic response. In many instances the sequence appears to be the following: The catecholamine (a so-called first messenger) stimulates the enzyme adenylate cyclase, which is located on the internal surface of the plasma membrane of the target cell. This enzyme then accelerates the intracellular generation of a cyclic nucleotide (the so-called second messenger), which in turn activates enzymes known as protein kinases; the kinases then phosphorylate a wide variety of important substrates that appear to mediate the characteristic responses attributed to the catecholamines.

β-Adrenergic responses are usually accompanied by an increase in the formation of cyclic AMP, which is thought to mediate the cellular response. In contrast, α-adrenergic stimulation is usually associated with a decrease or no change in cyclic AMP (with the exception of the brain, where increases have been reported in some regions). Therefore the responses to α- and β-receptor stimulation appear to be evoked by different biochemical mechanisms (Williams and Lefkowitz, 1978).

The number of functional receptors can be influenced by hormonal, genetic, and developmental factors. Changes in the number of receptors may profoundly alter sensitivity and responsiveness to catecholamines (Williams and Lefkowitz, 1978). Prolonged exposure of receptors to their agonists attenuates the biologic response to that agonist. This desensitization (which actually is never complete) has been demonstrated with a variety of hormones and drugs. It is reversible, since resensitization occurs when receptor exposure to an agonist is terminated. Studies with β-adrenergic receptors revealed that desensitization was accompanied by a reduction in a number of receptor sites and a decrease in responsiveness of

TABLE IV

Effects of Circulating Norepinephrine (NE) and Epinephrine (E) and Receptors Stimulated[a]

Effector system	Response and type of receptor stimulated[b]	
	NE	E
Isolated heart	Positive inotropic β and chronotropic β	Positive inotropic β and chronotropic β
Heart frequency *in vivo*	Bradycardia (vagal reflex)	Tachycardia β
Mean arterial blood pressure	Increase	Slight increase or decrease
Skeletal muscle	Vasoconstriction α	Vasodilatation β
Liver	Vasoconstriction α	Vasodilatation β
Skin	Vasoconstriction α	Vasoconstriction α
Kidneys	Vasoconstriction α	Vasoconstriction α
Sweat glands (localized[c] secretion)	Activation α	Activation α
Intestinal smooth muscle (decrease of motility and tone)	Relaxation α,β	Relaxation α,β
Pupils	Weak dilatation α	Dilatation α
Central nervous system	Slight or no effect?	Apprehension, excitation?
Blood sugar (glycogenolysis)	Slight increase β	Increase β
Free fatty acids (lipolysis)	Increase β	Increase β
Basal metabolic rate (with increased heat production)	Slight increase (mainly due to increased FFA)	Increase (mainly due to increased FFA?)
Blood eosinophils	Slight fall?	Fall?

[a] From Manger and Gifford, (1977), taken partially from von Euler and Ström (1957), by permission of the American Heart Association.
[b] The receptors on which NE and E act can be classified as α and β receptors, depending on the reaction of the effector organs to contact with these amines. β receptors have been subdivided into β_1 and β_2 (Furchgott, 1972). For example, cardiac inotropy and lipolytic effects of the catecholamines are β_1 responses whereas bronchodilatation and vasodilatation appear to be β_2 responses. Evidence suggests that in distal coronary resistance vessels there are α- and β-adrenergic receptors that on stimulation may, under some circumstances, cause vasoconstriction and vasodilatation, respectively (Mudge *et al.*, 1976).
[c] Stimulation accounts for activation of sweat glands on palms and a few other regions but generalized sweating in patients with pheochromocytoma remains unexplained. ? = Mechanism uncertain.

adenyl cyclase to the agonist. Although this apparent loss of receptor sites may be explained by an increased avidity of the agonist for binding, which thereby blocks further physiological response (Snyder, 1979), there is little reason at the present time to believe that this is necessarily a general principle (personal communication from Dr. R. J. Lefkowitz). It is noteworthy that antagonists, such as propranolol, do not desensitize β-adrenergic receptors.

The precise mechanism responsible for desensitization remains unclear; however, the process of desensitization of cells exposed to β-adrenergic agonists appears to be an important means of suppressing cellular responsiveness in the face of chronic and excess exposure to β-adrenergic agonists. Although much less is known about α-adrenergic receptors, desensitization to epinephrine has clearly been demonstrated in one model system where membrane voltage appeared to be critically involved (Williams and Lefkowitz, 1978).

As stated by Snyder (1979), manipulations that could reverse desensitization would have important clinical implications. It is interesting that guanine nucleotides (guanosine triphosphate and guanosine diphosphate) can reverse the decreased β-adrenergic binding that follows prolonged exposure to catecholamines. These nucleotides appear selectively to reverse the formation of a high-affinity receptor complex of agonists for β-adrenergic receptors, as well as receptors for glucagon, prostaglandin, dopamine, opiates, and α-adrenergic agonists. Other nucleotides (e.g., GMP, ATP, ADP, or AMP) do not alter receptor–agonist affinity. Snyder points out that "alpha adrenergic receptors and opiate receptors are regulated by guanine nucleotides in the same way as beta adrenergic and glucagon receptors, but they are linked to decreases rather than increases in cyclic AMP" (Snyder, 1979). It should be emphasized that the phenomenon whereby guanine nucleotides resensitize desensitized receptors has only been demonstrated in isolated membranes and does not appear to be a general mechanism in terms of reversing desensitization that is induced in intact cells (personal communication from Dr. R. J. Lefkowitz).

In contrast to the decreased sensitivity resulting from receptor exposure to agonists, supersensitivity of β-adrenergic receptors occurs when blood or tissue catecholamines are significantly lowered. This supersensitivity was related to an increased number of β-adrenergic receptors without any increase in affinity for the receptor site. Depletion of catecholamines in the rat heart resulted in a 50–100% increase in β-adrenergic receptor number, and this was associated with increased generation of cyclic AMP in response to catecholamine stimulation in the perfused rat heart (Williams and Lefkowitz, 1978). It is noteworthy that chronic treatment of rats with the β-adrenergic antagonist, propranolol, caused a 100% increase in the number of β-adrenergic receptors (Glaubiger and Lefkowitz, 1977). The intriguing question has been raised by Williams and Lefkowitz (1978) as to whether an increased number of β-adrenergic receptors due to propranolol treatment might account for the "propranolol withdrawal syndrome" observed clinically after cessation of treatment.

Hormones can significantly influence the receptor number and responsiveness to catecholamines in a number of different target cells. For example, adrenalectomy in the rat is accompanied by a three- to fivefold increase in β-adrenergic receptor number and an increased responsiveness to catecholamines; these changes are reversed by administration of cortisone. Steroids can also influence myometrial function. Catecholamines induce contraction of the myometrium via an α-adrenergic mechanism, whereas inhibition of contraction or relaxation of the myometrium occurs via a β-adrenergic mechanism. When the uterus is under the influence of estrogen, the α-mechanism predominates and catecholamines cause contraction; however, administration of progesterone significantly inhibits the contraction effect caused by α-adrenergic stimulation. It seems probable that alteration of the α-receptor number accounts for these results. α-Receptor number is markedly reduced in the myometrium under the influence of progesterone when compared with the uterus predominantly under the influence of estrogen. No change in β-receptors is induced by either of these hormones, nor is there any change in the affinity of catecholamines for receptor sites (Williams and Lefkowitz, 1978).

With regard to the heart, it is noteworthy that triiodothyronine can increase the sensitivity of the fetal mouse heart to the chronotropic effect of β-adrenergic stimulation. Furthermore, a marked hyperresponsiveness of rat myocardial phosphorylase to catecholamines in hyperthyroidism has been observed. Administration of triiodothyronine or thyroxine to induce hyperthyroidism resulted in a very significant increase in the number of β-receptors without a change in receptor affinity for agonists or antagonists. Williams and Lefkowitz (1978) have found no change in receptor sites in adipose cells from hyperthyroid rats; therefore it is not clear whether receptor alteration occurs in tissues other than the myocardium in hyperthyroidism. The mechanism whereby hormones alter receptors remains unclear.

A. Adrenergic Receptors in the Myocardium

Catecholamine receptors in the heart consist of those in the myocardium and those in the coronary vessels.

The dominant adrenergic receptors in the heart appear to be of the β_1 type and are located on the cardiac sarcolemma. These receptors are recognized and activated by catecholamines to varying degrees, depending on the affinity and binding at the receptor site. Activation of these myocardial receptors augments myocardial contraction and heart rate as well as the demand for oxygen in the heart. However, in addition to β-receptors, the sinoatrial node appears to possess α-receptors that when stimulated exert a negative chronotropic response (James *et al.*, 1968). Some investigators have also proposed the existence of atrial myocardial α-receptors that may subserve a negative inotropic function (Imai *et al.*, 1961). Others have suggested that the atria contain both α- and β-receptors that respond, respectively, to stimulation by increasing or decreasing action potential duration (Grovier *et al.*, 1966).

Adrenergic agonists and glucagon stimulate the enzyme adenyl cyclase in the sarcolemma and thereby increase generation of cyclic AMP (the so-called second messenger). The enhanced myocardial contractility results from an increased calcium influx across the sarcolemma. In addition, there is an accompanying acceleration of relaxation that appears to be brought about by activation of the calcium pump in the sarcoplasmic reticulum (Katz, 1977). Accelerated relaxation (i.e., an abbreviated systole) is, of course, essential for adequate diastolic filling and an efficient cardiac output during conditions of enhanced myocardial contractility and tachycardia (Katz, 1977).

Figure 5 schematically depicts the interrelationships between calcium and cyclic AMP within the myocardium. The β-adrenergic agonists stimulate the generation of $3',5'$-cyclic AMP, which is then converted by the enzyme phosphodiesterase to $5'$-AMP (a biologically inactive substance) and inorganic phosphate. It is noteworthy that phosphodiesterase inhibitors can

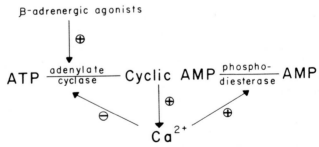

Fig. 5. Interrelationships between Ca^{2+} and cyclic AMP within the myocardium. β-Adrenergic agonists activate adenylate cyclase, thereby causing cyclic AMP levels to rise. This in turn increases intracellular Ca^{2+}, which tends to reverse these effects by promoting a reduction in cyclic AMP levels through the ability of Ca^{2+} to inhibit adenylate cyclase and to activate phosphodiesterase. (From Tada *et al.*, p. 15, 1976, by permission of the American Heart Association.)

exert catecholaminelike effects on the heart. The level of cyclic AMP in the cell is thus controlled by the rate of its synthesis and degradation. An increased intracellular concentration of cyclic AMP is associated with an enhanced influx of calcium ions into the cell. However, an increased concentration of intracellular calcium both inhibits adenyl cyclase and activates phosphodiesterase. Hence the enhanced flow of calcium ions into the cell caused by cyclic AMP can ultimately lead to a decline in the level of this cyclic nucleotide by a negative feedback mechanism (Katz, 1977).

Recently it has become apparent that before a cellular response can be achieved, cyclic AMP must react with additional enzymes (protein kinases) to form still another messenger, the cyclic AMP-dependent protein kinases. Activation of the enzyme protein kinase then results in phosphorylation of the sarcoplasmic reticulum, thereby causing stimulation of calcium transport and an accelerated relaxation of the myocardium. This cascade of reactions is schematically represented in Fig. 6.

Dephosphorylation, which appears to limit and terminate the physiological effects caused by the cascade of reactions, is attributed to hydrolysis induced by a class of enzymes known as phosphoprotein phosphatases. Although cyclic AMP seems to be involved in the electrophysiological re-

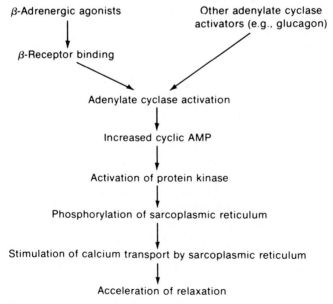

Fig. 6. Cascade of reactions by which agents that increase cyclic AMP levels can accelerate relaxation in the heart. (From Katz, 1977, p. 156, reprinted by permission.)

sponses of the heart to catecholamines, evidence for membrane dephosphorylation is inconclusive (Katz, 1977).

The precise mechanism of the excitation–contraction coupling is complex and incompletely understood. However, it appears that depolarization of the sarcolemma by an action potential initiates an influx of calcium into the interior of the myocardial cell. Calcium finally binds to troponin c, the calcium receptor of cardiac contractile protein, and contraction occurs (Katz, 1977). The effects of norepinephrine that can be released from the sympathetic nerve terminals in all parts of the heart and of epinephrine and norepinephrine released into the circulation from the adrenal gland or elsewhere are similar. The role of the catecholamines becomes particularly important under conditions of physiological and pathological stress and under some circumstances of myocardial damage and congestive heart failure.

Braunwald and co-workers (1976, p. 279) stated that "the quantity of norepinephrine released by the sympathetic nerves in the heart is probably the most important mechanism regulating the position of the force–velocity and ventricular performance curves under physiological conditions." They pointed out that almost instantaneous changes in myocardial contractility are affected by variations in impulse traffic in cardiac adrenergic nerves. Drugs that block these nerves or deplete catecholamine stores in the heart can block or reduce the myocardial response to stimulation of these nerves. Conversely, postganglionic denervation or drugs that block or impair neuronal reuptake of norepinephrine can increase the amount of norepinephrine at myocardial adrenergic receptor sites and thereby augment the response of the heart.

An infusion of isoproterenol, a synthetic catecholamine, stimulates the β-adrenergic receptors of the heart in a manner quite similar to that of exercise (i.e., a reduction in afterload, and end-diastolic and end-systolic dimensions, accompanied by an increase in myocardial contractility, cardiac index, heart rate, and ventricular force–velocity relation). β-Blockade with propranolol "reduced the endurance for maximal activity, the cardiac output, the mean arterial pressure, the left ventricular minute work, and the maximal oxygen uptake and increased the arteriovenous oxygen difference and the central venous pressure in normal human subjects" (Braunwald *et al.*, 1976). Ventricular end-diastolic dimension did not decrease during β-blockade, in contrast to the decrease noted in the unblocked state.

The effects of β-adrenergic blockade on four circulatory variables during maximal exercise are indicated in Fig. 7.

Various forms of stress can cause liberation of catecholamines into the circulation from the adrenal medulla and other portions of the adrenergic system. The response of the myocardium to these circulating catecholamines

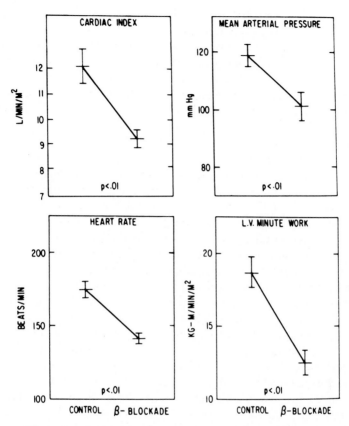

Fig. 7. Effects of β-adrenergic blockade on four circulatory variables during maximal exercise in normal subjects. The mean values (±SEM) are shown for each variable. (From Epstein *et al.,* 1965, p. 1750, reprinted by permission.)

is less rapid in onset than the response following cardiac adrenergic nerve stimulation; however, it is identical to that caused by the neurotransmitter released from the adrenergic nerves in the heart.

B. Adrenergic Receptors in the Coronary Circulation

Regulation of the coronary circulation and the coronary artery response to catecholamines is difficult to study and interpret. Administration of catecholamines can induce (1) an increase in systemic blood pressure and coronary artery perfusion pressure that may be accompanied by myogenic autoregulation in the coronary arteries that elevates coronary resistance; (2)

an augmented myocardial contractility, due to β_1-receptor stimulation, which increases myocardial oxygen consumption and metabolism and release of metabolites that cause coronary vasodilatation; (3) an increase or decrease in extravascular compression of the intramyocardial coronary vessels, depending on whether the heart rate is increased or decreased; (4) stimulation of α- and β_2-adrenergic receptors that cause vasoconstriction and vasodilatation, respectively. As pointed out by Braunwald and co-workers (1976, pp. 223–224), it is difficult if not impossible to predict the net effect of these various actions of the catecholamines on the coronary circulation and its bloodflow.

Both α- and β-adrenergic receptors have been identified in coronary arteries. Although most studies suggest that the β-adrenergic receptor is β_2 (Braunwald *et al.*, 1976), some evidence suggests it could be a β_1-receptor (Baron *et al.*, 1972). Furthermore, it is possible that dopaminergic receptors also exist in the coronary arteries, since in the presence of both α- and β-blockade, dopamine causes coronary vasodilatation (Vatner *et al.*, 1973).

Identification of receptors can be facilitated by using isolated segments of coronary arteries and thus avoiding the influence on the coronary circulation of alterations in myocardial contractility and metabolism. Stimulation of α-receptors of an isolated coronary segment causes vasoconstriction, whereas β_2-receptor stimulation induces vasodilatation (Zuberbuhler and Bohr, 1965; Baron *et al.*, 1972). The neurotransmitter, norepinephrine, which stimulates both α- and β-receptors, causes relaxation in small coronary arteries; β-blockade will prevent this relaxation and permit only vasoconstriction because of α-receptor stimulation. In larger coronary segments norepinephrine usually causes an initial vasoconstriction followed by vasodilatation. The vasoconstriction can be prevented with an α-receptor blocker such as phenoxybenzamine (Zuberbuhler and Bohr, 1965).

Stimulation of the stellate ganglion in the dog, which causes release of norepinephrine from cardiac sympathetic nerves, or intracardiac administration of norepinephrine, causes α-receptor stimulation and a short period of vasoconstriction followed by vasodilatation, which results from the increased metabolic activity of the heart (Berne, 1958; Berne *et al.*, 1965; Braunwald *et al.*, 1976). Following β_1-adrenergic blockade (which prevents increments in heart rate, in myocardial contraction, and in myocardial metabolism), stimulation of the sympathetic nerves to the heart produces only α-stimulation and coronary vasoconstriction. The latter effect can be inhibited by α-adrenergic blockade (Feigl, 1967). Some evidence suggests that the coronary arteries are normally under a tonic constriction that is mediated by the sympathetic nerves (Vatner *et al.*, 1970).

In summary, it appears that the coronary vasodilatation that follows administration of norepinephrine or sympathetic nerve stimulation is caused by the increased myocardial metabolism that accompanies β_1-receptor stimulation of the myocardium. In the absence of increased myocardial metabolism, the α-constrictor response of the coronary arteries to the neuronally released or injected norepinephrine appears to be dominant (Braunwald *et al.*, 1976). Braunwald and co-workers (1976) have pointed out that the coronary vascular responses to catecholamines and drugs may be markedly different in the unanesthetized as compared with the responses in anesthetized animals. Undoubtedly many conflicting results reporting the effect of catecholamines and drugs on the coronary circulation may depend on whether or not the animal was anesthetized.

IV. Neural Regulation of the Heart

A. Innervation

Randall has emphasized the importance of correlating function with neural structure innervating the heart at the time when the structure is identified. By so doing, errors in identifying cardiac nerves and in interpreting their function will be minimized (Randall, 1977, Chapter 2). However, this approach of study is only possible in the experimental animal. For that reason we have described below the effects that Randall and his associates observed when various cardiac nerves in the dog were electrically stimulated. For a detailed description of the nervous connections to the heart, the reader is referred to Chapters 2, 3, and 4 in "Neural Regulation of the Heart" (Randall, 1977).

1. Cardiac Nerves on the Right in the Dog

In the dog two vagi (parasympathetic) nerves descend from the nodose ganglia through the neck, where they become intermingled with sympathetic nerve fibers connecting the superior cervical and middle (caudal) cervical ganglia. Sympathetic preganglionic nerves leave the spinal cord from the second, third, and fourth (and occasionally the first and fifth) anterior thoracic roots and join the stellate and middle cervical ganglia before going to the heart. Fibers from the middle cervical ganglia extend caudally and posteriorly to connect with the stellate ganglia. The latter connect with the sympathetic chains that extend caudally. The distribution of upper thoracic anterior roots to the dog myocardium and their contribution to inotropic responses are indicated in Fig. 8.

The *right stellate cardiac nerve* arises from the stellate ganglion (or its branches) and innervates the right atrium and provides a major innervation of the sinoatrial (S-A) nodal region. Stimulation of the right stellate nerve

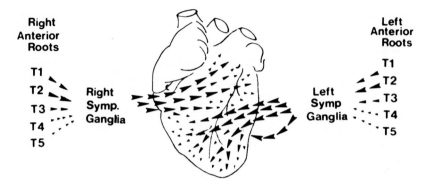

Fig. 8. Distribution of upper thoracic anterior roots to the dog myocardium. The size of the arrow heads indicate the relative contribution of anterior roots to regional inotropic cardiac responses. The right anterior roots dominate in the basal regions of the heart whereas the left roots dominate in the apical regions. (From Wurster, 1977, p. 226. Copyright © 1977 by Oxford University Press, Inc. Reprinted by permission.)

can markedly augment sinus node pacemaker activity and induce near maximal obtainable heart rates. It can also augment inotropism in the atria, but it exerts little if any effect on the ventricles.

The *right recurrent cardiac nerve* arises from the recurrent laryngeal nerve, the middle cervical ganglion, and the vagus. It contains vagal and sympathetic efferent fibers and many afferents that arise from all four heart chambers; it has a mixed efferent and afferent function.

Two major cardiac branches, the *craniovagal and caudovagal nerves,* arise from the right thoracic vagus and innervate the right atrium. Stimulation of these nerves causes mainly a parasympathetic response, although both vagal and sympathetic effects (especially on the right side of the heart) may occur.

Randall and associates found that stimulating various *cardiac branches of the vagus nerve* on the right caused a wide variety of results. For example, stimulation at one level below the middle cervical ganglion caused a greater negative inotropism in the right than in the left atrium and a suppression of conduction through the atrioventricular (A-V) node but no atrial slowing (i.e., no effect on the S-A node). On the other hand, with stimulation of an adjacent level atrial suppression was more prompt and more profound in both atria and was accompanied by complete A-V blockade; sometimes complete inhibition of S-A nodal discharge was induced and asystole occurred. At other times atrial fibrillation occurred during or following stimulation. They concluded that different responses were due to different contents of parasympathetic and sympathetic nerve fibers innervating localized portions of the heart.

2. Cardiac Nerves on the Left in the Dog

The *innominate nerve* arises mainly from the middle cervical ganglion; it also receives a branch from the vagus and it may connect with the adjacent ansae-ganglion region. In addition, it contains afferent fibers from cardiac receptors. Stimulation induces both sympathetic and parasympathetic effects.

The *ventromedial nerve* arises from the vagus but receives a connection from the middle cervical ganglion. Stimulation causes parasympathetic and sympathetic cardiac effects—the latter accounting for enhanced cardiac contractility, particularly on the left side of the heart.

The *dorsal cardiac nerve* arises from the middle cervical ganglion and may connect with the vagus and a few small sympathetic branches. It sends only minor connections to the heart, and it terminates in a fanlike distribution to the aortic arch and descending aorta. Although stimulation of this nerve may augment myocardial contractility, it appears that it contains numerous afferent fibers that reveal bursts of action potentials synchronous with the aortic pressure pulse.

The *ventrolateral cardiac nerve* arises from the middle cervical ganglion and sometimes partly from the adjacent ansa. It also has a few connections with the vagus and it receives a few branches from the recurrent laryngeal nerve. Its branches penetrate the pericardium to splay out on the left atrium, and a major portion extends over the ventral and dorsolateral left ventricular surfaces. It also forms a dorsal ventricular plexus near the coronary sinus. It has few afferent fibers and is considered primarily a sympathetic nerve that affects a large portion of the ventricular mass and the A-V nodal region.

The *left stellate cardiac nerve* arises from the ansa and/or stellate ganglion and may become incorporated in the ventrolateral cardiac nerve. The nerve appears to contain primarily afferent fibers from the left atrium but occasionally a few from the ventricles; however, rarely, it may augment force of contraction or heart rate in the left atrium.

In addition to the large cardiac nerve fibers on the left, described previously, small branches of the left vagus connect with the heart. Stimulation of these elicit profound parasympathetic effects (e.g., negative chronotropic effects on the heart and/or dromotropic changes involving the S-A and/or A-V nodal regions). Some afferents are also present in these nerves. As on the right side, no functional efferent cardiac nerves were found arising from the sympathetic chain below the stellate ganglion.

3. Peripheral Distribution of Cardiac Nerves

Although the myocardium is not anatomically a syncytium, the concept of a physiological syncytium remains, since excitation spreads throughout the entire heart (Randall, 1977, p. 78). However, it has been demonstrated that stimulation of individual thoracic cardiac nerves results in contraction of localized myocardial segments. It appears, therefore, that specific nerves innervate specific muscle segments (Szentiványi *et al.*, 1967). The effects of nerve stimulation on patterns of contractile force and changes in refractory periods in various parts of the myocardium have permitted identification and mapping of regional cardiac nerve distribution (Randall, 1977, pp. 78–85; Randall *et al.*, 1972).

4. Intracardiac Nerves

There are some neural elements present between myocardial cells that persist after extrinsic cardiac denervation. These elements appear to be primarily postganglionic parasympathetic elements, although some may be sympathetic nerves that are associated with intrinsic ganglion cells. The atria, the S-A and A-V nodal regions, and the bundle of His receive a rich supply of excitatory adrenergic fibers and inhibitory cholinergic fibers. It is established that the S-A node is supplied by sympathetic and parasympathetic nerves on the right side, whereas the A-V node is innervated by sympathetic nerves and the vagus on the left. The S-A node contains perhaps the richest network of fibers in the heart (Anderson and del Castillo, 1972), and there is evidence suggesting that each myocardial fiber in this region receives a separate innervation (Dahlström *et al.*, 1965). In addition, very high concentrations of catecholamines (Shindler *et al.*, 1968) and cholinesterase (James and Spence, 1966) are present in the S-A node.

Elsewhere in the heart it appears that one cholinergic nerve terminal supplies a single effector muscle cell, whereas one adrenergic nerve fiber releases neurotransmitter for several muscle cells. Nerves with vesicles containing granules have been considered adrenergic because they release norepinephrine. Agranular vesicles are characteristic of cholinergic fibers, which release acetylcholine. However, unequivocal differentiation of cardiac afferent and efferent nerve types is difficult on a histological basis. Some controversy still exists as to whether nerves terminate directly on myocardial cells. Although most investigators believe there is a synaptic cleft and that the neurotransmitter must diffuse from the nerve terminal to the myocardial effector cells, some studies have demonstrated neuromuscular contacts in some parts of the heart (e.g., A-V nodal tissue). Detailed reviews of the fine structure of cardiac innervation have been presented elsewhere (Borchard, 1978; Yamauchi, 1973).

The ventricles are richly innervated by adrenergic nerves (more so in the basal portions than in the apex), but the density of these nerves is much less than that in the atria. Cholinergic innervation is sparse to moderate except in the proximal ventricular conducting system. Kent and associates concluded from their studies that the rich cholinergic innervation of the ventricular conduction system in canine and human hearts may protect against spontaneous ventricular fibrillation during myocardial infarction. They also found that the increased ventricular fibrillation threshold caused by vagal stimulation was independent of adrenergic innervation (Kent *et al.*, 1974). The anatomic arrangement of cardiac nerves in man is quite similar to that of the dog except that in man the sympathetic and vagal nerves are anatomically separate. However, a major connection between the vagus and middle cervical ganglia may occur (Randall, 1977, p. 28).

B. Sympathetic Regulation

As pointed out by Randall (1977, p. 45), autonomic innervation of the heart permits rapid and highly specialized adjustments in cardiac action. He stated that "there is compelling evidence that these neural mechanisms exercise greater control than hormonal (adrenal medulla) or intrinsic (heterometric) length–tension relationships."

Exercise is accompanied by activation of the sympathetic nerves, augmentation of myocardial contractile force, and an elevated heart rate. An increased rate of myocardial tension development, a faster ejection velocity, and a shorter systole occur without a reduction in stroke volume. Ventricular contraction is much more rapid and the rates of change in pressure (dP/dt) are much greater than those at rest. Augmentation of ventricular contraction causes an elevation of pressure pulse.

More intense exercise can invoke the Frank–Starling mechanism (Randall, 1977, p. 48). Siegel and associates (1961) reported elevations in the concentrations of catecholamines in coronary sinus blood that were related to increased activation of the sympathetic nerves innervating the myocardium. Depletion of cardiac catecholamines (which can occur in congestive heart failure or can be induced with a drug such as reserpine) results in a decreased inotropic response to sympathetic nerve stimulation; improvement of ventricular performance, which normally characterizes exercise, does not occur or is attenuated (Randall, 1977, p. 48).

As mentioned earlier, stimulation of the sympathetic cardiac nerves in the dog augment ventricular contraction, heart rate, and arterial pressure. Stimulation of these nerves also influences the atria such that A-wave duration is decreased and atrial pulse pressure is augmented (Ulmer and Randall, 1961). A change in carotid sinus pressure can reflexly (via the central nervous system and cardiac nerves) influence the activity of the heart. A lowering of blood pressure activates the efferent sympathetic nerves and decreases vagal activity; as a result, atrial and ventricular contraction are augmented. Increasing carotid sinus pressure causes opposite effects (Sarnoff *et al.*, 1960; Sarnoff and Mitchell, 1962). The effects on ventricular ejection dynamics of stimulating sympathetic cardiac nerves are indicated in Table V.

There is evidence that increased sympathetic nerve activity improves synchrony of excitation and contraction within each chamber of the heart. Synchrony is critical to the ability of cardiac ejection to keep pace when the demands for cardiac output increase. Stimulation of the sympathetic cardiac nerves can also cause alterations in the location of the pacemaker. For example, stimulation of the left stellate frequently causes a shift of the pacemaker to points in or around the coronary sinus or A-V node (Randall, 1977, pp. 55–56).

Randall has pointed out that it is difficult to depict accurately the precise alterations in the electrocardiogram that may emerge during generalized sympathetic nerve stimulation, presumably because of a differential nerve distribution to various regions of the myocardium. He has summarized concisely some of the electrocardiographic changes that may be provoked by sympathetic excitation and has stated that "sympathetic excitation is often accompanied by marked alterations in cardiac rate and rhythm with associated changes in ECG (and His bundle electrocardiogram) morphologies." Such changes include sinus tachycardia (most commonly during right-side stimulations); atrial and ventricular premature systoles; and atrial, junctional, and ventricular tachycardias. However, when changes in rate are prevented (as by atrial pacing), reasonably predictable changes may be observed. During left stellate stimulation (LSS) the pacemaker frequently shifts from the S-A nodal (or high right atrial) region to junctional (or low atrial) regions with accompanying changes in configuration of the P wave and shortened P-R interval. The RS-T segment is frequently depressed and the terminal phase of the T wave becomes markedly elevated. The Q-T interval may also be significantly prolonged. During right stellate ganglion stimulation (RSS), sinus tachycardia is the most frequently encountered alteration. Because of S-A nodal predominance, the P wave almost invariably remains upright and of normal configuration, appearing to become more prominent in those instances in which the pacemaker was not in the S-A node before stimulation. P-R intervals may decrease, particularly in those instances in which the heart rate accelerates, but also in the absence of such acceleration caused by increased conduction velocity through the A-V node. RS-T segment elevation is sometimes prolonged and is often accompanied by T wave flattening or even inversion. Q-T prolongation may or may not occur (Randall, 1977, p. 57). Randall cited evidence that right stellate ganglionectomy or left stellate stimulation prolonged the Q-T interval and increased T wave amplitudes, whereas left stellate ganglionectomy or right stellate stimulation increased T wave negativity with or without Q-T interval changes. These changes could be correlated with changes

TABLE V

Sympathetic Influences upon Cardiac Dynamic Events (Heart Rate Kept Constant)[a]

Ascending Aortic Flow
  1. Acceleration (increased) (index of contractility)
  2. Peak flow (increased, and occurs earlier)
  3. Deceleration (increased)
  4. Ejection time (decreased)
  5. Stroke volume (increased)
  6. Cardiac output (increased)
Ventricular Pressure
  1. Atrial contraction (increased)
  2. Max dP/dt (increased) (index of contractility)
  3. Min dP/dt (increased) (reflects elevated peripheral resistance)
  4. Systolic pressure (increased)
  5. Peak systolic pressure occurs later in systole because of the increase in impedance (i.e., resistance is increased and the aorta is stiffer)
  6. Diastolic pressure (decreased)
  7. Diastolic period (increased)
Aortic Pressure
  1. Upslope (increased)
  2. Systolic pressure (increased)
  3. Diastolic pressure (increased)
  4. Pulse pressure (increased)
Ventricular Volume
  1. Ejection rate (increased)
  2. Ejection volume (increased)
  3. Systolic volume (decreased)
  4. Diastolic volume (increased ?)
  5. Filling rate (increased)

[a] From Randall (1977, Chapter 3, p. 53). Summary by Dr. W. Nichols. Copyright © 1977 by Oxford University Press, Inc. Reprinted by permission.

in ventricular refractory period, right stellate ganglionectomy being associated with refractory period prolongation over the anterior ventricular surface and left ganglionectomy producing prolongation on the posterior surface" (Randall, 1977, p. 58). It is pertinent that right stellectomy causes a greater decrease in norepinephrine concentration in the right ventricle and anterior wall of the left ventricle, whereas left stellectomy produces a maximal decrease in the posterolateral areas of the left ventricle (Kimata, 1965). Randall interpreted alterations in amplitude of the T wave in terms of improved synchrony or greater rate of repolarization of individual segments within the ventricle. He stated that "the more synchronous contraction of individual elements of the ventricle during systole, and the more nearly simultaneous relaxation of these elements during diastole imply similar alterations in electrical depolarization and repolarization, respectively" (Randall, 1977, p. 58).

It is noteworthy that following excision of the S-A node, supraventricular, positive chronotropic effects can be elicited by stimulation of the cardiac sympathetic nerves, thus indicating a regulation of heart rate independent of the S-A nodal mechanism.

The effect of sympathetic stimulation on the atrial refractory period remains controversial; however, the ventricular refractory period is clearly shortened. The marked reduction in ventricular fibrillation threshold during stellate stimulation has been attributed to the shortened refractory period induced by sympathetic activation. Ventricular tachycardia can be induced by stimulation of sympathetic nerves, especially those on the left; however, it is unclear whether the sympathetic nerves to the heart play an important role in the genesis of ventricular tachycardias encountered. Although sympathetic activation accompanied by a pronounced increase in mechanical performance of the heart increases ventricular automaticity, it is unlikely that ventricular dysrhythmia would develop except perhaps in the presence of A-V block (Randall, 1977, p. 68).

A-V conduction time is shortened by sympathetic nerve stimulation; the effect of left stellate stimulation is more pronounced than stimulation on the right—minimal effects occur in the His Purkinje and ventricular muscle conduction. Randall (1977, p. 63) points out that an important tonic sympathetic influence on A-V conduction, combined with an autonomic action on the S-A node, indicates a homeostatic role for the sympathetic nervous system on dromotropic, chronotropic, and inotropic mechanisms.

There is evidence of cardiotonic influences of the sympathetic nerves; even at rest and under anesthesia nerve impulses at low frequencies can be detected. These tonic discharges change synchronously with arterial pulsation, presumably because of the baroreceptor reflex mechanism.

Sympathetic nerve innervation of the heart can significantly influence the excitability of the myocardium. Skelton reported that cardiac sympathectomy in the dog protected against ventricular fibrillation and reduced mortality rate following occlusion of the left circumflex coronary artery from 80 to 0% (Skelton et al., 1962).

Ebert (1969) has shown that cardiac denervation markedly reduced or prevented the release of potassium from the heart after coronary ligation; he concluded that potassium flux was important in the genesis of ventricular fibrillation in the ischemic myocardium.

Coronary occlusion stimulates cardiac afferent fibers (Malliani et al., 1973), which reflexly activate efferent cardiac sympathetic fibers (Malliani et al., 1969) and thereby induces ventricular arrhythmias (Gillis et al., 1974). Complete cardiac denervation causes a marked depletion of catecholamines in the heart (Ebert *et al.*, 1970; Goodall and Kirshner, 1956). Despite functional reinnervation the catecholamine concentration in the heart remains markedly reduced (Hageman *et al.*, 1973b).

Spurgeon and associates (1974) reported that the interesting finding that cardiac denervation decreased the norepinephrine concentration in the atria and ventricles to 1–3% of control concentrations, whereas epinephrine concentrations were reduced only to 40–60%. The epinephrine concentration in conductile tissue (except for the S-A node) did not decrease significantly below control values; however, the norepinephrine concentration in the right and left bundle branches and S-A and A-V nodal conductile tissue decreased markedly to almost zero. These results indicate that a substantial amount of epinephrine is nonneuronal, since denervation is accompanied by degeneration of the sympathetic cardiac innervation with a concomitant disapparance of the norepinephrine-containing vesicles normally present in these nerves. Hoffman (1967) demonstrated that catecholamines increased diastolic depolarization in Purkinje fibers and pacemaker cells, which resulted in increased firing. Han and associates (1964) also studied the adrenergic effects on ventricular vulnerability and presented evidence that a homogeneous distribution of catecholamines throughout the myocardium tends to reduce vulnerability to arrhythmias.

It is not surprising, therefore, that conditions (e.g., sympathetic nerve stimulation, myocardial ischemia or infarction) that alter sympathetic activity and catecholamine content in a region of the myocardium enhance the chance of developing cardiac dysrhythmias. As pointed out by Randall (1977, p. 67), such changes, coupled with alterations in recovery of myocardial excitability and disorganized conduction may lead to multiple reentry circuits and fibrillation. The value of using adrenergic blocking agents, particularly some of the β-blockers, to control and prevent hazardous dysrhythmias must be considered in a variety of clinical situations afflicting the heart.

C. Parasympathetic–Sympathetic Interaction Involving the Myocardium

A few remarks should be made regarding the parasympathetic control of myocardial function and the interactions of the sympathetic and parasympathetic innervation of the heart. Recent advances regarding this subject have been reviewed by Levy (1977a) and will be considered in this section. It should be appreciated that cholinergic and adrenergic interactions are complex and that their effects on cardiac function may be synergistic or antagonistic. Apparently, parasympathetic influences are modulated to some extent by the degree of sympathetic activity. With a high level of sympathetic tone, the vagal center in the medulla is inhibited. Under certain circumstances activation of sympathetics may exaggerate the cardiovascular response to parasympathetic stimulation, whereas under other conditions the response is markedly blunted (Higgins *et al.*, 1973). Elevation of blood pressure can produce reciprocal effects and reduce sympathetic traffic and augment parasympathetic activity, whereas an increase in arterial CO_2 will stimulate both the vagus and sympathetic nerves (Armour *et al.*, 1977). For a comprehensive review concerning parasympathetic control of the heart the reader is referred elsewhere (Higgins *et al.*, 1973).

Vagal and sympathetic activity are constantly varying; however, even moderate vagal stimulation can overshadow strong cardiac sympathetic activity and mask sympathetic influences on the myocardium. Furthermore, the response to vagal stimulation is more rapid than that due to sympathetic stimulation. Time dependency of the pacemaker response to vagal stimulation depends partly on high concentrations of acetylcholinesterase in the S-A nodal region and consequent rapid hydrolysis of acetylcholine released in this region by vagal terminals; inactivation of norepinephrine released by sympathetic nerve terminals in the same region is less rapid. A-V conduction is depressed by vagal impulses, whereas the cardiac sympathetic nerves have the opposite effect. Behavior of A-V conduction differs from activity in the S-A node with respect to autonomic interactions, since change in activity of one division of the autonomic nervous system is independent of the background level of the other division.

Vagal stimulation reduces heart rate, automaticity, contractile force, and maximal left ventricular dP/dt; however, diminution of contractile force evoked by vagal stimulation or acetylcholine infusion is accentuated if myocardial contractility is first augmented by an infusion of norepinephrine or by cardiac nerve stimulation (Stanton and Vick, 1968; Hollenberg *et al.*, 1965). Levy (1977a) termed the latter phenomenon "accentuated antagonism" and has indicated that the principle sympathetic–parasympathetic interactions on the heart can be subdivided into two major categories: reciprocal excitation and accentuated antagonism.

Additional evidence of accentuated antagonism can be demonstrated. For example, immediately following cessation of supramaximal stimulation of the vagi, there is a transient increase in left ventricular pressure caused by a "rebound" enhancement in myocardial contractility. Also, the greater the background of sympathetic activity, the more profound the depressant effect of a given level of vagal activity (Levy, 1977a).

Both interneuronal and intracellular processes appear to be involved in the mechanism responsible for accentuated antagonism. Postganglionic cholinergic vagal activity can decrease nerve traffic in cardiac sympathetic nerves and thereby reduce the quantity of norepinephrine released in the

heart. This inhibitory effect of acetylcholine on the release of norepinephrine, which has been identified as a muscarinic effect, can be blocked with
atropine. On the other hand, nicotinic agents can release norepinephrine in
the heart. Many studies have shown that acetylcholine and cholinergic
stimulation may release norepinephrine from the heart. The effect of cardiac sympathetic stimulation, alone and in combination with vagal stimulation, on norepinephrine overflow into the coronary sinus blood is shown in
Fig. 9. It is evident that vagal stimulation suppresses the release of
norepinephrine induced by sympathetic stimulation; however, atropine
blocks this suppressive effect of vagal stimulation. The mechanism whereby
acetylcholine diminishes the release of norepinephrine in the heart during
sympathetic stimulation remains unclear. Prostaglandins of the E series are
released into coronary sinus blood by acetylcholine or vagal activation.
Whether or not prostaglandins subserve an intermediary role in suppressing
norepinephrine secretion at a given level of cardiac sympathetic activity
remains controversial (Levy, 1977a).

In addition to the muscarinic inhibition of norepinephrine release, accentuated vagal–sympathetic antagonism depends on an intracellular
mechanism that reduces the cardiac response to norepinephrine. Acetylcholine produces a greater reduction in left ventricular contractile force and
maximum dP/dt during a simultaneous norepinephrine infusion than when
it is given alone. As indicated by Levy (1977a), it appears that cyclic nucleotides are involved in the actions of the sympathetic and parasympathetic
nerves on the myocardium and in the interactions between these autonomic

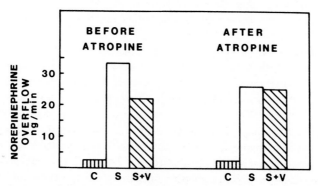

Fig. 9.   The rate of norepinephrine overflow into the coronary sinus during the control
state (C), during cardiac sympathetic stimulation (S), and during combined sympathetic and
vagal stimulation (S + V). The heights of the bars indicate the mean values for six anesthetized
dogs. The data on the left were obtained before atropine; those on the right after atropine
sulfate, 1 mg/kg. (From Levy, 1977a, p. 121. Copyright © 1977 by Oxford University Press,
Inc. Reprinted by permission.)

nerves. Norepinephrine increases intracellular levels of cyclic AMP and thereby enhances glycogen phosphorylase activity in the myocardium. Acetylcholine has no effect or causes a slight reduction of basal levels of cyclic AMP; yet if cyclic AMP levels are elevated by adrenergic stimulation, then acetylcholine profoundly depresses the intracellular level of this cyclic nucleotide. Contrariwise, acetylcholine increases the intracellular level of another cyclic nucleotide, cyclic GMP. It is probable that this latter nucleotide acts as an intermediary by which acetylcholine and cholinergic drugs elicit some of their cardiac effects—responses opposite to those produced by adrenergic stimuli where cyclic AMP is the intermediary. There is evidence that cyclic GMP accelerates hydrolysis of cyclic AMP and may thereby lower the intracellular level of the latter nucleotide (Beavo *et al.*, 1971).

From the foregoing, Levy (1977a) has proposed that vagal stimulation may suppress myocardial cyclic AMP in two ways: (1) by opposing the tendency for adrenergic stimuli to elevate intracellular levels of cyclic AMP and (2) by raising the concentration of cyclic GMP, which may accelerate the hydrolysis of cyclic AMP. Figure 10 schematically depicts the inhibitory influence of terminal vagal fibers on postganglionic sympathetic neurons in the heart; it represents the interneuronal and intracellular mechanisms responsible for accentuated antagonism between cardiac autonomic nerves.

D. Cardiac Reflexes

Reflex mechanisms play a major role in regulating heart function by their influence on autonomic cardiac nerve activity. The following remarks are based mainly on the review of cardiac reflex mechanisms by Armour *et al.* (1977).

The central nervous system is continuously monitoring the instant-to-instant status of the heart via afferent cardiac nerves. In addition to the well-known baroreceptor reflexes, which are so important in autonomic modulation of blood pressure changes, preganglionic sympathetic nerve activity is modulated by other structures, such as receptors in the heart, great vessels, and lungs, which respond to mechanical pressure and distortion. Bursts of sympathetic activity appear with each systole, whereas sympathetic activity decreases with inspiration. Powerful reflexes arising from cardiopulmonary receptors can activate cardiac sympathetic and parasympathetic nerves simultaneously (Armour *et al.*, 1977).

Afferent nerves can also be activated by increases in coronary flow and/or pressure, coronary occlusion, or myocardial ischemia, and this activation can reflexly cause cardiac sympathetic nerve discharge (Brown and Malliani, 1971). Even stimulation of sciatic, brachial, and saphenous nerves can evoke

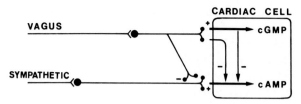

Fig. 10. The interneural and intracellular mechanisms responsible for accentuated antagonism between the cardiac sympathetic and vagal nerves. (Modified from Levy, p. 367, 1977b, by permission of MIT Press.)

excitation of cardiac sympathetic nerves while simultaneously inhibiting vagal activity (Iriuchijima and Kumada, 1963); these are known as somatosympathetic reflexes. It has been proposed that local cardiac reflexes can activate postganglionic sympathetic nerves via thoracic ganglia (Williams, 1967). Hence it is evident that reflex activation of sympathetic efferent cardiac nerves can occur via afferent as well as efferent fibers.

Kezdi and associates (1974) observed a decreased cardiac output, blood pressure, heart rate, and postganglionic sympathetic neural activity following occlusion of the circumflex coronary artery in the dog. Administration of atropine mainly increased the heart rate, whereas transection of the vagi increased sympathetic nerve activity, cardiac output, and mean systemic blood pressure. These investigators recommended that cardiogenic shock secondary to myocardial infarction be treated by administering atropine to decrease bradycardia and also by administering isoproterenol and norepinephrine to increase cardiac output and peripheral resistance. However, as pointed out by Armour and associates (1977), therapy with agents that increase cardiac output and peripheral resistance represent a "double-edged sword," since they increase cardiac work and coronary blood flow demand.

Hypertension and tachycardia occur in some patients during angina, and vasoconstrictor responses and increased cardiac output have been observed after myocardial infarction as well as following coronary occlusion. Such pressor reflexes may compensate for the decreased contractility of injured myocardium and thus help prevent cardiogenic shock due to myocardial infarction (Malliani *et al.*, 1969). James and associates (1975) suggested that serotonin released from platelets in the region of atherosclerotic plaques or infarcts may reflexly cause some of the blood pressure changes associated with myocardial infarction. They observed that injections of small amounts of serotonin into proximal segments of the left coronary artery caused hypertension, whereas injection into the distal segments caused hypotension.

In summary, Armour, Wurster, and Randall (1977) have schematically depicted the known reflex connections of the heart and a number of hypothetical pathways (Fig. 11). Preganglionic sympathetic fibers leave the spinal cord and make synaptic connections with postganglionic sympathetic cardiac nerves in the stellate but more often in the caudal ganglia. Preganglionic parasympathetic fibers travel in the vagi and terminate on postganglionic nerves in or near the heart.

Some vagal and sympathetic cardiac efferent nerves show cyclic activity with cardiac rhythm, whereas other efferent fibers do not exhibit this activity. The autonomic efferent cardiac nerves are modulated by reflexes that originate in the carotid and aortic baroreceptors. Excitatory impulses are conveyed from these receptors by afferent nerves to the medulla, where they inhibit descending reticulospinal tracts to preganglionic cell bodies and thereby reduce postganglionic sympathetic outflow to the heart. Usually, when sympathetic activity increases, vagal activity decreases. This reciprocal relationship (indicated in Fig. 11) does not always occur, since coactivation of both sympathetic and parasympathetic systems may occur under some conditions.

Nonbaroreceptor afferent nerves also influence autonomic nerves to the heart. Cardiopulmonary afferents may excite or inhibit sympathetic outflow to the cardiovascular system. Sympathetic afferent fibers from the heart travel to the spinal cord via sympathetic nerves and dorsal roots; visceral afferents may reach the spinal cord via ventral roots. Stimulation of these afferent nerves primarily activates sympathetic efferents to the heart.

Many cardiac reflexes are cardiocardiac reflexes, i.e., impulses that arise in the heart, are relayed to the central nervous system, and then return to the heart. Some evidence suggests that certain cardiocardiac reflexes may occur in extrinsically denervated hearts. These reflexes release norepinephrine in response to weak beats and acetylcholine in response to strong beats (Kositzky, 1971).

Reflexes from coronary arteries or myocardial infarcts may be depressor or pressor and cause hypotension or hypertension. It is noteworthy that these reflex pathways may be interrupted by coronary bypass surgery. Cardiac reflexes and activation of sympathetic nerves appear to be important in producing several types of arrhythmias. For example, excessive sympathetic activity in humans with the prolonged QT syndrome may cause lethal cardiac arrhythmias (Schwartz and Malliani, 1975).

E. Intracranial Mechanism of Cardiac Regulation

Manning (1977) has recently reviewed the intracranial mechanisms involved in cardiac regulation. The central nervous system can exert influences on the cardiovascular system. Autonomic activity evoked by dience-

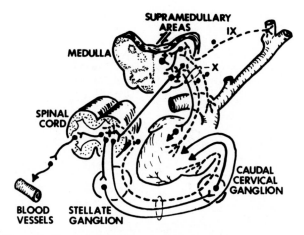

Fig. 11. Diagram of hypothetical reflex connections of the canine heart. Afferent fibers are indicated by dashed lines and efferent fibers by solid lines. Sympathetic cardiac afferent fibers may have excitatory influences on cardiac sympathetic efferent fibers at the spinal level or via supraspinal connections (not shown). Baroreceptor afferent fibers may travel to the medulla from the carotid sinus by way of the glossopharyngeal nerve (IX) or from the aortic arch by way of the vagus nerve (X). These baroreceptors reflexly excite (+) cardiac vagal efferent fibers and inhibit (−) descending spinal sympathoexcitatory pathways to preganglionic neurons that are destined to the heart and blood vessels. Other cardiopulmonary afferents traveling in the vagus nerve may excite or inhibit (±) the descending spinal sympathoexcitatory pathways. Sympathetic cardiac preganglionic fibers may synapse with postganglionic neurons in the stellate ganglion or more commonly in the caudal cervical ganglion. (From Armour *et al.*, 1977, p. 180. Copyright © 1977 by Oxford University Press, Inc. Reprinted by permission.)

phalic stimulation can cause a variety of arrhythmias. Electrocardiographic changes that may be associated with intracranial lesions appear related to alterations in the interplay of the sympathetic and parasympathetic nervous systems. Although confusion exists regarding the precise location of bulbar synaptic stations of some cardiac reflexes, efferent nerves that cause vagal cardioinhibitory effects probably reside in the nucleus ambiguus. Hypothalamic pressor areas suppress sinus reflex bradycardia; the limbic forebrain, limbic hindbrain, and hypothalamus may be interrelated with baroreceptor reflex pathways. A corticohypothalamic sympathoinhibitory system involves efferent fibers that inhibit sympathetic discharge and stimulate vagal activity.

Manning (1977) has indicated that a preeminent vasomotor center in the medulla governing cardiovascular control is too simplistic a concept. He states that the "addition of a hypothalamic loop to the controller provides that organ with greater flexibility in regulating basic reflex activity" (Manning, 1977). According to his schema (see Fig. 12), the "basic homeostatic

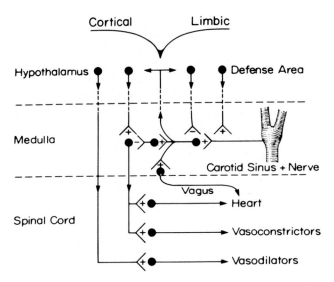

Fig. 12. A schema depicting a hypothalamic-medullary loop whereby descending hypothalamic systems can inhibit components of the carotid sinus medullary input by either presynaptic or postsynaptic mechanisms. Such inhibition permits full development of hypothalamic activity on spinal sympathetic neurons. In addition, an ascending system of the IX nerve engages diencephalic neurons. (From Manning, 1977, p. 204. Copyright © 1977 by Oxford University Press, Inc. Reprinted by permission.)

reflexes are represented by the IX nerve input which makes synaptic connection in the medullary reticular formation. . . . These medullary synaptic stations are impinged upon by neural systems of diencephalic origin which offer tonic as well as phasic adjustment to cardiomotor and vasomotor spinal outflow."

F. Spinal Sympathetic Control of the Heart

For a detailed account of the spinal sympathetic control of the heart the reader should consult the review by Wurster (1977) on which most of the following discussion is based.

Cardiac changes and alterations in control mechanisms may occur in a number of diseases that involve the spinal cord (e.g., multiple sclerosis, amyotrophic lateral sclerosis, poliomyelitis, tabes dorsalis, Shy Dragger syndrome, tetanus). Severe tetanus may be accompanied by pronounced hypertension, vasoconstriction, tachycardia, and arrhythmias—manifestations resulting from sympathetic hyperactivity (Corbett *et al.*, 1969). This sympathetic overactivity results from a reduction in mechanisms that normally inhibit sympathetic neurons in the spinal cord (Paar and Wellhöner, 1973). Trauma or mechanical or electrical stimulation of the cord may also markedly affect neural regulation of the heart. For example, increased intracranial pressure can cause marked hypertension by a reflex in which the spinal cord participates (Manger *et al.*, 1959; Meyer and Winter, 1970). Cardiovascular effects are induced by stimulation of the adrenergic nervous system with release of catecholamines from the sympathetic nerves and adrenal medulla (Manger *et al.*, 1959).

Spinal animals and patients with lesions above the T_5 level exhibit marked cardiovascular responses during afferent nerve stimulation. Some responses (e.g., marked increase in blood pressure, vasoconstriction, increased cardiac contractility) are due to activation of the adrenergic system; other responses (e.g., bradycardia and vasodilatation of the face, neck, and shoulders) result from reflex activation of the vagus induced by the hypertension (Frankel and Mathias, 1979; Manger *et al.* 1979). From studies of patients with spinal cord lesions, Wurster and Randall (1975) concluded that in high spinal lesions (T_5 or above) afferent nerve stimulation (by bladder distension) caused vasoconstriction and also increased cardiac contractility and elevated mean and pulse pressure. The latter indicated inotropic effects of the sympathetic cardiac innervation. In patients with lesions below T_5, marked increases in pulse pressure did not occur (Fig. 13).

A number of investigators have reported spinal reflexes that especially involve the heart. In spinal animals increased coronary artery pressure, occlusion of the coronary sinus, and myocardial ischemia cause increased sympathetic activity accompanied by cardiac arrhythmias. These cardiocardiac reflexes can be alleviated by sectioning T_1 to T_5 dorsal roots (Wurster, 1977).

There is evidence that the sympathetic nervous system to the heart and vascular system may be differentially controlled; that is, activation or inhibition of the sympathetic nerves to one organ or area can occur without a similar response to others. As stated by Wurster (1977), "The monolithic view of mass sympathetic discharge has fallen."

Somatic and visceral afferent nerves can excite and inhibit postganglionic nerves to the heart and blood vessels. The afferent excitatory and inhibitory impulses ascend to the brain in pathways located respectively in the dorsolateral sulcus and dorsolateral funiculus regions of the spinal cord; excitatory fibers activate pressor pathways in the reticular formation of the brain stem that descend in the dorsolateral funiculus. The inhibitory afferents may suppress descending excitatory pathways and activate descending inhibitory pathways (Wurster, 1977).

HIGH LESION

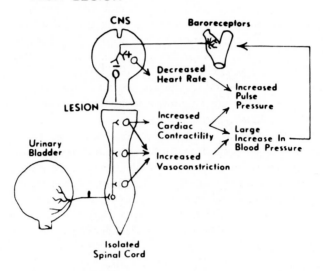

LOW LESION

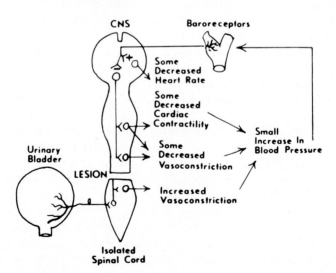

Fig. 13. Diagram of cardiovascular reflexes in response to bladder distension in patients with high (above T_5) and low (below T_5) spinal cord transection. (From Wurster and Randall, 1975, p. 1291, reprinted by permission.)

G. Autonomic Control of Nodal Tissue

Urthaler and James (1977) have reviewed the cholinergic and adrenergic control of the sinus node and atrioventricular (A-V) junction. Formation, integration, and conduction of cardiac impulses all occur in specialized myocardial cells that are profoundly influenced by autonomic cardiac nerves and a variety of blood-borne substances, including the catecholamines. The normal pacemaker is the sinus node, and resting heart rate results from synchronous impulses generated spontaneously from these cells. If sinus node activity fails, alternate pacemakers become available—the major substitute being in the region of the A-V node and His bundle. Except for the sinus node, the A-V junction has the richest adrenergic and cholinergic nerve supply in the heart. Cholinesterase is also heavily concentrated in these areas and in the bundle of His (Urthaler and James, 1977). Urthaler and associates (1973, 1974) have shown that there is a mathematical relationship between automaticity in the sinus node and in the A-V junction.

The sinus node is exposed to norepinephrine that is released as the neurotransmitter from the cardiac sympathetic nerves; it is also exposed to catecholamines that are released elsewhere (i.e., epinephrine and norepinephrine from the adrenal medulla and norepinephrine from other sympathetic nerves) and reach the heart through the blood. Perfusion of the sinus node with epinephrine or norepinephrine mimics adrenergic stimulation of the node (e.g., by electrical stimulation of the right stellate ganglion). Immediate sinus tachycardia occurs on perfusing with epinephrine, norepinephrine, or isoproterenol; however, isoproterenol hydrochloride is about 10 times more potent (on a weight basis) than the naturally occurring catecholamines. Following administration of maximally effective doses of these agents, tachycardia rarely exceeds 3 min (Urthaler and James, 1977). Dopamine also causes an immediate tachycardia but is less potent by weight than norepinephrine. On the other hand, L-dopa (the precursor of dopamine) produces a prolonged tachycardia that is slow in onset and less marked than that produced by norepinephrine. The effect of L-dopa may be due to synthesis of dopamine and norepinephrine. Neither tyrosine nor phenylalanine exert any chronotropic effect on perfusion (James *et al.*, 1970).

A positive chronotropic effect can result from (1) a direct accelerating effect of an agent on sinus node cells; (2) release of intranodal catecholamine stores; (3) inhibition of reuptake mechanism for catecholamines in the heart; (4) inhibition of catabolism of the catecholamines; or (5) anticholinergic action on the vagus or on the local response to acetylcholine. Negative chronotropic responses are chiefly augmented cholinergic effects; however, bradycardia may be mediated through antiadrenergic mechanisms (e.g., blockade of β-adrenergic receptors, local norepinephrine depletion, or neural inhibition of norepinephrine release (Urthaler and James, 1977).

It appears that norepinephrine in the sinus node exists in at least two pools—that released by neural stimulation and that which can be released by tyramine (James *et al.,* 1970).

Perfusion of the A-V junction with epinephrine, norepinephrine, or iso-proterenol causes a junctional tachycardia that is almost immediate in onset and of brief duration. Perfusion with tyramine or quanethidine causes a release of norepinephrine and produces an immediate onset of tachycardia; however, the tachycardia is prolonged—similar to that seen following sinus node perfusion with these agents.

β-Adrenergic blockade of the sinus node of the dog diminishes heart rate by about 20% whereas blockade of the A-V junction reduces the rate by 45%.

Positive and negative chronotropic effects of certain drugs can be mediated by mechanisms independent of the adrenergic and cholinergic systems. For example, perfusion of the sinus node or A-V junction with glucagon or guanosine will produce tachycardia despite β-receptor blockade or pretreatment with drugs that block adrenergic neural transmission. Also, theophylline and aminophylline have chronotropic and inotropic effects that are not abolished by β-receptor blockade. Adenosine perfusion of the sinus node or A-V junction causes a profound bradycardia despite the presence of a cholinergic muscarinic blockade; bradycardia is not altered by β-receptor blockade, catecholamine depletion, or sympathetic nerve block-ade (Urthaler and James, 1977). Although there is some evidence that cyclic AMP may be the mediator for the chronotropic and inotropic effects of the catecholamines (Sutherland *et al.,* 1968), the mechanisms whereby the catecholamines and other substances cause changes in heart rate and contractile force remain uncertain. It is noteworthy that perfusion of the sinus node with cyclic AMP produces only a bradycardia that is unaltered by pretreatment with atropine or a β-receptor blocker (James, 1965).

H. Autonomic Control of the Coronary Circulation

The adrenergic receptors and their influence on coronary blood flow have been discussed earlier in this chapter. In this section the autonomic control of the coronary circulation will be considered in more detail. The following is based primarily on the recent review of autonomic control of the coronary circulation by Pace (1977).

Metabolic activity of the heart is crucial in the control of its blood supply. Coronary blood flow is closely related to myocardial oxygen consumption.

Recent evidence suggests that adenosine, which is released from myocardial cells when oxygen demand is increased, may play a key role in causing vasodilatation and thus augmenting coronary blood flow and oxygen delivery. Despite the central role exerted by metabolic factors in controlling myocardial perfusion (Berne and Rubio, 1977), there is no doubt that the autonomic nervous system also influences coronary blood flow. β-Adrenergic blockade unmasks vasoconstriction resulting from cardiac sympathetic nerve activity; parasympathetic stimulation causes coronary vasodilatation (Pace, 1977).

Sympathetic nerves have close contact with the muscular layer of arteries in the heart, although these nerves do not appear to penetrate the media to any extent (Ehinger et al., 1966). There is evidence for innervation of coronary arteries by sympathetic and parasympathetic nerves, whereas capillaries appear uninnervated. The media of large coronary vessels are not in close approximation with nerve terminals, and it has been suggested that these vessels may only be under moderate or mild control by the autonomic system. In contrast, nerves become more numerous and in closer association with smooth muscle as the coronary vessels become smaller—probably indicating a greater autonomic control of the coronary vessels as they become smaller. Since the neurotransmitter released at these nerve terminals has to diffuse a certain distance before it reaches the media, it is possible that only the outer cells of the muscular wall are stimulated to contract, whereas cells near the lumen remain unaffected (Pace, 1977).

As mentioned previously, the cardiodynamic metabolic effects dominate the coronary blood flow response during sympathetic nerve stimulation. Granata and co-workers (1965) found that immediately after the onset of electrical stimulation, vasoconstriction occurred and was accompanied by a decreased coronary flow while heart rate and blood pressure remained unchanged; with subsequent augmentation of heart rate and contractility, the vasoconstriction was converted to vasodilatation.

In some species immediate coronary vasodilatation may be induced by electrical stimulation of sympathetic nerves to the heart. In the cat, such vasodilatation can be abolished and converted to vasoconstriction by β-adrenergic blocking agents (Brown, 1968). This latter finding suggests that immediate coronary vasodilatation during sympathetic stimulation is due to a β-adrenergic effect. Furthermore, the vasoconstriction (which occurs following β-adrenergic blockade) can, in turn, be abolished by α-adrenergic blockade with dibenzyline. It appears, therefore, that during sympathetic stimulation α-adrenergic vasoconstrictor activity becomes manifest if coronary vasodilatation and cardiac metabolic effects are prevented by β-adrenergic blockade with propranolol. If only the metabolic effects are prevented by administration of practolol (which selectively blocks only the metabolic effects on the heart caused by sympathetic stimulation), then stimulation of cardiac sympathetic nerves will not significantly diminish coronary blood flow. The latter finding suggests that α-adrenergic constrictor effects may be inhibited in the presence of a β-adrenergic dilator system (Nayler and Carson, 1973; Pace, 1977).

It is noteworthy that β-adrenergic blockade in the anesthetized dog results in a significant decrease in myocardial oxygen consumption and an increase in cardiac efficiency (Nayler and Carson, 1973); however, during β-blockade, cardiac sympathetic nerve stimulation causes coronary artery vasoconstriction and a mean reduction in coronary sinus blood P_{O_2} of 6 mm Hg. The latter effect can be prevented by α-adrenergic blockade (Feigl, 1975a,b). Feigl has suggested that coronary α-adrenergic receptors may play a role in controlling myocardial oxygen consumption by retarding microvascular flow, thereby permitting increased oxygen extraction by the heart. Others have presented evidence that the coronary vasoconstriction due to α-receptor activity may increase nutritive flow to myocardial tissue (Juhász-Nagy and Szentiványi, 1973).

Studies by Gregg and co-workers (1972) revealed that cardiac denervation reduced the mean circumflex coronary blood flow in anesthetized dogs to about 50% of that in the innervated heart; resting cardiac oxygen consumption also decreased in a manner parallel to the reduction in coronary flow. Following cardiac denervation, coronary blood flow and myocardial function appear adequate even during moderate stress; however, cardiac sympathetic innervation may be of value for optimal control of blood flow and myocardial performance under conditions of mild to moderate stress. Certainly during severe stress, sympathetic innervation of the heart is mandatory for maximal performance of the heart. (See discussion in Section IV,I.)

In vivo studies, therefore, support the concept that both β- and α-adrenergic receptors are present in the coronary arteries; under appropriate conditions such as those previously cited, β-receptor stimulation produces smooth muscle relaxation and vasodilatation, whereas α-receptor stimulation causes muscle contraction and vasoconstriction.

Furthermore, as mentioned previously (Section III,B), *in vitro* studies revealed that catecholamines caused segments of small coronary arteries (250–500 μm) to relax, whereas large arteries (1.5–2.5 mm) were caused to contract. In small arteries relaxation responses were abolished by β-adrenergic blockers and often converted to contraction, whereas contraction responses in large arteries were abolished by α-adrenergic blockers (Zuberbuhler and Bohr, 1965). It should be mentioned that α- and β-adrenergic receptors have been pharmacologically identified in coronary arteries of the unanesthetized dog. Pitt and associates (1967) found only coronary dilatation during the initial 20–30 sec following intracoronary infusion of norepinephrine. Vatner and co-workers (1975) demonstrated that intravenous administration of norepinephrine resulted in a decrease in coronary vascular resistance for the initial 20–30 sec followed by a prolonged coronary vasoconstriction. This constrictor response occurred despite increases in left ventricular pressure and contractility. Failure of previous investigators to demonstrate the latter response probably resulted from the effects of anesthesia on coronary vascular reactivity (Vatner and Braunwald, 1975). When propranolol was administered to unanesthetized dogs, adrenergic activity appeared to be minimal, since no significant alterations in coronary or systemic hemodynamics occurred (Pitt et al., 1970).

It is noteworthy that although some forms of stress, such as hypoxic hypoxia, may enhance β-adrenergic activity, the latter is not essential for the coronary vasodilatation that occurs (Erickson and Stone, 1972) under conditions of hypoxic stress.

With regard to reflex control of the coronary circulation, it appears that bilateral carotid occlusion following bilateral vagotomy evokes an increased heart rate, blood pressure, and circumflex coronary artery blood flow. Feigl (1967) found that a marked decrease in coronary artery resistance accompanied these changes. In the presence of β-blockade, diastolic resistance in the coronary arteries increased; however, bilateral upper thoracic sympathectomy abolished this rise in resistance. The results suggest that α-adrenergic coronary vasoconstriction may participate in the reflex induced by carotid sinus hypotension (Feigl, 1975a). Conversely, simulation of carotid sinus hypertension (by electrically stimulating the carotid sinus nerves) in the conscious dog resulted in a decreased mean and late coronary resistance, heart rate, and aortic pressure. Neither β-blockade nor atropine administration altered the coronary dilator response; however, the response was prevented by α-receptor blockade (Vatner et al., 1970). Apparently, carotid sinus nerve stimulation results in a reduction in the resting sympathetic constrictor tone (Abboud, 1972; Pace, 1977).

Carotid chemoreceptor stimulation by intracarotid administration of nicotine causes a decrease in coronary vascular resistance and an increase in coronary blood flow. Studies by Vatner and McRitchie (1975) in conscious dogs indicate that this coronary vasodilatation induced by nicotine is caused to a minor degree by reflex activation of vagal cholinergic fibers; however, the major cause appeared to be withdrawal of α-adrenergic constrictor tone, which seemed related to the onset of hyperventilation initiated by chemoreceptor stimulation.

Finally, it is noteworthy that activation of intracardiac receptors may result in reflex coronary dilatation through a vagal pathway (Feigl, 1975a).

It has been speculated that activation of α-adrenergic receptors (which occurs in the presence of β-blockade during baroreceptor hypotension) may be responsible for precipitating anginal pain in some patients with coronary insufficiency who are being treated with β-blocking drugs (Pace, 1977).

Pace has summarized points of importance regarding autonomic control of the coronary circulation: Synaptic association of sympathetic and parasympathetic nerves becomes closer as the arteriolar level is approached, thus providing more control of the smaller vessels, which are especially involved in nutritive blood flow. Vagal cholinergic excitation produces coronary vasodilatation, whereas adrenergic excitation causes either vasoconstriction or vasodilatation. α-Adrenergic constriction can only be demonstrated after β-blockade, which prevents both the metabolic cardiac effects and the coronary vasodilatation caused by sympathetic stimulation. Therefore, as Pace has pointed out, it is difficult to evaluate the functional significance of the α-receptors in the presence of augmented myocardial metabolism, which is associated with the release of metabolites causing vasodilatation.

Pace has concisely stated that

the coronary circulation, therefore, appears to possess two possible but relatively weak mechanisms for vasodilatation, e.g., cholinergic parasympathetic and beta adrenergic sympathetic. Based on preliminary evidence it may be surmised that each may participate selectively under different physiological conditions. It is probably fair to assume that active coronary vasodilatation via beta adrenergic mechanisms accompanies generalized myocardial augmentation via the sympathetic nerves, enhancing the subsequent coronary vasodilatation. Conversely, active cholinergic dilatation may arise as a sequela from reflex activation of vagal cholinergic fibers to the myocardium without specific vasomotor regulator functions. A third physiologic mechanism potentially responsible for coronary vasodilatation is the inhibition of tonic vasoconstrictor activity in the alpha receptor system. Thus, while evidence may be marshalled for each of at least three neurogenic mechanisms for regulation, it is probable that all are subsidiary to the direct action of adenosine, or comparable metabolites, acting in consort with varying levels of blood oxygen during widely varying metabolic demands upon the myocardium [Pace, 1977].

I. Cardiac Denervation and Reinnervation

Chemical denervation of the heart by the use of atropine with β-adrenergic blockade, reserpine, 6-hydroxydopamine, or immunosympathectomy lacks specificity, since it affects the autonomic nervous system in areas other than the heart. On the other hand, surgical denervation of the heart provides a more precise means of evaluating the role of cardiac innervation on myocardial performance at rest and during stress; however, it has been emphasized that the method of denervation can radically influence results. The denervation must be complete but without disturbance of other viscera (e.g., the lungs and gastrointestinal tract). The effect of anesthesia on cardiovascular responses and the fact that reinnervation may occur as early as 20–30 days following cardiac denervation in the subhuman species must be appreciated (Kaye, 1977; Donald, 1974). An understanding of the effects of complete or partial cardiac denervation is important with regard to its clinical implications in heart transplantation (Shaver *et al.*, 1969; Stinson *et al.*, 1970); in autonomic neuropathies, which may accompany diabetes mellitus (Lloyd-Mostyn *et al.*, 1974); and in Chagas' disease (Amorium *et al.*, 1973). Apparently, diabetic autonomic neuropathy can result in complete cardiac denervation with a fixed rate and a heart that is unresponsive to sympathetic or parasympathetic stimuli (Lloyd-Mostyn *et al.*, 1974). For a thorough account of denervation and reinnervation of the heart the reader is referred to a recent review by Kaye (1977).

Donald, Shepherd, and associates have performed a series of studies that have clarified the functional ability of the denervated heart and the influence of sympathetic innervation on myocardial performance (Donald, 1974; Donald and Samueloff, 1966; Donald and Shepherd, 1963; Donald *et al.*, 1964, 1968). Total cardiac denervation in the mongrel dog resulted in an absence of sinus arrhythmia and a very regular R-R interval.

The heart rates were between 90 and 120 beats/min (quite similar to rates in the normal dog) if the animal was not disturbed. At rest, values for cardiac output, stroke volume, left ventricular systolic pressure, left ventricular dP/dt, and left ventricular maximal ejection rate were similar to values in normal dogs. The immediate and marked tachycardia observed in normal dogs that were startled or exposed to emotional excitement was absent in dogs with cardiac denervation. Intravenous administration of atropine or tyramine to denervated dogs did not cause a change in heart rate, in contrast to the tachycardia seen in normal dogs. Intravenous administration of catecholamines induced a more pronounced elevation of heart rate in the denervated dog than in the intact dog. The denervated heart was more responsive to norepinephrine than to epinephrine.

Mild exercise caused a modest tachycardia and an increased cardiac output; however, the latter was almost entirely due to an increased stroke volume that accompanied the increased left ventricular end diastolic pressure and the increased fiber length. (Similar hemodynamic alterations have been observed in man following cardiac transplantation.) On the other hand, the increased cardiac output in the normal dog during exercise resulted almost entirely from the increased heart rate. With severe exercise the heart rate increased slowly and reached a much reduced peak value during the first 2 min of running as compared to the peak value in the normal dog. The pattern of oxygen uptake during and immediately following exercise was similar in the normal and in the dog with cardiac denervation; oxygen uptake and cardiac output were as high before as after denervation. These investigators also demonstrated that even with the extreme effort of racing performed by greyhounds (which probably required some anaerobic metabolism) there was only a very minor reduction in the ability of the denervated heart to meet the circulatory demands of maximal exercise (Donald *et al.,* 1964).

Bilateral adrenalectomy in mongrel dogs maintained on cortisone replacement did not alter the response of the denervated heart to exercise; therefore, since the technique of total cardiac denervation depletes myocardial catecholamines (Cooper *et al.,* 1961), Donald and Shepherd concluded that the tachycardia observed in their denervated animals could not be ascribed to catecholamines released from the heart or adrenal glands. Furthermore, the increase in cardiac rate was not dependent on changes in right atrial transmural pressure or blood temperature (Donald and Shepherd, 1963).

Subsequently it was shown that moderate exercise of dogs with chronic cardiac denervation liberated a substance (presumably catecholamines) into the blood, which in turn accelerated the heart rate of an isolated denervated heart. This acceleration could be prevented by β-adrenergic blockade with propranolol. On the other hand, it was found that β-adrenergic blockade with a similar dose of propranolol administered to mongrel dogs with chronic cardiac denervation did not alter the response of the heart rate to moderate exercise (Guyton *et al.,* 1972). These findings indicated that circulating catecholamines were not responsible for the tachycardia accompaning moderate exercise in dogs with chronic cardiac denervation (Donald and Samueloff, 1966). From the foregoing it was concluded that exercise tachycardia in dogs with chronic denervation resulted from an intrinsic property of the heart rather than from a blood-borne agent.

As demonstrated by Donald and associates (1964), there was very little reduction in myocardial performance in the dog with cardiac denervation, even with severe exercise. [Supersensitivity of the denervated heart to circulating catecholamines (Donald and Shepherd, 1965) may be an important factor in augmenting performance of the denervated heart during intense exercise (Guyton *et al.,* 1972).] Furthermore, β-adrenergic blockade in the normal greyhound only slightly increased racing time and maximal heart rate (apparently, β-adrenergic blockade abolishes the effects of circulating catecholamines on the heart but only partially blocks the reflex stimulation of cardiac sympathetic nerves evoked by exercise) (Donald *et al.,* 1968). However, in the presence of both cardiac denervation and β-adrenergic blockage, the capability of performing severe work (Donald and Samueloff, 1966) or racing (Donald *et al.,* 1968) was markedly curtailed. Most of the mongrel dogs failed to complete a heavy workload, and in the greyhounds cardiac acceleration was markedly limited, racing time was prolonged, and animals finished in a state of collapse. Donald and associates concluded that the cardiostimulant action of both the sympathetic innervation of the heart and circulating catecholamines was necessary for maximal myocardial performance. Interruption of one of these mechanisms (by cardiac denervation or β-adrenergic blockade) reduced maximal performance only slightly; however, withdrawal of both support mechanisms severely limited performance of maximal exercise. In the presence of cardiac denervation and β-adrenergic blockade, the heart must depend solely on the Frank–Starling length–tension mechanism to increase its power of contraction. The latter mechanism is sufficient to handle a moderate workload but incapable of sustaining adequate myocardial function during maximal exercise (Donald *et al.*, 1968). It is noteworthy that similar hemodynamic alterations have been observed during mild exercise in man following cardiac transplantation (Shaver *et al.*, 1969; Stinson *et al.*, 1970).

Studies on the metabolism of the denervated heart have been few and controversial. Although there appear to be no major alterations in myocardial metabolism, Gregg and associates found that in denervated conscious dogs at rest and during exercise the coronary blood flow and myocardial oxygen consumption were about half that of normal dogs under similar conditions (Gregg *et al.*, 1972).

In summary, Donald stated that,

> Animal studies and later clinical experience seem to have satisfied that initial question of the competence of the transplanted heart to meet the demands of everyday activity. The heart derprived of extrinsic cardiac nerves adequately meets the demand of pressure and volume loading by the length-tension mechanism and a limited intrinsic tachycardia or, if the stress is sufficiently severe, by the additional excitatory effect of circulating catecholamines [Donald, 1974].

As previously mentioned, the myocardial content of catecholamines and the sympathetic nerves to the heart appear to be involved in the genesis of arrhythmias and ventricular fibrillation that develop following acute occlusion of the coronary artery in the normal dog. Arrhythmias and ventricular fibrillation induced by coronary occlusion or a potassium releasing agent in the normal dog can be prevented by cardiac denervation (Ebert *et al.*, 1968, 1970; Schaal *et al.*, 1969; Vanderbeek and Ebert, 1970).

Other studies involving the stress of hypertension, hypotension, anemia, or hypoxia in animals and man with cardiac denervation indicated that the neurally induced tachycardia is an important part of the cardiac response to stress; the denervated or transplanted heart responds less than normally to these forms of stress (Kaye, 1977). Studies on the transplanted human heart after β-adrenergic blockade suggest that the heart has an intrinsic ability to increase its rate in addition to the acceleration caused by circulating catecholamines (Shaver *et al.*, 1969). Studies also indicate that the denervated or transplanted heart becomes almost totally deplete of catecholamines (Cooper *et al.*, 1961, 1962; Goodall and Kirshner, 1956) and that it obeys Cannon's "laws of denervation" (Cannon, 1939) and becomes supersensitive to circulating catecholamines (Cooper *et al.*, 1964; Dempsey and Cooper, 1968; Donald and Samueloff, 1966; Donald and Shepherd, 1965; Ebert, 1968; Priola, 1969). As a result, the denervated or transplanted heart responds with increases in heart rate, force of contraction, and cardiac output to infusions of even minute concentrations of catecholamines. Supersensitivity may be explained by a loss of intraneuronal binding of circulating catecholamines (Dempsey and Cooper, 1968). Evidently, the ability of the transplanted heart to synthesize, bind, and store catecholamines is dependent on its content of sympathetic nerves (Potter *et al.*, 1965).

Uptake, retention, and synthesis of catecholamines by the transplanted heart were found to be only a few percent of those in the normal intact heart; however, little change occurred in the *in vitro* activity of the enzymes (monoamine oxidase and catechol O-methyltransferase) that metabolize the catecholamines. Since catecholamines coming in contact with the myocardium of the transplanted heart are not taken up by neurons, they are metabolized largely by COMT, as are the circulating catecholamines (Potter *et al.*, 1965).

Recent investigations by Palmer and associates (1975) indicated that denervation causes changes in the postjunctional adrenergic receptor as well as the prejunctional uptake mechanism. Since adenylate cyclase activity from the atria and ventricles of denervated hearts exhibited a two- to threefold greater increase in response to norepinephrine than normal hearts, it was suggested that denervation supersensitivity might depend on both prejunctional and postjunctional changes.

The response of the denervated heart to sympathomimetic drugs (e.g., tyramine, metaraminol, ephedrine, and mephentermine), which normally displace and release catecholamines, is attenuated, whereas the responses to ouabain, calcium chloride, and glucagon are similar to those in the normal heart (Kaye, 1977).

Reinnervation of the heart may occur in the subhuman species but not in the human after cardiac transplantation. Functional responses to reflex and electrical stimulation of the nervous system return to normal within 1–3 years following cardiac denervation (Kaye, 1977). It is noteworthy that functional reinnervation of various segments of the heart, the return of reflexes, and decrease in supersensitivity of segments of the myocardium have been correlated with the return of local myocardial catecholamine content (Kaye, 1977). Kaye has demonstrated that the atria (particularly the left atrium) recover their norepinephrine first and that it subsequently returns to the base of the ventricles and finally to the apical area. In his experience, sympathetic reinnervation of the heart occurred in a base-to-apex direction and was complete about 9 months after denervation. Although return of function (which appeared complete by 9–12 months) parallels return of measurable quantities of myocardial norepinephrine, it is interesting that concentrations of norepinephrine were only a fraction of normal concentrations even 26 months after denervation (Kaye, 1977). (Normal concentrations are greater than 2 $\mu g/g$ for atrial tissue and 1 $\mu g/g$ for ventricular tissue.)

J. Neural Influences on Cardiac Electrical Activity

Not only do the autonomic nerves to the heart alter mechanical and metabolic function, but they also influence electrical activity. All these effects are caused by actions of norepinephrine and acetylcholine, which alter sarcolemmal ionic conductances and thereby produce changes in membrane properties and transmembrane potential.

Modest hyperpolarization is induced by norepinephrine and is probably caused either by an activation of the sodium pump or a change in the sodium/potassium ratio. If an action potential is induced by sympathetic nerve activation, it reduces transmembrane potential and augments an influx of calcium and probably some other ions. Calcium is the essential stimulus for excitation–contraction coupling and is also important in regulating intracellular calcium stores (Hoffman, 1977).

Norepinephrine alters the action potential duration to varying degrees. The explanation for this variability is unclear. However, there is evidence for the existence of both β- and α-adrenergic receptors: The former increase and the latter decrease atrial and idioventricular pacemaker rate (Rosen *et al.,* 1977). Activation of β-receptors causes action potential shortening, whereas activation of α-receptors causes prolongation (Giotti *et al.,* 1973). The magnitude of the change is small and masked by rate-dependent changes in action potential duration, since catecholamines usually accelerate heart rate (Hoffman, 1977). The actions of catecholamines on β- and α-cardiac adrenergic receptors, as summarized by Reder and Rosen (1978), appear in Table VI.

Catecholamines exert an important effect on the myocardium by increasing automaticity; i.e., they increase rate of spontaneous firing of specialized cardiac fibers. Studies on cardiac Purkinje fibers indicate that catecholamines increase the slope of the slow diastolic phase of depolarization (phase 4) so that the transmembrane potential reaches the threshold more rapidly. This effect occurs consistently with relatively high concentrations of norepinephrine; however, with very low concentrations of this catecholamine, a slight decrease in the slope of phase 4 invariably occurs,

TABLE VI

Actions of Catecholamines on α and β Cardiac Adrenergic Receptors[a]

β-Effects

   An increase in the sinus rate

   Increased conduction velocity through the A-V node (thereby resulting in shortening of the A-H interval in His bundle electrograms and the P-R interval in ECGs)

   A decrease in both the functional and effective refractory periods of the A-V node, permitting an increase in ventricular rate during A-V block due to a decrease in the degree of block

   A slight shortening of the relative refractory period of the ventricular specialized conducting system

   Changes in ventricular vulnerability to arrhythmias, as reflected in a decreased ventricular fibrillation threshold and altered Q-T intervals in the ECG

α-Effects

   Depression of spontaneous automaticity of Purkinje fibers and atrial specialized conducting fibers

   An increase in cardiac action-potential duration

   A decrease in potassium uptake by Purkinje fibers

   Conduction block in partially depolarized Purkinje fibers

---

[a] Table compiled from data of Reder and Rosen (1978).

which diminishes the rate of autonomic firing. Extremely high concentrations of epinephrine may cause incomplete repolarization and a series of oscillatory depolarizations before repolarization is finally complete. It appears that a slowing of automaticity is due to stimulation of α-adrenergic receptors, whereas an acceleration is caused by β-receptor activation (Hoffman, 1977). Recently it has been shown that the effects of β-adrenergic amines on automaticity are greater in neonates than in adults (Rosen *et al.*, 1977; Mary-Rabine *et al.*, 1978). Figure 14 reveals modifications of the transmembrane action potential recorded from the S-A node that result in altered automaticity.

Experimental evidence suggests that the effects of catecholamines on transmembrane potentials may result from activation of adenylate cyclase and the generation of cyclic AMP. Exposure of Purkinje fibers to dibutyryl cyclic AMP produces effects similar to those caused by the catecholamines on phases 2, 3, and 4 of the transmembrane potential. Furthermore, intracellular injection of cyclic AMP mimics the effects of catecholamines on phase 4 and shortens the action potential (Tsien *et al.*, 1972).

The effect of stimulating β-adrenergic receptors in various cells of the heart varies. Activation of β-receptors of cells in the sinus node augments the slope of phase 4 depolarization and thereby increases the frequency with which they generate action potentials. Exogenous catecholamines and

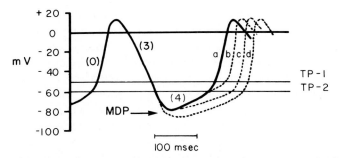

Fig. 14. Diagrammatic representation of the transmembrane potentials of a fiber in the sinoatrial node showing the changes responsible for alterations in the normal automatic mechanism. MPD = maximum diastolic potential; (4) indicates phase 4 of the transmembrane potential; TP = threshold potential. The diagram indicates that a decrease in the slope of phase 4 (upstrokes a to c), a shift of threshold potential from TP-2 to TP-1 (upstrokes a to b) or an increase in maximum diastolic potential (from c to d) all can decrease the rate of automatic firing. (From Hoffman, 1977, p. 292. Copyright © by Oxford University Press, Inc. Reprinted by permission.)

sympathetic nerve stimulation may also shift the pacemaker site within the sinus node. Stimulation of β-receptors of atrial cells has little effect on action potentials in the working myocardium, although high catecholamine concentrations accelerate repolarization of normal human atrial cells. Specialized cells in the crista terminalis of the atrium, however, respond to β-adrenergic stimulation by the appearance of enhancement of spontaneous diastolic depolarization.

The mitral valve leaflets are richly innervated with sympathetic fibers; catecholamines increase pacemaker activity in these leaflets but by a mechanism different from that in the atrium or sinus node. Catecholamines initiate a delayed after-depolarization, which responds to an increased rate of stimulation by an increase in spontaneous action potentials.

β-Adrenergic stimulation of atrioventricular (A-V) cells improves and accelerates conduction through the A-V node. Catecholamines increase the rates of depolarization in cells of the upper (AN) and middle (N) region of the A-V node. Cells of the lower nodal region (NH) are capable of spontaneous impulse formation; in these cells catecholamines enhance spontaneous diastolic depolarization and impulse initiation. However, catecholamines do not appear to cause firing in the AN and N regions of the A-V node.

Stimulation of β-adrenergic receptors of ventricular muscle cells has little effect on transmembrane potentials and conduction velocity; spontaneous depolarization and automatic impulse formation are not induced, but repolarization may be slightly accelerated (Hoffman, 1977).

The response to catecholamines of cells with abnormal electrical properties (due to disease, drugs, or experimental intervention) may differ dramatically from that of normal myocardial cells. Sometimes catecholamines may restore electrical activity of depressed cells toward normal; at other times they may facilitate or cause unusual electrical phenomena. By sufficiently hyperpolarizing transmembrane potential of depressed cells, abnormal automatic firing frequently ceases and normal electrical activity is restored. If cells are markedly depressed by adrenergic β-blockade, catecholamines may increase resting potential or maximum diastolic potential and restore transmembrane potential toward normal. The effect of catecholamines on rate, rhythm, and conduction of abnormal cells altered by drugs or disease is difficult to predict; sometimes catecholamines restore electrical activity toward normal, but other times they may cause afterpotentials and "slow" responses (i.e., action potentials with remarkably low rates of depolarization, which are small in amplitude and propagate extremely slowly) (Hoffman, 1977).

The effects of vagal stimulation or acetylcholine administration on electrical activity of normal and abnormal myocardial cells will not be considered here. Recent discussions of this topic appear elsewhere (Urthaler and James, 1977; Hoffman, 1977). However, for simplicity of comparing and understanding differences between the effects of catecholamines and acetylcholine on the physiological response and action potential in various regions of the heart, Tables VII and VIII have been included.

Normally, changes in cardiac activity caused by the sympathetic or parasympathetic nerves result from increased activity in one of these components of the autonomic system and from decreased activity in the other. Sympathetic stimulation increases sinus rate, and since A-V conduction is enhanced and the sinus normally fires at the most rapid rate, sympathetic stimulation does not cause arrhythmias despite vagal withdrawal. However, failure of the sinus to respond to the liberated norepinephrine or impairment of impulse transmission from sinus to atrium may be accompanied by emergence of ectopic atrial or ventricular rhythm; under these circumstances, sympathetic stimulation increases normal automaticity of specialized cells at ectopic sites. Even if the sinus responds normally to the liberated norepinephrine, enhanced responsiveness to catecholamines elsewhere in the heart can lead to arrhythmias and conduction disturbances. If A-V conduction does not permit a one-to-one transmission of a rapid atrial rate, ventricular escape may occur.

Abnormal cells in the conduction system may respond to normal concentrations of norepinephrine with an excessive rate and escape from sinus control. Activation of some efferent sympathetic nerves may change condi-

TABLE VII

Effects of Catecholamines on the Electrophysiological Properties of the Heart[a]

Region	Physiological response	Effects on action potential
S-A node	Acceleration of pacemaker, shortened refractory period	Accelerated diastolic depolarization,[b] Accelerated repolarization[c] (Hyperpolarization)[c]
Atrial myocardium	Shortened refractory period (enhanced contractility)[b]	Accelerated repolarization[c]
A-V node	Accelerated conduction	Increased amplitude[b] Increased rate of depolarization[b]
His–Purkinje system	Promotion of pacemaker activity, shortened refractory period	Accelerated diastolic depolarization[d] Accelerated repolarization[c] (Hyperpolarization)
Ventricular myocardium	Shortened refractory period (enhanced contractility)[b]	Accelerated repolarization[c] (Hyperpolarization)[c]

[a] From Katz (1977, p. 368), reprinted by permission.
[b] Possibly or probably due to increased calcium conductance.
[c] Probably due to increased potassium conductance.
[d] Probably due to accelerated decrease in i_{K_2} (outward potassium current).

TABLE VIII

Effects of Acetylcholine on the Electrophysiological Properties of the Heart[a]

Region	Physiological response	Effects on action potential
S-A node	Slowing of pacemaker	Hyperpolarization[b] Slowed diastolic depolarization[b]
Atrial myocardium	Shortened refractory period (depressed contractility)	Acceleration of repolarization[b] Reduced slow inward current
A-V node	Slowed conduction	Reduced "summation" of impulses in AN region (acceleration of repolarization and decreased amplitude)[c]
His–Purkinje system and ventricular myocardium	Little or none	Acceleration of repolarization only at extremely high concentrations[b]

[a] From Katz (1977, p. 365), reprinted by permission.
[b] Probably due to increased potassium conductance.
[c] Possibly due to increased potassium conductance.

tions in only one area of the heart and alter impulse conduction, impulse generation, or repolarization.

Changes in electrophysiological properties of cardiac muscle that occur in various diseases and during therapy with some drugs may markedly influence the response of the heart to sympathetic activation. For example, in the presence of a segment of ischemic myocardium the inotropic and chronotropic effects caused by augmented sympathetic tone will increase perfusion requirements and intensify ischemia. The latter may then evoke arrhythmias and conduction disturbances. Electrophysiological alterations occur with some drugs; digitalis may modify the response of myocardial fibers to catecholamines and thereby induce arrhythmias during sympathetic nerve activation.

Sympathetic activity may also improve A-V conduction, reduce heart block, eliminate an ectopic ventricular focus, and restore cardiac rhythm. Similar effects may be exerted on supraventricular rhythm in the presence of sinoatrial conduction defects. An increased sinus rate may actually reduce the likelihood of atrial and ventricular ectopic impulses.

The interplay of the autonomic nervous system and its effects on abnormal electrophysiology of the heart is complex and the myocardial responses are variable and sometimes unpredictable. For a detailed account of neural influences on cardiac electrical activity and rhythm the reader is referred to the review by Hoffman (1977), on which the preceding discussion is based.

K. The Autonomic Nervous System in Relation to Electrocardiographic Waveform and Cardiac Rhythm

Electrocardiographic waveform abnormalities may occur in patients with central nervous system disease (e.g., trauma, tumor, infections, cerebrovascular accidents). Such abnormalities appear to be caused by altered autonomic influence on ventricular recovery and cardiac rhythm (Abildskov and Vincent, 1977); they consist of prolonged Q-T intervals, prominent U waves, and large T waves (of either polarity). Low T waves and/or S-T segment displacement may also be observed but are less marked and less characteristic. Of major significance is the enhanced susceptibility of the heart to cardiac arrhythmias that occur in some patients with central nervous system disease.

Sympathetic nerve stimulation can alter T wave amplitude and cause S-T segment displacement, and stellate ganglion stimulation can cause electrocardiographic and vectorcardiographic changes (Rothberger and Winterber, 1910; Ueda et al., 1964; Yanowitz et al., 1966). Furthermore, right ganglionectomy can cause a greater T wave positivity and a prolonged refractory period of the anterior ventricular walls, whereas left ganglionectomy can cause a greater T wave negativity and prolonged refractory periods principally in the posterior wall (Yanowitz *et al.*, 1966). From the electrophysiological effects of stimulating various cardiac nerves, it appears that there is localized rather than diffuse cardiac distribution of sympathetic nerves (Abildskov and Vincent, 1977).

Central nervous system disease is associated not only with electrophysiological abnormalities in waveforms but also with ventricular arrhythmias. Experimental procedures (e.g., stimulation of the hypothalamus or stellate ganglia) result in both waveform abnormalities and arrhythmias such as sinus and junctional tachycardia and ventricular arrhythmias. The fact that sympathetic nerve blockade can sometimes eliminate these abnormalities supports the view that autonomic dysfunction is the cause of the abnormalities.

Prolongation of the Q-T interval can be induced by left stellate ganglion stimulation and by right stellate ganglionectomy. Also, it has been reported that the rapid intravenous injection of catecholamines as a bolus caused transient Q-T prolongation, whereas slow infusion shortened the Q-T interval. It was suggested that administration of catecholamines in a bolus may not permit complete intravascular mixing; therefore the catecholamine effect on different parts of the heart may have been unequal. Prolonged Q-T interval syndromes have been described in man, and in this condition, ventricular fibrillation, particularly after exertion or emotional stress, may result in syncope. This condition has been successfully treated by left stellate ganglionectomy and left sympathectomy, and propranolol has also been employed successfully to diminish episodes of ventricular fibrillation. Evidence suggests that prolonged Q-T interval syndromes involve "a local imbalance of cardiac responses to the sympathetic nervous system" (Abildskov and Vincent, 1977).

Experimental sympathetic stimulation reduces threshold and increases vulnerability of the heart to ventricular fibrillation (Kliks, *et al.*, 1975). If both sympathetic stimulation and coronary occlusion are induced simultaneously, then the fibrillation threshold is reduced even further. On the other hand, sympathectomy raises fibrillation threshold and protects against fibrillation. Vagal stimulation also elevates fibrillation threshold and decreases the occurrence of spontaneous fibrillation induced by coronary occlusion. Excess parasympathetic activity can account for the reflex bradycardia and atrioventricular conduction disorders associated with some types of myocardial infarction (Abildskov and Vincent, 1977).

Increased adrenergic activity may accompany myocardial infarction as a result of fear, reduced cardiac output, and decreased blood pressure; evidence of increased adrenergic activity is reflected by increased plasma and urinary catecholamine concentrations (Gazes *et al.,* 1959; Hingerty and O'Boyle, 1972; Jewitt *et al.,* 1969; McDonald *et al.,* 1969; Nelson, 1970). The effectiveness of adrenergic β-blockade in reducing the occurrence of arrhythmias further supports the concept that adrenergic activity plays an important role in the genesis of arrhythmias in ischemic heart disease and myocardial infarction. Whether the antiarrhythmic action of propranolol is due primarily to its β-adrenergic blocking effect or its quinidinelike effect on membrane stabilization is uncertain (Lemberg *et al.,* 1970). However, since cardioselective β-blockers (e.g., practolol and satalol), which have minimal quinidinelike actions, are effective in suppressing some types of arrhythmias due to ischemic heart disease, it seems probable that their antiarrhythmic action results from β-blockade (Khan *et al.,* 1972). The arrhythmogenic threshold of the myocardium may be reduced by either the norepinephrine released as the neurotransmitter from the sympathetic nerves directly innervating the myocardium or the circulating catecholamines released from the adrenal medulla or sympathetic nerves elsewhere in the body. It is noteworthy that practolol has been reported to have adrenergic nerve depressant properties (Roberts and Kelliher, 1970) and that it is more effective in treating arrhythmias occurring early, when plasma catecholamine concentrations are usually highest, rather than late, after myocardial infarction (Allen *et al.,* 1975). Some studies on digitalis and ouabain-induced toxicity suggest that practolol exerts its antiarrhythmic effect not only by β-adrenergic receptor blockade but by depressing adrenergic nerve activity (Kelliher and Roberts, 1974).

Finally, it has been pointed out that increased sympathetic activity to the heart can increase the magnitude of ischemic injury in the experimental animal and thereby enhance the genesis of arrhythmias (Abildskov and Vincent, 1977). The degree of ischemic injury and the occurrence of arrhythmias may be reduced by propranolol, which has been shown to improve myocardial oxygenation and hemodynamics in some patients following myocardial infarction (Mueller *et al.,* 1974).

V. Adrenergic Involvement in Cardiac Pathophysiology

From the foregoing it seems well established experimentally that the sympathetic innervation of the heart and circulating catecholamines can play an important role in the alteration of the electrophysiology of the myocardium and in the genesis of arrhythmias. Although the role of the adrenergic system is less clearly defined, it appears that in the human it can also play a significant or key role in some types of cardiac pathophysiology.

A. Arrhythmias in Myocardial Ischemia and Infarction

Earlier in this chapter studies were cited that indicate that an augmented adrenergic activity to the heart facilitates the induction of ventricular arrhythmias, including fibrillation. Ventricular tachycardia is frequently induced by electrical stimulation of sympathetic nerves to the heart (Armour *et al.*, 1972; Gillis *et al.*, 1974; Hageman *et al.*, 1973a; Urthaler and James, 1973; Van Citters *et al.*, 1966). Electrophysiological evidence indicates that coronary occlusion can activate cardiac sympathetic afferent fibers (Malliani *et al.*, 1973), which in turn can excite efferent cardiac sympathetics (Malliani *et al.*, 1969) and result in ventricular arrhythmias (Gillis *et al.*, 1974). Bilateral cardiac sympathectomy reduces the incidence of ventricular fibrillation and the mortality rate that usually follows experimental coronary occlusion (Cox and Robertson, 1936; Ebert, 1969; Ebert *et al.*, 1970; Fowlis *et al.*, 1974; Harris, 1964; Harris *et al.*, 1951; Skelton *et al.*, 1962). Furthermore, β-adrenergic blockade exerts a protective effect in reducing ventricular fibrillation following coronary occlusion (Khan *et al.*, 1972). Ebert (1969) showed that in dogs with cardiac sympathectomy, the release of potassium from the myocardium was absent or attenuated following coronary ligation. Therefore activity of the sympathetic innervation of the heart may be an important determinant of potassium flux and may be involved in the genesis of ventricular arrhythmias accompanying a coronary occlusion. It is noteworthy that the infarcts resulting from coronary occlusion were similar in size whether the cardiac nerves were intact or not (Randall, 1977).

Fowlis and associates demonstrated that cardiac sympathectomy provided significant protection against postocclusion mortality, particularly in the first 15 min following occlusion. Thereafter the difference in mortality following coronary occlusion between control dogs and dogs with cardiac sympathectomy became progressively less significant with the passage of time. Although the reasons for the protective effect of sympathectomy are unknown, these investigators pointed out that removal of sympathetics may result in depletion or impaired release of myocardial norepinephrine, a diminished stimulus to the release of adrenal catecholamines into the circulation, interruption of cardiocardiac excitatory spinal reflexes, or a combination of these mechanisms (Fowlis *et al.*, 1974).

In accord with the findings of others (Ebert *et al.*, 1970; Goodall and Kirshner, 1956), Fowlis and co-workers (1974) demonstrated that myocardial norepinephrine was significantly reduced (0.13 ± 0.08 μg/g of myocardium, wet weight) 4 weeks after cardiac sympthectomy but returned to normal (0.66 ± 0.3 μg/g) at 6 months. [The explanation for this return to normal concentration of norepinephrine is unclear. Others have reported that cardiac sympathectomy results in a marked depletion in myocardial catecholamines for as long as 12 months, despite reinnervation (Hageman *et al.*, 1973b).] Slightly higher norepinephrine concentrations were found in the nonischemic myocardium of the left ventricle of dogs that succumbed within 15 min of the coronary occlusion as compared to ventricles of dogs surviving more than 48 hr; the lower norepinephrine concentration in the latter group may have resulted from some degree of heart failure. Norepinephrine concentrations in infarcted areas of the ventricles gradually decreased over 48 hr to relatively low levels; this finding is similar to results reported by others (Russell *et al.*, 1961). Table IX reveals the effect of coronary occlusion on norepinephrine concentrations in intact dogs and those subjected to cardiac sympathectomy.

Fowlis and associates found no correlation between myocardial norepinephrine content and postocclusion heart rate and ventricular arrhythmias. Hence they could not implicate the absolute norepinephrine concentration in the genesis of arrhythmias and death. Whether coronary occlusion in dogs with cardiac sympathectomy may be associated with impaired release of myocardial norepinephrine and/or an impaired reflex release of catecholamines into the circulation from the adrenal and elsewhere remains uncertain. Although the precise mechanism whereby sympathectomy protects agsinst fatal arrhythmias following occlusion is unclear, a suppression of the adrenergic effect on the heart appears to be implicated.

Spurgeon and co-workers (1974) reported that cardiac denervation resulted in a reduction of atrial and ventricular epinephrine to 40–60% of

TABLE IX

Myocardial Norepinephrine[a]

	BSTG-4 wk	BSTG-6 mo	Control
Left atrium mean		0.89 ± 0.28 (9)	1.0 ± 0.4 (7)
Nonischemic ventricle			
Mean	0.13 ± 0.08 (3)	0.66 ± 0.3 (11)	0.68 ± 0.4 (15)
<15 min		0.75 ± 0.33 (4)	0.86 ± 0.5 (6)
>48 hr		0.51 ± 0.25 (5)	0.59 ± 0.33 (8)
Infarcted ventricle			
Mean		0.59 ± 0.38 (7)	0.58 ± 0.5 (10)
<15 min		0.69 ± 0.37 (4)	0.94 ± 0.63 (4)
>48 hr		0.21 ± 0.06 (2)	0.3 ± 0.23 (5)

[a] Values in micrograms per gram of myocardium (wet weight ± standard deviation). BSTG: Bilateral stellate ganglionectomy and thoracic sympathectomy. 4 wk: Four weeks duration. 6 mo: Six months duration. <15: Animals dying in less than 15 min. >48: Animals surviving more than 48 hr. Number of dogs in each group in parentheses. Mean values for BSTG-4 wk were significantly less than mean values for control and for BSTG-6 mo ($p < 0.005$, derived by Student t-test) for the nonischemic ventricle. No other significant differences were found. From Fowlis *et al.* (1974, p. 753), reprinted with permission.

control concentrations, whereas norepinephrine was reduced to 1–3% of control levels. They also found that the norepinephrine in conductile tissue (i.e., the bundle branches, S-A and A-V nodal tissue) was reduced to levels approaching zero, whereas epinephrine concentrations in conductile tissue (except for the S-A node) were not significantly reduced. These results suggested that, in contrast to the intraneuronal location of myocardial norepinephrine, epinephrine appears to be present in a nonneuronal location, since it persists after denervation.

Catecholamines can increase diastolic depolarization in Purkinje fibers and pacemaker cells and thereby can induce repetitive firing (Hoffman, 1967). As pointed out by Randall (1977), these changes induced by catecholamines, coupled with the nonuniform recovery of ventricular muscle excitability (Han and Moe, 1964), can result in disorganized conduction and lead to multiple reentry circuits and fibrillation. Randall (1977) has stated that

> the high incidence of premature beats and ventricular tachycardia in normal dogs subjected to major coronary vessel occlusion and the marked attenuation of such disrhythmias following denervation, suggest an important association between local catecholamine content of the myocardium and the development of arrhythmias after infarction. A homogeneous distribution of catecholamines throughout the myocardium, on the other hand, tends to decrease vulnerability to such dysrhythmia [Han et al., 1964].

Opie and associates (1979) have recently reviewed the biochemical aspects of arrhythmogenesis and ventricular fibrillation. They indicated that any biochemical event that (1) decreases resting potential, (2) produces the slow response, (3) shortens the action potential duration, or (4) enhances phase 4 depolarization could be important in the genesis of arrhythmias. They proposed that acute myocardial ischemia is accompanied by an abrupt increase in extracellular potassium (within seconds of coronary occlusion), which causes a loss of membrane potential and a shortened action potential duration. Furthermore, localized hyperkalemia can block the fast response (i.e., the fast inward current caused by sodium ions passing through inward channels in myocardial cells) and unmask or evoke a slow response (i.e., the slow inward current caused predominantly by calcium ions passing through slow inward channels). If hyperkalemia is sufficiently severe it can prevent normal depolarization, and under such circumstances a slow response may be provoked by catecholamines via the generation of cyclic AMP in myocardial cells. In experimental coronary occlusion, increased cyclic AMP has been linked to ventricular arrhythmias and fibrillation. This hypothesis is supported by experiments in which perfusion of an isolated heart preparation with cyclic AMP, β-adrenergic agonists, or theophylline caused a decreased ventricular fibrillation threshold. Also, increased automaticity occurs in partially depolarized Purkinje fibers, especially when there is stimulation by catecholamines or cyclic AMP in the presence of a low external potassium level (Opie et al., 1979). It is noteworthy that at supposed antiarrhythmic concentration of propranolol the following effects are exerted on Purkinje fibers: (1) decreased action potential amplitude, (2) decreased maximal slope of phase-0 depolarization; (3) decreased membrane responsiveness; (4) decreased conduction velocity; (5) decreased action potential duration; and (6) decreased automaticity (Hoffman and Bigger, 1971). Propranolol also slows sinus automaticity and increases the effective refractory period of atrial and A-V nodal tissue and thus antagonizes the electrophysiological effects of β-adrenergic stimulation. The P-R interval is prolonged by propranolol's action on the A-V node (increasing the A-H but not the H-V interval). A high degree of A-V nodal block by propranolol must be avoided clinically, since subsidiary pacemakers may be suppressed and asystole result (Arnsdorf and Hsieh, 1978, p. 1955). It should be appreciated that in addition to its action as a β-adrenergic blocker, propranolol (at relatively high concentrations) also exerts a direct membrane effect somewhat similar to that of quinidine [e.g., propranolol inhibits sodium entry and increases potassium flux and potassium content in myocardial cells (Arnsdorf and Hsieh, 1978)].

B. Myocardial Ischemia and Infarction

Maroko, Braunwald, and associates have presented convincing evidence that indicates that a variety of metabolic and pharmacological interventions can alter myocardial infarct size following coronary occlusion (Braunwald, 1978a; Maroko and Braunwald, 1976). Their findings support the concept that the extent of ischemic myocardial damage following coronary occlusion is importantly influenced by the balance between myocardial oxygen supply and demand. Furthermore, it appears that myocardial damage can be reduced or minimized by interventions that (1) reduce oxygen demand, (2) increase myocardial oxygen supply, (3) augment anaerobic metabolism, (4) enhance transport of energy substrates, or (5) protect against autolytic or heterolytic damage (Maroko and Braunwald, 1976).

Maroko and associates also demonstrated that pacing-induced tachycardia or administration of agents causing a positive inotropic or chronotropic effect on the heart (e.g., isoproterenol, glucagon, bretylium, digitalis) will elevate myocardial oxygen consumption and will increase the extent of myocardial injury following experimental coronary occlusion. Therefore it is conceivable that in some patients following myocardial infarction a significant activation of the adrenergic system may increase the extent of myocardial injury. Contrariwise, reducing oxygen consumption by β-adrenergic blockade with propranolol (Maroko and Braunwald, 1976; Maroko *et al.*, 1969, 1971) or practolol (Libby *et al.*, 1973) reduced myocardial ischemic injury following experimental coronary occlusion.

Intraaortic balloon counterpulsation reduces myocardial oxygen needs by lowering systolic pressure and augmenting coronary artery flow (by increasing aortic diastolic pressure); this mechanical intervention was found to reduce markedly the extent of myocardial ischemic injury (Maroko *et al.*, 1972a; Braunwald and Maroko, 1972). In addition, Spotnitz and associates (1977) have observed that intraaortic balloon counterpulsation appears to reduce adrenergic activity and minimize release of catecholamines into arterial and coronary sinus blood; this limitation of adrenergic activity may play an additional role in reducing ischemic injury by intraaortic balloon counterpulsation.

It is pertinent that in some patients who develop S-T segment elevation (as a consequence of arterial hypotension, anginal pain, or ventricular fibrillation), a reduction in the S-T elevation may occur after propranolol administration (Maroko *et al.*, 1972a,b) and during intraaortic balloon counterpulsation (Maroko *et al.*, 1972a). In addition, propranolol administration (Gold *et al.*, 1974) and intraaortic balloon counterpulsation (Leinbach *et al.*, 1973) reduced the S-T segment elevations and improved metabolism in patients with acute myocardial infarction (Mueller *et al.*, 1971, 1974).

Despite the potentially harmful effects that may be caused by epinephrine and norepinephrine on an ischemic area of myocardium, dopamine (Intropin) has been employed therapeutically in the treatment of cardiogenic shock resulting from myocardial infarction. Dopamine exerts an inotropic effect on the heart, usually without a significant increase in heart rate, and thereby causes a rise in systolic blood pressure and improves peripheral blood flow. Dopamine causes vasoconstriction of skeletal muscle vasculature; however, the unique ability of this catecholamine to dilate renal, mesenteric, cerebral, and coronary arteries (as mentioned in Section III) are distinct virtues in the treatment of cardiovascular shock, particularly when the blood pressure is not at a critically low level that may initially require a potent vasoconstrictor.

It is particularly intriguing and significant that a recent study of patients with "preinfarction" angina documented a vasospastic origin of their anginal attacks (Maseri *et al.*, 1978). Maseri and his associates observed a reduction in myocardial blood supply and coronary vasospasm during angina, independent of the severity of coronary atherosclerosis. They further demonstrated that angina at rest with S-T segment depression was not preceded by increased myocardial metabolic demand but was associated with reduced myocardial perfusion and coronary vasospasm. It is also noteworthy that other investigators have demonstrated that coronary vasoconstriction can be reflexly induced in patients with effort angina by the cold pressor test (Mudge, *et al.*, 1976).

Maseri and co-workers (1978) emphasized that coronary artery spasm has been established as the cause of Prinzmetal's angina and that this mechanism may be extended to include a significant number of other forms of angina. They concluded that coronary vasospasm may be an important cause of myocardial infarction and thrombosis, in the absence or presence of a variable degree of coronary athersclerosis.

Hills and Braunwald (1978) recently reviewed the current understanding of coronary artery spasm. They pointed out that in anesthetized animals coronary blood flow is regulated primarily by the metabolic demands of the heart and that neural influences are relatively unimportant in the control of myocardial blood flow.

On the other hand, experiments in conscious animals have demonstrated that coronary blood flow not only is influenced by metabolic requirements of the heart but also can be greatly influenced by neural mechanisms. As mentioned earlier, both α- and β-adrenergic receptors have been identified in the coronary arteries of the unanesthetized dog (Pitt *et al.*, 1967). The initial large segments of the coronary arteries are richly supplied with α-adrenergic receptors but are termed "conductance" vessels, since vascular resistance is mainly regulated by changes in the lumen of the smaller coronary branches, which have been termed "resistance" vessels (Braunwald *et al.*, 1976). Under normal circumstances the large "conductance" coronary arteries contribute very little to vascular resistance; however, with adrenergic stimulation these arteries constrict markedly and increase vascular resistance (Hills and Braunwald, 1978). There seems to be no question that in normal conscious animals and human beings neurogenic influences on the heart are potentially of great importance.

Catheter-induced coronary artery spasm has been demonstrated to occur occasionally during coronary arteriography, presumably because of mechanical stimulation of the coronary ostia. The coronary artery spasm that causes Prinzmetal's variant angina is usually accompanied by pain at rest (which usually occurs at about the same time each day) and is usually accompanied by S-T elevations (indicating transmural ischemia) rather than the S-T segment depressions (indicating subendocardial ischemia) occurring with typical angina. Hills and Braunwald (1978) point out that although β-adrenergic blockade is usually beneficial to patients with typical angina pectoris, it may be detrimental in patients with Prinzmetal's variant angina, since such a blockade permits α-receptor-mediated coronary vasoconstriction to occur unopposed. On the other hand, α-adrenergic blockade or β-adrenergic stimulation may be beneficial (Hills and Braunwald, 1978). It is noteworthy that partial cardiac sympathectomy in association with coronary artery grafting has proved beneficial to two patients with Prinzmetal's angina (Grondin and Limet, 1977).

The precise cause and mechanism for the coronary artery spasm in Prinzmetal's syndrome remain unclear. Some attention has been focused on α-adrenergic response in the large coronary arteries resulting from sympathetic nerve stimulation or circulating catecholamines (Yasue *et al.*, 1976). Some evidence suggests that increased sympathetic activity may result from increased parasympathetic activity; however, any interrelationship between the parasympathetic nervous system, the adrenergic nervous system, and circulating catecholamines remains to be elucidated (Hurst *et al.*, 1978, p. 1194).

Hills and Braunwald have briefly reviewed the accumulating evidence that coronary artery spasm may be a cause of typical angina pectoris and myocardial infarction. Although the frequency with which coronary spasm plays a role in the genesis of typical angina pectoris and myocardial infarction is unknown, these investigators have indicated the need to assess the efficacy of α-adrenergic blockade in alleviating the occurrence of angina and myocardial infarction. It is interesting that α-adrenergic blockade with phenoxybenzamine can prevent the reflex coronary vasoconstriction elicited in patients with coronary artery disease (Mudge *et al.*, 1976). Braunwald made the intriguing speculation that circulating catecholamines may stimulate the α-adrenergic receptors of human platelets and thereby enhance their ability to produce and release thromboxane A_2, a potent vasoconstrictor. It is conceivable that α-adrenergic blockade can also prevent release of thromboxane A_2 from platelets. Braunwald has further emphasized that in patients in whom ischemia is due to coronary spasm with impaired oxygen delivery (rather than to augmented myocardial oxygen needs) blockade of β_2-adrenergic receptors may be detrimental. Propranolol produces a nonselective β-adrenergic blockade of both β_1-receptors in the myocardium (which reduces oxygen need) and β_2-receptors in the coronary arteries. Since β_2-receptor stimulation induces coronary vasodilatation, blockade of this receptor will permit the unopposed influence of coronary constrictor influences (Braunwald, 1978b).

Finally, Hills and Braunwald (1978) have pointed out the possibility that coronary artery denervation and interruption of adrenergic vasoconstrictor fibers may play a role in the relief of angina in patients who have undergone surgical revascularization, particularly if relief persists despite occlusion of the graft.

C. Adrenergic Nervous System Alterations in Heart Failure

The adrenergic system provides a means for rapid cardiovascular circulatory adjustments—i.e., changes in myocardial contractility, heart rate, and vascular tone. Under normal circumstances activation of cardiac adrenergic nerves and/or an increase in circulating catecholamines subserve a function of "boosting" (augmenting) cardiac function. The adrenergic system also plays an important compensatory (supportive) role in circulatory adjustments of patients to congestive heart failure. Therefore caution must be exercised in using antiadrenergic drugs in patients with a limited cardiac reserve (Braunwald *et al.,* 1977, p. 1177). The concentration of plasma catecholamines has been used as an index of adrenergic activity; however, it must be appreciated that plasma catecholamine elevations after adrenergic activation reflect not only the magnitude of sympathetic stimulation and catecholamine release, but also the effectiveness of inactivating mechanisms and the extent of catecholamine overflow into the circulation (Manger *et al.,* 1975). Furthermore, it is noteworthy that physical training can markedly decrease the rate of catecholamine turnover and may, therefore, influence the adrenergic response to stress. Östman and associates (1972) have reported that cardiac norepinephrine and adrenal catecholamines are significantly increased in trained rats. With acute prolonged exercise cardiac norepinephrine decreased in untrained but not in trained rats. Cardiac norepinephrine turnover was markedly slower in trained rats than in untrained ones. During exercise norepinephrine turnover increased but remained slower in trained rats, and the urinary excretion of catecholamines was greater in the untrained animals. They concluded that chronic physical training induces a functional adaptation of the adrenergic system that results in a better transmitter economy during exercise. The bradycardia of the "athlete's heart" may be due to a decreased cardiac sympathetic nerve activity caused by training (Östman-Smith, 1979).

In normal persons very little change in the concentration of arterial plasma catecholamines occurs during moderate muscular exercise; Chidsey and co-workers (1962a) found that average plasma norepinephrine concentrations rose from 0.28 μg/liter to 0.46 μg/liter. These results were similar to those found in patients with heart disease but without heart failure. On the other hand, in patients with congestive heart failure, the average plasma norepinephrine concentration was 0.63 μg/liter at rest and significantly increased to 1.73 μg/liter during exercise. Since no consistent change in plasma concentrations of epinephrine occurred in patients with heart failure, it appears that the adrenal medulla did not participate in the increased adrenergic activity. Chidsey and co-workers (1962b) concluded that increased adrenergic activity may have an important supportive role in patients with congestive heart failure. Elevated urinary excretion of norepinephrine provides additional evidence of augmented sympathetic nerve activity in patients with congestive heart failure (Chidsey *et al.,* 1965).

Chidsey and associates (1963, 1965) also demonstrated a significant depletion of norepinephrine in myocardial tissue removed during cardiac surgery from patients with heart failure. The norepinephrine concentration in atrial tissue removed from patients with congestive heart failure averaged 0.49 $\mu g/g$, whereas it averaged 1.77 $\mu g/g$ in patients who had not had congestive heart failure—a highly significant difference ($p < 0.01$). The norepinephrine concentration in left ventricular papillary muscle of patients who had heart failure averaged 0.52 $\mu g/g$. Furthermore, there was a significant ($p < 0.05$) correlation between norepinephrine concentrations in atrial and ventricular tissue (e.g., when atrial concentrations were less than 0.40 $\mu g/g$, ventricular concentrations averaged 0.27 $\mu g/g$; when atrial concentrations exceeded 0.40 $\mu g/g$, ventricular concentrations averaged 0.73 $\mu g/g$).

Rutenberg and Spann (1976) concisely reviewed the alterations of cardiac sympathetic neurotransmitter activity in congestive heart failure. Much of the following discussion is based on this review. Spann, Chidsey, and co-workers demonstrated that in the dog (Chidsey *et al.*, 1964) and in the cat (Spann *et al.*, 1964, 1965) a profound reduction in cardiac norepinephrine occurred in experimentally induced heart failure (left or right) or in right ventricular hypertrophy with or without heart failure (Spann *et al.*, 1967a,b) (Fig. 15). Reduced concentrations of norepinephrine occurred in both ventricles, regardless of which ventricle was subjected to a hemodynamic strain.

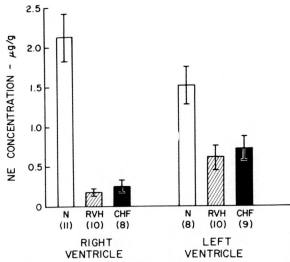

Fig. 15. The average norepinephrine concentration of the right and left ventricles of normal cats and cats with right ventricular hypertrophy (RVH) and congestive heart failure (CHF). Vertical lines with cross bars equal ± 1 standard error of the mean. Numbers in parentheses equal number of animals in each group. (From Spann *et al.*, 1967b, p. 348, reprinted by permission of the American Heart Association, Inc.)

Total norepinephrine content was also markedly diminished, reflecting a true depletion rather than a "dilution" effect of a normal amount of norepinephrine by myocardial hypertrophy (Rutenberg and Spann, 1976). The time course of changes in ventricular norepinephrine concentration and content following experimental production of congestive heart failure is indicated in Fig. 16. It is noteworthy that there was usually no remarkable change in the concentration of norepinephrine in tissues other than the heart during congestive failure (Spann et al., 1965).

The finding of an increased rate of norepinephrine efflux from the coronary sinus when left ventricular pressure was acutely increased to 100 mm Hg suggests that the significant increases in ventricular pressure may be involved in the mechanism of cardiac norepinephrine depletion. Studies

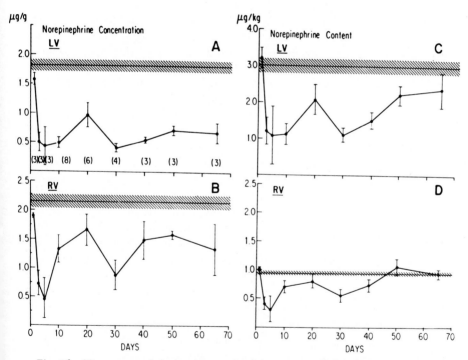

Fig. 16. Time course of changes in norepinephrine concentration in μg/g (A and B) and time course of changes in total norepinephrine content in each ventricle expressed as μg/kg body weight (C and D). Solid circles and vertical bars represent the mean values ± 1 standard error of the mean obtained from animals with congestive heart failure. Horizontal lines and hatched areas represent the mean ± 1 standard error of the mean obtained from 15 normal animals. Numbers in parentheses at the bottom of panel A refer to the number of animals sacrificed at each point in time that provided the data shown in all four panels. (From Spann et al., 1965, p. 315, reprinted by permission of the American Heart Association, Inc.)

revealed that there was a significantly diminished uptake and/or binding of infused norepinephrine in guinea pigs with experimentally induced congestive heart failure as compared to control animals. This impairment in uptake or binding or both, was evident in the heart but not the kidney of animals with congestive failure (Fig. 17). Additional studies indicated that the myocardial norepinephrine depletion occurring in these animals with congestive heart failure could not be explained by a more rapid net turnover of norepinephrine. Furthermore, the depleted norepinephrine stores in the presence of a normal net turnover suggest that the rate of norepinephrine formation is reduced (Spann *et al.*, 1965).

Pool and associates (1967) found a marked reduction in cardiac tyrosine hydroxylase (the rate-limiting enzyme for norepinephrine biosynthesis) activity in dogs with experimentally induced heart failure; average enzyme activity was 3.3 nmole/g per hour in normal dogs compared to 0.4 nmole/g per hour in dogs with congestive heart failure. Also, a highly significant positive correlation was evident between the concentration of norepinephrine and tyrosine hydroxylase in various portions of the myocardium in both the failing and normal heart. They concluded that the available evidence taken together supports the hypothesis of a parallel reduction in synthesis, uptake, and binding of norepinephrine rather than a specific disturbance of one of these functions (Pool *et al.*, 1967). Furthermore, it was subsequently established that any alterations in the enzymes (COMT and MAO) responsible for inactivating the catecholamines could not account for the severe depletion of cardiac norepinephrine occurring in heart failure (Krakoff *et al.*, 1968).

Evidence indicates that in one type of experimental heart failure, there is a reduction in myocardial norepinephrine that parallels the absence of fluorescence in adrenergic nerve terminals of the heart (Vogel *et al.*, 1969). Vogel and associates found that in some animals recovery from heart failure was associated with a return toward normal of both norepinephrine concentration and adrenergic nerve fluorescence within 4 weeks. This interesting observation suggests that the adrenergic abnormality occurring with heart failure may be a reversible metabolic dysfunction of the neuron rather than a permanent malfunction or an actual loss of adrenergic nerves.

It is interesting that experimental Chagas' disease, produced by inoculating *Trypanosoma cruzi* into rats, caused a temporary disappearance of cardiac norepinephrine as determined by histochemical fluorescence and fluorometric quantitation (Machado *et al.*, 1978). Machado and associates suggested that norepinephrine depletion, by impairing the positive inotropic effect of the cardiac sympathetic nerves, was probably the main factor causing congestive heart failure in the acute phase of Chagas' disease. However, it must be appreciated that undoubtedly other factors, such as the

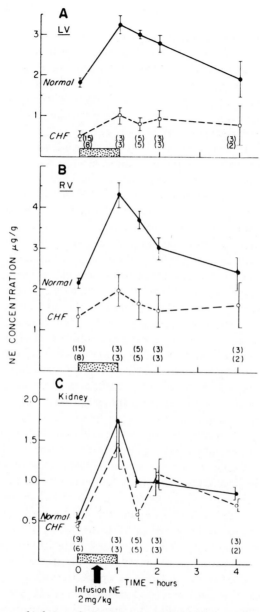

Fig. 17. Effects of infusion of norepinephrine (NE) on the concentrations of norepine-phrine in the (A) left ventricles (LV), (B) right ventricles (RV), and (C) kidneys of normal guinea pigs (solid lines and circles) and guinea pigs with congestive heart failure (CHF) (open circles and broken lines). Vertical bars represent ±1 standard error of the mean. Stippled areas represent duration of infusion, and the numbers in parentheses refer to the number of animals in each group sacrificed at the various times. (From Spann *et al.,* 1965, p. 316, reprinted by permission of the American Heart Association, Inc.)

acute myocarditis, are also necessary to cause heart failure, since sympathetic denervation will not by itself produce congestive failure.

Experimental myocardial infarction is accompanied by a marked depletion or complete disappearance of norepinephrine in the infarcted areas and also a significant decrease in the concentration of norepinephrine in the noninfarcted myocardium—more so in ventricular than in atrial tissue (Mathes and Gudbjarnason, 1971; Mathes *et al.*, 1971). Repletion of myocardial norepinephrine started 2 weeks after infarction and normal concentrations of norepinephrine were found after 6 weeks. No correlation was noted between the concentration of myocardial norepinephrine and the first derivative of left ventricular function (dP/dt); it was concluded that alterations in left ventricular (contractile function) were not related to changes in norepinephrine concentrations.

Studies relating cardiac contractile function to myocardial norepinephrine concentrations were performed on ventricular papillary muscle isolated from normal cats and from those with congestive heart failure or with chronic cardiac denervation (Spann *et al.*, 1967b). Cardiac norepinephrine concentrations were profoundly depleted in the animals with congestive failure and even more so in those with cardiac denervation. However, the contractile function of the muscle was only depressed in the cats with congestive failure; function was normal in the muscle isolated from the denervated hearts (Fig. 18). It was concluded that cardiac stores of norepinephrine are not fundamental for maintaining basic myocardial contractility and that norepinephrine depletion is not responsible for the intrinsic depression or myocardial contractility in the failing heart. Similar observations and conclusions have been reported by others (Dhalla *et al.*, 1971).

The fact that norepinephrine-depleted heart muscle is supersensitive to the positive inotropic effect of norepinephrine (Spann *et al.*, 1967b) suggests that the circulating catecholamines may play an important role in supporting myocardial function in the failing heart. This conclusion seems particularly reasonable, since the circulating catecholamines are increased in patients with congestive heart failure (Chidsey *et al.*, 1962b). The conclusion gains support from evidence that congestive heart failure can appear or be aggravated when propranolol (Stephen, 1966) or guanethidine (Gaffney and Braunwald, 1963) is administered to patients with advanced heart disease. It is noteworthy that Covell and co-workers (1966) found that despite increased adrenergic activity and the increased release of catecholamines from extracardiac sources that accompany congestive heart failure, the response (i.e., increments in heart rate and contractile force) to stimulation of the cardiac sympathetic nerves is markedly reduced in dogs with heart failure as compared to normal animals. Hence these authors concluded that the release of norepinephrine from sympathetic nerves innervating the

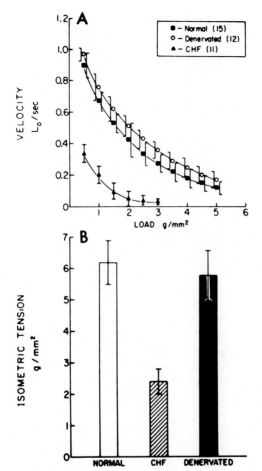

Fig. 18. Ventricular contractile state. (A) Average force and velocity in right ventricular papillary muscles isolated from normal cats and from cats with congestive heart failure (CHF) or denervation. Velocity is expressed on the ordinate as muscle lengths (L_0)/sec and total load is expressed on the abscissa as g/mm². (B) Average maximal active tension developed at the apex of the length–tension curve in isolated right ventricular papillary muscles from the three groups of cats, expressed as g/mm². All vertical bars equal ±1 standard error of the mean, and each number in parentheses represents the number of animals in that group. (From Rutenberg, and Spann, 1976, p. 91, reprinted with permission.)

heart must be profoundly reduced in experimental heart failure accompanied by norepinephrine depletion.

Finally, it should be mentioned that there is evidence for a reduced degree of parasympathetic influence on sinoatrial node automaticity in patients with heart failure; furthermore, the baroreceptor-induced slowing of the heart appears markedly attenuated (Eckberg *et al.*, 1971). On the other hand, in experimental heart failure, accompanied by a marked depletion of cardiac norepinephrine, a normal content of myocardial acetylcholine and a normal response to vagal stimulation has been reported (Meirson, 1969).

D. Adrenergic Nerves and the Hypertrophied Heart

Borchard (1978) reported an interesting study on the adrenergic nerves of normal and hypertrophied hearts of experimental animals and humans that combined biochemical, histochemical, electron microscopic, and morphometric analyses. At the time of cardiac operations, specimens were obtained from the auricles of 46 patients with a variety of diagnoses and varying degrees of cardiac hypertrophy. The mean concentrations of catecholamines in these specimens are given in Table X. A statistically highly significant decrease in norepinephrine content with increasing hypertrophy of muscle fibers was evident. In some cases of moderate hypertrophy, norepinephrine concentrations were not depressed; however, with severe hypertrophy, norepinephrine levels decreased to about 30% of "control values" (not more than 15% of this loss could be attributed to scarring). With a norepinephrine concentration below 0.6 μg/g wet weight, clinical heart failure was invariably present. Borchard suggests that there may be an adaptive augmentation of the adrenergic nerves in the early phase of hypertrophy but that subsequently in the later chronic phase the nerves become less dense and reduced in number. Signs of nerve degeneration also become apparent, but the cause for this remains obscure.

In a recent elegant thesis by Östman-Smith (1979) the conclusion was drawn that the "adaptive cardiac hypertrophy produced by chronic exercise is not caused by a direct effect of the increased workload on the cardiac

TABLE X

Human Myocardial Tissue[a]

Group	Norepinephrine (μg/g)	Epinephrine (μg/g)
Right auricle		
Without failure	1.29 ± 0.13	0.11 ± 0.03
With failure	1.06 ± 0.18	0.02 ± 0.00
Left auricle		
Without failure	0.77 ± 0.08	0.06 ± 0.02
With failure	0.43 ± 0.08	0.01 ± 0.00

[a] Table compiled from data of Borchard (1978). Values represent mean concentrations of catecholamines (μg/g wet weight).

muscle cell, but is instead mediated by release of noradrenaline from cardiac sympathetic nerves. Furthermore, increased activity of cardiac sympathetic nerves may be the final common pathway in all forms of compensatory cardiac hypertrophy."

E. Cardiac Pathophysiology Associated with Excessive Adrenergic Activity or Excessive Circulating Catecholamines

The effects and significance of excessive adrenergic activity in arrhythmias, myocardial ischemia, and heart failure have already been discussed. A number of clinical conditions are associated with augmented adrenergic activity, and it is conceivable that if the activity is profoundly increased and/or prolonged, the electrophysiology and function of the heart may be significantly influenced. Furthermore, cardiopathology may appear.

A fascinating recent experimental development is the demonstration by Witzke and Kaye (1976) that nerve growth factor (a glycoprotein) enhances sympathetic nerve growth, increases cardiac adrenergic innervation, and elevates myocardial norepinephrine. When nerve growth factor was administered to newborn puppies, changes in structure and function occurred that were similar to those seen in human idiopathic hypertrophic subaortic stenosis. The hypothesis that nerve growth factor might be involved in the pathogenesis of this disease is a most intriguing idea.

By far the most informative condition for studying the effects of excessive circulating catecholamines on the heart is pheochromocytoma. In this disease concentrations of circulating catecholamines are often markedly elevated. In addition to the large number of pathologic and metabolic complications caused by circulating catecholamines, chronic exposure of the heart to elevated plasma concentrations of catecholamines can cause a cardiomyopathy and pronounced electrophysiological alterations (Manger and Gifford, 1977).

1. Cardiomyopathy in Pheochromocytoma

Cardiomyopathy has been noted at autopsy in some patients who died from complications of pheochromocytoma (Kline, 1961; Rose, 1974; Van Vliet *et al.,* 1966). Van Vliet and co-workers (1966) reported that of 26 patients at the Mayo Clinic who died with pheochromocytoma, 15 (58%) had active myocarditis that these authors believed resulted from excessive catecholamines. Examples of active myocarditis in two of their patients are evident in Fig. 19. Focal areas of degeneration and necrosis of myocardial fibers, with foci of inflammatory cells (predominantly histiocytes, but some plasma cells and occasional polymorphonuclear leukocytes) were present

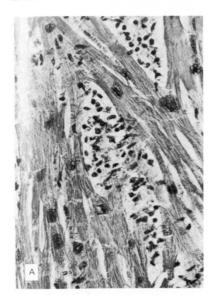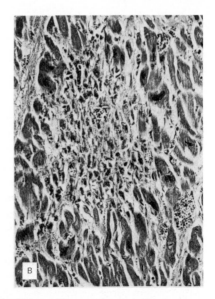

Fig. 19.   (A) Left ventricular myocardium of a 45-year-old man, who died with an unsuspected pheochromocytoma 5 days after removal of the left kidney, showing active myocarditis,
with focal degeneration of myocardial fibers and inflammation (hematoxylin and eosin stain,
320X). Delicate collagenous fibers were present in these foci. (Note: This patient's ECG is
shown in Fig. 20.) (B) Left ventricular myocardium of a 38-year-old man, who died of congestive heart failure that was thought to be due to a myocarditis (hematoxylin and eosin stain,
170X). An unsuspected phechromocytoma was present. The myocardium showed active
myocarditis consisting of foci of degenerated myocardial fibers and inflammation. (From Van
Vliet *et al.*, 1966, p. 1105, reprinted by permission.)

and most numerous in the left ventricle. In addition, increased fibrosis in
these foci and diffuse edema of the myocardium were observed. In a few
cases of hearts with active myocarditis, there was thickening of small and
medium-sized arteries because of edema of the intima and media and some
fibrous replacement of the media. A moderately severe degree of coronary
sclerosis was found in 14 of the 26 patients.

The pathological changes of active myocarditis were found in patients
with pheochromocytoma who had sustained or paroxysmal hypertension;
they were similar to lesions seen in the myocardium of some patients who
had received therapeutic infusions of norepinephrine and to lesions found
in various laboratory animals after injections of catecholamines. No active
catecholamine myocarditis was evident in four patients with pheochromocytomas that were apparently nonfunctioning (Van Vliet *et al.*,
1966).

Eleven of the 15 patients with active myocarditis had left ventricular failure with pulmonary congestion, which was frequently accompanied by a period of hypotension (refractory to treatment) prior to death. In one patient a diagnosis of active myocarditis had been made on the basis of cardiomegaly, dyspnea, tachycardia, and palpitations. Signs and symptoms had been present for 13 years before a pheochromocytoma was discovered at autopsy (Van Vliet *et al.*, 1966). Engelman and Sjoerdsma (1964) reported a patient whose cardiomyopathy, presumably related to excess catecholamine, subsided after resection of the pheochromocytoma. Significant left ventricular failure may occur in the absence of longstanding or severe hypertension (Yankopoulos *et al.*, 1974).

2. Electrocardiographic Changes in Pheochromocytoma

a. CLINICAL EVIDENCE

Electrocardiographic changes, particularly sinus tachycardia, may be frequently observed in patients with pheochromocytoma. Atrial or ventricular premature contractions or tachycardia are not infrequent during hypertensive crises. Supraventricular tachycardia up to 200/min in two patients and 160/min in a third patient has been recorded (Saint-Pierre *et al.*, 1970). Ectopic beats may result from stimulation of the myocardium by increased circulating catecholamines (Durante and Soloff, 1962). Furthermore, myocardial "irritability" is increased if its concentration of catecholamines is excessive. In their review of alterations in the electrocardiogram of patients with pheochromocytoma, Sayer and associates (1954) have categorized these as abnormalities of rhythm or abnormalities suggesting myocardial ischemia, damage, or strain. Disorders of rhythm consisted of the following: (1) wandering pacemaker, (2) sinoauricular dissociation, (3) Auricular tachycardia, (4) auricular premature contractions, (5) auricular flutter, (6) auricular fibrillation, (7) nodal tachycardia, (8) ventricular premature contractions, (9) ventricular tachycardia.

Sayer and associates found that arrhythmias occurred most frequently during paroxysms of hypertension and sometimes persisted after the blood pressure had returned to normal levels. All reported arrhythmias disappeared after the tumors were removed (Sayer *et al.*, 1954). Following administration of benzodioxane or phenoxybenzamine to one of their patients with pheochromocytoma and sustained hypertension, Sayer and co-workers observed a reversion toward normal of T waves. prolongation of the Q-T interval, and a clockwise rotation of the heart, with a shift to a more vertical position. ECG abnormalities suggesting myocardial damage included the following: (1) left axis deviation; (2) right axis deviation [occasionally with patterns similar to those seen in acute cor pulmonale and related to a marked increase in pulmonary artery pressure and a disproportionate increase in right ventricular work, which can be produced by catecholamine infusions (Witham and Fleming, 1951)]; (3) abnormally high or peaked P waves; (4) low or inverted T waves (often diffusely distributed); (5) S-T segment deviations and prolongation of Q-T interval. Sayer and co-workers (1954) reported that these changes occurred transiently during or between paroxysms of hypertension, and continuously in some patients with sustained hypertension. They stated that disappearance of these abnormalities sometimes occurred spontaneously, during hypertension paroxysms or during a low-sodium regimen. Partial or complete reversal of these abnormalities to normal was noted in patients after tumor removal. It must be kept in mind, however, that evidence of irreversible myocardial damage [e.g., that associated with catecholamine cardiomyopathy as described by Kline (1961) and Van Vliet and co-workers (1966) or with coronary atherosclerosis and/or myocardial infarction] may persist after a hypertensive crisis caused by pheochromocytoma or after tumor removal.

Sayer and co-workers emphasized that in the absence of any demonstrable etiologic factors the ECG abnormalities described earlier should alert the clinician to consider the possibility of pheochromocytoma. They appropriately stated that the pathogenesis of the abnormal electrocardiogram produced by a

> pheochromocytoma is a complex interplay of the relative amounts of epinephrine and norepinephrine secreted by the tumor, the duration of the secretion, whether intermittent or sustained, and the net effects of these pressor amines upon the cardiac rate, rhythm, output, oxygen demand and supply, as well as the coronary circulation, pulmonary and peripheral arterial resistance, and perhaps the body electrolyte distribution [Sayer *et al.*, 1954].

It is well to remember, as indicated by Futterweit and associates (1962) and noted by others, that a singularly striking feature of the ECG of some patients with pheochromocytoma is a diffuse distribution of T and S-T changes (Cahill and Monteith, 1951; Iseri *et al.*, 1951; Sayer *et al.*, 1954; Shapiro *et al.*, 1951). These changes are in contrast to those observed in patients with other forms of hypertension exhibiting a "strain pattern."

More recently, Saint-Pierre and co-workers (1970) have reviewed the electrocardiographic findings in patients with pheochromocytoma reported in the literature and have also presented the findings in 21 of their own patients. They noted that ventricular extrasystoles were particularly common and were recorded in about 50% of the reports in the literature. Auricular extrasystoles occurred less frequently.

Of the patients recently reported by Saint-Pierre and colleagues (1974), the following ECG abnormalities were noted: (1) left ventricular hypertrophy patterns; (2) arrhythmias (occurring sometimes without hypertension and liable to be induced by effort); (3) coronary insufficiency patterns;

(4) variable and transient repolarization disturbances (probably related to functional or autonomic disturbances caused by high concentrations of blood catecholamines); (5) disturbances of repolarization accompanying clinical, roentgenologic, and hemodynamic manifestations of myocardial involvement (catecholamine cardiomyopathy).

None of the preceding changes in the ECG can be considered specific, but when they occur in association with the onset of palpitations, hypertension, and other symptoms and signs of increased circulating catecholamines, they take on greater diagnostic significance. The extent to which an associated coronary atherosclerosis might have contributed to some of the ECG abnormalities encountered is difficult to assess, especially since the effects of pheochromocytoma may facilitate coronary atherogenesis (Perrin *et al.,* 1960).

A particularly fascinating electrocardiographic pattern, consistent with that observed in acute anterior myocardial infarction (note S-T elevations in precordial leads and Q wave in aVL), was observed in one of the patients with pheochromocytoma studied at the Mayo Clinic (Fig. 20). These ECG changes apparently were not the result of myocardial infarction but were probably related to the effects of excessive circulating catecholamines.

Electrocardiographic changes consistent with acute anteroseptal myocardial infarction have recently been reported in another patient with an adrenal pheochromocytoma studied at the Mayo Clinic (Fig. 21). This 59-year-old woman never experienced chest pains, and because of rapid reversal of the changes, they were attributed to a toxic myocarditis resulting from catecholamines rather than to a transmural infarction (Radtke *et al.,* 1975). Others have reported a similar case (Pelkonen and Pitkanen, 1963).

Chang and Bashour have recently reported the case of a 51-year-old black woman with pheochromocytoma who presented with striking cardiographic changes mimicking ischemic heart disease at one time and acute pulmonary embolism at other times. Paroxysmal episodes were accompanied by abnormalities of repolarization of the Q-T interval and deep and wide symmetrically inverted T waves without changes in the QRS complex. Prominent P waves in Leads II, III, and aVF were frequently observed with no significant change in the QRS axis. The Q-T interval remained prolonged even when T waves were upright. Normal ECGs were recorded during several attacks of paroxysmal hypertension. These investigators pointed out that symmetric T wave inversion with or without a prolonged Q-T interval is not specific for coronary artery disease; similar ECG changes have been seen in acute pancreatitis, gallbladder disease, acute cerebrovascular accidents, during administration of quinidine, atypical angina with normal coronary arteriograms, and diencephalic discharges. Although the mechanism whereby these changes induce repolarization abnormalities is not well un-

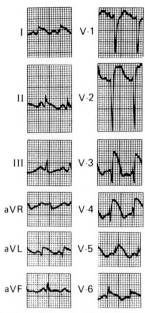

Fig. 20. This ECG was recorded about 24 hr before death in a 45-year-old man with a right adrenal pheochromocytoma who was in circulatory shock. He had not been recognized as having a pheochromocytoma and, following a left nephrectomy for transitional cell carcinoma of the kidney pelvis, was found to be in circulatory collapse. Postmortem examination revealed no evidence of acute myocardial infarction, no mural thrombosis, and no significant coronary atherosclerosis; an incidental finding was an atrial septal defect. However, scattered throughout the myocardium were focal areas of necrosis associated with myocardial fiber degenerative changes and inflammatory cell infiltrations. It was felt by Dr. A. L. Brown (pathologist at the Mayo Clinic) that these pathological legions could best be explained on the basis of excessive circulating catecholamines from his pheochromocytoma. (Note: This patient's myocardial pathology is shown in Fig. 19A.) (Courtesy of Dr. H. B. Burchell, Senior Consultant in Cardiology, University of Minnesota. From Manger and Gifford, 1977, reprinted by permission.)

derstood, a diencephalic discharge of catecholamines has been implicated in some of these conditions. Finally, Cheng and Bashour (1976) cite evidence for the toxic effects of excessive levels of catecholamines on the myocardium. They also noted that reversible T wave inversions have been induced in normal man by intravenous infusion of norepinephrine.

It is interesting that electrocardiographic changes similar to those that occurred in the patient of Cheng and Bashour were observed in a patient who inadvertently received an overdose of norepinephrine and developed circulatory shock (personal communication from Dr. Howard B. Burchell, Senior Consultant in Cardiology, University of Minnesota).

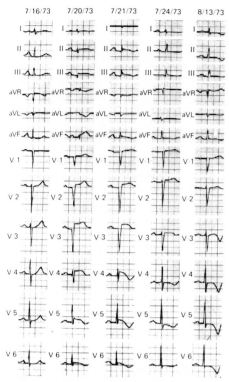

Fig. 21. Serial electrocardiograms. The S-T segment elevation and loss of R wave voltage over anterior precordial leads on July 20, 1973, suggested acute anteroseptal infarction. There is S-T segment elevation in leads II, III, and aVF. Note also the rapid resolution of these changes: by July 24, 1973, R wave voltage was returning to normal and by August 13, 1973, it was normal and only widespread T wave inversion was evident. The ECG was that of a 59-year-old white woman who developed a paroxysm of hypertension (250/105 mm Hg) and became apathetic, disoriented, and transiently blind. A left hemisensory deficit, dysesthesia of the left leg, and a left Babinski were noted and shortly therafter she became unresponsive and diaphoretic and showed signs of peripheral vasoconstriction. The ECG became abnormal at this time and thereafter sequential changes were observed, as shown in the figure. She regained her sight in a few hours but peripheral vasoconstriction persisted and the sensory deficits improved only gradually. She was treated with α- and β-adrenergic blocking agents, and subsequently a pheochromocytoma was successfully removed from the region of the left adrenal gland. (From Radtke *et al.*, 1975, p. 702, reprinted with permission from *Am. J. Cardiol.*)

Occasionally bradycardia instead of tachycardia occurs in patients with pheochromocytoma (Forde *et al.*, 1968: Hamilton *et al.*, 1953; Hegglin and Holtzmann, 1937; Sode *et al.*, 1967). Vagal response to elevated blood pressure during hypertensive crises in some of these patients evidently causes sinus slowing instead of the usual sinus tachycardia, premature beats, and ectopic tachycardias that result from β-adrenergic stimulation of the myocardium (Forde *et al.*, 1968). Rarely, reflex bradycardia with depression of the sinus node and escape of lower pacemakers have been recorded in patients with pheochromocytoma during a severe hypertensive crisis (Burgess *et al.*, 1936; Esperson and Dahl-Iverson, 1946; Forde *et al.*, 1968). Nodal escape and A-V dissociation have been observed during hypertensive crises in association with both bradycardia (Burgess *et al.*, 1936; Esperson and Dahl-Iversen, 1946; Forde *et al.*, 1968) and tachycardia (Futterweit *et al.*, 1962).

Forde and co-workers (1968) have reported two patients with intermittent chest pain and arrhythmia who were initially suspected of having acute myocardial infarction. Constant ECG and blood pressure monitoring revealed that episodically severe hypertension (associated with anterior chest pressure or pain, palpitations, and other clinical manifestations) occurred coincidentally with reflex bradycardia and nodal escape rhythm and A-V dissociation (Fig. 22, 23). With subsidence of the hypertensive crises, the ECG reverted to normal sinus rhythm. The rise in blood pressure always preceded the onset of the arrhythmia. In case 1 (Fig. 22) it was found that only the plasma epinephrine became markedly elevated during a spontaneous hypertensive crisis, whereas in case 2 (Fig. 23) both epinephrine and norepinephrine plasma concentrations reached very high levels when hypertension was induced by massage of the right upper abdomen (Table XI). It is noteworthy that sinus bradycardia and occasionally complete A-V dissociation have been produced by intravenous infusion of norepinephrine into human subjects (Barnett *et al.*, 1950).

As emphasized by Forde and co-workers (1968), the diagnosis of pheochromocytoma should be considered in any patient with periodic bradycardia and escape of lower pacemakers. Careful documentation of the blood pressure before and during such arrhythmias is mandatory, and if it is disclosed that these electrocardiographic abnormalities are induced by hypertensive crises, a pheochromocytoma must be strongly suspected. To date, reflex bradycardia with nodal escape rhythm in patients with pheochromocytoma has almost invariably been described in those who have paroxysmal and not persistent hypertension. One 44-year-old woman with slight hypertension (160/108 mm Hg recumbent) had isoelectric T waves in leads I and aVL, diphasic T waves in leads V3-4, and inverted T waves in leads II, III, and V5-6. Slight S-T depression in leads V5-6 and a prominent P wave in lead II were also present (Futterweit *et al.*, 1962). She developed a blood pressure rise of 80/46 mm Hg above the basal level following a histamine (0.025 mg iv) provocative test, and simultaneously the ECG revealed further peaking of the P-waves, A-V dissociation, and supraventricular and ventricular extrasystoles. The ECG returned to the prestimulation state 20 min after

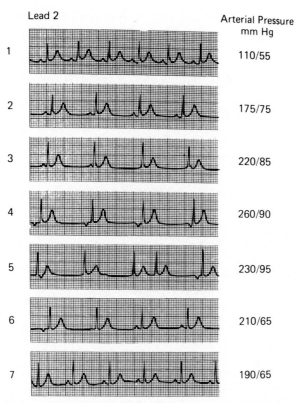

Fig. 22. Sequential changes in cardiac rhythm during an episode of hypertension in case 1, demonstrating slowing of the sinus pacemaker and nodal escape rhythm with A-V dissociation as the blood pressure rises, and restoration of sinus rhythm, culminating in sinus tachycardia, as the blood pressure falls toward normal (paper speed 25 mm/sec). Note the initial drop in blood pressure (shown in Table XI) at the outset of this attack when the epinephrine became elevated. On one occasion the blood pressure rose from 120/80 to 250/100 mm Hg during the development of A-V dissociation and then fell to 80/60 mm Hg. This is particularly interesting since hypotensive periods have occasionally been reported in patients harboring a pheochromocytoma which secretes predominantly epinephrine. This is patient No. 30. described in Chapter 7 of "Pheochromocytoma" by Manger and Gifford (1977). Numbers on the left-hand margin indicate time in minutes. (From Forde *et al.,* 1968, p. 389, reprinted with permission from *Am. Heart J.*)

histamine administration. Three days following pheochromocytoma extirpation no ECG abnormalities were evident.

An electrocardiographic finding that has been noted (Burgess *et al.,* 1936; French and Campagna, 1961; Pincoffs, 1929) in patients with pheochromocytoma, but not previously emphasized was observed in case 2, mentioned earlier (Manger and Yormak, 1977). Figure 24 reveals a continuous

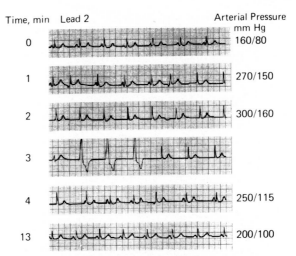

Time, min   Lead 2   Arterial Pressure
                                              mm Hg
   0   160/80
   1   270/150
   2   300/160
   3
   4   250/115
  13   200/100

Fig. 23. Sequential changes in cardiac rhythm during an episode of hypertension precipitated by message of right upper abdominal quadrant in case 2. Note depression of sinus pacemaker and appearance of lower foci as blood pressure rises. When blood pressure declines, sinus mechanism is restored (paper speed 25 mm/sec). This is patient No. 32 described in Chapter 7 of "Pheochromocytoma" by Manger and Gifford (1977). (From Forde *et al.,* 1968, p. 391, reprinted with permission from *Am. Heart J.*)

recording from Lead II in this patient during a paroxysmal attack of hypertension. During the periods of bradycardia and nodal escape, the T waves became exceptionally high and decreased toward normal when the blood pressure returned to normal and the bradycardia subsided. Also, there was a slight and transient depression of the S-T segment. The finding of a huge T wave is in no way specific for pheochromocytoma. Enlarged T waves may be seen in myocardial infarction or hyperkalemia; however, one would usually expect other typical ECG changes to occur concomitantly with these latter conditions.

The ECG of a patient with pheochromocytoma reported by French and Campagna revealed a prolonged Q-T interval, prominent U waves, depressed S-T segments, and high, peaked T waves (French and Campagna, 1961)—abnormalities that were clearly reversible.

A summary of the electrocardiographic abnormalities that may be seen in patients with pheochromocytomas that are actively secreting catecholamines is given in Table XII.

b. Experimental Evidence

Tenzer (1954) stated that epinephrine injected into the normal man increases cardiac frequency and the amplitude of the P waves, shortens the

TABLE XI

Plasma Levels of Epinephrine and Norepinephrine in Two Cases of Pheochromocytoma with Reflex Bradycardia and Nodal Escape Rhythm[a]

	Blood pressure (mm Hg)	Plasma epinephrine[b] (μg/liter plasma)	Plasma norepinephrine[b] (μg/liter plasma)
Normal concentrations (upper limit)		<1.5	<6.6
Case 1			
Control	154/80	1.3[c]	3.8[c]
During spontaneous hypertensive attack			
Onset	80/50	2.6	3.5
Rising	205/68	26.7	3.6
Peak	240/130		
Falling	198/73	2.9	3.4
Case 2			
Control	158/80	3.1[c]	8.2[c]
During hypertensive attack induced by pressure in right upper quadrant			
Peak	300/160	28.5[c]	27.3[c]

[a] Modified from Forde et al. (1968, p. 391).
[b] Performed by Dr. W. M. Manger, New York University Medical Center.
[c] Average of two rapid sequence samples. From Manger and Gifford (1977, p. 189), reprinted by permission.

A. Onset of attack (BP = > 300/115, normal BP = 130/65).
   Nodal escape rhythm—heart rate = 58/min.

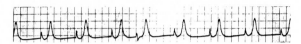

B. Symptoms subsiding. Nodal escape with some sinus
   rhythm—heart rate = 51-63/min.

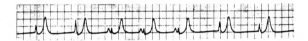

C. 3-5 minutes after onset, symptoms gone (BP = 135/60).
   Regular sinus rhythm—heart rate = 82/min.

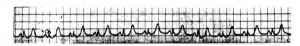

Fig. 24. Continuous recording from lead II (coronary care unit monitoring electrodes) in a 58-year-old white male with pheochromocytoma during paroxysmal attack of hypertension. This is the same patient whose ECG appears in Fig. 23. (From Manger and Yormak, 1977, reprinted by permission.)

TABLE XII

ECG Abnormalities Sometimes Seen in Patients with Pheochromocytoma[a,b]

Atrial, nodal, or ventricular tachycardia
Atrial or ventricular premature contractions (with or without bigeminy)
Bradycardia with or without complete A-V dissociation with or without T wave elevation and peaking
Wandering pacemaker
Atrial flutter or fibrillation
Left or right axis deviation
Abnormally high or peaked P waves
Low or inverted T waves
S-T segment deviations
Prolonged Q-T interval

[a] From Manger and Gifford (1977, p. 191), reprinted by permission.
[b] Reversibility of ECG abnormalities plus absence of etiologic explanation suggests pheochromocytoma.

P-R interval, increases myocardial excitability, and provokes alterations in rhythm. In addition, he mentions that therapeutic doses of epinephrine can cause elevation of T waves, whereas larger doses will cause T wave inversion. When moderate doses of norepinephrine were injected, bradycardia and depression of the P wave occurred; in addition, nodal rhythm sometimes appeared, and frequently the T waves became elevated.

It is noteworthy that infusions of epinephrine or norepinephrine into the coronary artery of dogs produced high, upright, peaked T waves with depressed S-T segments (Barger *et al.,* 1961). Large upright T waves, associated with prominent U waves, prolonged Q-T interval, and T-U fusion have not infrequently been observed as an electrocardiographic manifestation of intracranial disease (Burch and Phillips, 1968).

Experimental animal studies on the effect of hypothalamic or stellate ganglion stimulation, and stellate ganglionectomy, suggest that sympathetic pathways are involved in some of these ECG alterations (Melville *et al.,* 1963; Yanowitz *et al.,* 1966). Increased concentrations of circulating catecholamines may conceivably cause disturbances in the myocardium in a manner similar to those induced by activation of the sympathetic innervation of the heart. Intravenous administration of epinephrine or norepinephrine to healthy subjects leads to reversible ECG alterations. Sjöstrand (1951) found that epinephrine invariably caused the appearance of a positive afterpotential following the T wave that was coupled with an associated depression of the T wave and S-T segment. After vagal block, the ECG changes caused by epinephrine were augmented. On the other hand, administration of norepinephrine caused the reverse of the epinephrine effect; i.e., norepinephrine in the same dose produced a slight rise in the T wave, whereas the positive afterpotential was either decreased or unchanged and the heart rate was slowed. ECG changes similar to those evoked by epinephrine were encountered in seven of eight patients with pheochromocytoma by Cannon and Sjöstrand (1952). They emphasized that marked and variable reversible ECG changes occurring in a very short time should suggest the possibility of pheochromocytoma.

Watkins (1957) had commented that ECG alterations could be related to shifts in cellular potassium accompanying hyperglycemia caused by increased circulating catecholamines. Consistent with this concept, French and Campagna (1961) suggested that altered potassium metabolism, with subsequent development of hypokalemia, could account for prolonged Q-T intervals, S-T depression, and prominent U waves in addition to the positive afterpotential (where the U or T wave descends and merges with the P wave before reaching the base line) noted in their patient and described by Cannon and Sjöstrand. They further pointed out that although the upright, peaked T wave in their patient was not consistent with hypokalemia, catecholamines can secondarily cause a marked vagal effect, which could account for the T wave peaking (Cannon, 1955). Dr. Howard B. Burchell (personal communication) suggested the possibility that a disparate flow of catecholamines into the myocardium might occur and result in local differences in sympathetic "drive" that could produce large T waves; he felt, however, that a transient ischemia of the subendocardial zone was a more likely explanation for the huge T waves.

It should be pointed out that concentration of serum potassium during paroxysms of hypertension in patients with pheochromocytoma have not been adequately studied. During a constant intravenous infusion of epinephrine (10–18 μg/min) in 12 normal young men, the mean serum potassium decreased very significantly by 17.3% without any remarkable change in serum sodium or chloride (Jacobson et al., 1951). Concomitantly, there was a decrease in urinary sodium, chloride, and potassium. The alteration in serum potassium was thought to reflect an intracellular shift. Keys (1938) noted a similar decrease in potassium in normal men following intravenous injection of 0.005–0.3 mg of epinephrine chloride but a return to levels slightly above preinjection values within 40–60 min. More recently, Massara and co-workers (1970) demonstrated that intravenous infusion of epinephrine (0.01 mg/min) into healthy volunteers caused approximately a 20% decrease in serum potassium, which could be prevented by propranolol. The latter finding suggested that epinephrine-induced hypokalemia was mediated by β-adrenergic receptors (Massara et al., 1970). These findings were in contrast to the immediate marked rise in plasma potassium caused by intravenous injections of epinephrine in dogs, cats, and rabbits (Keys, 1938). A number of other investigators have found that administration of epinephrine causes a decrease in serum potassium (Brewer et al., 1939; Castelden, 1938; Dury, 1951; Rogoff et al., 1950).

Graded intravenous infusions of norepinephrine in six normal young men caused a sharp fall in potassium clearance by the kidney without remarkably affecting clearance of sodium chloride (Pullman and McClure, 1952); also, there was a slight but statistically significant rise in serum potassium concentration (which averaged 5.2%) without any remarkable change in serum sodium or chloride. These results suggested that norepinephrine might cause a migration of potassium from intracellular to extracellular fluid. MacKeith (1944), however, reported one patient with pheochromocytoma who had very elevated serum potassium between hypertensive attacks; he pointed out that intravenous epinephrine may produce an 86% rise in blood potassium. Only rarely has the serum potassium been reported elevated in patients with pheochromocytoma (McCullagh and Engel, 1942). Serum electrolytes are nearly always within normal limits in those patients with pheochromocytoma who have sustained hypertension; they are also normal between the hypertensive crises in those patients who have paroxysmal hypertension with pheochromocytoma.

In the final analysis, we must recognize how totally imprecise are the contributions made by the electrocardiogram to the diagnosis of pheochromocytoma. After kindly reviewing this section on electrocardiography, Dr. Raymond Pruitt emphasized the desirability of pointing out the near total lack of specificity of the electrocardiographic changes occurring in patients with pheochromocytomas. He pointed out that the origin of ECG changes may be more readily identified from clinical phenomena that suggest the presence of pheochromocytoma than from the ECG changes themselves (personal communication from Dr. Raymond D. Pruitt, Emeritus Dean, Mayo Medical School).

VI. Concluding Remarks

In the preceding account an attempt has been made to demonstrate clearly that the adrenergic nervous system and circulating catecholamines can play an important role in normal physiology and pathophysiology of the heart. It should also be mentioned that a vast array of experimental physiological and pharmacological manipulations [including administration of certain drugs—e.g., drugs that influence the adrenergic neural transmission and the synthesis and inactivation of catecholamines—and alterations in sodium (Doyle, 1968) and hormonal balance (de Champlain *et al.,* 1968)] can change the concentrations and turnover rate of catecholamines in the heart and elsewhere; however, space does not permit their consideration in this review.

A recent comprehensive account of current concepts of cardiac function (including neural control of the heart and biochemical mechanisms of adrenergic and cholinergic regulation of myocardial contractility) has been presented elsewhere (Berne *et al.,* 1979) and may be of additional interest to the reader.

Acknowledgment

The extraordinarily fine assistance of my research associate, Mildred Hulse, in preparing, editing, and measurably improving this manuscript was invaluable. The assistance of Richard Seides, Richard Sussman, and Reverend Don Bundy in proofreading, referencing, and editing was also extremely helpful. I am particularly grateful to Drs. Howard B. Burchell, Brian F. Hoffman, Michael P. Kaye, Robert J. Lefkowitz, Michael R. Rosen, and John T. Shepherd for their helpful comments and constructive suggestions regarding the manuscript.

This review was supported by the National Hypertension Association, Inc.; the Pew Memorial Trust; and the Hypertension Fund of the Institute of Rehabilitation Medicine.

References

Abboud, F. M. (1972). *Fed. Proc., Fed. Am. Soc. Exp. Biol.* **31**, 1226–1239.

Abildskov, J. A., and Vincent, G. M. (1977). *In* "Neural Regulation of the Heart" (W. C. Randall, ed.), pp. 409–424. Oxford Univ. Press, London and New York.

Allen, J. D., Pantridge, J. F., and Shanks, R. G. (1975). *Am. J. Med.* **58**, 199–208.

Amorim, D. S., Mello de Oliveira, J. A., Manço, J. C., Gallo, L., Jr., and Meira de Oliveira, J. S. (1973). *Acta Cardiol.* **28**, 431–440.

Anderson, M., and del Castillo, J. (1972). *In* "Electrical Phenomena in the Heart" (W. C. DeMello, ed.), Chapter 9, pp. 236–257. Academic Press, New York.

Armour, J. A., Hageman, G. R., and Randall, W. C. (1972). *Am. J. Physiol.* **223**, 1068–1075.

Armour, J. A., Wurster, R. D., and Randall, W. C. (1977). *In* "Neural Regulation of the Heart" (W. C. Randall, ed.), Chapter 6, pp. 159–186. Oxford Univ. Press, London and New York.

Arnsdorf, M. F., and Hsieh, Y.-Y. (1978). *In* "The Heart" (J. W. Hurst, R. B. Logue, R. C. Schlant, and N. K. Wenger, eds.), 4th ed., pp. 1943–1963. McGraw-Hill, New York.

Avakian, O. V., and Gillespie, J. S. (1967). *J. Physiol. (London)* **191**, 71P–72P.

Avakian, O. V., and Gillespie, J. S. (1968). *Br. J. Pharmacol. Chemother.* **32**, 168–184.

Axelrod, J. (1957). *Science* **126**, 400–401.

Axelrod, J. (1962). *J. Biol. Chem.* **237**, 1657–1660.

Axelrod, J. (1963). *In* "Symposium on the Clinical Chemistry of Monoamines" (H. Variey and A. H. Gowencock, eds.), pp. 5–18. Elsevier, Amsterdam.

Axelrod, J. (1973). *Harvey Lect.* **67**, 175–197.

Axelrod, J., Inscoe, J. K., Senoh, S., and Witkop, B. (1958). *Biochim. Biophys. Acta* **27**, 210–211.

Axelrod, J., Kopin, I. J., and Mann, J. D. (1959). *Biochim. Biophys. Acta* **36**, 576–577.

Barger, A. C., Herd, J. A., and Liebowitz, M. R. (1961). *Proc. Soc. Exp. Biol. Med.* **107**, 474–477.

Barnett, A. J., Blacket, R. B., DePoorter, A. E., Sanderson, P. H., and Wilson, S. M. (1950). *Clin. Sci.* **9**, 151–179.

Baron, G. D., Speden, R. N., and Bohr, D. F. (1972). *Am. J. Physiol.* **223**, 878–881.

Beavo, J. A., Hardman, J. G., and Sutherland, E. W. (1971). *J. Biol. Chem.* **246**, 3841–3846.

Berne, R. M. (1958). *Circ. Res.* **6**, 644–655.

Berne, R. M., and Rubio, R. (1977). *Adv. Cardiol.* **12**, 303–317.

Berne, R. M., DeGeest, H., and Levy, M. N. (1965). *Am. J. Physiol.* **208**, 763–769.

Berne, R. M., Sperelakis, N., and Geiger, S. R., eds. (1979). "Handbook of Physiology," Sect. 2, Vol. I. Am. Physiol. Soc., Bethesda, Maryland.

Bloom, G., Östlund, E., von Euler, U. S., Lishajko, F., Ritzén, M., and Adams-Ray, J. (1961). *Acta Physiol. Scand.* **53**, Suppl. 185, 1–34.

Borchard, F. (1978). *Norm. Pathol. Anat.* **33**, 1–68.

Braunwald, E. (1978a). *Harvey Lect.* **71**, 247–282.

Braunwald, E. (1978b). *N. Engl. J. Med.* **299**, 1301–1303.

Braunwald, E. and Maroko, P. R. (1972). *Ann. Intern. Med.* **76**, 659–691.

Braunwald, E., Harrison, D. C., and Chidsey, C. A. (1964). *Am. J. Med.* **36**, 1–4.

Braunwald, E., Ross, J., Jr., and Sonnenblick, E. H. (1976). "Mechanism of Contraction of the Normal and Failing Heart." Little, Brown, Boston, Massachusetts.

Braunwald, E., Ross, J., Jr., and Sonnenblick, E. H. (1977). *In* "Harrison's Principles of Internal Medicine" (G. W. Thorn, R. D. Adams, E. Braunwald, K. J. Isselbacher, and R. G. Petersdorf, eds.), 8th ed., pp. 1167–1177. McGraw-Hill, New York.

Brewer, G., Larson, P. S., and Schroeder, A. R. (1939). *Am. J. Physiol.* **126**, 708–712.

Brown, A. M. (1968). *J. Physiol. (London)* **198**, 311–328.

Brown, A. M., and Malliani, A. (1971). *J. Physiol. (London)* **212**, 685–705.

Burch, G. E., and Phillips, J. H. (1968). *South. Med. J.* **61**, 331–336.

Burgess, A. M., Waterman, G. W., and Cutts, F. B. (1936). *Arch. Int. Med.* **58**, 433–447.

Buu, N. T., and Kuchel, O. (1977). *J. Lab. Clin. Med.* **90**, 680–684.

Cahill, G. F., and Monteith, J. C. (1951). *N. Engl. J. Med.* **244**, 657–661.

Cannon, P. (1955). *Ir. J. Med. Sci.* **359**, 499–511.

Cannon, P., and Sjöstrand, T. (1952). *Scand. J. Clin. Lab. Invest.* **4**, 266–267.

Cannon, W. B. (1939). *Am. J. Med. Sci.* **198**, 737–750.

Cannon, W. B., and Lissak, K. (1939). *Am. J. Physiol.* **125**, 765–777.

Cannon, W. B., and Rosenblueth, A. (1933). *Am. J. Physiol.* **104**, 557–574.

Castelden, J. I. M. (1938). *Clin. Sci.* **3**, 241–245.

Chapman, C. B., Jensen, D., and Wildenthal, K. (1963). *Circ. Res.* **12**, 427–440.

Cheng, T. O., and Bashour, T. T. (1976). *Chest* **70**, 397–399.

Chidsey, C. A., Harrison, D. C., and Braunwald, E. (1962a). *N. Engl. J. Med.* **267**, 650–654.

Chidsey, C. A., Harrison, D. C., and Braunwald, E. (1962b). *Proc. Soc. Exp. Biol. Med.* **109**, 488–490.

Chidsey, C. A., Braunwald, E., Morrow, A. G., and Mason, D. T. (1963a). *N. Engl. J. Med.* **269**, 653–658.

Chidsey, C. A., Kaiser, G. A., and Braunwald, E. (1963b). *Science* **139**, 828–829.

Chidsey, C. A., Kaiser, G. A., Sonnenblick, E. H., Spann, J. F., and Braunwald, E. (1964). *J. Clin. Invest.* **43**, 2386–2393.

Chidsey, C. A., Braunwald, E., and Morrow, A. G. (1965). *Am. J. Med.* **39**, 442–451.

Christensen, N. J. (1973). *Scand. J. Clin. Lab. Invest.* **31**, 343–346.

Cooper, T., Gilbert, J. W., Jr., Bloodwell, R. D., and Crout, J. R. (1961). *Circ. Res.* **9**, 275–281.

Cooper, T., Willman, V. L., Jellinek, M., and Hanlon, C. R. (1962). *Science* **138**, 40–41.

Cooper, T., Willman, V. L., and Hanlon, C. R. (1964). *Dis. Chest* **45**, 284–287.

Corbett, J. L., Kerr, J. H., Prys-Roberts, C., Smith, A. C., and Spalding, J. M. K. (1969). *Anaesthesia* **24**, 198–212.

Covell, J. W., Chidsey, C. A., and Braunwald, E. (1966). *Circ. Res.* **19**, 51–56.

Cox, W. F., and Robertson, H. F. (1936). *Am. Heart J.* **12**, 285–300.

Dahlström, A., Fuxe, K., Mya-Tu, M., and Zetterström, B. E. M. (1965). *Am. J. Physiol.* **209**, 689–692.

de Champlain, J., Krakoff, L. R., and Axelrod, J. (1968). *Circ. Res.* **23**, 479–491.

de Champlain, J., Farley, L., Cousineau, D., and van Amerigen, M.-R. (1976). *Circ. Res.* **38**, 109–114.

Dempsey, P. J., and Cooper, T. (1968). *Am. J. Physiol.* **215**, 1245–1249.

Dhalla, N. S., Naidu, K. J., and Bhagat, B. (1971). *Cardiovasc. Res.* **5**, 376–382.

Donald, D. E. (1974). *Circ. Res.* **34**, 417–424.

Donald, D. E., and Samueloff, S. L. (1966). *Am. J. Physiol.* **211**, 703–711.

Donald D. E., and Shepherd, J. T. (1963). *Am. J. Physiol.* **205**, 393–400.

Donald, D. E., and Shepherd, J. T. (1965). *Am. J. Physiol.* **208**, 255–259.

Donald, D. E., Milburn, S. E., and Shepherd, J. T. (1964). *J. Appl. Physiol.* **19**, 849–852.

Donald, D. E., Ferguson, D. A., and Milburn, S. E. (1968). *Circ. Res.* **22**, 127–134.

Douglas, W. W. (1968). *Br. J. Pharmacol.* **34**, 451–474.

Doyle, A. E. (1968). *Lancet* **1**, 1399–1400.

Durant, J., and Soloff, L. A. (1962). *Lancet* **2**, 124–126.

Dury, A. (1951). *Endocrinology* **49**, 663–670.

Ebert, P. A. (1968). *J. Cardiovasc. Surg.* **9**, 414–419.

Ebert, P. A. (1969). Personal communication cited by Schaal *et al.* (1969).

Ebert, P. A., Allgood, R. J., and Sabiston, D. C., Jr. (1968). *Ann. Surg.* **168**, 728–735.

Ebert, P. A., Vanderbeek, R. B., Allgood, R. J., and sabiston, D. C., Jr. (1970). *Cardiovasc. Res.* **4**, 141–147.

Eckberg, D. I., Drabinsky, M., and Braunwald, E. (1971). *N. Engl. J. Med.* **285**, 877–883.

Ehinger, B., Falk, B., and Sparrong, B. (1966). Symp. Elec. Activ. Innervation Blood Vessels, Cambridge, 1966; *Bibl. Anat.* **8**, 35–45.

Engelman, K., and Sjoerdsma, A. (1964). *Ann. Intern. Med.* **61**, 229–241.

Epstein, S. E., Robinson, B. F., Kahler, R. L., and Braunwald, E. (1965). *J. Clin. Invest.* **44**, 1745–1753.

Erickson, H. H., and Stone, H. L. (1972). *Aerosp. Med.* **43**, 422–428.

Esperson, T., and Dahl-Iversen, E. (1946). *Acta Chir. Scand.* **94**, 271–290.

Evarts, E. V., Gillespie, L., Fleming, T. C., and Sjoerdsma, A. (1958). *Proc. Soc. Exp. Biol. Med.* **98**, 74–76.

Feigl, E. O. (1967). *Circ. Res.* **20**, 262–271.

Feigl, E. O. (1975a). *Circ. Res.* **37**, 88–95.

Feigl, E. O. (1975b). *Circ. Res.* **37**, 175–182.

Fölklow, B. (1971). *Clin. Sci. Mol. Med.* **41**, 1–12.

Forde, T. P., Yormak, S. S., and Killip, T., III (1968). *Am. Heart J.* **76**, 388–392.

Fowlis, R. A. F., Sang, C. T. M., Lundy, P. M., Ahuja, S. P., and Colhoun, H. (1974). *Am. Heart J.* **88**, 748–757.

Frankel, H. L., and Mathias, C. J. (1979). *Paraplegia* **17**, 46–51.

French, C., and Campagna, F. A. (1961). *Ann. Intern. Med.* **55**, 127–134.

Furchgott, R. F. (1972). *In* "Catecholamines" (H. Blaschko and E. Muscholl, eds.), pp. 283–335. Springer-Verlag, Berlin and New York.

Futterweit, W., Allen, L., and Moser, M. (1962). *Metab. Clin. Exp.* **11**, 589–599.

Gaffney, T. E., and Braunwald, E. (1963). *Am. J. Med.* **34**, 320–324.

Gaffney, T. E., Braunwald, E., and Cooper, T. (1962a). *Circ. Res.* **10**, 83–88.

Gaffney, T. E., Morrow, D. H., and Chidsey, C. A. (1962b). *J. Pharmacol. Exp. Ther.* **137**, 301–305.

Gazes, P. G., Richardson, J. A., and Woods, E. F. (1959). *Circulation* **19**, 657–661.

Gillis, D., Pearle, L., and Hoekman, T. (1974). *Science* **185**, 70–72.

Giotti, A., Ledda, F., and Mannaioni, P. F. (1973). *J. Physiol. (London)* **229**, 99–113.

Glaubiger, G., and Lefkowitz, R. J. (1977). *Biochem. Biophys. Res. Commun.* **78**, 720–725.

Gold, H. K., Leinbach, R. C., and Maroko, P. R. (1974). *Circulation* **50**, Suppl. III, 33 (abstr.).

Goldberg, H. C., and Marsden, C. A. (1975). *Pharmacol. Rev.* **27**, 135–206.

Goldberg, L. I. (1972). *Pharmacol. Rev.* **24**, 1–29.

Goldberg, L. I. (1974). *N. Engl. J. Med.* **291**, 707–710.

Goldberg, L. I., Kohli, J. D., Kotake, A. N., and Volkman, P. H. (1978a). *Fed. Proc., Fed. Am. Soc. Exp. Biol.* **37**, 2396–2402.

Goldberg, L. I., Volkman, P. H., and Kohli, J. D. (1978b). *Annu. Rev. Toxicol.* **18**, 57–79.

Goldenberg, M., and Rapport, M. M. (1951). *J. Clin. Invest.* **30**, 641–642.

Goodall, McC. (1950). *Acta Physiol. Scand.* **20**, 137–152.

Goodall, McC., and Kirshner, N. (1956). *J. Clin. Invest.* **35**, 649–656.

Granata, L., Olsson, R. A., Huvos, A., and Gregg, D. E. (1965). *Circ. Res.* **16**, 114–120.

Gregg, D. E., Khouri, E. M., Donald, D. E., Lowensohn, H. S., and Stanislaw, P. (1972). *Circ. Res.* **31**, 129–144.

Grondin, C. M., and Limet, R. (1977). *Ann. Thorac. Surg.* **23**, 111–117.

Grovier, W. C., Mosal, N. C., Whittington, P., and Broom, A. H. (1966). *J. Pharmacol. Exp. Ther.* **154**, 255–263.

Guyton, R. A., Bianco, J. A., Ostheimer, G. W., Shanohan, E. H., and Daggett, W. M. (1972). *Am. J. Physiol.* **223**, 1021–1028.

Hageman, G. R., Goldberg, J. M., Armour, J. A., and Randall, W. C. (1973a). *Am. J. Cardiol.* **32**, 822–830.

Hageman, G. R., Geis, W. P., and Kaye, M. P. (1973b). *Fed. Proc., Fed. Am. Soc. Exp. Biol.* **32**, 344.

Hamilton, M., Litchfield, J. W., Peart, W. S., and Sowry, G. S. C. (1953). *Br. Heart J.* **15**, 241–249.

Han, J., and Moe, G. K. (1964). *Circ. Res.* **14**, 44–60.

Han, J., de Jalon, G., and Moe, G. K. (1964). *Circ. Res.* **14**, 516–524.

Harris, A. (1964). *In* "Mechanisms and Therapy of Cardiac Arrhythmias" (L. S. Dreifus and W. Likoff, eds.), Chapter 12, pp. 345–378. Grune & Stratton, New York.

Harris, A. S., Estandia, A., and Tillotson, R. F. (1951). *Am. J. Physiol.* **165**, 505–512.

Harrison, D. C., Chidsey, C. A., Goldman, R., and Braunwald, E. (1963). *Circ. Res.* **12**, 256–263.

Hegglin, R., and Holzmann, M. (1937). *Dtsch. Arch. Klin. Med.* **180**, 681–691.

Higgins, C. B., Vatner, S. F., and Braunwald, E. (1973). *Pharmacol. Rev.* **25**, 119–155.

Hillarp, N.-Å. (1959). *Acta Physiol. Scand.* **46**, Suppl. 157, 1–38.

Hills, L. D., and Braunwald, E. (1978). *N. Engl. J. Med.* **299**, 695–702.

Hingerty, D., and O'Boyle, A. (1972). *In* "Clinical Chemistry of the Adrenal Medulla" (I. N. Kugelmass, ed.), Chapter 9, pp. 78–88. Thomas, Springfield, Illinois.

Hoffman, B. F. (1967). *Ann. N.Y. Acad. Sci.* **139**, 914–939.

Hoffman, B. F. (1977). *In* "Neural Regulation of the Heart" (W. C. Randall, ed.), Chapter 10, pp. 291–312. Oxford Univ. Press, London and New York.

Hoffman, B. F., and Bigger, J. T., Jr. (1971). *In* "Drill's Pharmacology in Medicine" (J. R. DiPalma, ed.), 4th ed., pp. 824–852. McGraw-Hill, New York.

Hoffmann, F., Hoffmann, E. J., Middleton, S., and Talisnik, J. (1945). *Am. J. Physiol.* **144**, 189–198.

Hökfelt, B. (1951). *Acta Physiol. Scand.* **25**, Suppl. 92, 1–134.

Hollenberg, M., Carriere, S., and Barger, A. C. (1965). *Circ. Res.* **16**, 527–536.

Hurst, J. W., Logue, R. B., and Walter, P. F. (1978). *In* "The Heart" (J. W. Hurst, R. B. Logue, R. C. Schlant, and N. K. Wenger, eds.), 4th ed., Chapter 62E, pp. 1156–1290. McGraw-Hill, New York.

Imai, S., Shigei, T., and Hashimoto, K. (1961). *Circ. Res.* **9**, 552–560.

Iriuchijima, J., and Kumada, M. (1963). *Jpn. J. Physiol.* **13**, 599–605.

Iseri, L. T., Henderson, H. W., and Derr, J. W. (1951). *Am. Heart J.* **42**, 129–136.

Iversen, L. L. (1975a). *In* "Handbook of Physiology" (H. Blaschko, G. Sayers, and D. A. Smith, eds.), Vol. VI, pp. 713–722. Am. Physiol. Soc., Washington, D.C.

Iversen, L. L. (1975b). *Science* **188**, 1084–1089.

Jacobson, W. E., Hammarsten, J. F., and Heller, B. I. (1951). *J. Clin. Invest.* **30**, 1503–1506.

James, T. N. (1965). *J. Pharmacol. Exp. Ther.* **149**, 233–247.

James, T. N., and Spence, C. A. (1966). *Anat. Rec.* **155**, 151–161.

James, T. N., Bear, E. S., Lang, K. F., and Green, E. W. (1968). *Am. J. Physiol.* **215**, 1366–1375.

James, T. N., Bear, E. S., Lang, K. F., Gree, E. W., and Winkler, H. H. (1970). *Arch. Intern. Med.* **125**, 512–547.

James, T. N., Isobe, J. H., and Urthaler, F. (1975). *Circulation* **52**, 179–192.

Jewitt, D. E., Mercer, C. J., Reid, D., Valori, C., Thomas, M., and Shillingford, J. P. (1969). *Lancet* **1**, 635.

Juhász-Nagy, A., and Szentiványi, M. (1973). *Arch. Int. Pharmacodyn. Ther.* **206**, 19–20.

Katz, A. M. (1977). "Physiology of the Heart." Raven, New York.

Kaufman, S., and Friedman, S. (1965). *Pharmacol. Rev.* **17**, 71–100.

Kaumann, A. J. (1972). *Naunyn-Schmiedeberg's Arch. Pharmacol.* **273**, 134–153.

Kaye, M. P. (1977). *In* "Neural Regulation of the Heart" (W. C. Randall, ed.), Chapter 12, pp. 345–378. Oxford Univ. Press, London and New York.

Kelliher, G. J., and Roberts, J. (1974). *Am. Heart J.* **87,** 458–467.

Kent, K. M., Epstein, S. E., Cooper, T., and Jacobowitz, D. C. (1974). *Circulation* **50,** 948–955.

Keys, A. (1938). *Am. J. Physiol.* **121,** 325–330.

Kezdi, P., Kordenat, R. K., and Misra, S. N. (1974). *Am. J. Cardiol.* **33,** 853–860.

Khan, M. F., Hamilton, J. T., and Manning, G. W. (1972). *Am. J. Cardiol.* **30,** 832–837.

Kimata, S. (1965). *Jpn. Circ. J.* **29,** 17–20.

Kliks, B. R., Burgess, M. J., and Abildskov, J. A. (1975). *Am. J. Cardiol.* **36,** 45.

Kline, I. K. (1961). *Am. J. Pathol.* **38,** 539–552.

Kopin, I. J. (1964). *Pharmacol. Rev.* **16,** 179–191.

Kositzkey, G. I. (1971). *Proc. Int. Union Physiol. Sci.* **9,** 319 (abstr.).

Krakoff, L. R., Buccino, R. A., Spann, J. F., Jr., and Champlain, J. (1968). *Am. J. Physiol.* **215,** 549–552.

Kuchel, O., Buu, N. T., Fontain, A., Hamet, P., Unger, T., and Genest, J. (1977). *Eur. J. Clin. Invest.* **7**(1), 75–76.

LaBrosse, E. H., and Hertting, G. (1964). *Fed. Proc., Fed. Am. Soc. Exp. Biol.* **19,** 398–404.

LaBrosse, E. H., Axelrod, J., and Kety, S. S. (1958). *Science* **128,** 593–594.

Langer, S. Z. (1974). *Biochem. Pharmacol.* **23,** 1793–1800.

Lefkowitz, R. J. (1976). *N. Engl. J. Med.* **295,** 323–328.

Leinbach, R. C., Gold, H. K., Buckley, M. J., Austen, W. G., and Sanders, C. A. (1973). *Circulation* **48,** Suppl. IV, 100 (abstr.).

Lemberg, L., Catellanos, A., Jr., and Arcebal, A. G. (1970). *Am. Heart J.* **80,** 479–487.

Levitt, M., Spector, S., Sjoerdsma, A., and Udenfriend, S. (1965). *J. Pharmacol. Exp. Ther.* **148,** 1–8.

Levy, M. N. (1977a). *In* "Neural Regulation of the Heart" (W. C. Randall, ed.), Chapter 4, pp. 97–129. Oxford Univ. Press, London and New York.

Levy, M. N. (1977b). *In* "Cardiovascular System Dynamics," p. 365–370. MIT Press, Cambridge, Massachusetts.

Libby, P., Maroko, P. R., Covell, J. W., Malloch, C. I., Ross, J., Jr., and Braunwald, E. (1973). *Cardiovasc. Res.* **7,** 167–173.

Lloyd-Mostyn, R., Watkins, P. J., and Oram, S. (1974). *Br. Heart J.* **36,** 397.

Loewi, O. (1921). *Pflueger's Arch. Gesamte Physiol. Menschen Tiere* **189,** 239–242.

Machado, C. R. S., Machado, A. B. M., and Chiari, C. A. (1978). *Am. J. Trop. Med. Hyg.* **27,** 20–24.

McCullagh, E. P., and Engel, W. J. (1942). *Ann. Surg.* **116,** 61–75.

McDonald, L., Baker, C., Bray, C., McDonald, A., and Restieaux, N. (1969). *Lancet* **2,** 1021–1023.

MacKeith, R. (1944). *Br. Heart J.* **6,** 1–12.

Malliani, A., Schwartz, P. J., and Zanchetti, A. (1969). *Am. J. Physiol.* **217,** 703–709.

Malliani, A., Ricordati, G., and Schwartz, P. J. (1973). *J. Physiol. (London)* **229,** 457–469.

Manger, W. M., and Gifford, R. W., Jr. (1977). "Pheochromocytoma." Springer-Verlag, Berlin and New York.

Manger, W. M., and Yormak, S. S. (1977). *In* "Pheochromocytoma" (W. M. Manger and R. W. Gifford, Jr.), p. 190. Springer-Verlag, Berlin and New York.

Manger, W. M., Wakim, K. G., and Bollman, J. L. (1959). "Chemical Quantitation of Epinephrine and Norepinephrine in Plasma." Thomas, Springfield, Illinois.

Manger, W. M., von Estorff, I., Davis, S. W., Chu, D., Wakim, K., and Dufton, S. (1975). *Fed. Proc., Fed. Am. Soc. Exp. Biol.* Abstr. 2853, 723.

Manger, W. M., Davis, S. W., and Chu, D. (1979). *Arch. Phys. Med. Rehabil.* **60**, 159–161.

Manning, J. W. (1977). *In* "Neural Regulation of the Heart" (W. C. Randall, ed.), Chapter 7, pp. 189–209. Oxford Univ. Press, London and New York.

Maroko, P. R., and Braunwald, E. (1976). *Circulation* **53**, Suppl. I, 162–168.

Maroko, P. R., Braunwald, E., Covell, J. W., and Ross, J., Jr. (1969). *Circulation* **40**, Suppl. III, 130 (abstr.).

Maroko, P. R., Kjekshus, J. K., Sobel, B. E., Wantanabe, T., Covell, J. W., Ross, J., Jr., and Braunwald, E. (1971). *Circulation* **43**, 67–82.

Maroko, P. R., Bernstein, E. F., Libby, P., DeLaria, G. A., Covell, J. W., Ross, J., Jr., and Braunwald, E. (1972a). *Circulation* **45**, 1150–1159.

Maroko, P. R., Libby, P., Covell, J. W., Sobel, B. E., Ross, J., Jr., and Braunwald, E. (1972b). *Am. J. Cardiol.* **29**, 223–230.

Mary-Rabine, L., Hordof, A. J., Bowman, F. O., Malm, J. R., and Rosen, M. R. (1978). *Circulation* **57**, 84–90.

Maseri, A., L'Abbate, A., Baroldi, G., Chierchia, S., Marzilli, M., Ballestra, A. M., Severi, S., Parodi, O., Biagini, A., Distante, A., and Pesola, A. (1978). *N. Engl. J. Med.* **299**, 1271–1277.

Massara, F., Tripodina, A., and Rotunno, M. (1970). *Eur. J. Pharmacol.* **10**, 404–407.

Mathes, P., and Gudbjarnason, S. (1971). *Am. Heart J.* **81**, 211–219.

Mathes, P., Cowan, C., and Gudbjarnason, S. (1971). *Am. J. Physiol.* **220**, 27–32.

Meirson, F. Z. (1969). *Circ. Res.* **25**, Suppl. II, 143.

Melville, K. I., Blum, B., Shister, H. E., and Silver, M. D. (1963). *Am. J. Cardiol.* **12**, 781–791.

Meyer, G. A., and Winter, D. L. (1970). *J. Neurosurg.* **33**, 662–675.

Moskowitz, M. A., and Wurtman, R. J. (1975a). *N. Engl. J. Med.* **292**, 274–280.

Moskowitz, M. A., and Wurtman, R. J. (1975b). *N. Engl. J. Med.* **292**, 332–338.

Mudge, G. H., Jr., Grossman, W., Mills, R. M., Jr., Lesch, M., and Braunwald, E. (1976). *N. Engl. J. Med.* **295**, 1333–1337.

Mueller, H. S., Ayres, S. M., Conklin, E. F., Gianelli, S., Jr., Mazzara, J. T., Grace, W. T., and Neal, T. F., Jr. (1971). *J. Clin. Invest.* **50**, 1885–1900.

Mueller, H. S., Ayres, S. M., Religa, A., and Evans, R. G. (1974). *Circulation* **49**, 1078–1087.

Nagatsu, T., Levitt, M., and Udenfriend, S. (1964). *J. Biol. Chem.* **239**, 2910–2917.

Nayler, W. G., and Carson, V. (1973). *Cardiovasc. Res.* **7**, 22–29.

Nelson, P. G. (1970). *Br. Med. J.* **3**, 735–737.

Opie, L. H., Nathan, D., and Lubbe, W. F. (1979). *Am. J. Cardiol.* **43**, 131–148.

Östman, I., Sjöstrand, O., and Swedin, G. (1972). *Acta Physiol. Scand.* **86**, 299–308.

Östman-Smith, I. (1979). *Acta Physiol. Scand., Suppl.* **477**, 1–118.

Otten, U., and Theonen, H. (1975). *Proc. Natl. Acad. Sci. U.S.A.* **72**, 1415–1419.

Outschoorn, A. S., and Vogt, M. (1952). *Br. J. Pharmacol. Chemother.* **7**, 319–324.

Paar, G. H., and Wellhöner, H. H. (1973). *Naunyn-Schmiedeberg's Arch. Pharmacol.* **276**, 437–445.

Pace, J. B. (1977). *In* "Neural Regulation of the Heart" (W. C. Randall, ed.), Chapter 11, pp. 315–344. Oxford Univ. Press, London and New York.

Palmer, G. C., Spurgeon, H. A., and Priola, D. V. (1975). *J. Cyclic Nucleotide Res.* **1**, 89–95.

Pelkonen, R., and Pitkanan, E. (1963). *Acta Med. Scand.* **173**, 41–44.

Perrin, A., Normand, J., Mornex, R., and Froment, R. (1960). *Rev. Atheroscler.* **2**, 211–221.

Pincoffs, M. C. (1929). *Trans. Assoc. Am. Physicians* **44**, 295–299.

Pitt, B., Elliot, E. C., and Gregg, D. E. (1967). *Circ. Res.* **21**, 75–84.

Pitt, B., Green, H. L., and Sugishita, Y. (1970). *Cardiovasc. Res.* **4**, 89–92.

Pool, P. E., Covell, J. W., Levitt, M., Gibb, J., and Braunwald, E. (1967). *Circ. Res.* **20**, 349–353.

Potter, L. T., and Axelrod, J. (1963). *J. Pharmacol. Exp. Ther.* **442**, 299–305.

Potter, L. T., Cooper, T., Willman, V. L., and Wolfe, D. E. (1965). *Circ. Res.* **16**, 468–481.

Priola, D. V. (1969). *Am. J. Physiol.* **216**, 604–614.

Pullman, T. N., and McClure, W. W. (1952). *J. Lab. Clin. Med.* **39**, 711–719.

Raab, W., and Gigee, N. (1955). *Circulation* **11**, 593–603.

Radtke, W. E., Kazmier, F. J., Rutherford, B. D., and Sheps, S. G. (1975). *Am. J. Cardiol.* **35**, 701–705.

Randall, W. C., ed. (1977). "Neural Regulation of the Heart." Oxford Univ. Press, London and New York.

Randall, W. C., Armour, J. A., Geis, W. P., and Lippincott, D. B. (1972). *Fed. Proc., Fed. Am. Soc. Exp. Biol.* **31**, 1199–1208.

Reder, R. F., and Rosen, M. R. (1978). *Drug Ther. (Hosp. Ed.)* **3**, No. 7, 43–55.

Renkin, E. M., and Rosell, S. (1962). *Acta Physiol. Scand.* **54**, 223–240.

Roberts, J., and Kelliher, G. (1970). *Fed. Proc., Fed. Am. Soc. Exp. Biol.* **32**, 780.

Rogoff, J. M., Quashnock, J. M., Nixon, E. N., and Rosenberg, A. W. (1950). *Proc. Soc. Exp. Biol. Med.* **73**, 163–169.

Rose, A. G. (1974). *S. Afr. Med. J.* **48**, 1285–1289.

Rosen, M. R., Hordof, A. J., Ilvento, J. P., and Danilo, P., Jr. (1977). *Circ. Res.* **40**, 390–400.

Rothberger, J., and Winterberger, H. (1910). *Pflueger's Arch. Gesamte Physiol. Menschen Tiere* **135**, 506.

Russell, R. A., Crafoord, J., and Harris, A. S. (1961). *Am. J. Physiol.* **200**, 995–998.

Rutenberg, H. L., and Spann, J. F., Jr. (1976). *In* "Congestive Heart Failure Mechanisms, Evaluation and Treatment" (D. T. Mason, ed.), Chapter 7, pp. 85–95. Yorke Medical Books, Dun-Donnelley, New York.

Saavedra, J. M., Grobecker, H., and Axelrod, J. (1976). *Science* **191**, 483–484.

Saint-Pierre, A., Perrin, A., Mornex, R., and Pouzeratte, J.-P. (1970). *Coeur Med. Interne* **9**, 3–11.

Saint-Pierre, A., Lejosne, C., and Perrin, A. (1974). *Coeur Med. Interne* **13**, 59–73.

Sarnoff, S. J., and Mitchell, J. H. (1962). *In* "Handbook of Physiology" (W. F. Hamilton and P. Dow, eds.), Sect. 2, Vol. I, pp. 489–532. Am. Physiol. Soc., Washington, D.C.

Sarnoff, S. J., Gilmore, J. P., Brockman, S. K., Mitchell, J. H., and Linden, R. J. (1960). *Circ. Res.* **8**, 1123–1136.

Sayer, W. J., Moser, M., and Mattingly, T. W. (1954). *Am. Heart J.* **48**, 42–53.

Schaal, S. F., Wallace, A. G., and Sealey, W. C. (1969). *Cardiovasc. Res.* **3**, 241–244.

Schuelke, D. M., Mark, A. I., Schmid, P. G., and Eckstein, J. W. (1971). *J. Pharmacol. Exp. Ther.* **176**, 320–327.

Schwartz, P. J., and Malliani, A. (1975). *Am. Heart J.* **89**, 45–50.

Shapiro, A. P., Baker, H. M., Hoffman, M. S., and Ferris, E. B. (1951). *Am. J. Med.* **10**, 115–130.

Shaver, J. A., Leon, D. F., Graw, S., III, Leonard, J. J., and Bahnson, H. T. (1969). *N. Engl. J. Med.* **281**, 822–827.

Shindler, R., Harakal, C., and Sevy, R. W. (1968). *Proc. Exp. Biol. Med.* **128**, 789–800.

Siegel, J. H., Gilmore, J. P., and Sarnoff, S. J. (1961). *Circ. Res.* **9**, 1336–1350.

Simeone, F. A., and Sarnoff, S. J. (1947). *Surgery* **22**, 391–401.

Sjöstrand, T. (1951). *Acta Physiol. Scand.* **24**, 247–260.

Skelton, R. B., Gergely, N., Manning, G. W., and Coles, J. C. (1962). *J. Thorac. Cardiovasc. Surg.* **44**, 90–96.

Snyder, S. H. (1979). *N. Engl. J. Med.* **300**, 465–472.

Sode, J., Getzen, L. C., and Osborne, D. P. (1967). *Am. J. Surg.* **114**, 927–931.

Spann, J. F., Jr., Chidsey, C. A., and Braunwald, E. (1964). *Science* **145**, 1439–1441.

Spann, J. F., Jr., Chidsey, C. A., Pool, P. E., and Braunwald, E. (1965). *Circ. Res.* 17, 312–321.
Spann, F. J., Jr., Buccino, R. A., and Sonnenblick, E. H. (1967a). *Proc. Soc. Exp. Biol. Med.* 125, 522–524.
Spann, J. F., Jr., Buccino, R. A., Sonnenblick, E. H., and Braunwald, E. (1967b). *Circ. Res.* 21, 341–354.
Spector, S., Sjoerdsma, A., Zaltzman-Nirenberg, P., Levitt, M., and Udenfriend, S. (1963). *Science* 139, 1299–1301.
Spotnitz, H. M., Beach, P. M., Brigman, D., Truccone, N., Parodi, E. N., Manger, W. M., and Malm, J. R. (1977). *J. Surg. Res.* 22, 453–462.
Spurgeon, H. A., Priola, D. V., Montoya, P., Weiss, G. K., and Alter, W. A. (1974). *J. Pharmacol. Exp. Ther.* 190, 466–471.
Stanton, H. O., and Vick, R. I. (1968). *Arch. Int. Pharmacodyn. Ther.* 176, 233–248.
Starke, K., Taube, H. D., and Borowski, E. (1977). *Biochem. Pharmacol.* 26, 259–268.
Stephen, S. A. (1966). *Am. J. Cardiol.* 18, 463–472.
Stinson, E. B., Griepp, R. B., Clark, D. A., Dong, E., and Shumway, N. E. (1970). *J. Thorac. Cardiovasc. Surg.* 60, 303–319.
Stjärne, L., and Brundin, J. (1975). *Acta Physiol. Scand.* 94, 139–141.
Sutherland, E. W., Robison, G. A., and Butcher, R. W. (1968). *Circulation* 37, 279–306.
Szentiványi, M., Pace, J. P., Wechsler, J. S., and Randall, W. C. (1967). *Circ. Res.* 21, 691–702.
Tada, M., Kirchberger, M. A., Iorio, J. M., and Katz, A. M. (1976). *Circ. Res.* 36, 8–17.
Tenzer, C. (1954). *Acta Cardiol.* 9, 532–541.
Tsien, R. W., Giles, W. R., and Greengard, P. (1972). *Nature (London), New Biol.* 240, 181–183.
Ueda, H., Yanai, Y., Marav, S., Haruine, K., Mashima, S., Kuroiwa, A., Sugimoto, T., and Shimomura, K. (1964). *Jpn. Heart J.* 5, 359–372.
Ulmer, R. H., and Randall, W. C. (1961). *Am. J. Physiol.* 201, 134–138.
Urthaler, F., and James, T. N. (1973). *Am. J. Physiol.* 224, 1155–1161.
Urthaler, F., and James, T. N. (1977). *In* "Neural Regulation of the Heart" (W. C. Randall, ed.), Chapter 9, pp. 247–288. Oxford Univ. Press, London and New York.
Urthaler, F., Katholi, C. R., Macy, J., Jr., and James, T. N. (1973). *Am. Heart J.* 86, 189–195.
Urthaler, F., Katholi, C. R., Macy, J., Jr., and James, T. N. (1974). *Cardiovasc. Res.* 8, 173–186.
Van Citters, R. L., Smith, O. A., and Ruttenberg, H. D. (1966). *Am. J. Physiol.* 211, 293–300.
Vanderbeck, R. B., and Ebert, P. A. (1970). *Am. J. Physiol.* 218, 803–806.
Vane, J. R. (1969). *Br. J. Pharmacol.* 35, 209–242.
Van Vliet, P. D., Burchell, H. B., and Titus, J. L. (1966). *N. Engl. J. Med.* 274, 1102–1108.
Vatner, S. F., and Braunwald, E. (1975). *N. Engl. J. Med.* 293, 970–976.
Vatner, S. F., and McRitchie, R. J. (1975). *Circ. Res.* 39, 664–673.
Vatner, S. F., Franklin, D., Van Citters, R. L., and Braunwald, E. (1970). *Circ. Res.* 27, 11–21.
Vatner, S. F., Millard, R. W., and Higgins, C. B. (1973). *J. Pharmacol. Exp. Ther.* 187, 280–295.
Vatner, S. F., Higgins, C. B., and Braunwald, E. (1975). *Circ. Res.* 34, 812–823.
Vendsalu, A. (1960). *Acta Physiol. Scand.* 49, Suppl. 173, 1–123.
Viveros, O. H., Arqueros, L., and Kirshner, N. (1968). *Life Sci.* 7, 609–618.
Vogel, J. H. K., Jacobowitz, D., and Chidsey, C. A. (1969). *Circ. Res.* 24, 71–84.
von Euler, U. S. (1946). *Acta Physiol. Scand.* 12, 73–97.
von Euler, U. S. (1956). "Noradrenaline." Thomas, Springfield, Illinois.
von Euler, U. S., and Strom, G. (1957). *Circulation* 15, 6.
von Euler, U. S., Franksson, C., and Hellström, J. (1954). *Acta Physiol. Scand.* 31, 1–5.
Watkins, D. B. (1957). *J. Chronic Dis.* 6, 510–527.
Weil-Malherbe, H., Axelrod, J., and Tomchick, R. (1959). *Science* 129, 1226–1227.

Weinshilboum, R. M., Thoa, N. B., Johnson, D. G., Kopin, I. J., and Axelrod, J. (1971). *Science* **174**, 1349–1351.

West, G. B., Shepherd, D. M., and Hunter, R. B. (1951). *Lancet* **2**, 966–969.

West, G. B., Shepherd, D. M., Hunter, R. B., and MacGregor, A. R. (1953). *Clin. Sci.* **12**, 317–325.

Whitby, L. G., Axelrod, J., and Weil-Malherbe, H. (1961). *J. Pharmacol. Exp. Ther.* **132**, 193–201.

Williams, L. T., and Lefkowitz, R. J. (1978). "Receptor Binding Studies in Adrenergic Pharmacology." Raven, New York.

Williams, T. H. (1967). *Nature (London)* **214**, 309–310.

Witham, A. C., and Fleming, J. W. (1951). *J. Clin. Invest.* **30**, 707–717.

Witzke, D. J., and Kaye, M. P. (1976). *Surg. Forum* **27**, 295–297.

Wurster, R. D. (1977). *In* "Neural Regulation of the Heart" (W. C. Randall, ed.), Chapter 8, pp. 213–246. Oxford Univ. Press, London and New York.

Wurster, R. D., and Randall, W. C. (1975). *Am. J. Physiol.* **228**, 1288–1292.

Wurtman, R. J. (1966). "Catecholamines." Little, Brown, Boston, Massachusetts.

Wurtman, R. J., Kopin, I. J., and Axelrod, J. (1963). *Endocrinology* **73**, 63–74.

Yamauchi, A. (1973). *In* "Ultrastructure of the Mammalian Heart" (C. E. Challice and S. Virágh, eds.), pp. 127–178. Academic Press, New York.

Yankopoulos, N. A., Montero, A. C., Curd, W. G., Jr., Kahil, M. E., and Condon, R. E. (1974). *Chest* **66**, 585–587.

Yanowitz, F., Preston, J. B., and Abildskov, J. A. (1966). *Circ. Res.* **18**, 416–428.

Yasue, H., Touyama, M., Kato, H., Tanaka, S., and Akiyama, F. (1976). *Am. Heart J.* **91**, 148–155.

Zumerbuhler, R. C., and Bohr, D. F. (1965). *Circ. Res.* **16**, 431–440.

5

Emotion and the Heart

Henry I. Russek and Linda G. Russek

Every affection of the mind that is attended with either pain or pleasure, hope or fear, is the cause of an agitation whose influence extends to the heart.

William Harvey, 1628

Twentieth-century man has inherited the benefits of technological progress and social mobility, but he has also had to pay the price for unfulfilled adaptation to a rapidly changing environment. Rushing to make deadlines, the accumulation of debts, responsibilities and moral compromises, unhygienic practices, and the drive for power and prestige have led to the burgeoning of diseases that every day threaten his well-being. Chief among these maladies is coronary heart disease.

HEARTS AND HEART-LIKE ORGANS, VOL. 2

Until recently the authoritative view considered such variables as elevated blood pressure, elevated serum cholesterol, cigarette smoking, obesity, diabetes, and a family history of coronary disease to be the major factors predictive of increased coronary risk. It has become increasingly evident, however, that coronary heart disease incidence in American men cannot be adequately explained by these traditional risk factors and that "something of great importance is being missed" (Keys *et al.*, 1972). That the missing variable may be the elusive factor of emotional stress is supported by a wide range of research studies indicating that certain psychological, social, and behavioral conditions do place persons at increased risk of acquiring manifest coronary disease. Indeed, consistent and persuasive findings appear to link this disorder to prolonged emotional stress, a specific behavior pattern, sociocultural mobility, and stressful life events.

Whether or not emotional stress is eventually confirmed as a major risk factor in coronary heart disease, there can be no denial of its profound significance once the cardiac disorder has become clinically manifest. Emotional arousal is commonly found as a precipitating influence in anginal episodes, acute myocardial infarction, congestive heart failure, arrhythmias, and sudden death. Even during sleep, when the emotions stem from the unconscious, the patient remains vulnerable to these unfortunate consequences. Similarly, anxiety and psychic tension may not only aggravate cardiovascular symptoms but also seriously impede rehabilitation in patients with rational or distorted fears concerning the consequences of their disease. In extreme cases cardiac neurosis or anxiety–depression may be more disabling than the cardiac disorder itself.

I. Emotional Stress as a Major Risk Factor in Coronary Heart Disease

A. Occupational Influences

In recent years efforts to define the role of psychic stress in the etiology of coronary atherosclerosis have been more productive than earlier attempts by astute clinicians employing largely anecdotal evidence. In a study of young coronary patients it has been noted that differentiation from healthy control subjects could be more readily made by the dimensions of occupational (emotional) stress than by differences in heredity, diet, obesity, tobacco consumption, or exercise (Table I) (Russek, 1959). Thus it was found that at the time of their attack 91% of 100 patients as compared with only 20% of healthy controls had been holding down two or more jobs, working more than 60 hr per week, or experiencing unusual insecurity,

TABLE I

Incidence of Various Factors in Coronary and Control Groups

Group	No.	Heredity (positive)	High-fat diet	Stress and strain (occupational)	Obesity	Tobacco (30 cigs.)	Exercise
Coronary	100	67%	53%	91%	26%	70%	58%
Control	100	40%	20%	20%	20%	35%	60%
Ratio		1.7 to 1	2.7 to 1	4.6 to 1	1.3 to 1	2 to 1	1 to 1

discontent, or frustration in relation to employment. Buell and Breslow (1960) have also reported findings that support a relationship between hours of work and death from coronary disease. In a study of the registered mortality rate of men in California, they observed that light workers under the age of 45 who are on the job more than 48 hr a week have twice the risk of death from coronary heart disease that other light workers of similar age do. To test the validity of these observations, we decided to compare the prevalence of coronary artery disease in various occupational categories in which obvious differences exist with respect to "tensions" created by routine demands of the job (Russek, 1960). For this purpose physicians themselves appeared uniquely suited for survey by questionnaire. This seemed to be so not only because of greater reliability of the anticipated data, but also because of striking differences in the demands of professional life among those engaged in various segments of medical practice. Although premedical and undergraduate medical education in the United States is essentially similar for all physicians, it is chiefly in specialty practice that distinct differences prevail among the emotional stresses that develop at work. Obviously, the burdens and responsibilities of the general practitioner, the consultant, and the specialist provide as marked a contrast as may be found among other occupational categories more difficult to study.

On the basis of rankings by eight independent judges, four professional groups were selected, of which two were prejudged to be in a "high-stress" area of medical practice (general practitioners and anesthesiologists) and two in a "low-stress" area (pathologists and dermatologists). Questionnaires were sent out to 4000 physicians, 1000 in each of the four categories under study, in order to determine the prevalence of coronary heart disease in each of these groups (Russek, 1960). From an analysis of the 2587 replies (64.7%), it was evident that general practitioners and anesthesiologists have distinctly higher coronary heart disease prevalence rates than dermatologists and pathologists.

The prevalence of coronary disease was lowest among dermatologists 40–69 years of age and highest among general practitioners in the same age group (3.2% as compared with 11.9%) (Table II). Among English physicians a greater vulnerability among general practitioners has also been noted. Morris et al. (1952) have reported that full-time general practitioners, aged 40–64, had about twice as high an incidence of coronary heart disease as other members of the profession. If emotional stress of occupational origin is a major influence in the etiologic spectrum of coronary artery disease, certainly the practitioner of medicine, whose routine duties encompass responsibility not only for health but also for life itself, should be found among the most vulnerable in our society. The high frequency of the disease among members of the medical profession as a group has indeed

TABLE II

Percentage Prevalence of Coronary Heart Disease in Four Specialty Categories Ranked by Stressfulness

Specialty	Age at survey				Stress rank
	40–49	50–59	60–69	40–69	
Dermatology	0.9	5.1	7.8	3.2	least
Pathology	1.8	5.2	11.7	4.1	
Anesthesiology	2.6	13.7	30.0	8.9	
General practice	6.0	12.0	23.3	11.9	most
Average	2.8	8.6	18.4	7.0	
		Trend of prevalence rates and stress ranks			
Chi-square	11.6	7.6	8.2	36.4	
Probability	<0.001	<0.01	<0.01	<0.001	

attracted attention for many years and has led to the designation "morbus medicorum" for angina itself. In 1910 Sir William Osler, commenting on the high prevalence of the disease among doctors, wrote the following:

> In a group of 20 men, every one of whom I knew personally, the outstanding feature was the incessant treadmill of practice; and yet if hard work—that "badge of all our tribe"—was alone responsible, would there not be a great many more cases? Every one of these men had an added factor—worry; in not a single case under 50 years of age was this feature absent. . . . Listen to some of the comments which I jotted down of the circumstances connected with the onset of attacks: "A man of great mental and bodily energy, working early and late in a practice, involved in speculations in land"; "domestic infelicities"; "worries in the Faculty of Medicine"; "troubles with the trustees of his institution"; "law suits"; "domestic worries." . . . At least 6 or 7 men of the 6th decade were carrying loads light enough for the 5th, but too much for a machine with an ever lessening reserve.

As in our survey of doctors, we have conducted similar studies of coronary disease prevalence among members of various specialties in the dental and legal professions (Russek, 1962), among personnel at the New York Stock Exchange, and among members of other professions. Our survey of 25,000 professional men in 20 occupational categories has clearly demonstrated that a marked gradient exists in the distribution of coronary disease that appears strikingly related to the prejudged stressfulness of occupational activity (Fig. 1).

B. Anxiety and Depression

Data from a population of male subjects studied while undergoing selective coronary angiography suggest that anxiety and depression may be directly related to the atherosclerotic process (Zyzanski et al., 1975). The degree of reported atherosclerosis showed a striking correlation with scores on self-administered scales for anxiety and depression, with the higher scores significantly discriminating those men having two or more coronary vessels with luminal obstructions of 50% or greater from those with lesser degrees of abnormality. The hypochondriasis scale of the MMPI, a measure of somaticizing, has also been found associated both prospectively and retrospectively with angina pectoris (Jenkins, 1971) but not with the amount of coronary atherosclerosis (Friedman et al., 1974). The theory of "emotional drain," a state both of physical and mental exhaustion, as prodromal to myocardial infarction (Bruhn et al., 1969) has recently received support from other observers (Kavanaugh and Shephard, 1973), who noted increased fatigue and poor general health in the week preceding the coronary attack in 102 survivors of this event.

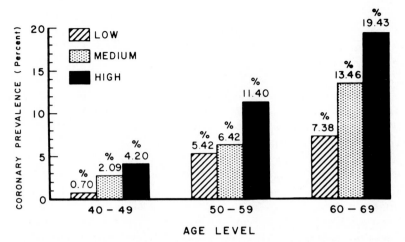

Fig. 1.   Coronary prevalence by age and stress group. Classification according to stress is as follows: *low:* dermatologists, orthodontists, patent lawyers, and periodontists; *medium:* oral surgeons, other lawyers, pathologists, security analysts, and trial lawyers; *high:* anesthesiologists, general practice dentistry, general practice law, general practice medicine, and security traders.

C. The Coronary Personality

The concept of a coronary-prone behavior pattern is also not new. Even before the turn of the century, Osler (1896) described the pernicious combination of a certain configuration of personality traits and the mounting pressures of environment. In his experience the typical patient with coronary disease was "a keen and ambitious man, the indicator of whose engines is always set at 'full speed ahead.'" This description was later supported by the independent observations of Arlow (1945), Kemple (1945), and others and more recently by Wolf (1958) and Russek (1959). Arlow observed "a compulsive striving for achievement and mastery which never seems to end." Kemple found the coronary patient to be an aggressive, ambitious individual with intense physical and emotional drive, unable to delegate authority or responsibility with ease, possessing no hobbies, and concentrating all his thoughts and energy in the narrow groove of his career. Wolf similarly described the coronary-prone individual as one who not only meets a challenge by expending extra effort, but who takes little satisfaction from his accomplishments. This unrelenting striver who seemingly meets with frustration and lack of rewards for his efforts (Sisyphus reaction) may be suffering from debilitated ego defenses that culminate in psychic exhaustion and emotional drain (Bruhn *et al.,* 1969). We also found the young coronary patient frequently to have been a victim of overwork, often as a result of his excessive drive, intense desire for recognition, or profound sense of obligation to his employer, his family, or others, but more commonly, simply as a consequence of meeting life's challenges with maximum and unstinting effort. Compulsive about time and overmeticulous, these patients were often concerned about trivia, impatient with subordinates, and worrisome. As perfectionists, they generally chose to do the work themselves rather than delegate it to others. It was their usual practice to take on more responsibilities at an occupational, social, or domestic level than good judgment would dictate. Many had never learned to say "no." They minimized their symptoms and neglected prudent rules of health. Perhaps most characteristic was a restlessness during leisure hours and a sense of guilt during periods of "relaxation." Consequently, the young coronary patient rarely took vacations, and such leisure time as he did possess was frequently regimented by obligatory participation in an assortment of social, civic, or educational activities. It seemed evident, therefore, that behavior patterns, quite independently of the demands of the job itself, could generate high degrees of emotional stress.

Because of the retrospective nature of these studies, others have challenged the existence of a coronary-prone behavior pattern, asserting that its alleged characteristics may follow rather than precede the coronary event. Negating this claim are the findings of Friedman and Rosenman (1959) and Rosenman *et al.* (1966) in a long-term prospective study of more than 3500 male subjects. Thus these authors observed a significantly higher coronary morbidity and mortality among men previously identified as possessing a certain well-defined action–emotion complex that has been designated and now popularized as the Type A behavior pattern.

Such behavior is observed in individuals who are engaged in a relatively chronic struggle to obtain an unlimited number of poorly defined things from their environment in the shortest period of time and, if necessary, against the opposing resistance of other persons or things in this same environment. In addition to intense ambition, competitive drive, sense of urgency, and preoccupation with deadlines, more than 80% were alleged to manifest "excessively rapid body movement, tense facial and bodily musculature, explosive conversational intonations, hand or teeth clenching, excessive unconscious gesturing, and a general air of impatience." These visible manifestations were not frequently encountered in our own series of young patients. Such features would appear to represent a caricature rather than a portrait of the average coronary patient under the age of 40 in our experience. In fact, most of the young patients seemed to show a striking degree of self-control, dignified reserve, and outward complacency during interrogation. in many of these subjects, psychological factors would have remained unrecognized had we not made a special inquiry regarding their presence.

Despite such differences, it is now widely acknowledged that subjects possessing the Type A behavior pattern suffer twice as frequently from coronary attacks as individuals with the converse behavior pattern B, who are defined as being free from Type A characteristics and who therefore experience no pressing conflict with either time or other individuals. In confronting life situations they are also free of any habitual sense of time urgency. The value of such classification is evident from the fact that the predictive strength of the Type A behavior pattern for the risk of developing coronary heart disease was found to be at least as potent as that of the other major risk factors, including serum cholesterol, cigarette smoking, and high blood pressure (Rosenman *et al.,* 1966).

It has been found in both clinical and epidemiologic studies that anxiety, depression, and neurotic defenses are linked with the risk of developing angina pectoris and possibly also with the risk of myocardial infarction. However, the presence of Type A behavior pattern and its association with coronary heart disease appears to be quite independent of these factors. Correlational studies of several different groups of coronary patients and healthy individuals have sought to measure anxiety, depression, and neurosis. Distinction therefore has been made between the Type A individual and the subject suffering from anxiety. The Type A person is said rarely to despair of approaching failure, although he strongly strives to win. On the other hand, the subject with a classic anxiety state is commonly thought to seek assistance when the demands appear overwhelming. Similarly, Type As advance while subjects with anxiety tend to retreat in comparably challenging situations.

The divergent styles of living associated with Type A and Type B behavior have been correlated with different patterns of response to acute stress and differing predisposition to coronary attacks. Type A men exhibited a larger increase in plasma norepinephrine before, during, and after a problem-solving task than Type B men, who are relatively resistant to coronary heart disease (Rosenman *et al.,* 1966). This suggests that Type A individuals overreacted to the situation in comparison with reactions of Type B subjects. Of further significance is the ability or inability of Type A or Type B individuals to master a continuing emergency situation, which is the important determinant of whether or not a sustained fight or flight reaction takes place. This will be dealt with in sections to follow.

D. Social Mobility and Stressful Life Events

One of the important observations from recent stress research studies pertains to social and cultural mobility. In one investigation (Syme *et al.,*

1964) coronary heart disease rates were found to be over two times higher among men who had experienced several lifetime job changes and geographic moves than among men with no such changes; the rates were three times higher among men reared on farms who later moved to the city to take white-collar jobs compared with men who either remained on the farm or who took blue-collar jobs in the city. The differences were not attributable to variations in diet, smoking habits, physical activity, obesity, blood pressure, age, or familial longevity. These findings have been confirmed in other investigations. In a long-term prospective study conducted in Evans County, Georgia, Kaplan and associates (1971) found twice the prevalence of coronary heart disease among lower-status persons who had moved upward in social status during the period as among those who had remained at the same level. A number of additional studies are also consistent with the view that risk of coronary heart disease increases with major changes in place of residence, major changes in occupation, and discrepancies between culture of origin and the current cultural situation. It would appear that as persons move into unfamiliar social circumstances or into a social environment for which they have not previously been prepared, the rates of coronary heart disease increase.

Similarly, new studies are in keeping with the view that stress, American-style, is a major contributing factor in heart disease. In an extensive study in San Francisco, Marmot and associates (1975) have reported that Japanese-Americans who adhere to their traditional cultural values have the same low incidence of heart disease as do men in Japan. In contrast, Japanese-Americans who become westernized in their habits have a heart disease rate two and one-half times higher than that of those who live in the more traditional manner. Competition and haste seemed to account for the differences among groups more than the other major heart disease factors such as diet, smoking, and lack of exercise. Interestingly, the traditional group of Japanese were found to maintain the Japanese cultural mores of staying within a close-knit family, living quiet lives, and being noncompetitive. As indicated by Marmot, groups in Japan may compete, but individuals generally do not. These observations are important because they open to question the conclusions of other migration studies that have failed to deal with the stresses of sociocultural mobility.

Another hypothesis now beginning to gain support from the social–psychological research in this area concerns the relationship of stressful life events to coronary heart disease. Holmes and Rahe (1967) have developed a social readjustment rating scale to measure such life events as change in residence, injury, job changes, death of a loved one, and birth of a child. From this, many studies have been carried out showing an association between a wide spectrum of life events and a variety of disease outcomes. In one prospective study (Parkes *et al.,* 1969) 4486 widowers 55 years of age and older were followed for 9 years after the death of their wives. During the first 6 months of bereavement, the mortality rate was found to be 40% higher than would be expected for married men of the same age. Significantly, the greatest component in this excess death rate was mortality due to coronary heart disease.

II. Emotional Stress and Standard Coronary Risk Factors

From these findings it is difficult to comprehend the sustained apathy toward the possible significance of emotional factors in the etiology of coronary heart disease on the part of many authorities in the cardiovascular and epidemiologic fields. High cholesterol, elevated blood pressure, and cigarette smoking, although constantly mentioned, are completely absent in more than half of all new cases of coronary heart disease encountered in clinical practice (Jenkins, 1971). Indeed, most patients do not have high blood cholesterol and only a fraction have high blood pressure (Rosenman, 1968). Data from pooled prospective studies in the United States actually show that of men with two or more of these alleged risks, only about 10% develop coronary heart disease over a 10-year period, while the remainder do not (Syme, 1975). Similarly, preventive measures directed against these etiologic influences appear to have met with little success. For example, although more than 100,000 American physicians have allegedly given up smoking and no segment of our society is more aware of the potential dangers of hypercholesterolemia and hypertension than are members of the medical profession, there has been no significant change either in longevity or in average age at death from coronary heart disease among doctors in the United States over the past 20 years (Table III) (Russek and Russek, 1977). Furthermore, it is axiomatic that the greater the importance of the standard risk factors in the etiology of coronary heart disease, the greater must be the role of emotional stress in its causation. Certainly, anxiety and tension are unrivaled in their ability to elevate blood pressure and serum cholesterol, to increase the consumption of tobacco, to augment obesity through dietary indiscretion, to aggravate diabetes, and to interfere with a regimen of regular exercise. Even these indirect effects of psychic stress, barring all others, would seem adequate to ensure its pathogenetic significance in coronary heart disease (Russek, 1965).

TABLE III

Deaths among United States Physicians

	Jan.–April 1955	Jan.–April 1965	Jan.–April 1967	Jan.–April 1970
Average age at death (years)	69.6	68.9	69.6	67.2
Average age, coronary deaths only (< 70 years)	61.0	60.8	60.6	59.4
Total no. of deaths	1148	1091	1251	1013

III. Pathogenetic Interrelationship between Psychic Stress and Dietary Fat

Much evidence now suggests that most of the lethality of a high-fat diet in Western society may actually be dependent on the "catalytic" influence of stressful living (Russek, 1959, 1962). Moreover, it is equally apparent that the atherogenicity of emotional stress must be appreciably diminished, if not nullified, by subsistence on a diet low in fat. Snapper (1941) also came to the conclusion that stress has little or no effect if the diet is poor in animal fat, following his studies of the Chinese population under the severe stress of Japanese invasion. Racial groups in other geographical areas such as Korea, Yemen, and Japan have also exhibited a distinct immunity to coronary disease, despite obvious emotional stress in their pattern of life. Since this "immunity" seems to be lost when high-fat diets are ingested, the role of the emotions has often been assigned a position of secondary significance. The fallacy in such reasoning is made apparent by the striking pathogenetic interrelationship that exists between psychic stress and dietary fat. This phenomenon is observed both in the animal kingdom and in man.

A. Stress and Atherosclerosis in Animals

Inasmuch as dietary habits among various population groups reflect profound differences in patterns of living, "diet cannot be readily isolated from the matrix of man's total transaction with his environment" (Lown and Stare, 1959). In the animal kingdom, however, major environmental factors have been identified and controlled far more readily and more completely than is possible with corresponding factors in human society. For example, at the Philadelphia zoo, mammals and birds who have been on a constant diet were reported to have had a tenfold increase in arteriosclerosis of the coronary arteries within a decade (Ratcliffe *et al.,* 1960). Their increased susceptibility to vascular degenerative lesions has been ascribed to the psychological disturbances caused by social interactions resulting from increased population densities in the zoo. Man's response to population density appears to correspond closely to that of other animals. This is reflected in the significantly higher death rate from clinical coronary heart disease that has been found in metropolitan communities as compared with rural areas (Rikli *et al.,* 1960).

Experimentally, the profound but dependent role of stress in atherogenesis has been clearly confirmed. It has been shown that hypercholesterolemia and aortic atherosclerosis in cholesterol-fed rabbits may be augmented or reduced by drugs that stimulate or depress the central nervous system (Myasnikov, 1958). Greater degrees of hypercholesterolemia and coronary atherosclerosis have also been evoked in rats fed an atherogenic diet and exposed to a particular form of stress, than in their unstressed controls (Uhley and Friedman, 1959). Recently, similar observations have been made in monkeys (Gutstein, 1978). It is of further interest that although intimal changes are rare in the coronary arteries of wild immature monkeys, changes in the intima observed in immature caged rhesus monkeys are common after 1.5–3 months of captivity, and have been interpreted as a response to emotional stress (Vlodaver *et al.*, 1968). Additional experiments were needed, however, to determine whether such stresses alone are capable of initiating atherosclerosis when the diet is low in fat. Clear answers were provided by the careful studies of Gunn *et al.* (1960) in rabbits. These authors found that on a cholesterol-rich diet, hypothalamic stimulation, like other forms of stress, increased the atherogenicity of diet alone. More important was the observation that hypothalamic stimulation in controls on a low-cholesterol diet left the vascular system unimpaired. As will be shown, these experimental studies seem to correlate with epidemiologic data obtained in man. Thus, like "stressed" animals in the laboratory, "stressed" human beings do not appear to manifest an increased susceptibility to atherosclerosis unless the composition of the diet has been relatively high in animal fat.

B. Emotional Stress and Diet in Man

The findings of Groen *et al.* (1959) in a study of Benedictine and Trappist monks provide insight into the role of fat, as related to stress, in the genesis of coronary disease. Both of these groups live in rural areas removed from the stresses of urban life and, in the monastic environment, are free from economic and family problems. The Benedictines have a diet substantially the same as other Europeans, whereas the Trappists do not eat fish, meat, eggs, or butter. Although there is a much higher level of blood cholesterol among the Benedictine monks, no striking differences were observed in coronary heart disease prevalence, and not a single instance of significant disease was encountered under the age of 65 in either group. Moreover, both groups showed a far smaller incidence of coronary disease than the general population. It seems significant, therefore, that although the "unstressed" Benedictine monk eats as much fat as the greatly harassed general practitioner of medicine, he suffers only about one-fifth as often from clinical coronary disease (Russek, 1960).

Similarly, it is noteworthy that Somali camel herdsmen are relatively free from clinical symptoms suggestive of coronary atherosclerosis, although they are known to subsist on a high-fat diet derived from approximately 5 liters of camel's milk per day (Lapiccirella *et al.*, 1962). Although many theories may be advanced to explain this seemingly paradoxical immunity, a major factor for these people, whose pastoral and patriarchal way of life has remained unchanged for centuries, could be their relative freedom from serious psychological stress. Similarly, although physical fitness as a result of arduous activity has been assumed to protect the East African Masai, freedom from coronary disease in this pastoral people, despite a diet rich in animal products and dairy fat (Mann *et al.*, 1965) also could be largely an outcome of the simplicity of their way of life.

In like manner, the unusually low incidence of death from myocardial infarction reported for the noncompetitive, content Italian-American community of Roseto, Pennsylvania (Stout *et al.*, 1964), also suggests that lifestyle may be an important determinant of the atherogenicity of a high-fat diet. *Thus, although both habitual diet and stressful living appear to be implicated in the pathogenesis of clinical coronary disease, mounting evidence suggests that each is dependent on the other for pathological significance.*

IV. Emotional Stress and Tobacco Consumption

Despite the statistical relationship between tobacco smoking and clinical coronary heart disease, our studies suggest that smoking may often be a manifestation of underlying emotional stress rather than, of itself, a potent etiologic factor in atherogenesis (Russek, 1964, 1973). We observed a rising frequency of the smoking habit with increased occupational stress and a *lower* coronary heart disease prevalence *among persons who stopped smoking* than *among those who had never smoked.* Since our survey was undertaken before the national campaign against the smoking habit, those who stopped smoking in our study did so of their own free will without medical indication or other coercion. The data indicated that whereas the smoking of tobacco may be implicated in the pathogenesis of coronary heart disease, the relationship is not clear. No explanation is at hand to account for the *low prevalence* of coronary heart disease *among persons who once smoked* (Fig. 2). Interestingly, this finding was overlooked in the earlier Framingham and Albany studies and later rejected as having no paradoxical significance. It is possible, nonetheless, that the ability to stop smoking without duress implies a resilient personality response to stress and thereby a diminished vulnerability to atherogenic influences (Russek, 1964, 1973).

V. Emotional Stress and the Pathogenesis of Atherosclerosis

At present, there is no clear understanding of the manner in which emotional stress may hasten the advent of clinical coronary artery disease. Eleva-

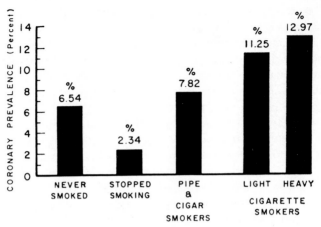

Fig. 2.   Coronary prevalence by smoking habit.

tion in blood cholesterol level, metabolic changes in the vascular wall leading to an increase in its lipid receptiveness, augmentation of myocardial
oxygen requirements, and increase in the coagulability and viscosity of the
blood all appear to be implicated. Thus, prolonged emotional stress, acting
through the cerebral cortex and hypothalamus via neurohormonal and hormonal mechanisms, may contribute not only to the initiation and progression of atheromatosis but to its clinical complications as well.

A. Influence of Emotional Stress on Homeostasis

Numerous investigators have shown that stressful life experiences are
capable of evoking hypercholesterolemia despite constant diet and exercise.
Bogdonoff *et al.* (1959) have also shown that emotional episodes cause a
rapid mobilization of nonesterified fatty acids from the body tissues into the
circulation; these authors have obtained similar results with infusions of
epinephrine and norepinephrine. Steinberg and Shafrir (1960) and others
have shown in animals that it is cortisone that enhances the ability of
epinephrine to trigger sharp blood lipid increases under the influence of
psychic stress. They observed a marked and almost immediate rise in the
nonesterified fatty acids, followed by a slower but definite rise in serum
cholesterol. According to Sabin (1959), free fatty acids are irritating and, in
excess, may cause subendothelial hemorrhage and small mural thrombi.
Whatever the exact mechanisms underlying such responses may be, hyper-
lipemia so evoked is believed to "provide metabolic substrate for the
aroused organism."

As a result of emotional arousal, sympathetic adrenergic effects on vascular tissue metabolism may prepare the soil for subsequent lipid depositions primarily by damaging the intima. Prolonged vasoconstriction could reduce blood flow in vasa vasorum and produce vascular wall ischemia, leading to increased permeability and intramural edema. Raab and Humphreys (1947) have shown that catecholamines also diminish myocardial efficiency by wasting oxygen in a disproportionate fashion. Through this action the hormones are capable not only of increasing myocardial vulnerability in the presence of coronary atherosclerosis but of inducing severe, potentially necrotizing myocardial hypoxia in animals with perfectly normal coronary vessels. Indeed, Raab and associates (1964) have produced myocardial necroses in rats solely by subjecting these animals to sensory and emotional stresses. Groover *et al.* (1963) have also reported myocardial infarction without demonstrable atherosclerosis in baboons subjected to the emotional storm induced by trapping and caging. It seems probable, therefore, that occult disease in man may surface to clinical view solely or prematurely as a result of stressful life experiences.

The blood clotting elements have also been found to be susceptible to emotional stresses. Dreyfuss and Czaczkes (1959) measured clotting time and found it to be accelerated in 36 medical students on the morning of a final examination in medicine. Still and Heiffer (1958) observed sharp increases in viscosity, mediated through the action of the sympathetic nervous system, as the result of emotional stimuli in animals. Similarly, Haft (1974) has demonstrated that microvascular platelet aggregation, often associated with necrosis, may occur in the hearts of animals receiving prolonged epinephrine infusion. More significantly, stress-induced platelet elevation, with reduction in blood clotting time, has been reported in human subjects (Hames, 1975). Such changes appear to be part of an adaptive response to combat designed to prevent blood loss. When this mechanism reacts excessively over a prolonged period of time, blood with increased coagulability and decreased fluidity may slow sufficiently, in passing through narrowed coronary or cerebral arteries, to produce thrombosis. Even when coronary atherosclerosis is not present, microcirculatory platelet aggregation and/or catecholamine-induced myocardial hypoxia due to emotional stress could conceivably account for the instances of "unexplained" angina pectoris and myocardial infarction observed clinically.

B. Stress and the Candidate for a Coronary Attack

Obviously not all persons subjected to prolonged emotional stress will develop coronary heart disease. Reference has already been made to the apparent immunity of "stressed" populations subsisting on a low-fat diet. What is more difficult to understand, however, is the varying susceptibility that appears to exist between persons in different socioeconomic groups and within specific groups themselves. The studies of Hames (1975) have shed important light on determinants of individual as well as group susceptibility. In a long-term study of the prevalence of coronary heart disease in Georgia, Hames observed that there were genetic differences in the capacity of individuals to mount a physiological response to challenge, and that these differences may account for the varied susceptibility to coronary attacks. The coronary prone were found to be involved in changing roles, requiring an ability for new adaptation or coping. They were found to be less physically active; smoked more; had recently acquired more of the status symbols, such as education or ownership of property, and had less internal strength as reinforcement from the family structure. *Their physiological forces for coping with change were accelerated.* The more prone produced twice as much epinephrine as the less prone in a 24-hr period. At the same time their platelets were more sticky and the fibrinolytic activity of their blood was decreased.

Endocrinologic profiles revealed that in coping with similar growing demands, the less coronary prone did not marshall the full array of physiological responses observed in the more coronary prone. Such genetic differences in "fight or flight" response appear to assume major significance when augmented by increasing responsibility and challenge. In a period of less than 10 years, Hames (1975) found that the difference in social class in coronary heart disease prevalence in white males had disappeared. Thus, as lower socioeconomic white males became more competitive and assumed greater responsibility, the incidence of coronary episodes increased primarily by claiming its victims from the "hyperreactors" to stress. It must be concluded therefore that although the magnitude of the stressors in our environment may influence group susceptibility to coronary heart disease, the adaptive capacity of each person in coping with stress may be a major determinant of individual susceptibility.

VI. The Mastery of Stress

There is mounting evidence to support the belief that vulnerability to coronary heart disease, mental and emotional disorders, and other psychosomatic syndromes may be correlated with the ability or inability of the individual to handle stress in continuum. All individuals have a characteristic manner of responding to an acute threat in keeping with the "basic disposition" of the personality, but it is only in those who fail in the mastery of stress in continuum that sustained reactions occur and predispose to subsequent disease. Cannon (1932) was among the first to show the relation of behavioral and emotional changes to physiological responses. With the term "fight or flight reaction" he characterized a set of responses attributed to the adrenal medulla. Later, studies by Selye (1950) and Thorn (1951) placed more emphasis on the sustained nature of the stress reaction, which they considered to be mediated through the action of the adrenal cortex. Since the ability or inability of individuals to master a continuing emergency situation is the important determinant of whether or not a sustained reaction takes place, methods have been devised to record responses that may shed light on the predisposition to subsequent disease.

Funkenstein and associates (1957) have clearly shown in studies of young college students that many individuals fail to adapt to recurrent exposure to stressful stimuli. In experiments with laboratory-induced frustration at three weekly testing sessions, they were able to identify those subjects in whom the degree of physiological response was either minimal throughout or of diminishing intensity with repetitive exposures. In contrast, others were found to display a significant response initially, which either did not diminish or actually became accentuated in subsequent tests. Prospective studies are necessary to determine the validity of such methods for identifying future candidates for coronary heart disease. For the present, the hypothesis is most attractive and consistent with clinical and experimental observations.

VII. Stress, Adaptation, and Evolution

If man is subject to the same evolutionary forces that Darwin observed in the lower animals a century ago, then he is participating in a process of natural selection that is determining who shall survive in the complex and changing society he has created. Since his appearance on this planet, Homo sapiens has spent some 3.75 million years in the forest, 10,000 years on the farm, and only 300 years in the factory. Because adaptation to changing environment is a process that may require hundreds of thousands of years, modern man may have far to go in his continuing evolutionary development before acquiring the capacity to cope adequately with the relatively unfamiliar problems that now confront him. In this new environment of industrialized and mechanized society, many individuals actually appear to be responding to the symbolic and real challenges of daily urban living in the same manner as primitive man once reacted to the far greater threat to survival itself while inhabiting the forest and the cave. Moreover, although the fight or flight mechanism was apparently designed for short-term emergency needs, it would appear that coronary-prone subjects often possess homeostatic mechanisms that remain chronically mobilized in response to the demands of a rapidly changing environment. By sustained general autonomic arousal such persons manifest a failure to master stress in continuum. From the resulting chronic activation of the defense center in the hypothalamus, cholesterol levels in the blood are maintained at a higher range, circulating catecholamines are present in increased concentration, and clotting mechanisms are adversely affected. A high-fat diet, cigarette smoking, lack of exercise, and diabetes could readily exert a harmful influence by exaggerating certain components of these physiological expressions of fight or flight. Similarly, prolonged emotional stress, sociocultural mobility, or stressful life events could also bridge the gap between subclinical genetic predisposition and premature maturation of coronary artery disease.

VIII. Augmented Sympathetic Arousal and Ischemic Heart Disease

Although designed to be beneficial when danger threatens, catecholamines can also be detrimental. Their effects may lead to sudden rises in blood pressure, dangerous arrhythmias, and increased oxygen requirements for the heart. Aggregation of platelets in the microcirculation and diffuse myocardial necrosis are also well-known consequences of stress or prolonged catecholamine infusions (Haft, 1974). Of even greater interest is the role of augmented sympathetic arousal in the etiology of ischemic heart disease.

Reference has already been made to laboratory studies showing that there are significant differences in the capacity of normal individuals to mount a physiological response to recurrent challenge (Funkenstein et al., 1957). These observations take on added importance when considering the evidence that the pattern of reaction to stress may be a major determinant of susceptibility to future disease. There are now abundant data to indicate that patients with coronary disease respond to a variety of stresses with augmented catecholamine release when compared with control subjects. Nestel et al. (1967) demonstrated a statistically higher vanilmandelic acid excretion in such patients after mildly painful stimuli or after the stress of doing arithmetic problems. Similarly, one of the major characteristics of the Type A coronary-prone individual is his excessive secretion of norepinephrine in response to a nonphysical competitive task (Rosenman et al., 1966). Even more conclusive is the finding in prospective studies that those developing clinical coronary disease tend to produce twice as much epinephrine in a 24-hr period as the less coronary prone (Kaplan et al., 1971).

The possible importance of the sympathetic nervous system in the pathogenesis of clinical coronary heart disease is also suggested by the finding that rise in diastolic pressure in the cold pressor test was the single most important variable for coronary heart disease prediction in a 23-year longitudinal prospective investigation conducted by Keys *et al.* (1971). The relative risk ratio for coronary heart disease death or myocardial infarction of the hyperreactor group was 2.4 times that of the men who showed a rise of less than 20 mm in diastolic pressure in the test. Although Type A behavior is associated with heightened response to psychological stimuli whereas hyperreaction to cold represents an augmented response to physical challenge, one of us (LGR) has found no significant relationship between hyperreactivity to cold and Type A behavior pattern (Russek, 1977). If significant at all, therefore, hyperreactivity to cold must be an independent variable completely divorced from the psychosocial Type A/B paradigm.

Although considerable data attest to the significance of stress and augmented sympathetic activity in the etiology of coronary heart disease, certain conclusions concerning the extent of their influence can be drawn from natural experiments within the framework of human history. For example, the rarity of coronary episodes in German concentration camps and in the occupied Scandinavian countries during World War II indicates that morbidity and mortality are determined by the nature of the nutritional substrate upon which the psychological and physiological responses operate. In other words, stress and cholesterol appear to be dependent on each other for pathogenetic significance (Russek, 1959, 1962). In this connection we have repeatedly emphasized that high-fat diet and stressful living represent an exceptionally lethal combination; and this is undoubtedly true for those without the genetic endowment to master stress.

Indirect confirmation of the importance of excessive and disproportionate sympathetic responses in the causation and progression of coronary heart disease has recently been obtained from long-term studies employing beta adrenergic blocking agents. In one controlled trial of approximately 3000 postinfarction patients in the United Kingdom, cardiac deaths were reduced by more than one-third in patients receiving the cardioselective β-adrenergic blocker, practolol. Although serious consideration is now being given to the use of such drugs *after* anterior myocardial infarction, there may also be good rationale for their use in selected coronary-prone subjects and those with known disease as prophylactic therapy *before* the advent of infarction.

IX. Primary and Secondary Prevention in Ischemic Heart Disease

Stress research has clearly shown that every person inherits a genetically determined pattern of response to both emotional and physical demands. In some the physiological consequences of exposure to challenge reflect an augmented alarm reaction indicative of the inability of the individual to master stress. This genetic weakness may lie dormant or may be brought to clinical recognition by the struggle to survive in a competitive environment, by stressful life events, or by social and cultural mobility. Sustained arousal for "fight or flight" may be further aggravated by acquired behavioral characteristics that create the atmosphere for repetitive crises in confronting life situations (Type A behavior pattern). Ideal therapy would allow an alarm reaction proportionate to the challenge, with rapid return to a state of "relaxation" when the threat has passed; it would confer "diminishing responses to repetitive crises" as an indication of the mastery of stress.

At present, a determined effort is being made by the medical and psychotherapeutic communities to mobilize a holistic treatment approach to stress management and to promote a new model of well-being called "wellness." This concept of wellness, different from the disease model, which states that one is well if he is without physical signs and symptoms, goes beyond the classical concept. Wellness includes higher levels of health derived from spiritual, mental, and emotional growth, education, and self-actualization. It encompasses an integration and complex combination of mind, body, and spirit in contrast with the disease model, which relates to only one part, the body. Our increasing understanding of the interaction between mind and body and its role in the causation and exacerbation of psychosomatic diseases has engendered mounting interest in the wellness model. In our own program as in others across the country, a multidimensional approach is followed in an effort to provide, through experience and education, new and appropriate channels by which each individual can responsibly choose what proves most effective for him. The ability to make self-informed and responsible choices is considered to be the keynote of any desired outcome. The most notable therapeutic modalities and educational skills in use for this purpose are the following: (a) assertiveness training, (b) prescribed exercise, (c) cognitive restructuring therapies, (d) biofeedback with visual imagery, (e) meditation (relaxation response), (f) progressive Jacobsonian relaxation, (g) autogenic hypnosis, (h) individual and group psychotherapy, (i) body awareness training, (j) dietary regulation. The failure to master stress has been attributed to the rigidity of the response repertoire when evoked by challenges of varying magnitude. It is manifested by the inability to create, choose, and adapt expectations and beliefs, coping skills, and problem-solving techniques to meet the demands of the situation.

Cognitive restructuring therapies are concerned primarily with the psychological aspects of language and communication. Whereas some cognitive restructuring therapists emphasize problem solving, others are more concerned with coping skills. The problem-solving approach teaches the individual to stand back and systematically analyze a problem situation in the absence of any acute stress; the coping skills approach concentrates on what the individual must do when immediately confronted with an acute stressful situation. The problem-solving treatment is designed to have the person learn how to identify problems, generate alternative solutions, tentatively select a solution and then test and verify the efficacy of that solution. In contrast, Ellis's Rational Emotive Therapy (RET) attempts to make the individual aware of negative self-statements and images and of the anxiety-engendering, self-defeating, and self-fulfilling prophecy aspects of such thinking.

Assertiveness training has proven to be most effective in providing a process and structure for thinking, feeling, and behaving that still allows for individuation in its use. Based on the theory of reciprocal inhibition, anxiety or anger cannot be present when assertive behavior is being utilized. We believe that assertiveness may be a civilized means of defusing the fight–flight mechanism while still allowing the individual to defend himself in a manner appropriate to the perceived degree of threat.

Exercise would appear to be another valuable technique for neutralizing the cumulative effects of stress. Since the original purpose of the fight or flight mechanism was to activate the musculoskeletal system, regular exercise by recoupling the muscular component of the stress response may serve to neutralize the alarm reaction. Exercise may also divert attention from higher psychological processing to more primitive bodily function, thereby alleviating anxiety and tension.

The simplicity and potential of methods for obtaining the "relaxation response," which is the reverse of the "fight or flight" phenomenon and which also appears to have a center of control within the hypothalamus, have stimulated wide public interest in this approach. The many techniques of meditation seem to have a common basis, namely, "restriction of attention to an unchanging source of stimulation." The result is essentially the same: predominance of alpha EEGs and a physiological pattern of relaxation. Autogenic hypnosis, progressive Jacobsonian relaxation, and biofeedback with visual imagery are also effective modalities for redirecting one's attention to our internal environment by cognitive mediation, using pictures and internal auditory dialogue.

Individual and group therapy are also valuable treatment modalities for both supporting and directing the course of emotional and behavioral change.

Whereas behavior modification and cognitive restructuring therapies may reduce the buildup of stress and meditation and exercise may encourage its discharge, there are also pharmacological agents that are valuable in blunting its final expression. Thus the use of propranolol may prevent some of the important pathophysiological consequences of the stress reaction by blocking chronotropic and inotropic effects, the aggregation of platelets in the microcirculation of the heart, the development of diffuse cardiac necrosis and other responses, and sedatives and tranquilizers are useful in diminishing central autonomic hyperactivity.

Acknowledgment

Supported by The Russek Foundation, Inc., New York, N.Y., and Boca Raton, Florida.

References

Arlow, J. A. (1945). Identification of mechanisms in coronary occlusion. *Psychosom. Med.* **7**, 195.

Bogdonoff, M. D., Estes, E. H., Jr., and Harlan, W. (1959). Psychophysiologic studies of fat metabolism. Read before the American College of Physicians, Chicago, April 21.

Bruhn, J. G., Chandler, B., and Wold, S. (1969). A psychological study of survivors of myocardial infarction. *Psychosom. Med.* **31**, 8.

Buell, P., and Breslow, L. (1960). Mortality from coronary heart disease in California men who work long hours. *J. Chronic Dis.* **2**, 615.

Cannon, W. B. (1932). "The Wisdom of the Body." Norton, New York.

Dreyfuss, F., and Czaczkes, J. W. (1959). Blood cholesterol and uric acid of healthy medical students under stress of an examination. *Arch. Intern. Med.* **103**, 708.

Friedman, G. D. *et al.* (1974). A psychological questionnaire predictive of myocardial infarction. *Psychosom. Med.* **36**, 327.

Friedman, M., and Rosenman, R. H. (1959). Association of specific overt behavior pattern with blood and cardiovascular findings: Blood cholesterol level, blood clotting time, incidence of arcus senilis, and clinical coronary artery disease. *J. Am. Med. Assoc.* **169**, 1286.

Funkenstein, D. H., King, S. H., and Drolette, M. (1957). "Mastery of Stress." Harvard Univ. Press, Cambridge, Massachusetts.

Groen, J. J. *et al.* (1959). Influence of nutrition, individuality and different forms of stress on blood cholesterol. *Proc. Int. Cong. Diet.,* 1959 p. 19.

Groover, M. R., Jr., Seljeskog, E. L., Haglin, J. J., and Hitchcock, C. R. (1963). Myocardial infarction in the Kenya baboon without demonstrable atherosclerosis. *J Angiol.* **14**, 409.

Gunn, C. G., Friedman, M., and Byers, S. O. (1960). Effect of chronic hypothalamic stimulation upon cholesterol induced atherosclerosis in the rabbit. *J. Clin. Invest.* **39**, 1963.

Gutstein, W. H. (1978). Can emotional stress cause atherosclerosis? *11th Annu. Cardiovasc. Symp.,* 1978 p. 000.

Haft, J. I. (1974). Microcirculatory platelet aggregation in the heart with epinephrine infusion. *In* "Cardiovascular Problems: Perspectives and Progress" (H. I. Russek, ed.), p. 257. Univ. Park Press, Baltimore, Maryland.

Hames, C. (1975). "Most likely to succeed" as a candidate for a coronary attack. *In* "New Horizons in Cardiovascular Practice" (H. I. Russek, ed.), p. 129. Univ. Park Press, Baltimore, Maryland.

Holmes, T. H., and Rahe, R. H. (1967). The social readjustment rating scale. *J. Psychosom. Res.* **11**, 213.

Jenkins, C. D. (1971). Psychologic. and social precursors of coronary disease. *N. Engl. J. Med.* **284**, 244.

Kaplan, B. H. *et al.* (1971). Occupational mobility and coronary heart disease. *Arch. Intern. Med.* **128**, 938.

Kavanaugh, T., and Shepherd, R. J. (1973). The immediate antecedents of myocardial infarction in active men. *Can. Med. Assoc. J.* **109**, 19.

Kemple, C. (1945). Rorschach method and psychosomatic diagnosis: Personality traits of patients with rheumatic disease, hypertensive cardiovascular disease, coronary occlusion and fracture. *Psychosom. Med.* **7**, 85.

Keys, A. *et al.* (1971). Mortality and coronary heart disease among men studied for 23 years. *Arch. Intern. Med.* **128**, 201.

Keys, A., *et al.* (1972). Probability of middle-aged men developing coronary disease in five years. *Circulation* **45**, 815.

Lapiccirella, V. *et al.* (1962). Enquète clinique, biologique et cardiographique parmi les tribus nomades de le Somalie qui se nourrissent seulement de lait. *Bull. W.H.O.* **27**, 681.

Lown, B., and Stare, F. J. (1959). Atherosclerosis, infarction and nutrition. *Circulation* **20**, 161.

Mann, G. V., Schaffer, R. D., and Rich, A. (1965). Physical fitness and immunity to heart diseases in Masai. *J. Atheroscler. Res.* **2**, 1308.

Marmott *et al.* (1975). Report in the New York Times, October 28.

Morris, J. N., Heady, J. A., and Barley, R. G. (1952). Coronary heart disease in medical practitioners. *Br. Med. J.* **1**, 503.

Myasnikov, A. L. (1958). Influence of some factors on development of experimental cholesterol atherosclerosis. *Circulation* **17**, 99.

Nestel, P. G. *et al.* (1967). *Am. Heart J.* **73**, 227.

Osler, W. (1896). Lectures on angina pectoris and allied states. *N. Y. Med. J.* **4**, 224.

Osler, W. (1910). Angina pectoris. *Lancet* **1**, 697.

Parkes, C. M., Benjamin, B., and Fitzgerald, R. G. (1969). Broken heart: A statistical study of increased mortality among widowers. *Br. Med. J.* **1**, 740.

Raab, W., and Humphreys, R. J. (1947). Drug action upon myocardial epinephrine-sympathin concentration and heart rate. *J. Pharmacol. Exp. Ther.* **89**, 64.

Raab, W., Chaplin, J. P., and Bajusz, E. (1964). Myocardial necroses produced in domesticated rats and in wild rats by sensory and emotional stresses. *Proc. Soc. Exp. Biol. Med.* **116**, 665.

Ratcliffe, H. L. *et al.* (1960). Changes in the character and location of arterial lesions in mammals and birds in the Philadelphia Zoological Garden. *Circulation* **21**, 730.

Rikli, A. E. *et al.* (1960). "U. S. Public Health Survey," Public Health Reports, U.S.P.H.S., Washington, D.C.

Rosenman, R. H. (1968). Prospective epidemiological recognition of the candidate for ischemic heart disease. *Psychother. Psychosom.* **16**, 189.

Rosenman, R. H., Friedman, M. *et al.* (1966). Coronary heart disease in the western collaborative group study. *J. Amer. Med. Assoc.* **195**, 86.

Russek, H. I. (1959). Role of heredity, diet and emotional stress in coronary heart disease. *J. Am. Med. Assoc.* **171**, 503.

Russek, H. I. (1960). Emotional stress and coronary heart disease in American physicians. *Am. J. Med. Sci.* **240**, 711.

Russek, H. I. (1962). Emotional stress and coronary heart disease in American physicians, dentists and lawyers. *Am. J. Med. Sci.* **243**, 716.

Russek, H. I. (1964). Tobacco consumption and emotional stress and emotional stress in the etiology of coronary heart disease. *Geriatrics* **19**, 425.

Russek, H. I. (1965). Stress, tobacco and coronary disease in North American professional groups: Survey of 12,000 men in 14 occupational groups. *J. Am. Med. Assoc.* **192,** 189.

Russek, H. I. (1973). Emotional stress as a cause of coronary heart disease. *J. Am. Coll. Health Assoc.* **22,** 120.

Russek, H. I., and Russek, L. G. (1977). Behavior patterns and emotional stress in the etiology of coronary heart disease: Sociological and occupational aspects. *In* "Stress and the Heart" (D. Wheatley, ed.), Raven, New York.

Russek, L. G. (1977). Relationship between two major risk factors in coronary heart disease: Type A behavior pattern and response to the cold pressor test. Dissertation, School of Human Behavior, United States International University, San Diego, California.

Sabin (1959). In Page, I. H. Atherosclerosis—a commentary. *Fed. Proc., Fed.* **18,** 47. *Am. Soc. Exp. Biol.*

Selye, H. (1950). "Stress." Acta, Inc., Montreal.

Snapper, L. (1941). "Chinese Lessons to Western Medicine: A Contribution to Geographical Medicine from the Clinics of Peiping Union Medical College," p. 29. Wiley (Interscience), New York.

Steinberg, D., and Shafrir, E. (1960). Cortisone held "vital" to lipid rise in stress. *Med. News* **6,** 1.

Still, J. W., and Heiffer, M. H. (1958). Blood viscosity in response to various stimuli. Reported at Fed. Am. Soc. Exp. Biol., April 26.

Stout, C., Morrow, J., Brandt, E. N., Jr., and Wolf, S. (1964). Unusually low incidence of death from myocardial infarction: Study of an Italian-American community in Pennsylvania. *J. Am. Med. Assoc.* **188,** 845.

Syme, S. L. (1975). Social and psychological risk factors in coronary heart disease. *Mod. Concepts Cardiovasc. Dis.* **44,** 17.

Syme, S. L. *et al.,* (1964). Some social and cultural factors associated with the occurrence of coronary heart disease. *J. Chronic Dis.* **17,** 277.

Thorn, G. W. (1951). "Diagnosis and Treatment of Adrenal Insufficiency." Thomas, Springfield, Illinois.

Uhley, H. N., and Friedman, M. (1959). Blood lipids, clotting and coronary atherosclerosis in rats exposed to a particular form of stress. *Am. J. Physiol.* **197,** 396.

Vlodaver, Z., Medalie, J., and Neufeld, N. H. (1968). Coronary arteries in immature monkeys, preliminary report of the relationships to activity and diet. *J. Atheroscler. Res.* **8,** 923.

Wolf, S. G. (1958). Cardiovascular reactions to symbolic stimuli. *Circulation* **18,** 287.

Zyzanski, S. J., Jenkinds, C. D., Ryan, T. J. *et al.* (1975). Emotions, behavior pattern and atherosclerosis. Presented at Annual Meeting of the American Psychosomatic Society, New Orleans, March 21.

The Nature of Stress and Its Relation to Cardiovascular Disease

Hans Selye

I. Stress and Adaptation

A. Stress: Definition and Description

Much confusion has arisen in the lay and even in the scientific literature because the term "stress" means different things to different people. Stress is part of our daily life, but it is associated with a great variety of essentially dissimilar problems, such as surgical trauma, burns, emotional arousal, mental or physical effort, fatigue, pain, fear, the need for concentration, the humiliation of frustration, the loss of blood, intoxication with drugs or environmental pollutants, or even the kind of unexpected success that requires an individual to reformulate his life-style.

Stress is present in the businessman under constant pressure; in the athlete straining to win a race; in the air-traffic controller who bears continuous responsibility for hundreds of lives; in the husband helplessly watching his wife's slow, painful death from cancer; in a race horse, its jockey, and the spectator who bets on them. Medical research has shown that, although all these face quite different problems, they respond with a stereotyped pattern of biochemical, functional, and structural changes essentially involved in coping with any type of increased demand on vital activity, particularly adaptation to new situations. All endogenous or exogenous agents that make such demands are called stressors. Distinguishing between their widely differing specific effects and the nonspecific (common) biologic response that they elicit is the key to a proper understanding of biologic stress.

From the point of view of its stressor activity, it is even immaterial whether the agent or situation being faced is pleasant or unpleasant; all that counts is the intensity of the demand for readjustment or adaptation that it creates. The mother who is told that her only son died in battle suffers a terrible mental shock; if years later it turns out that the news was false and the son unexpectedly walks into her room alive and well, she experiences extreme joy. The specific results of the two events, sorrow and joy, are completely different, in fact they are opposite to each other, yet their stressor effect—the nonspecific demand for readjustment to a new situation—is the same.

It is difficult to see at first how such essentially different things as cold, heat, drugs, hormones, sorrow, and joy could provoke an identical biologic reaction. Nevertheless this is the case; it can now be demonstrated by highly objective, quantitative biochemical and morphological parameters that certain reactions are totally nonspecific and common to all types of agents, whatever their superimposed specific effects may be.

The conceptual distinction between the specific and the nonspecific consequences of any demand made on the body was the most important step in the scientific analysis of stress phenomena.

Contrary to previously widely held opinion, stress is not identical to nervous tension. It occurs in experimental animals even after total surgical deafferentation of the hypothalamus, which eliminates all neurogenic input. It can occur during anesthesia in man as well as in lower animals. It can occur even in plants, which have no nervous system.

If one seeks to understand the field of stress one must first realize that the word "stress" is often used very loosely, not only by the lay public but by professionals as well. I myself have been guilty, in some of my earlier writings, of implying, as was pointed out by the *British Medical Journal,* that stress is its own cause(!).

The best way to conceive of stress is in its most specific sense, that of a *state* which is recognizable by the presence of an organized set or sequence of bodily changes, which I will shortly describe. The experimental data lead to the inescapable conclusion that any demand (i.e., any agent, situation, or environmental change that necessitates adaptation in order to maintain healthy life) will evoke this standard set of responses, which I call the "stress syndrome." Note that, strictly speaking, the syndrome is *not* stress: it is merely the manifestation of it.

Stress is the state manifested by a specific syndrome which consists of all the nonspecifically induced changes within a biologic system. Thus, stress has its own characteristic form and composition, but its cause is a demand as such, not any particular demand.

With regard to nonspecificity, the concept of stress is not without precedent. All machines, whether animate or inanimate, require energy for any of their activities, be these constructive or destructive. In fact, we shall see that biologic stress is closely linked to, though not identical with, energy utilization. This explains its apparently paradoxical yet inseparable combination with the specific effects of the particular agent that creates a need for adaptive work. Any demand made on the body must be for some particular, that is, specific activity and yet is inseparably associated with nonspecific phenomena (i.e., energy utilization), just as in the inanimate world specific demands made on machines to increase or decrease room temperature, to produce light or sound, to accelerate or decrease motion are invariably dependent on energy utilization. Figure 1 illustrates this.

The bodily changes produced, whether a person is exposed to nervous tension, physical injury, infection, cold, heat, X-rays, or anything else, are what we call stress. This is what is left when we abstract from the specific changes that are produced only by one or few among these agents. In my earlier writings I had defined stress, somewhat more simply but less precisely, as *the sum of all nonspecific changes caused by function or damage,* or *the rate of wear and tear in the body.* Its simplest and most generally accepted definition is *the nonspecific response of the body to any demand.*

Therefore stress is not something to be avoided. Indeed, it cannot be avoided, since just staying alive creates some demand for life-maintaining energy. Even while man is asleep, his heart, respiratory apparatus, digestive tract, nervous system, and other organs must continue to function. Complete freedom from stress can be expected only after death. However, in

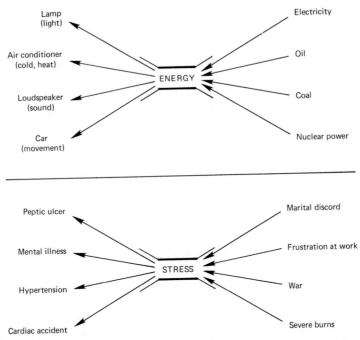

Fig. 1. Each result (*on the left*) is specific, each causative agent (*on the right*) is specific. Yet they are all nonspecific results and agents in that they must go through a common pathway. No direct connection is possible between a result (*on the left*) and a cause (*on the right*).

everyday life we must distinguish between two types of stress effects, namely, *eustress* (from the Greek *eu,* or "good"—as in "euphony," "euphoria," "eulogy") and *distress* (from the Latin *dis,* or "bad"—as in "dissonance," "disease," "dissatisfaction"). Depending on conditions, stress is associated with desirable or undesirable effects.

The presence of stress is evidenced by certain observable and measurable adjustments going on in the body. The workings of stress are extremely complex (see Fig. 2). Apart from specific stimuli, which need not be discussed here, the first effect of any agent or demand made on the body—be it running up a flight of stairs, dealing with a viral infection, or performing a dance—is to produce a nonspecific stimulus (the agent's "stressor effect"). This may be a nervous impulse, a chemical substance, or lack of an indispensable metabolic factor; it is referred to simply as the "first mediator," because we know nothing about its nature. We are not even certain that it has to be an excess or deficiency of any particular substance; it is possible that various derangements of homeostasis can activate the stress mechanism. Undoubtedly, in man, with his highly developed central nervous system (CNS), emotional arousal is one of the most frequent activators. Yet it cannot be regarded as the only factor, since typical stress reactions can occur in patients exposed to trauma, hemorrhage, and so on, while under deep anesthesia. Indeed, anesthetics themselves are commonly used in experimental medicine to produce stress, and "stress of anesthesia" is a serious problem in clinical surgery.

We have still to identify the first mediator(s), but we do know that eventually stress acts on the hypothalamus and particularly on the median eminence (ME). This action seems largely to be mediated through or modified by nervous stimuli coming from the cerebral cortex, the reticular formation, and the limbic system (especially the hippocampus and amygdala). The incoming nervous stimuli reach certain neuroendocrine cells, most of which are located in the ME. These act as "transducers," transforming nervous signals into a humoral messenger, the corticotropic hormone releasing factor (CRF), which can be demonstrated histochemically in the ME region and can also be extracted from it (see Fig. 2). Oddly enough, the posterior pituitary contains the highest concentration of CRF, and it has been isolated from this source in relatively pure form, thus permitting the approximate determination of its chemical formula as a polypeptide that subsequently was allegedly synthesized. Yet we have no conclusive proof that the CRF-active material extracted from the hypothalamus is identical with that obtained from the posterior lobe, since only the existence of the latter has been definitely ascertained. Although vasopressin (antidiuretic hormone) possesses considerable CRF activity, it is not identical with CRF; this has been shown by the well-documented differences in their chemical structure and physiological activity.

CRF reaches the anterior lobe through the hypothalamo–hypophseal portal system that originates in the ME region within a network of capillaries into which CRF is discharged by the local neuroendocrine cells. It is then carried down through the larger veins of the pituitary stalk to a second capillary plexus in the pituitary. A flow in the opposite direction is supposedly also possible.

The adrenocorticotropic hormone (ACTH) secretion of the anterior lobe is not stimulated by the hypothalamus through nervous pathways descending in the pituitary stalk but rather through blood-borne substances carried by way of the portal veins. That is why transection of the stalk inhibits the ACTH secretion only before vascular connections between the hypothalamus and the gland are reestablished; if regeneration of these vessels is prevented by interposing a plate between the cut ends of the stalk, this pathway is permanently blocked.

In vivo and *in vitro* experiments have both proved that CRF elicits a discharge of ACTH from the adenohypophysis into the general circulation.

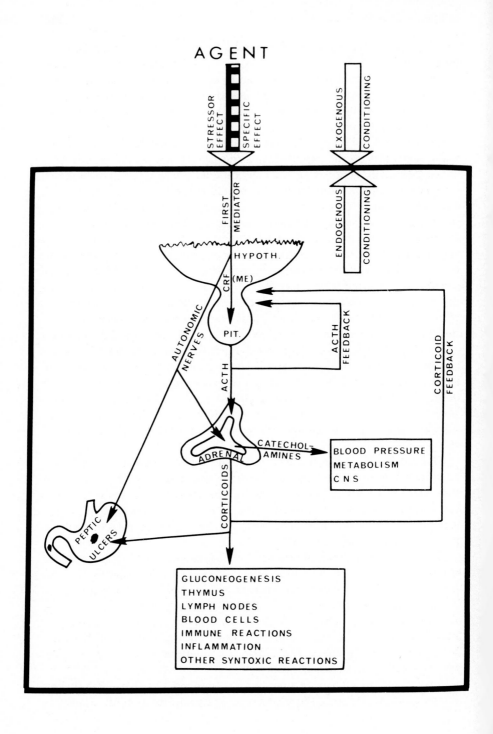

On reaching the adrenal cortex, it causes secretion of corticoids, mainly glucocorticoids such as cortisol or corticosterone. These induce glyconeogenesis, thereby supplying a readily available source of energy for the adaptive reactions necessary to meet the demands faced by the body. In addition, they facilitate various other enzymatically regulated adaptive metabolic responses and suppress immune reactions as well as inflammation, assisting the body to coexist with potential pathogens (syntoxic reactions). Furthermore, the glucocorticoids are responsible for the thymicolymphatic involution, eosinopenia, and lymphopenia characteristic of acute stress. Curiously, glucocorticoids are needed for the acquisition of adaptation primarily during the alarm reaction, but not so much to maintain the adjustment during the stage of resistance. ACTH plays a comparatively minor role in the secretion of mineralocorticoids, such as aldosterone, which is regulated mainly by the renin–hypertensin system and the blood electrolytes, whose homeostasis is in turn influenced by them.

This chain of events is cybernetically controlled by several biofeedback mechanisms. Whether an excess of CRF can inhibit its own endogenous secretion is still doubtful because its lifespan in the circulating blood is very short. On the other hand, there is definite proof of an ACTH feedback (short-loop feedback) by a surplus of the hormone, which returns to the hypothalamo–pituitary system and inhibits further ACTH production. We have even more evidence to substantiate the existence of a corticoid feedback mechanism (long-loop feedback) in that a high blood corticoid level similarly inhibits ACTH secretion. It is still not quite clear to what extent these feedbacks act on the neuroendocrine cells of the hypothalamus, the adenohypophysis, or both. (Hence in Fig. 2 the corresponding arrowheads merely point toward the hypothalamo–hypophyseal region in general, without specifying exactly where their target areas are situated.)

Another major pathway involved in the stress mechanism is carried through the catecholamines liberated under the influence of an acetylcholine discharge, at autonomic nerve endings and in the adrenal medulla.

Fig. 2. *Principal pathways mediating the response to a stressor agent and the conditioning factors that modify its effect.* When an agent acts on the body (*thick outer frame of the diagram*), the effect will depend on three factors (*broad vertical arrows pointing to the upper horizontal border of the frame*). All agents possess both nonspecific stressor effects (*solid part of arrow*) and specific properties (*interrupted part of arrow*). The latter are variable and characteristic of each individual agent; they are not discussed here other than to state that they are inseparably attached to the stressor effect and invariably modify it. The other *two heavy vertical arrows pointing toward the upper border of the frame* represent the exogenous and endogenous conditioning factors that largely determine the reactivity of the body. It is clear that since all stressors have some specific effects, they cannot elicit exactly the same response in all organs; furthermore even the same agent will act differently on different individuals, depending on the internal and external conditioning factors that determine their reactivity. (After Selye, 1976.)

The chromaffin cells of the latter secrete mainly epinephrine, which is of considerable value in that it stimulates mechanisms of general utility to meet various demands for adaptation. Thus it provides readily available sources of energy by forming glucose from glycogen depots and free fatty acids from the triglyceride stores of adipose tissue; it also quickens the pulse, raises the blood pressure to improve circulation into the musculature, and stimulates the central nervous system (CNS). In addition, epinephrine accelerates blood coagulation and thereby protects against excessive hemorrhage should wounds be sustained in conflicts. All of this is helpful in meeting the demands, whether they call for fight or flight.

B. The General Adaptation Syndrome (G.A.S.)

This *alarm reaction,* however, is evidently not the entire response. On continued exposure of an organism to any noxious agent capable of eliciting this reaction, a *stage of adaptation or resistance* ensues. In other words, no organism can be maintained continuously in a state of alarm. If the agent is so damaging that continued exposure becomes incompatible with life, the animal dies during the alarm reaction within the first hours or days. If it can survive, this initial reaction is necessarily followed by the stage of resistance. The manifestations of this second phase are quite different from—indeed, often the exact opposite of—those characterizing the alarm reaction. For example, during the alarm reaction, the cells of the adrenal cortex discharge their secretory granules into the bloodstream and thus become depleted of corticoid-containing lipid storage material, but in the stage of resistance the cortex becomes particularly rich in secretory granules. Whereas in the alarm reaction there is hemoconcentration, hypochloremia, and general tissue catabolism, during the stage of resistance there is hemodilution, hyperchloremia, and anabolism, with a return toward normal body weight.

Surprisingly, after still more exposure to the noxious agent, the acquired adaptation is lost and the animal enters a third phase, the *stage of exhaustion,* which follows inexorably if the stressor is severe enough and is applied for a sufficient length of time. Unless interrupted, this stage ends in death.

The development of all three stages is not necessary before we can speak of a G.A.S. Only the most severe stress leads rapidly to the stage of exhaustion and death. Most of the physical or mental exertions, infections, and other stressors that act on us during a limited period produce changes corresponding only to the first and second stages.

The triphasic nature of the G.A.S. gave us the first indication that the body's adaptability, or *adaptation energy,* is finite. Animal experiments have shown quite convincingly that exposure to cold, muscular effort, hemorrhage, and other stressors can be withstood for just so long. After the initial alarm reaction, the body becomes adapted and begins to resist, the length of the resistance period depending on the body's innate adaptability and the intensity of the stressor. Yet, eventually, exhaustion ensues.

Exactly what is lost, we cannot yet say, except that it is not merely caloric energy. Food intake is normal during the stage of resistance, and so caloric energy is amply available. Apparently, just as any machine gradually wears out, even if it has enough fuel, so does the human body sooner or later become the victim of constant wear and tear.

C. Objections to the Concept

Even though experiments were extremely suggestive, there remained two apparently insurmountable obstacles in the way of formulating the concept of a single, standard response to stress: (1) Different stimuli of equal toxicity (or stressor potency) do not necessarily elicit exactly the same syndrome in different people; (2) the same stimulus may produce different lesions in different individuals.

1. It was eventually shown that though qualitatively distinct stimuli do differ only in their specific actions, their nonspecific stressor effects are essentially the same. (But it must be noted that even the nonspecific effects can be modified by the superimposed specific effects of a particular stimulus.)

2. The occurrence of different lesions in individuals subjected to the same stressors has been traced to "conditioning factors" that can selectively enhance or inhibit one or the other stress effect. The conditioning may be internal (e.g., genetic predisposition, age, or sex) or external (e.g., treatment with certain hormones and drugs, dietary factors, our society, and traditions). Under the influence of such conditioning factors a normally well-tolerated degree of stress can become pathogenic and cause "diseases of adaptation" affecting the predisposed body area.

To sum up: the stressor effects of an agent are nonspecific (i.e., common to diverse stimuli), whereas the specific effects are variable and characteristic of each individual agent. But the response does not depend exclusively on these two actions of the stimulus; the reactivity of the target also plays a role, and this can be modified by numerous internal or external conditioning factors.

Since all stressors have some specific effects, they cannot always elicit exactly the same response, and even the same stimulus will act differently in different individuals, depending on the internal and external conditioning factors.

Although any kind of adaptive activity sets our stress apparatus in motion, it will depend largely on such conditioning factors whether the heart, stomach, brain, kidney, or liver will break down. They will determine what part of the body is the "weakest link" in a given situation. The concept of conditioning just outlined and the hypothesis that certain diseases are caused by derangements of the G.A.S. mechanism have clarified the relations between the physiology and pathology of stress in many fields.

D. Stress and Disease in General

Of course, every disease causes a certain amount of generalized stress, since it imposes demands for adaptation on the organism. Hence stress plays some role in the development of every disease; its effects—for better or worse—are added to the specific changes characteristic of the disease in question. The effect of stress may be curative (as illustrated by various forms of externally induced stress, such as shock therapy, physical therapy, and occupational therapy) or damaging, depending on whether the biochemical reactions characteristic of stress (e.g., stress hormones or nervous reactions to stress) combat or accentuate the trouble.

Stress is able to combat disease because of the phenomenon of cross-resistance. Thus pretreatment with one stressor may induce resistance by mobilizing the body's nonspecific adaptive system. For example, syntoxic hormones (glucocorticoids) liberated during systemic stress can protect against various excessive and harmful inflammatory or immune reactions. This principle has been applied clinically in the treatment of inflammatory diseases and the suppression of graft rejection. However, there probably exist other forms of cross-resistance.

Even before we knew anything about the mechanism of stress reactions, nonspecific treatments were in use that relied on the exposure of patients to stressors (cold, heat, hydrotherapy, bloodletting, exercise, fever therapy, electroshock, and so on). Some of them had been in use for centuries; it was not known how these agents acted, but there could be no doubt that in many cases they were beneficial. And it is still not clear why some nonspecific therapeutic procedures are more valuable in certain diseases than in others, but probably their specific effects are superimposed on—in some cases, even more important than—their nonspecific effects.

In any case, all these treatments do produce stress and often act through the liberation of stress hormones such as ACTH, corticoids, and catecholamines (adrenaline, noradrenaline). Whenever this is true, it is of course much more acceptable to the patient to receive the hormones from outside (i.e., by prescription) than to count on their production by exposure of the patient to drastic types of nonspecific treatments.

E. The Diseases of Adaptation (Stress Diseases)

Diseases in whose development the nonspecific stressor effects of the eliciting pathogen play a major role are called diseases of adaptation or stress diseases. But just as there is no pure stressor (i.e., an agent that causes only the nonspecific response and has no specific action), so there are no pure diseases of adaptation. Some nonspecific components participate in the pathogenesis of every malady, but no disease is due to stress alone. The justification for placing a malady in this category is directly proportional to the role that maladjustment to stress plays in its development. In some instances (e.g., surgical shock), stress may be by far the most important pathogenic factor. However, in other cases (instantly lethal intoxications, traumatic injuries to the spinal cord, most congenital malformations) it plays little or no role, either because the damage is inflicted so rapidly that there is no time for any adaptive process or because the pathogen is highly specific. In the latter event, whatever develops represents a secondary result and is not the primary component. Typical diseases of adaptation are due to insufficient, excessive, or faulty reactions to stressors, as in inappropriate hormonal or nervous responses.

Some diseases in which stress usually plays a particularly important role are high blood pressure, heart accidents, gastric or duodenal ulcers (the "stress ulcers"), and various types of mental disturbances. Yet there is no disease that can be attributed exclusively to maladaptation, since the cause of nonspecific responses will always be modified by various "conditioning factors" that enhance, diminish, or otherwise alter disease proneness. Most important among these are the specific effects of the primary pathogen and the factors influencing the body's reactivity by endogenous (heredity, previously sustained damage to certain organs) or by exogenous (concurrent exposure to other pathogens and environmental agents, diet) conditioners. Hence the diseases of adaptation cannot be ascribed to any one pathogen but only to "pathogenic constellations"; they belong to what we have called the pluricausal diseases ("multifactorial maladies"), which depend on the simultaneous effect of several potentially pathogenic factors that alone would sometimes not produce disease.

F. Syntoxic and Catatoxic Responses

Biochemical analysis of the stress syndrome showed that homeostasis depends mainly on two types of reactions: syntoxic (from the Greek *syn*, meaning "together") and catatoxic (from the Greek *cata*, meaning "against"). In order to resist different toxic stressors, the body apparently can regulate its reactions through chemical messengers and nervous stimuli that either pacify or incite to fight. The syntoxic stimuli act as tissue tranquilizers, creating a state of passive tolerance that permits a kind of symbiosis, or peaceful coexistence with aggressors.

The catatoxic agents cause chemical changes (mainly through the production of hepatic microsomal enzymes) that lead to an active attack on the pathogen, usually by accelerating its metabolic degradation.

Presumably, in the course of evolution the body learned to defend itself against all kinds of aggressors (whether arising in the organism or the environment) through mechanisms that help it tolerate the aggressor (syntoxic) or destroy it (catatoxic). Among the most effective syntoxic hormones are the glucocorticoids. These inhibit inflammation and many other essentially defensive immune reactions and are being effectively used in the treatment of diseases in which inflammation itself is the major cause of trouble (e.g., certain types of inflammation of the joints, eyes, or respiratory passages). Likewise, they have a marked inhibitory effect on the immunologic rejection of grafted foreign tissues (e.g., a heart or kidney transplant).

It is not immediately evident why it should be advantageous to inhibit inflammation or interfere with the rejection of foreign tissues, since both phenomena are essentially useful defense reactions. The main purpose of inflammation is to localize irritants (e.g., microbes) by putting a barricade of inflammatory tissue around them to prevent their spread into the blood, which could lead to sepsis and even death. The suppression of this basic defense reaction is an advantage, however, when a foreign agent is in itself innocuous and causes trouble only by inciting inflammation. In such cases, inflammation itself is what we experience as a disease. Thus in many patients who suffer from hay fever or extreme inflammatory swelling after an insect sting, suppression of defensive inflammation is essentially a cure, because the invading stressor agent is not in itself dangerous or likely to spread and kill. In the case of grafts, it may even be lifesaving.

It is illuminating to distinguish between direct and indirect pathogens. Direct pathogens cause disease regardless of the body's reaction, whereas indirect pathogens cause damage only because they provoke exaggerated defensive responses.

If a man accidentally exposes his hand to a strong acid, alkali, or boiling water, damage will occur regardless of his reactions, because these are all direct pathogens. They would damage even the hand of a dead man, who obviously could not put up any defense reactions. Most common inflammatory irritants, including allergens, are essentially indirect pathogens: They cause disease only through the purposeless defense reactions that they stimulate.

Immunologic reactions, which lead to the destruction of microbes, grafts, and other foreign tissues, undoubtedly developed during evolution as useful defensive mechanisms against potentially dangerous foreign materials. When the attack against the foreign agent is unnecessary or even harmful—as in the case of many allergens, heart transplants, and so on—man can improve on the wisdom of Nature by suppressing this hostility. When the aggressor is dangerous, the defensive reaction should not be suppressed but if possible increased beyond the normal level, which can be achieved, for example, by catatoxic substances that carry the chemical message to the tissues to destroy the invaders even more vigorously than would normally be the case.

Although we know a great deal about the body's capacity to produce its own syntoxic hormones, such as corticoids, we know substantially less about its ability to produce catatoxic substances. Some natural hormones do possess such activities, but they are weak. The most active catatoxic compounds are synthetics, among which the most powerful so far examined is a hormone derivative designated by the chemical name "pregnenolone 16α-carbonitrile," commonly called PCN. This is also the most nonspecific catatoxic substance in that it exhibits the greatest destructive ability against the largest number of poisons.

G. Homeostasis and Heterostasis

Natural homeostatic mechanisms are usually sufficient to maintain a normal state of resistance; however, when the organism is faced with unusually heavy demands, ordinary homeostasis is not enough. The "thermostat of defense" must be raised to a heightened level. For this process I proposed the term "heterostasis" (from the Greek *heteros,* or "other") as the establishment of a new steady state by treatment with agents that stimulate the physiological adaptive mechanisms through the development of normally dormant defensive tissue reactions. Both in homeostasis and in heterostasis the *milieu intérieur* participates actively.

We can stimulate the production of natural protective agents by treatment with chemicals that augment the induction of catatoxic or syntoxic enzymes or by immunization with bacterial products (e.g., vaccination) that increase the body's manufacture of serologic antibodies to combat infections.

In homeostatic defense the potential pathogen (which threatens the fixity of the *milieu intérieur*) automatically activates usually adequate catatoxic or syntoxic mechanisms; when these do not suffice, such natural catatoxic or syntoxic agents can also be administered readymade by the physician.

Heterostasis depends on treatment with artificial remedies that have no direct curative action but that can precipitate the production of unusually high amounts of the body's own natural catatoxic or syntoxic agents so as to achieve fixity of the *milieu intérieur,* despite abnormally high demands that could not be met without outside help.

The most salient difference between homeostasis and heterostasis is that the former maintains a normal steady state by physiologic means whereas the latter "resets the thermostat" of resistance to a heightened defensive capacity by artificial interventions from the outside. By chemical treatment this process induces the body to raise the production of its own natural nonspecific (multipurpose) remedies. However, each type of planned or enforced training of the body through outside interventions also raises resistance from the homeostatic to the heterostatic level.

Heterostasis differs essentially from treatment with drugs (e.g., antibiotics, antacids, antidotes, pain killers) that act directly and specifically rather than by strengthening the body's own natural nonspecific defenses; in treatment with drugs the *milieu intérieur* is passive.

II. Stress and Cardiovascular Disease

A. Generalities

Many of the cardiovascular diseases in the pathogenesis of which stress appears to play an important role usually occur in combination (e.g., hypertension, arteriosclerosis, myocardial infarcts), and so it is difficult to discuss them separately. Furthermore, it is hard to classify the factors involved in the causation of stress-induced cardiovascular disease because of complexities in their interrelations (not to mention the fact that lesions of the cardiovascular system furnish some of the most clear-cut examples of pluricausal diseases). For example, stressors may result in hypertension or cardiac infarction, yet psychogenic stress plays such a preponderant role that it deserves to be discussed in a special section. Also, the conditioning factors that predispose to cardiovascular disease overlap. Undoubtedly, genetic factors are important in determining behavior, the choice of an occupation, the site of residence (urban, rural), or even the type of diet. On the other hand, age, at least the chronologic age of an individual, though a highly important conditioning factor determining predisposition for cardiovascular disease, is largely independent of those just mentioned. Finally, the various indicators of stress and cardiovascular disease (pathologic anatomy, chemical changes, blood coagulability) not only have diagnostic value but also furnish significant data on probably important pathogenetic factors.

B. History

As early as 1812, Corvisart expressed the view that all heart diseases stem "from the action of the organ and from passions of man." He noted that the heart can be injured by crying in infancy, wrestling, fencing, playing wind instruments, laughing, weeping, reading, declamation, anger, madness, fear, jealousy, terror, love, despair, joy, avarice, cupidity, ambition, revenge, and every kind of effort. However, "to conceive man without passions, is to conceive a being without his attributes."

Only in recent times has special attention been given to statistical studies that would prove the relationship between the stressors of daily life (especially extreme muscular effort), traumatic injuries or intense emotional arousal, and cardiac disease.

Animal experiments have shown that, following suitable pretreatment, exposure to virtually any severe stressor can precipitate myocardial necroses or hypertensive vascular disease. For example, Raab et al. (1964) have noted that, "Wild rats exposed after periods of isolation to frightening noises (tape recording of hissing cat and squealing rat) displayed myocardial necroses in nearly 70% of the experiments." Sharma and Barar (1966) have observed that in rats, "restraint stress" produces depletion of glycogen from the myocardium with round cell infiltration, edema, focal necrosis, and fragmentation of fibers. Hauss (1973) has found that in rats, the emotional stress produced by restraint elicits typical mesenchymal reactions in the blood vessel walls with increased [^{35}S]sulfate and [^{3}H]thymidine incorporation. Essentially similar changes occur after exposure to other stressors, and these are considered to be the first step in the arteriosclerotic process characteristic of aging. "The deformation of the structure of the arterial wall participates essentially in the development of lipidosis, fibrinosis, and cell necroses. Aggregation of thrombocytes and thrombosis in the arterial wall results from the frequent reduplication of intima cells."

In other words, here again we are dealing with complex pathogenic situations in which both the conditioning or predisposing factors that induce disease proneness and the eliciting stressors play equally important roles.

C. Stressors in General

Evaluation of the literature suggests that various stressors may play a pathogenic role in cardiovascular disease. In predisposed patients myocardial infarcts can follow extracardiac surgical interventions (Vowles and Howard, 1958; Roseman, 1962) and a variety of other physical and mental stressors (White, 1961), though there may be a latency period between the stress and the myocardial infarction. Unaccustomed efforts are particularly harmful. In the years 1950–1959, 77% of all the claims for cardiac damage made in the state of Washington were for myocardial infarction or acute coronary insufficiency following unusual effort. This is borne out in both clinical practice and laboratory investigation. Yet a review of animal experiments and observations on man suggests that muscular work diminishes the severity and intensity of arteriosclerosis (Schlüssel, 1965).

Stressors in general are also involved in the development of hypertension. Even in workers exposed to continuous industrial noise, the blood pressure shows a great tendency to reach high values and ECG changes have been noted

> in persons exposed to the effect of continuous industrial medium-frequency and high-frequency noise of intensity 85 to 120 db, functional disturbances of the cardiovascular system were frequently observed. Very often the subjects exhibited an instability of the arterial blood pressure. The electrocardiographic data showed bradycardia with a tendency to retardation of the intravesicular conductivity, plus a depression of the T-wave that was most frequently observed after physical stress and at the end of the work-period [Shatalov *et al.*, 1962].

Stress may play a role in the production of endocarditis in that glucocorticoids decrease resistance to infection and both corticoids and catecholamines make increased demands on the cardiac valves by raising the blood pressure (Oka *et al.*, 1960).

D. Psychogenic Stressors

Psychogenic stressors are among the most frequent causes of cardiovascular disease, probably because of man's highly developed CNS. A large number of published observations suggest that tensions and threats arising from interpersonal relations in the family or at work are particularly apt to cause hypertension. For example, one review of the literature combined with personal observations (Wolf *et al.*, 1948) led to the conclusion that "hypertension may represent an atavistic protective reaction of mobilization, invoked inappropriately by these subjects to deal with day-to-day stresses and threats arising out of problems of interpersonal relation. It becomes harmful and leads to illness when this essentially emergency pattern is adopted as a way of life." Another such review (Reiser *et al.*, 1950) demonstrates how often emotionally stressful life situations worsen the course of the onset, associated symptoms, and complications of hypertension and how often relaxing situations improve the condition. Again, Hambling (1970) discussed the role of anxiety and other stressful interpersonal relations in the development of this disorder, and Pflanz (1974) reviewed hypertension as a disease largely dependent on stress, especially stress involved in social maladjustment.

On the other hand, cardiac infarcts are more often the result of acute, intense mental arousal due to life events and changes (Rahe *et al.*, 1974; Theorell, 1974; Lundberg *et al.*, 1975). In predisposed subjects, events causing anxiety and resentment increase the pulse rate, cardiac output, and blood pressure, and impair tolerance to exercise; whereas in the few cases where stress evokes dejection and despair, the cardiovascular response is hypodynamic with bradycardia, decreased blood pressure, and hypotension (Stevenson and Duncan, 1950). In this connection see also von Kerekjarto (1973) for statistical studies on psychosomatic complaints among patients suffering from arterial hypertension, hypotension, or chronic fatigue related to stress.

Arguing violently with superiors or members of the family, witnessing a serious car accident, or lifting a heavy weight may cause ventricular tachycardia, paroxysmal auricular tachycardia, complete heart block, and even sudden death; in fact, both physical and emotional exhaustion can provoke virtually all types of cardiac arrhythmias (and death) in the normal as well as the abnormal heart (Bernreiter, 1956). Presumably, the production by emotional stress in predisposed patients of arrhythmias is due to the release of catecholamines and cortisol (Bellet and Roman, 1970).

One excellent detailed review of the sociologic–demographic literature shows that the causes of sudden death in man may be classified into eight categories: "1) on the impact of the collapse or death of a close person; 2) during acute grief; 3) on threat of loss of a close person; 4) during mourning or on an anniversary; 5) on loss of status or self-esteem; 6) personal danger or threat of injury; 7) after the danger is over; 8) reunion, triumph, or happy ending" (Engel, 1971).

The many statistical studies in this area show that cardiovascular derangements (as well as other diseases of adaptation) depend not so much on the kind of demand made on an individual as on his reaction to it. One review of empirical findings indicates that personality characteristics and individual responses to stressors in life situations are related to coronary heart disease (Caffrey, 1967; experimental work is also considered in this study, especially relating to infarctoid necroses elicited by stress). Mai (1968) discussed the roles of personality and emotional stress in the pathogenesis of coronary disease, and one extensive review supported the hypothesis "of a link between perceived stress in the environment, a personality overreactive to stress and high blood pressure" (Cochrane, 1971).

Much debate has taken place about whether executives or subordinates are more subject to stress-induced cardiovascular disease, but there appears to be no uniformly applicable answer to this problem; the deciding factor is whether a person finds it more stressful to be responsible for giving orders or for having to obey them. Liesse *et al.* (1974), from various psychological tests, concluded that "patients with ischemic heart disease do not show an exclusive coronary-prone personality pattern. Different patterns can be identified among them. The common psychological coronary-prone component of these different patterns seems to be the incapacity to cope with anxiety or the inadequacy of their defense-mechanisms." Again, a statistical study based on questionnaires led to the inference that what counts in the production of CHD "may not be the amount of situational or intrapsychic stress a person is subjected to but the way he copes with it—his defensive style" (Wardwell and Bahnson, 1973).

In this respect two personality types have been distinguished by Friedman and Rosenman (1959): Type A, characterized by a behavior pattern of intense ambition, competitive drive, constant preoccupation with job deadlines, a sense of time urgency, restless motor mannerisms, and staccato-style verbal respones; and Type B, characterized by a converse behavior pattern. Sometimes a Type C is recognized as having essentially the characteristics of Type B, but with the added element of chronic anxiety. Type A subjects usually have a high cholesterol level, a shortened blood-clotting time, and an increased tendency to develop coronary artery disease, and arcus senilis (see also Rosenman, 1967; Friedman and Rosenman, 1974; Friedman et al., 1975). Allegedly, Type A people succumb to coronary artery disease six times more frequently than Type B people (Friedman et al., 1968).

Other studies have confirmed the findings of Friedman and Rosenman. One extensive review by Morris and Gardner (1969) notes that ischemic heart disease is particularly common among men "showing strong drive, competitiveness, time urgency and preoccupation with deadlines, and the frustrations attendant on these" (Type A). This is true especially in early middle age, and results in particularly fatal disease. The incidence is twice that among Type B patients, who do not exhibit such personality traits. Another review (Johns, 1973) suggests that the "long-term behavior arousal" associated with intense competitiveness interacts with such physical stressors as diet and cigarette smoking to produce coronary heart disease, noting, however, that the physiological mechanisms of this interaction have not been definitely established.

Statistical studies based mainly on questionnaires about subjective criteria and life habits lend credence to the "contention that a coronary-prone behavior pattern predicts the incidence of coronary heart disease in white males" (Wardwell, 1973). The decisive factor (again according to Wardwell) would appear to be that coronary candidates have an unusually strong tendency to manifest psychological and situational states in a variety of physical ways such as "restless activity, ambitious strivings, bodily symptoms of many different sorts, and pathogenic atherosclerotic and thrombotic processes." (For another discussion of the coronary-prone personality, see Zyzanski and Jenkins, 1970.)

It was Friedman and Rosenman who most recently and convincingly called attention to these two types, and they deserve the greatest credit for having clearly delineated them. However, they themselves are the first to point out that, during the nineteenth century, Sir William Osler described a behavior pattern typical of coronary-prone patients. If we accept the tenet that stress, like emotional responsiveness, is equally dependent on life events and on our reactions to them, it is evident that admitting the distinction of Types A and B is essentially equivalent to admitting that stress, especially emotional stress, plays a decisive role in the pathogenesis of cardiovascular disease and is more influential in those who respond to a given event intensely (i.e., with severe stress) than in unresponsive, phlegmatic persons. Of course, this concept is also very compatible with the hormonal theory, in that the tense, excitable Type A person responds more readily with catecholamine and corticoid secretion than does the Type B person.

In a survey of the literature, Carruthers (1969) suggests that among the stressors of modern life, fear, hatred, aggression, and frustration increase catecholamine and particularly norepinephrine secretion as well as the plasma levels of free fatty acids and triglycerides. They also augment platelet adhesiveness and hence can lead to thrombosis. Carruthers adds the comment that "in modern society wrath, reinforced by sloth and gluttony, is the deadliest of the seven sins." Job satisfaction has also been claimed to be inversely related to death from coronary heart disease.

Such activities as driving and public speaking can cause significant biochemical alterations, even in normal persons; according to Somerville (1973) a statistical study shows that experienced drivers who have suffered from coronary heart disease are subject to "angina, sinus tachycardia, ectopic beats and various arrhythmias" when driving. On the other hand, "healthy racing drivers stimulated by the emotions of competition and danger, develop high-grade sinus tachycardia, raised plasma catecholamines and free fatty acids immediately before and after a race." Similar alterations are induced in normal persons by public speaking. Taggart and Gibbons (1971) go so far as to say that angina due to emotional stress, and borderline left ventricular failure, "should be contraindications to holding a driving licence."

For a discussion of the most common emotional stressors and dietary factors involved in coronary accidents, see Russek (1973); and for a review on the stressors of modern life that contribute to cardiovascular disease, see Boulard (1973).

It has been so indubitably established that psychogenic stress is a risk factor in coronary heart disease that the American Academy of Psychosomatic Medicine formulated a resolution in 1973 "that psychosocial stresses must be included among the recognized high-risk factors in myocardial infarction" and suggested "that the psychiatrist and psychosocial team be formally incorporated as an integral part of the Coronary Care Unit for every patient" (Lenzner, 1974). For a discussion of empirical findings on the prevention of coronary heart disease by protection against excessive psychogenic stress, see Turner and Ball (1974).

E. Conditioning

1. Genetics

Undoubtedly, genetic predisposition plays an extremely important role in coronary heart disease. Evidence for this was presented in the previous section, in which the constitutional types of predisposed and comparatively resistant individuals were delineated from the psychologic point of view, but various other risk factors—such as a tendency to excessive eating, smoking, high cholesterol and free fatty acid levels, accelerated blood coagulation and disinclination to exercise—are also largely dependent on inherited constitutional factors. According to a follow-up study of 3,182 men 39–59 years old (Rosenman *et al.*, 1970), CHD appears to run in families, as do hypertension, the smoking habit, high cholesterol, triglyceride and β-lipoprotein levels, and Type A behavior.

See Gertler and White (1954) for an excellent multidisciplinary study conducted at the Massachusetts General Hospital with the cooperation of several experienced cardiologists, reviewing the indices characteristic of the "coronary candidate" and the precipitating agents of CHD, including heredity, athletic activity, endocrine factors, diet, and blood biochemistry. See also Kruse (1960) for an extensive review by a committee on cultural, societal, familial, psychological, and genetic influences on the development of cardiovascular disease, with special reference to stress and the G.A.S.

2. Diet

The dietary factors that predispose to cardiovascular disease in general exert the same conditioning effect on stress-induced hypertension or CHD. The most recognized among these nutritional factors are the foods with high saturated fat content (mainly animal fat) and cholesterol. However, Russek (1967), from a careful survey of the literature and from personal observations, concludes that "the concept of any disease arising from a single cause is obsolete and misleading. Much evidence now suggests that most of the lethalness of a high fat diet in Western society may actually be dependent on the 'catalytic' influence of stressful living." According to Russek, this is particularly true of CHD.

Excessive sodium intake is also harmful, especially in the presence of renal disease and hypertension, as is gluttony in general, because of the resulting adiposity, which makes increased demands on the circulatory system and at the same time augments the stressor effect of exercise.

For a discussion of the influence of diet on the development of cardiovascular disease, with special emphasis on nutritional factors determining predisposition to stress-induced experimental cardiac necroses, see Bajusz (1965).

Lipman (1960) gave a detailed description of a diet that was thought to alleviate stress-induced hypertension, especially when given in combination with an antihistaminic. Many other measures, such as life habits and exercise, have been recommended for the prevention of cardiovascular disease in man. Raab (1970) examines the interactions between corticoids, catecholamines, and diets, especially on the basis of corresponding animal experiments.

3. Occupation and Social Factors Including Urbanization

Statistical surveys show that the incidence of CHD has greatly increased during the present century, and that the relative immunity of primitive races disappears when they subject themselves to "civilized" life (Stewart, 1950). However, the effect on statistics of constantly improving diagnostic techniques and more accurate reporting of death from CHD must not be neglected (Master, 1960).

One study (Harburg et al., 1973) in high- and low-stress areas of Detroit revealed that social and economic stressors definitely predisposed to increased blood pressure, especially among blacks.

According to Syme et al. (1964), geographically and occupationally mobile subjects have a higher CHD incidence than others. This may be ascribed to their need for more frequent readjustment and adaptation to new circumstances.

There is general agreement that urban life is more conducive to hypertension and CHD than rural settings (e.g., see Marks, 1967; Smith, 1967; Gutmann and Benson, 1971), but here again it is difficult to distinguish between the relative role played by crowding, differences in diet, occupations, air pollution, and so on.

In any event, the occupational stressors of industrial society appear to play a dominant role in the high incidence of CHD as well as in establishing a predisposition for it through a rise in plasma lipids, altered hemodynamics, and accelerated blood clotting (Rosenman and Friedman,

1958). Also, according to Russek and Zohman (1958), who studied 100 young coronary patients, "severe emotional strain of occupational origin was observed in 91% of the test subjects as compared with 20% of normal controls. Emotional stress associated with job responsibility appears far more significant in the etiologic picture of coronary disease in young adults than heredity or a prodigiously high-fat diet." The authors add the comment that smoking "would appear to be an indication of heightened emotional tension rather than a predisposing or causative factor in coronary heart disease." Another study (Russek, 1959) noted that in 91 of 100 patients, prolonged emotional strain related to occupational responsibilities preceded a coronary attack. Smoking was particularly frequent among coronary patients, but again the habit may be a manifestation of inner stress rather than an etiologic factor. Furthermore, much of our envied leisure time is regimented by participation in social, educational, and civic events that "may represent a poor antidote for the emotional stresses of daily business competition."

There is significant statistical evidence against the popular idea that the high responsibility of top management positions entails a greater risk of coronary disease or death. In 1958 Lee and Schneider were surprised to learn that, among more than 1,000 subjects in business, hypertension and cardiovascular disease (arteriosclerosis, CHD, myocardial infarction) were disproportionately low in the executive group. Another statistical study (Mortensen *et al.*, 1959) showed that

> in the Bell Telephone System there is no material difference in coronary mortality between the top management group and the craftsmen and laborers group, but there is a marked difference between top management and middle management which is not explainable from presently available data. The popular notion that high executive positions are associated with high coronary mortality is likely due to the greater publicity connected with such deaths rather than to statistical facts.

Again, in a 6-year study of 1,356 cases (Pell and D'Alonzo, 1963), the age-adjusted incidence of myocardial infarction among male employees was inversely proportional to their annual income.

On the other hand, an extensive study on postal and telegraph workers (Reeder *et al.*, 1973) indicated that "a relatively low job level was related to a relatively high number of EKG abnormalities. These latter findings may be predictive of future coronary artery disease in this group." One possible explanation for these data is suggested by the observation, based on statistical studies, that "job satisfaction is negatively related to a group's rate of death from coronary heart disease" (Sales and House, 1971). Moreover, Pell and D'Alonzo (1963), cited earlier, state that "the demands of a top-management job may be no more stressful than situations commonly encountered by persons in lower job levels, at work and at home," and that men chosen for advancement may be those whose personal qualities are characteristic of both executive talent and resistance to coronary disease. It is conceivable, for example, that in selecting persons to assume greater responsibilities, supervisors and managers, knowingly or unknowingly, may tend to choose the better adjusted individuals, who by virtue of their personality and psychic state are better able to cope with life's stresses in general.

Lee and Schneider (1958), also cited earlier, note that "the disruption of the harmonious balance between a man and his environment can result from either the demands of the environment or the failure of the man to measure up to them. Success in a career goes hand in hand with good health. The executive, as part of his training, learns to judge the amount of occupational stress he can stand and to appreciate the value of outside avenues of expression."

Nevertheless, it should be kept in mind that other statistical studies give opposite results, which are attributed to the greater drive and willingness to accept stressful responsibilities among those who reach higher echelons. For example, one statistical study, which indicates a high probable correlation between CHD and social, cultural, and even religious factors, suggests that, although further proof is necessary, in the United States "coronary heart disease may be viewed as an alternative to certain personality disorders, particularly for native-born American middle class Protestants, who are culturally not permitted to be weak or to fail to compete successfully" (Wardwell *et al.,* 1964).

In an extensive epidemiologic study on 31,000 men in London (Morris *et al.,* 1953), CHD was found to be more frequent among those holding sedentary jobs. Bus conductors had less CHD than bus drivers, postmen less than telephonists, executives, and clerks. It is implied that these differences are determined by the amount of exercise required by their jobs. Extensive statistical studies among 12,000 members of 14 professional groups in the United States showed that CHD was strikingly related to occupational activity among physicians, lawyers, security analysts, and traders (Russek, 1965). Incidentally, these same studies disclosed that, though smoking was most frequent in stressful occupations, unexpectedly CHD was more common among nonsmokers than among persons who once smoked but gave it up. Possibly, "the ability to stop smoking may imply a resilient personality response to stress and diminished vulnerability to atherogenic influences."

According to Shirom *et al.* (1973), in Israeli kibbutzim, agricultural workers were most likely to experience stress associated with CHD, although the generally accepted predisposing factors among them did not significantly differ from those in managerial, professional, clerical, or factory workers.

In Japan the incidence of arteriosclerotic CHD is extremely low as compared to its incidence among the white North American population, says Matsumoto (1970). "Although the diet factor remains dominant in current thinking, the stress hypothesis merits the most intensive probing as alternate or associated explanations of observed relations and differentiations."

4. Age

Though it is a well-known fact that the incidence of arteriosclerosis and CHD increases with age, youth of itself is of course no guarantee of immunity. Extensive clinical and anatomical studies on coronary arteriosclerosis and cardiac infarcts in 866 patients 18–39 years of age, showed that a fatal coronary attack occurred most frequently during strenuous activity related to combat and other military duties (Yater et al., 1948).

Rats exposed to stressors undergo changes similar or identical to those of the first step in the arteriosclerotic process characteristic of aging. For example, the emotional stress produced by restraint elicits typical mesenchymal reactions in the blood vessel walls with increased [^{35}S]sulfate and [^{3}H]thymidine incorporation (Hauss, 1973).

According to Kappert (1952), in juvenile hypertension, excess production of mineralocorticoids—which activate hepatic hypertensinogen formation and catecholamine secretion—is especially important; however, these findings have not yet been confirmed.

In the literature there is a general impression, not supported by convincing statistical evidence, that fatal CHD occurs more frequently among young people now than some decades ago.

F. Diagnostic Indicators and Other Changes Characteristic of Stress-Induced Cardiovascular Disease

It is virtually impossible in practice to separate diagnostic indicators from other changes characteristic of stress-induced cardiovascular disease that are not particularly helpful in diagnosis. Since all these also help to analyze the pathogenesis of such maladies, they will be discussed here conjointly.

1. Stress Tests

Tests used to evaluate the stress resistance of patients with cardiovascular disease are based mainly on resistance to muscular exercise. Techniques commonly used are the bicycle orgometer, the treadmill, and step tests; isometric exercises are especially useful in the evaluation of left ventricular function (Payne et al., 1973; Helfant et al., 1974).

"Stress interviews" and cold pressor tests also have some diagnostic value (Wolf et al., 1955). Furthermore, in early hypertensive patients, psychogenic stress (e.g., arithmetic under time pressure) causes an unusual rise in pulse rate, blood pressure, blood glucose, oxygen consumption, muscular tone, plasma norepinephrine, free fatty acids, cortisol, and renin activity (Baumann et al., 1973).

The SRE (Schedule of Recent Experience) questionnaire seems to correlate fairly well with coronary heart disease (see Ander et al., 1974; Theorell and Rahe, 1974).

Both emotional and physical stress conditions considerably alter the ECG (Weiss, 1956; Sigler, 1961; Simonov et al., 1975). Several instruments have been devised to determine ECG changes, often in combination with other indices, such as blood pressure variations, by telemetry while patients are exercising on a treadmill (Ellestad, 1967). For the interpretation of various stress-induced ECG changes, the reader is referred to Simonson (1970), So and Oversohl (1974), Amsterdam et al. (1974), and Hiss et al. (1960), as well as to the preceding references.

ECG responses to isoproterenol have been recommended for the evaluation of myocardial efficiency in preference to arteriography or the treadmill test; however, the claims behind this recommendation require confirmation.

2. Morphology

In patients who died from CHD following severe stress, there was extensive fuchsinophilic degeneration of the myocardium (similar to that seen in experimental animals during the electrolyte steroid cardiopathy with necrosis [ESCN]), indicating a necrosis "of metabolic origin" (Danilova, 1963). A review of the literature also suggested that various nonvascular noxious factors interfering with myocardial metabolism play a decisive role in CHD. This is true especially of the production of microfocal necroses that coincide with or aggravate the pathogenic effects of primarily vascular disturbances (Myasnikov, 1964).

"Stress polycythemia" is manifested by a normal erythrocyte mass, but a high hematocrit reading secondary to contracted plasma volume. This condition can be elicited by a variety of stressors and may be related to certain types of hypertension (Emery et al., 1974).

Sosnierz and Wieczorek (1966) report that in 92 patients who died of various diseases, fuchsinophilic degeneration of the myocardium was constant among old people and absent in neonates; the intensity of fuchsinophilia was particularly high in patients who died under very stressful circumstances.

3. Blood Clotting

It is suggested by histologic evidence that the development of coronary thrombosis is often very gradual, taking several days before pain and occlusion become manifest. Therefore, events immediately preceding the attack are not of etiologic significance. "The pathologic appearances in a series of fatal cases of coronary thrombosis suggest strongly that excessive exercise and emotional stress are intimately concerned in the mechanism of coronary artery thrombosis" (Paterson, 1939).

The frequent lack of correlation between coronary thrombosis and myocardial infarction or "sudden coronary heart death," which was repeatedly emphasized in the earlier literature, has again been demonstrated on the basis of an extensive review. "In more than 50% of the examined acute-recent infarct and sudden coronary heart death cases, an acute-recent occlusion was not detected." In other patients it took place in an already almost completely stenotic vessel so that it could have little effect; hence special attention must be given to the "infarctoid myocardial necroses" such as have been produced in animals by combined treatment with steroids and stressors (Baroldi, 1969).

In conscious patients stressful procedures such as cardiac catheterization caused a rise in the platelet aggregation response to adenosine diphosphate, concurrently with an increase in plasma free fatty acids. It is suggested that catecholamines, released during emotional stress, may be responsible for enhanced platelet aggregation and the development of thrombosis as well as atherosclerosis (Gordon et al., 1973).

In rats immersion in cold water causes platelet aggregation in myocardial vessels, as shown by electron microscopy. "It is concluded that stress, probably via catecholamine secretion that enhances platelet stickiness, can induce intravascular platelet aggregation. It is possible that this mechanism plays a part in the relationship between stress and acute clinical myocardial infarction" (Haft and Fani, 1973; see also Levites and Haft, 1974).

4. Hormones

There is practically no doubt today that hormones participate in the development of stress-induced cardiovascular disease. Evidence in favor of this view has come from observations in man and from animal experiments. Here we shall limit ourselves to clinical findings, since a special section is devoted to experimental cardiovascular diseases.

Since catecholamines liberated from sympathetic nerve endings and the adrenal medulla cause a dramatic rise in blood pressure, their role in hypertension has long been suspected, and the production of what we have called "mineralocorticoid hypertension" in DOC-treated animals has led to many clinical studies on this and related steroids in patients with various forms of hypertension. [See *Experimental Cardiovascular Diseases* (Selye, 1970).]

The relevant literature has become too voluminous to be discussed here in detail; besides, a large part of it has already been analyzed in our earlier stress monographs (Selye, 1950, 1951; Selye and Horava, 1952, 1953; Selye and Heuser, 1954, 1956). Suffice it to say here that an increase in the plasma and urinary concentration of catecholamines, several mineralocorticoids (DOC, 18-OH-DOC, aldosterone), and renin has repeatedly, though not consistently, been noted in hypertensive patients (Raab, 1968; Palem-Vliers *et al.,* 1974; Esler and Nestel, 1973).

There is good reason to believe that both hypertension and CHD can be elicited during stress through a rise in the secretion of any of these humoral substances, and are often caused by the concurrent overproduction of several among them; one or the other can play the predominant role, depending on conditioning factors.

For a detailed discussion of hormonal participation in the pathogenesis of hypertension and other cardiovascular diseases, the reader must be referred to pertinent reviews and monographs, but it may be useful to summarize at least a few of the more salient facts.

Evidently, catecholamines and corticoids mutually enhance each other's pressor effects, and the hypertensive actions of mineralocorticoids are augmented by a high sodium intake. The latter also predisposes the kidney to damage, especially by mineralocorticoids, including renin-stimulated mineralocorticoid secretion. Thus a vicious circle may develop in which mineralocorticoids elicit renal injury and the resulting rise in renal pressor substances augments mineralocorticoid secretion, which further damages the kidney until fatal malignant hypertension ensues.

In predisposed persons almost any kind of stressor causes a rise in blood pressure as well as in catecholamine and corticoid secretion (Raab, 1966); furthermore, the therapeutic efficiency of both adrenergic blocking agents (e.g., propranolol) and antimineralocorticoids (e.g., spironolactone) supports this hypothesis (Kimura, 1974). It is still difficult, however, to explain the occasional instances of hypertension in which the blood level of renin is subnormal. According to some investigations, this "hyporeninemic hypertension" is probably a pluricausal disease of variable etiology, often dependent on increased production of some mineralocorticoid that decreases renin secretion (Distler, 1974).

A prolonged increase in blood pressure undoubtedly damages the vessel walls and contributes to the development not only of arteriosclerosis but even of the hyalinizing arterial lesions characteristic of malignant hypertension and periarteritis nodosa. All of this presumably can enhance the narrowing of cardiac arteries, and by damaging their endothelium, eventually results in thrombosis. The latter is further facilitated by the well-known decrease in blood-clotting time produced by catecholamines.

Nevertheless, an increasing body of evidence suggests that many types of myocardial necrosis are not due to coronary thrombosis but to metabolic necroses of the myocardium in which corticoids and sodium play decisive roles, as we shall see in Section G, "Experimental Cardiovascular Diseases." Furthermore, not all cases of sudden death produced by acute stress are due to myocardial necrosis; they may be of purely functional origin (e.g., ventricular fibrillation).

5. Nonhormonal Metabolites

The nonhormonal metabolic changes associated with stress-induced cardiovascular disease are often those characteristic of stress itself, such as a rise in serum FFA and cholesterol (Hammarsten *et al.,* 1957; Jolliffe, 1959; Wolf *et al.,* 1962); these changes are highly subject to the conditioning influence of the diet (Bajusz and Rona, 1972). Allegedly, hypertensive patients also tend to have especially high adrenal cholesterol levels.

In a study of the relationship of cholesterol levels to certain habit patterns under stress, a questionnaire showed marked individual differences in responses among medical students exposed to various psychogenic stressors. The blood cholesterol levels usually increased, but the reverse also occurred occasionally.

Subjects in the lower cholesterol group more often reported loss of appetite, exhaustion, nausea and anxiety when under stress; in addition, urge to be alone, tremulousness and depression were more frequent than expected, although these items only approached significance. The only item with a significant positive relationship to higher cholesterol levels was urge to eat [Thomas and Ross, 1963].

In another study the highest adrenal cholesterol concentrations were found in patients who committed suicide and in hypertensives, being much above those of persons who died in accidents (Hoch-Ligeti, 1966). Presumably, in both cases the changes are related to stress.

G. Experimental Cardiovascular Diseases

I shall limit myself here to a brief mention of the most salient facts and the citation of a few key references, since work on the role of stress in the production of experimental cardiovascular diseases has been reviewed extensively in the two-volume monograph *Experimental Cardiovascular Diseases* (Selye, 1970). It may be said in essence that, depending on conditioning factors (particularly previous exposure to stress, age, genetic predisposition, the hormonal and nutritional status of the subject), stress may produce or inhibit the development of cardiovascular diseases, but it almost always influences their course in some respect.

Most of the experimental work in this field has been done to establish the role of stress, or of hormones produced during stress, in *hypertension* with the associated renal and cardiovascular lesions. These include *arteriosclerosis* (of both the atheromatous and the purely calcifying type), and myocardial necroses (caused either by vascular occlusion or by disturbances of cardiac metabolism). It may be said that malignant hypertension with *hyalinizing* cardiovascular and renal disease is most easily reproduced in rats by chronic stress on high sodium diets, especially after sensitization by uninephrectomy. Indeed, in unilaterally nephrectomized rats kept on high-sodium diets, mineralocorticoids (deoxycorticosterone [DOC], aldosterone), somatotropic hormone (STH), or methylandrostenediol (MAD, which probably causes the adrenals to produce mineralocorticoids) easily induce such lesions by themselves, without exposure to stress.

Corticoids undoubtedly play a decisive role here, and a mutual feedback mechanism exists between mineralocorticoids (particularly aldosterone) and the renal pressor system in that renin stimulates aldosterone production whereas aldosterone inhibits renin secretion. This interplay helps to maintain pressor homeostasis under ordinary conditions. However, if the feedback mechanism is defective and intense nephrosclerosis is produced, the blood pressure rises to a level where it further damages the kidney and a vicious circle develops. Possibly, some corticoids can induce nephrosclerosis and hypertension without raising renin production ("hyporeninemic hypertension"); thus the rise in blood pressure is deprived of its self-inhibitory properties and becomes self-perpetuating and independent of renin.

Although this mechanism is far from being adequately proved by experimental evidence, it is obvious that the adrenal cortex plays a decisive role in the production of many types of hypertensive disease. Thus in adrenalectomized rats kept on a fixed dose of glucocorticoids just sufficient to maintain life, neither stress, MAD, nor STH can exert their usual hypertensive, vasotoxic, and nephrosclerotic effects, even if the animals are maximally sensitized by uninephrectomy and a high sodium chloride intake. Yet in adrenalectomized rats, under similar conditions, exogenous mineralocorticoids retain their pressor vasotoxic and nephrotoxic actions. Therefore it is postulated that stress, MAD, and STH do not act on the vascular system directly, but through the intermediary of the adrenals, in which they stimulate the synthesis of mineralocorticoids under certain conditions.

The so-called *adrenal regeneration hypertension* (ARH) has furnished us with another convenient tool for studying mineralocorticoid hypertension and proving that the production of excessive or abnormal adrenal corticoids may cause hypertensive disease. If one adrenal is removed and the other "demedullated" (an operation that also removes virtually the entire cortex except the glomerulosa), nephrosclerotic hypertension develops with vascular lesions that are indistinguishable from those produced by DOC. Unilateral nephrectomy in rats on a high sodium chloride intake sensitizes for this effect, just as it does for the comparable actions of mineralocorticoids. There is much evidence supporting the view that in rats subjected to this operation, the regenerating adrenal cells of the subcortical layer produce an excessive amount of DOC and related steroids which have a high vasotoxic effect.

The pressor actions of catecholamines are transitory and hardly ever conducive to self-perpetuating nephrosclerotic hypertension. Epinephrine and norepinephrine are effective even in the absence of the adrenals, but appear to potentiate the characteristic vasotoxicity of mineralocorticoids and hence probably play an important part in stress-induced hypertensive disease. Their increased secretion during stress may also raise the coagulability of blood and thereby predispose to stress-induced occlusive vascular thrombosis.

Infarctoid Necrosis

The electrolyte steroid cardiopathies with necrosis (ESCN) are produced in experimental animals, particularly in rats, by the conjoint administration of glucocorticoids and mineralocorticoids, or by steroids (e.g., fluorocortisol) that exert both gluco- and mineralocorticoid actions, but only if this treatment is combined with a high sodium diet or with exposure to sudden stress. A great variety of stressors have proved effective in eliciting this manifestation after conditioning with corticoids and sodium. On the other hand, diets poor in sodium or rich in potassium and/or magnesium, as well as potassium-sparing agents (spironolactone, amiloride) protect against this type of cardiac lesion. Many of these experimental observations have found clinical application in the therapeutic use of low-sodium, high-potassium, or high-magnesium diets, spironolactone and amiloride for cardiovascular disease.

It is also of interest that high-fat diets are particularly effective in causing cardiac necroses in rats pretreated with appropriate corticoids and high-sodium diets. In this respect they may replace stressors.

Finally, it should be mentioned that in rats under identical conditions, acute exposure to stress (forced muscular exercise, restraint, traumatic injuries) *may produce or prevent cardiac necrosis,* depending on circumstances. Gradual pretreatment with stressors, especially forced muscular exercise, can protect the fully conditioned rat (essentially a "coronary candidate") against the induction of cardiac necrosis by a subsequent extremely severe stress.

These findings further suggest close relationships between the experimental cardiopathies and their clinical equivalents. They may explain the long-puzzling paradox that exercise is considered to be dangerous and also to be of prophylactic value in patients prone to cardiac infarction. Presumably, keeping fit through gradual, comparatively mild exercise induces considerable resistance, whereas sudden extreme muscular effort may precipitate a cardiac accident, especially in persons used to sedentary life and unadapted to muscular effort.

It must be kept in mind, however, that unlike many patients who die from acute coronary accidents, the ESCN of the rat is not primarily due to coronary thrombosis, but to metabolic derangements in the cardiac muscle that predispose it to necrosis at times of increased demands for work. Only secondarily do thromboses tend to develop in necrotic areas of the heart, where the endothelium of the coronary vessels has lost its anticoagulant properties. In this connection, it is of particular interest that several investigators observed an inverse relationship between the incidence of detectable coronary thromboses and the rapidity with which a patient died after clinical manifestations of a heart attack. It has been deduced that probably sudden cardiac death in man is often due primarily to myocardial necrosis and that the occlusive thrombus develops only secondarily in the dead myocardial region. (See *The Chemical Prevention of Cardiac Necroses,* Selye, 1958.) So-called fuchsinophilic degeneration frequently precedes myocardial necrosis in man (as indicated by histologic investigations in patients who died very suddenly after an accident) and in experimental animals during the ESCN.

For the literature on each separate point, the reader is referred to *Experimental Cardiovascular Diseases* (Selye, 1970) and to the references listed and abstracted under separate headings in the encyclopedic treatise *Stress in Health and Disease* (Selye, 1976).

H. Prophylaxis through Coping with Psychogenic Stress

It may be worthwhile here to outline a model for coping with psychogenic stress, since stress-induced cardiovascular disease is evidently such a widespread danger in modern society. We may extend ourselves beyond our field of expertise in so doing, but the gap between the different disciplines that may have an effect on man's well-being needs to be bridged, and the results of basic work on stress should be made available. The following discussion is based on an article that has appeared in Spanish (Taché *et al.,* 1977).

1. Homeostatic Imbalance

Ever since Claude Bernard developed the concept of the *milieu intérieur* and Walter Cannon (1939) coined the term "homeostasis" to refer to the fluid stability of the *milieu intérieur,* scientists have used the notions— knowingly or not—to explain many phenomena that extend well beyond the limits of traditional physiology. We like to express man's daily encounter with the environment in terms of homeostasis. Since harmony within the internal milieu and with the external environment conditions survival, the individual fights to preserve or restore it. An event in the environment becomes a stimulus—or a stressor—whenever an individual's homeostatic equilibrium is disrupted by it.

Homeostasis can be endangered and restored with or without the participation of consciousness. For instance, on the physical level an important loss of blood is countered by vasoconstriction to help maintain adequate arterial tension. On the psychological level, however, stimuli are much more subject to interpretation by the individual. Man's needs being more complex than those of an amoeba, his network of communication with the environment is correspondingly much more elaborate, and the nervous system fulfills this function. Usually the brain is seen as an organ of thought that enables man to philosophize or enter into other highly regarded intellectual activities, but to a biologist the prime function of the nervous system is to allow the individual to deal with his environment, that is, to bring about perception and evaluation of events that may affect his well-being or survival and also to elicit certain types of activity to reestablish harmony when it has been lost.

2. The Adaptive Process

When the body has to adapt to an external event (Fig. 3), perception and interpretation of the stimulus lead to an assessment of the phenomenon and its implications; this may be considered the "input." On the other hand, specific responses are tested, and one or many will be chosen and utilized; this is the "output." If the response is adequate to the challenge, adaptation will follow as the stimulus is dealt with or a new level of homeostasis is reached.

Evaluation of the demand is based partly on an individual's background—genetic make-up, natural capacities, basic education, recent experiences—which he uses as points of reference in assessing the significance of the stimulus. These factors are in a way the cast that will mold certain events to become stimuli or the diffracting crystal that will give special colors to our experiences. The importance of such endogenous and exogenous factors is indicated in Fig. 3.

The behavioral responses may be somatic, intellectual, or emotional.

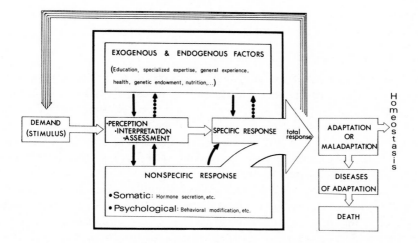

Fig. 3. Dealing with stressors usually entails finding the right specific response to the demand. Since endogenous and exogenous factors preside over the stimulus-to-response process, assessment may be modified by bringing a new outlook, by analyzing the situation from a different viewpoint. The nonspecifically secreted hormones are also meant to play a role in preparing for the specific response phase, but with man's evolved neocortex and with the variety of specific responses now available, these hormones may not help him to cope well with certain aspects of his environment. Dotted arrows indicate possible feedback.

Physiological reactions may arise all along the process, starting with perception; the intellectual response depends on individual predisposition, experience, and expertise, and these can be abetted through learning; the emotional arousal may begin with a growing awareness of the magnitude of the demand and subside once a specific countermeasure has been chosen.

These diagrams are very simple and do not comprise the various phases leading to assessment or specific responses. In reality, many feedback loops exist, through which requests may be made for additional information on the nature of the stimulus and the circumstances surrounding it, and a decision on a specific response may be arrived at after much internal dialogue and testing of possibilities. For the sake of simplicity, these details are not included here, since they are not essential for our discussion.

Stress (the nonspecific response of the body) is initiated at a very early stage: in fact, nonspecific physiological adaptation starts as soon as the body becomes aware of a demand (which could be physiological as well as psychological). The nonspecific response grows with the magnitude of the demand; moreover, if for some reason (such as internal conflict or lack of experience) the specific response is not easy to elicit, the stimulus-to-response process will be slowed down or stopped, and stress will increase while evaluation of the situation is prolonged, and while tentative, inadequate reactions are probed.

3. The Cost of Stress

The price that one has to pay for such unresolved situations may be quite significant. The psychological distress that usually accompanies internal conflicts is by no means the whole price; secondary physiological modifications may also occur in the body. Stress hormones (e.g., ACTH), of course, are secreted in response to a demand, and, as we have seen, may predispose to cardiovascular derangements; as well, the anterior hypophysis discharges other hormones that control various functions: FSH (follicle-stimulating hormone) and LH (luteinizing hormone), which in women regulate the sexual cycle and in men are responsible for the secretion of the male hormone, testosterone, and the development of spermatozoa; prolactin, which is involved in maintaining pregnancy and stimulating milk secretion after childbirth; and GH, the growth hormone.

In our experiments with rats, it was shown that, during prolonged and intense demands (immobilization), stress hormone concentrations are elevated well above normal values (Fig. 4). (Corticosterone was measured instead of ACTH for practical reasons, but the secretion of these two hormones is known to run parallel during stress.) Other pituitary hormone concentrations fall drastically (GH values drop below 40% of the norm within 24 hr) and, on the whole, stay around the 50% level until the 15th day (Taché et al., 1976).

4. Coping Mechanisms

Stress nowadays is not so much associated with physical survival as with a certain idea of survival. Society has identified new values that have been tagged as "necessary for survival," and in this "game," part of the nonspecific response is needlessly elicited. Sitting for an exam, applying for a job, the climate of competition using money and power as criteria of success—these are some of today's stressors that elicit the old physiological response in preparation for physical activity.

Broadly speaking, coping with stress in our society can be accomplished by (a) removing stressors from our lives; (b) nullifying potential stressors; (c) finding adequate specific responses in dealing with conditions we cannot or do not want to avoid; and (d) relaxing or finding diversion from the demand.

a. Removing Stressors

In some cases at least it would be easier to adjust social conditions to man's needs than to force him to waste his energy trying to adapt to changes

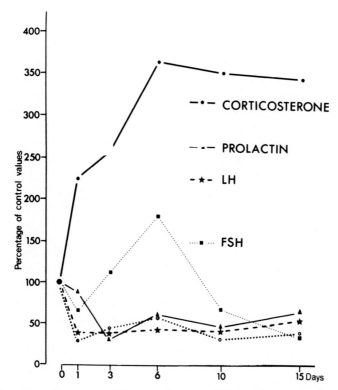

Fig. 4. Effect of chronic immobilization (8 hr daily during 1, 3, 6, 10, or 15 days) on the plasma levels of some sex hormones and the growth hormone in female rats: corticosterone, prolactin, luteinizing hormone (LH), growth hormone (GH same as STH), and follicle-stimulating hormone (FSH). (Tache *et al.*, 1976, by permission.)

in the environment that are of his own making anyway and that he could easily modify. Think of the uselessness of daily traffic jams, overpopulated housing projects, the irrelevance of much of our schooling. When society has a choice in determining certain parameters of the environment, it should not disregard certain needs of man that have been forgotten in recent times: the need to relate, to communicate, to exercise physically, and so on.

b. Nullifying Potential Stressors

Modifying one's perspective of things is an effective individual way of coping with stress. Very often, severe stress is induced unnecessarily, as there is no correspondence between the objective import of an event or circumstance (e.g., the boss's remarks) and the significance attached to it (the secretary's interpretation). It is not so much *to what* we react as *how* we react that is at the root of the problem.

Allergy is a parallel case in the field of pathology. Although most people will not react to common allergens, certain individuals will mobilize important immunologic defense mechanisms against them. In this case it is not the allergens (what they react to) but the response itself (how they react) that is the cause of disease. The allergen is not injurious to their health per se, but only through provoking unnecessary defense reactions. Taking an exam does not have the same survival significance as living through an epidemic or, as with prehistoric man, facing a pack of wolves. Yet we have not learned to respond in a different way to modern stressors.

Though man will always strive for values, his value system needs constant rethinking. For example, competition is not of the making of our society; it is a law of Nature, a condition of survival. Man has always competed against animals and other men for food, possession of territory, or shelter for his family. But these are basic necessities; without them man's survival is impossible. Today the problem seems to be that nonessentials are now proposed to man as being basic. From the two-family house of some years ago, we have evolved to the two-house family, which in itself would not be bad were it not for the fact that it has now become an "essential," a criterion of success. A new set of values needs to be proposed to man so that the inborn urge to compete will be more usefully gauged to the weight or consequence of the goal.

c. FINDING ADEQUATE SPECIFIC RESPONSES

In all cases where an event has become a stressor, an adequate specific response elicited as rapidly as possible will relieve stress. Barring quantitative overload, stress levels will decrease as one becomes an expert, develops the tools of the trade, and learns how to use them. In other words, when the capacity to elicit the specific response has been developed, the demand will be assessed differently. A typical case is that of a woman who once told us that she spent three days (and nearly as many nights) writing her first letter as special assistant to a deputy minister, but that now she could write important letters without becoming personally involved.

d. RELAXING OR FINDING DIVERSION FROM THE DEMAND

Relaxation is not as easy to achieve as is commonly believed. After a hard day's work, even highly trained persons will find that tension has accumulated and that they feel tired; although apparently the demand is no longer present, the mind and body keep responding to it.

Yet it is often said that if you can relax your muscles, the psychological cause of your tension will tend to disappear, and we cannot but be impressed by the number of persons who praise the numerous techniques now being publicized that are based on this idea, such as Transcendental Meditation (Bloomfield and Kory, 1976), the Relaxation Response (Benson *et al.,* 1974), Autogenic Training (Luthe, 1969), Transactional Analysis, Yoga, and even some kinds of physical exercise that induce relief from tension. Although such techniques do not seem to work equally well for all, it may still be worth the time and effort to take a close look at them.

5. Priorities for Coping

Reducing stress sometimes entails refusing to be placed under stress and, up to a point, refusing to meet challenges. Regular hours, good eating habits, physical exercise, and physical withdrawal from stressful situations are reported to be associated with fewer stress symptoms than other, more result-oriented techniques such as a change to a different work activity or a new strategy of attack on work (Howard *et al.,* 1975).

We have to realize clearly that work is a biological necessity. Just as our muscles become flabby and degenerate if not used, so our brain slips into chaos and confusion unless we constantly use it for some work that seems worthwhile to us. This in itself, as we have discussed, can cause significant psychogenic stress.

The great Canadian physician William Osler recognized the significance of work in this tribute:

> Though little, the master word looms large in meaning. It is the 'open sesame' to every portal, the great equalizer, the philosopher's stone which transmutes all base metal of humanity into gold. The stupid it will make bright, the bright brilliant, and the brilliant steady. To youth, it brings hope, to the middle-aged confidence, to the aged repose. It is directly responsible for all advances in medicine during the past twenty-five years. Not only has it been the touchstone of progress, but it is the measure of success in everyday life. And the master word is WORK.

We have all heard the sayings, "There is more to life than just work," or, "You should work to live, not live to work." These sound pretty convincing, but are they really? Our principal aim should be not to avoid work but to find the kind of occupation that, for us, is play. The best way to avoid harmful stress is to select an environment (wife, boss, friends) that is in line with our innate preferences—to find an activity we like and respect. Only thus can the need for frustrating constant readaptation that is the major cause of distress be eliminated.

Stress is inseparable from life. In prehistoric times it was the price that man had to pay to survive as an animal; now he pays the same price to accomplish what he considers great things. Those who are convinced that mere physical survival is not enough for them, must realize that there should be a proportion between what they *want* to do and what they *can* do, between the significance of the challenges they rise to meet and the price they will have to pay as a consequence, and their goals and priorities should be established accordingly.

6. A Code of Behavior

It is my belief that practical recommendations such as the preceding can be expressed as a scientifically based code of ethics. In the light of what my own laboratory and clinical study of somatic diseases has taught me concerning stress, I have tried to arrive at such a code, that is, one based not on the strictures and traditions of society, inspiration, or blind faith in the infallibility of a particular prophet, religious leader, or political doctrine, but on the verifiable laws that govern the body's reactions in maintaining homeostasis and living in satisfying equilibrium with its environment. I would summarize its most important principles briefly as follows:

a. FIND YOUR OWN STRESS LEVEL

The speed at which you can run toward your own goal. Make sure that both the stress level and the goal are really your own, and not imposed on you by society, for only you yourself can know what you want and how fast you can accomplish it. A turtle cannot run like a racehorse, nor can a racehorse be prevented from running faster than a turtle. The same is true of people.

b. BE AN ALTRUISTIC EGOIST

Do not try to suppress the natural instinct of all living beings to look after themselves first. Yet the wish to be of some use, to do some good to others, is also natural. We are social beings, and everybody wants somehow to earn respect and gratitude. You must be useful to others; this gives you the greatest degree of safety, because no one wishes to destroy such a person.

c. EARN THY NEIGHBOR'S LOVE

This is a contemporary modification of the maxim "Love thy neighbor as thyself." It recognizes that not all neighbors are lovable and that it is impossible to love on command.

Perhaps two short lines can encapsulate my philosophy:

Fight for *your* highest *attainable* aim,
But do not put up resistance in vain.

References

Amstersdam, E. A., Hughes, J. L., de Maria, A. N., Zelis, R., and Mason, D. T. (1974). Indirect assessment of myocardial oxygen consumption in the evaluation of mechanisms and therapy of angina pectoris. *Am. J. Cardiol.* **33**, 737–743.

Ander, S., Lindstrom, B., and Tibblin, G. (1974). Life changes in random samples of middle-aged men. *In* "Life Stress and Illness" E. K. E. Gunderson and R. H. Rahe, eds.), pp. 121–124. Thomas, Springfield, Illinois.

Bajusz, E. (1965). "Nutritional Aspects of Cardiovascular Diseases." Crosby Lockwood, London.

Bajusz, E., and Rona, G. (1972). "Recent Advances in Studies on Cardiac Structure and Metabolism. 1. Myocardiology" (3rd Annu. Meet. Int. Study Group Res. Cardiac Metab. 1970). Univ. Park Press, Baltimore, Maryland.

Baroldi, G. (1969). Lack of correlation between coronary thrombosis and myocardial infarction or sudden 'coronary' heart death. *Ann. N. Y. Acad. Sci.* **156**, 504–525.

Baumann, R., Ziprian, H., Gödicke, W., Hartrodt, W., Naumann, E., and Läuter, J. (1973). The influence of acute psychic stress situations on biochemical and vegetative parameters of essential hypertensives at the early stage of the disease. *Psychother. Psychosom.* **22**, 131–140.

Bellet, S., and Roman, L. (1970). Stress electrocardiography in the diagnosis of arrhythmias. *Geriatrics* **25**, 102–107.

Benson, H., Beary, J. F., and Carol, M. P. (1974). The relaxation response. *Psychiatry* **37**, 37–46.

Bernreiter, M. (1956). Cardiac arrhythmias in physical or emotional stress. *Mo. Med.* **53**, 19–20.

Bloomfield, H. H., and Kory, R. B. (1976). "Happiness. The TM Program, Psychiatry and Enlightenment." Dawn Press/Simon & Schuster, New York.

Boulard, P. (1973). Stress et maladies de couer (Stress and cardiac diseases). *In* L'Athérosclerose, pp. 161–166. Baillière et Fils, Paris.

Caffrey, B. (1967). A review of empirical findings. *Milbank Mem. Fund. Q.* **45**, No. 2, Part 2, 119–139.

Cannon, W. B. (1939). "The Wisdom of the Body." Norton, New York.

Carruthers, M. E. (1969). Aggression and atheroma. *Lancet*, 1170–1171.

Cochrane, R. (1971). High blood pressure as a psychosomatic disorder: a selective review. *Br. J. Soc. Clin. Psychol.* **10**, 61–72.

Corvisart, J. N. (1812). "An Essay of the Organic Diseases and Lesions of the Heart and Great Vessels." Branford & Read, Boston, Massachusetts.

Danilova, K. M. (1963). Morphological tests of the stress reaction in human myocardium. *Arkh. Patol.* **25**, No. 7, 42–49.

Distler, A. (1974). Ist die essentielle Hypertonie noch eine Krankheitseinheit? Abgrenzung der hypereninämischen Hypertonie" (Is essential hypertension still a disease entitty? Definition of hypo-reninemic hypertension). *Internist* **15**, 146–154.

Ellestad, M. H. (1967). Telemetry in monitoring stress electrocardiograms. *Biomed. Sci. Instrum.* **3**, 249–256.

Emery, A. C., Jr., Whitcomb, W. H., and Frohlich, E. D. (1974). 'Stress' polycythemia and hypertension. *J. Am. Med. Assoc.* **229**, 159–162.

Engel, G. L. (1971). Sudden and rapid death during psychological stress. Folklore or folk wisdom? *Ann. Intern. Med.* **74**, 771–782.

Esler, M. D., and Nestel, P. J. (1973) High catecholamine essential hypertension: clinical and physiological characteristics. *N. Z. J. Med.* **3**, 117–123.

Friedman, M., and Rosenman, R. H. (1959). Association of specific overt behavior pattern with blood and cardiovascular findings. Blood cholesterol level, blood clotting time, incidence of arcus senilis, and clinical coronary artery disease. *J. Am. Med. Assoc.* **169**, 1286–1296.

Friedman, M., and Rosenman, R. H. (1974). "Type A Behavior and Your Heart." Alfred A. Knopf, New York.

Friedman, M., Rosenman, R. H., Strauss, R., Wurm, M., and Kositchek, R. (1968). The relationship of behavior pattern A to the state of the coronary vasculature. A study of fifty-one autopsy subjects. *Am. J. Med.* **44**, 525–537.

Friedman, M., Byers, S. O., Diamant, J., and Rosenman, R. H. (1975). Plasma catecholamine response of coronary-prone subjects (Type A) to a specific challenge. *Meta., Clin. Exp.* **24**, 205–210.

Gertler, M. M., and White, P. D. (1954). Coronary Heart Disease in Young Adults. A Multidisciplinary Study." Harvard Univ. Press, Cambridge, Massachusetts.

Gordon, J. L., Bowyer, D. E., Evans, D. W., and Mitchinson, M. J. (1973). Human platelet reactivity during stressful diagnostic procedures, *J. Clin. Pathol.* **26**, 958–962.

Gutman, M. C., and Benson, H. (1971). Interaction of environmental factors and systematic arterial blood pressure: A review. *Medicine (Baltimore)* **50**, 543–553.

Haft, J. I., and Fani, K. (1973). Intravascular platelet aggregation in the heart induced by stress. *Circulation* **47**, 353–358.

Hambling, J. (1970). Psychodynamics of sustained high blood pressure. *Psychother. Psychosom.* **18**, 349–354.

Hammarsten, J. F., Cathey, C. W., Redmond, R. F., and Wolf, S. (1957). Serum cholesterol, diet and stress in patients with coronary artery disease. *J. Clin. Invest.* **36**, 897.

Harburg, E., Erfurt, J. C., Chape, C., Hauenstein, L. S., Schull, W. J., and Schork, M. A. (1973). Socioecological stressor areas and black-white blood pressure: Detroit. *J. Chronic Dis.* **26**, 595–611.

Hauss, W. H. (1973). "Tissue alterations due to experimental arteriosclerosis. *In* "Connective Tissue and Ageing" (H. G. Vogel, ed.), Int. Congr. Ser. No. 264, pp. 23–33. Excerpta Med. Found., Amsterdam.

Helfant, R. H., DeVilla, M. A., Meister, S. G., and Banka, V. S. (1974). Isometric handgrip stress in evaluation of left ventricular performance in patients with coronary heart disease. *Clin. Res.* **22**, 279A (abstr.).

Hiss, R. G., Smith, G. B., Jr., and Lamb, L. E. (1960). Pitfalls in interpreting electrocardiographic changes occurring while monitoring stress procedures. *Aerosp. Med.* **31**, 9–19.

Hoch-Ligeti, C. (1966). Adrenal cholesterol concentration in cases of suicide. *Br. J. Exp. Pathol.* **47**, 594–598.

Howard, J. H., Rechnitzer, P. A., and Cunningham, D. A. (1975). Coping with job tension. Effective and ineffective methods. *Public Pers. Manage.* Sept.–Oct., pp. 317–325.

Johns, M. W. (1973). Stress and coronary heart disease. *Ergonomics* **16**, 683–690.

Jolliffe, N. (1959). Fats, cholesterol, and coronary heart disease. A review of recent progress. *Circulation* **20**, 109–127.

Kappert, A. (1952). Der jugendliche Hochdruck (Juvenile hypertension). *Schweiz. Med. Wochenschr.* **82**, 821–825.

Kimura, K. (1974). Pathophysiological significance of sympathetic activity in cardiovascular diseases. *Jpn. Circ. J.* **38**, 181–194.

Kruse, H. (1960). Committee on cultural, societal, familial, psychological, and genetic influences. *Am. J. Public Health* **50**, Suppl., 71–104.

Lee, R. E., and Schneider, R. F. (1958). Hypertension and arteriosclerosis in executive and non-executive personnel. *J. Am. Med. Assoc.* **167**, 1447–1450.

Lenzner, A. S. (1974). Psychiatry in the coronary care unit. *Psychosomatics* **15**, 70–71.

Levites, R., and Haft, J. I. (1974) Effects of exercise-induced stress on platelet aggregation. *Clin. Res.* **22**, 285A (abstr.).

Liesse, M., van Imschoot, K., Mertens, C., and Lauwers, P. (1974). Caractéristiques psychologiques et reactions physiologiques au stress de sujets normaux et coronariens

(Psychologic characteristics and physiologic reactions to stress in normal and coronary-prone subjects). *J. Psychosom. Res.* **18**, 49–53.

Lipman, D. G. (1960). Stress and hypertension: Use of antistress diet and antihistamine. *J. Am. Geriatr. Soc.* **8**, 177–184.

Lundberg, U., Theorell, T., and Lind, E. (1975). Life changes and myocardial infarction: Individual differences in life change scaling. *J. Psychosom. Res.* **19**, 27–32.

Luthe, W. (1969). "Autogenic Therapy," 6 vols. Grune & Stratton, New York.

Mai, F. M. M. (1968). Personality and stress in coronary disease. *J. Psychosom. Res.* **12**, 275–287.

Marks, R. U. (1967). A review of empirical findings. *Milbank Mem. Fund Q.* **45**, No. 2, Part 2, 51–107.

Master, A. M. (1960). The role of effort and occupation (including physicians) in coronary occlusion. *J. Am. Med. Assoc.* **174**, 942–948.

Matsumoto, Y. S. (1970). Social stress and coronary heart disease in Japan. *Milbank Mem. Fund Q.* **48**, 9–36.

Morris, J. N., and Gardner, M. J. (1969). Epidemiology of ischaemic heart disease. *Am. J. Med.* **46**, 674–683.

Morris, J. N., Heady, J. A., Raffle, P. A. B., Roberts, C. G., and Parks, J. W. (1953). Coronary heart-disease and physical activity of work. *Lancet*, 1053, 1111, and 1120.

Mortensen, J. M., Stevenson, T. T., and Whitney, L. H. (1959). Mortality due to coronary disease analyzed by broad occupational groups. *Arch. Ind. Hyg.* **19**, 1–4.

Myasnikov, A. L. (1964). Myocardial necroses of coronary and noncoronary genesis. *Am. J. Cardiol.* **13**, 435–440.

Oka, M., Nakao, K., and Angrist, A. (1960). Nonspecific aspects of endocarditis. Clinical applications of an experimental study. *N. Y. State J. Med.* **60**, 669–678.

Palem-Vliers, M., Genard, P., and Eechaute, W. (1974). La détection de la 18-hydrox-11-désoxycorticosterone et de deux substances inconnues dans les urines de malades hyper-tendus. Isolement d'une de ces substances (Detection of 18-hydroxy-11-desoxycorticosterone and two unknown substances in the urine of hypertensive patients. Isolation of one of these substances). *Acta Clin. Belg.* **29**, 281–282.

Paterson, J. C. (1939). Relation of physical exertion and emotion to precipitation of coronary thrombi. *J. Am. Med. Assoc.* **112**, 895–897.

Payne, R. M., Horwitz, L. D., and Mullins, C. B. (1973). Comparison of isometric exercise and angiotensin infusion as stress tests for evaluation of left ventricular function. *Am. J. Cardiol.* **31**, 428–433.

Pell, S., and D'Alonzo, C. A. (1963). Acute myocardial infarction in a large industrial population. Report of a 6-year study of 1,356 cases. *J. Am. Med. Assoc.* **185**, 831–838.

Pflanz, M. (1974). Psychische und soziale Faktoren bei der Entstehung des Hochdrucks (Importance of mental and social factors in the genesis of hypertension). *Internist* **15**, 124–128.

Raab, W. (1966). Emotional and sensory stress factors in myocardial pathology. *Am. Heart J.* **72**, 538–564.

Raab, W. (1968). Correlated cardiovascular adrenergic and adrenocortical responses to sensory and mental annoyances in men. A potential accessory cardiac risk factor. *Psychosom. Med.* **30**, 809–818.

Raab, W. (1970). "Preventive Myocardiology. Fundamentals and Targets." Thomas, Springfield, Illinois.

Raab, W., Chaplin, J. P., and Bajusz, E. (1964). Myocardial necroses produced in domesticated rats and in wild rats by sensory and emotional stresses. *Proc. Soc. Exp. Biol. Med.* **116**, 665–669.

Rahe, R. H., Romo, M., Bennett, L., and Siltanen, P. (1974). Recent life changes, myocardial infarction, and abrupt coronary death. *Arch. Intern. Med.* **133**, 221–228.

Reeder, L. G., Schrama, P. G. M., and Dirken, J. M. (1973). Stress and cardiovascular health: An international cooperative study. I. *Soc. Sci. Med.* **7**, 573–584.

Reiser, M. F., Brust, A. A., Shapiro, A. P., Baker, H. M., Ranschoff, W., and Ferris, E. B. (1950). Life situations, emotions and the course of patients with arterial hypertension. *In* "Life Stress and Bodily Disease" (H. G. Wolff *et al.*, eds.), pp. 870–880. Williams & Wilkins, Baltimore.

Rosenman, M. D. (1962). Postoperative myocardial infarction. *Am. J. Proctol.* **13**, 372–376.

Rosenman, R. H. (1967). Emotional factors in coronary heart disease. *Postgrad. Med.* **42**, 165–172.

Rosenman, R. H., and Friedman, M. (1958). The possible relationship of occupational stress to clinical coronary heart disease. *Calif. Med.* **89**, 169–174.

Rosenman, R. H., Friedman, M., Straus, R., Jenkins, C. D., Zyzanski, S. J., and Wurm, M. (1970). Coronary heart disease in the Western Collaborative Group study. A follow-up experience of 4 ½ years. *J. Chronic Dis.* **23**, 173–190.

Russek, H. I. (1959). Role of heredity, diet, and emotional stress in coronary heart disease. *J. Am. Med. Assoc.* **171**, 503–508.

Russek. H. I. (1965). Stress, tobacco, and coronary disease in North American professional groups. Survey of 12,000 men in 14 occupational groups. *J. Am. Med. Assoc.* **192**, 189–194.

Russek, H. I. (1967). Role of emotional stress in the etiology of clinical coronary heart disease. *Dis. Chest.* **52**, 1–9.

Russek, H. I. (1973). The stress of life. *In* "The Paul D. White Symposium: Major Advances in Cardiovascular Therapy" (H. I. Russek, ed.), pp. 111–115. Williams & Wilkins, Baltimore, Maryland.

Russek, H. I., and Zohman, B. L. (1958). Relative significance of heredity, diet and occupational stress in coronary heart disease of young adults. Based on an analysis of 100 patients between the ages of 25 and 40 years and a similar group of 100 normal control subjects. *Am. J. Med. Sci.* **235**, 266–277.

Sales, S. M., and House, J. (1971). Job dissatisfaction as a possible risk factor in coronary heart disease. *J. Chronic Dis.* **23**, 861–873.

Schlüssel, H. (1965). Sport und Arteriosklerose" (Sports and arteriosclerosis). *Med. Welt* **28**, 1563–1569.

Selye, H. (1950). "Stress." Acta, Inc., Montreal.

Selye, H. (1951). "First Annual Report on Stress." Acta, Inc., Montreal.

Selye, H. (1958). "The Chemical Prevention of Cardiac Necroses." Ronald Press, New York.

Selye, H. (1970). "Experimental Cardiovascular Diseases," 2 vols. Springer-Verlag, Berlin and New York.

Selye, H. (1976). "Stress in Health and Disease." Butterworth, London.

Selye, H., and Heuser, G. (1954). "Fourth Annual Report on Stress." Acta, Inc., Montreal.

Selye, H., and Heuser, G. (1956). "Fifth Annual Report on Stress 1955–1956." Acta, Inc., Montreal.

Selye, H., and Horava, A. (1952). "Second Annual Report on Stress." Acta, Inc., Montreal.

Selye, H., and Horava, A. (1953). "Third Annual Report on Stress." Acta, Inc., Montreal.

Sharma, V. N., Barar, F. S. K. (1966). Restraint stress as it influences the myocardium of rat. *Indian J. Med. Res.* **54**, 1102–1107.

Shatalov, N. N., Saitanov, A. O., and Glotova, K. V. (1962). On the state of the cardiovascular system under conditions of exposure to continuous noise. *Gig. Tr. Prof. Zabol.* **6**, 10–14.

Shirom, A., Eden, D., Silberwasser, S., and Kellermann, J. J. (1973). Job stresses and risk factors in coronary heart disease among five occupational categories in kibbutzim. *Soc. Sci. Med.* 7, 875–892.

Sigler, L. H. (1961). Abnormalities in the electrocardiogram induced by emotional strain. Possible mechanism and implications. *Am. J. Cardiol.* 8, 807–814.

Simonov, P. V., Frolov, M. V., and Sviridov, E. P. (1975). Characteristics of the electrocardiogram under physical and emotional stress in man. *Aviat. Space Environ. Med.* 46, 141–143.

Simonson, E. (1970). Electrocardiographic stress tolerance tests. *Prog. Cardiovasc. Dis.* 13, 269–292.

Smith, T. (1967). A review of empirical findings. *Milbank Mem. Fund Q.* 45, No. 2, Part 2, 23–39.

So, C. S., and Oversohl, K. (1974). Die klinische Bedeutung des Kalium-Belastungs-EKG (The clinical significance of the potassium stress ECG). *Müench. Med. Wochenschr.* 116, 1657–1660.

Somerville, W. (1973). Emotions, catecholamines and coronary heart disease. *Adv. Cardiol.* 8, 162–173.

Sosnierz, M., and Wieczorek, M. (1966). The influence of stress on the pathomorphologic state of the heart. *Patol. Pol.* 17, 361–368.

Stevenson, I., and Duncan, C. H. (1950). Alterations in cardiac function and circulatory efficiency during periods of life stress as shown by changes in the rate, rhythm, electrocardiographic pattern and output of the heart in those with cardiovascular disease. *In* "Life Stress and Bodily Disease" (H. G. Wolff *et al.,* eds.), pp. 799–817. Williams & Wilkins, Baltimore, Maryland.

Stewart, I. McD. G. (1950). Coronary disease and modern stress. *Lancet* , 867–870.

Syme, S. L., Hyman, M. M., and Enterline, P. E. (1964). Some social and cultural factors associated with the occurrence of coronary heart disease. *J. Chronic Dis.* 17, 277–289.

Taché, J., Taché, Y., and Selye, H. (1977). "Integracion del estrés en trabajo individual diario" (Integration of stress in the individual's daily work). Editorial Karpos, Madrid.

Taché, Y., Du Ruisseau, P., Taché, J., Selye, H., and Collu, R. (1976). Shift in adenohypophyseal activity during chronic intermittent immobilization of rats. *Fed. Proc., Fed. Am. Soc.*

Taggart, P., and Gibbons, D. (1971). The motor-car and the normal and abnormal heart. *Triangle* 10, 63–68.

Theorell, T. (1974). Life events before and after the onset of a premature myocardial infarction. *In* "Stressful Life Events: Their Nature and Effects" B. S. Dohrenwend and B. P. Dohrenwend, eds.), pp. 101–117. Wiley, New York.

Theorell, T., and Rahe, R. H. (1974). Psychosocial characteristics of subjects with myocardial infarction in Stockholm. *In* "Life Stress and Illness" (E. K. E. Gunderson, and R. H. Rahe, eds.), pp. 90–104. Thomas, Springfield, Illinois.

Thomas, C. B., and Ross, D. C. (1963). Observations on some possible precursors of essential hypertension and coronary artery disease. VIII. Relationship of cholesterol level to certain habit patterns under stress. *Bull. Johns Hopkins Hosp.* 113, 225–238.

Turner, R., and Ball, K. (1974). Prevention of coronary heart-disease. *Lancet* , 411–412.

von Kerekjarto, M. (1973). Psychosomatische Beschwerden bei Hypotonie" (Psychosomatic disturbances in hypotension). *Internist* 14, 521–524.

Vowles, K. D. J., and Howard, J. M. (1958). Myocardial and cerebral infarctions as postoperative complications. *Br. Med. J.* May 10, 1096–1099.

Wardwell, W. I. (1973). A study of stress and coronary heart disease in an urban population. *Bull. N. Y. Acad. Med.* [2] 49, 521–531.

Wardwell, W. I., and Bahnson, C. B. (1973). Behavioral variables and myocardial infarction in the southeastern Connecticut heart study. *J. Chronic Dis.* **26,** 447–461.

Wardwell, W. I., Hyman, M., and Bahnson, C. B. (1964). Stress and coronary heart disease in three field studies. *J. Chronic Dis.* **17,** 73–84.

Weiss, B. (1956). Electrocardiographic indices of emotional stress. *Am. J. Psychiatry* **113,** 348–351.

White, P. D. (1961). The relation of heart disease to injury, stress and occupation. *In* "Cardiologia" (A. Bisteni *et al.,* eds.), pp. 43–47. Editorial Interamericana, Mexico.

Wolf, S., Pfeiffer, J. B., Ripley, H. S., Winter, O. S., and Wolff, H. G. (1948). Hypertension as a reaction pattern to stress: Summary of experimental data on variations in blood pressure and renal blood flow. *Ann. Intern. Med.* **29,** 1056–1076.

Wolf, S., Cardon, P. V., Jr., Shepard, E. M., and Wolff, H. G. (1955). "Life Stress and Essential Hypertension. A Study of Circulatory Adjustments in Man." Williams & Wilkins, Baltimore, Maryland.

Wolf, S., McCabe, W. R., Yamamoto, J., Adsett, C. A., and Schottstaedt, W. W. (1962). Changes in serum lipids in relation to emotional stress during rigid control of diet and exercise. *Circulation* **26,** 379–387.

Yater, W. M., Traum, A. H., Brown, W. G., FitzGerald, R. P., Geisler, M. A., and Wilcox, B. B. (1948). Coronary artery disease in men eighteen to thirty-nine years of age. Report of eight hundred sixty-six cases, four hundred fifty with necropsy examinations. *Am. Heart J.* **36,** 334–372, 481–526, and 683–722.

Zyzanski, S. J., and Jenkins, C. D. (1970). Basic dimensions within the coronary-prone behavior pattern. *J. Chronic Dis.* **22,** 781–795.

7

Hypoxia and the Heart

P. R. Moret

I. Introduction

A. Definition

The term "hypoxia" often leads to confusion, being linked with "ischemia." In order to differentiate between these two terms, some distinguish hypoxemic hypoxia (hypoxia due to insufficient oxygenation of arterial blood) from ischemic hypoxia (hypoxia due to decreased arterial flow). At the cellular level the consequences of these two forms of hypoxia are different. This chapter relates only to the different types of hypoxia of hypoxemic origin, a relatively less known condition than ischemia, which has been amply documented in various other reviews or books.

B. Hypoxic and Ischemic Heart

In hypoxia due to hypoxemia there is a lack of oxygen supply, but the supply of blood and other substrates vital to metabolism remains normal, or even increased dependent on whether chronic or acute hypoxia is involved. Ischemia, on the other hand, involves not only a decrease in oxygen, blood, and metabolite supply but also a decrease in "myocardial washout," that is, a difficulty in the elimination of toxic metabolic degradation products, particularly lactic acid and H^+ ions. Therefore in hypoxia, cellular pH and enzymatic activity have a greater likelihood of remaining within normal limits.

Hypoxia is a generalized phenomenon uniformly distributed throughout the myocardium, as opposed to ischemia, which is localized to the area perfused by a stenosed arteriosclerotic artery or to the subendocardial zone in cases of pressure overload as encountered in severe aortic stenosis. The inequalities in myocardial perfusion not only result in a loss of equilibrium in the membrane potential and, as a consequence, electrical instability and arrhythmias, but also provoke contractility disturbances associated with hypo- or akinetic zones.

C. Types of Hypoxic Heart

There are two conditions in which the hypoxic heart can be considered as being physiological: the fetal or newborn heart and the heart of high-altitude inhabitants. The most common and natural type of hypoxic heart is the fetal heart, which survives in a very hypoxic environment. The P_{O_2} of "arterial" fetal blood corresponds to that found in the mountaineer or astronaut at an altitude of 8000 m without a supplementary O_2 supply. The fetal, and newborn, heart is particularly resistant to anoxia (total deprivation of O_2 supply), but unfortunately these resistant properties are fairly rapidly lost after birth in populations living at low altitude. In high-altitude populations (more than 25 million people live at altitudes over 3500 m) this resistance to relative hypoxia is partially maintained. Studies on high-altitude populations are of particular interest for the physiologist or clinician. Angina pectoris, myocardial infarction, and systemic arterial hypertension have been noted to be rare at high altitude. Hypoxia, therefore, appears to protect the heart from ischemia.

Two pathological conditions are associated with hypoxemic hypoxia: chronic cor pulmonale of various origins and cyanotic congenital heart disease. These pathological conditions are also found at high altitude and are greatly aggravated by the lack of O_2 in atmospheric air. The type of chronic cor pulmonale found at high altitude is called chronic mountain sickness or Monge disease or Soroche cronico.

D. Hypoxia and Other Factors

The various types of chronic hypoxic heart (normal and pathological) have various factors uncommon: hypoxemia of a greater or lesser severity, modifications of pulmonary vasculature (vasoconstriction, alterations of intima and/or media), and pulmonary hypertension of a greater or lesser importance. Some hypoxic hearts have other associated factors. In the high-altitude heart the influences of the cold, of the decreased air density, of the dryness of the air, and of solar ultraviolet radiation are of importance. In addition, adrenergic and other hormonal regulations are different from those encountered in inhabitants of low altitudes. In chronic cor pulmonale, apart from the hypoxemia, there is often, particularly during the decompensation stage, an associated hypercapnia, respiratory and/or metabolic acidosis, and an infectious state that are of nonnegligible importance. These patients are often elderly, and undiagnosed coronary lesions may be present. In congenital malformations, hypoxemia due to a right–left shunt or to a serious pulmonary pathology is often complicated by a pressure overload (valvular stenosis or atresia) or a volume overload (shunts or valvular insufficiency).

E. Acute and Chronic Hypoxia

The cardiac repercussions: anatomy, histology, ultrastructure, metabolism, contractility, coronary circulation, and hemodynamics are totally different, depending on whether acute hypoxia (from a few minutes to a few hours or even days) or chronic hypoxia (a few months, years, even generations) is involved. Concerning the coronary flow or lactic acid production, for example, acute hypoxia provoked by inhalation of an oxygen-poor gaseous mixture results in an important increase in coronary flow and appearance of anaerobic metabolism with lactic acid production, whereas in high-altitude populations living permanently at over 3500 m, the coronary flow is less than that of low-altitude populations and there are no signs of anaerobic metabolism. The delimitation between the acute and chronic stage is difficult to determine, studies effected in acute hypoxic conditions being by no means applicable to conditions of chronic hypoxia of several years duration.

F. History

The first observations relative to the effects of hypoxia date back to Plutarch, in his accounts of the conquests of India by Alexander the Great in 326 B.C. He speaks of "cardiorespiratory" difficulties affecting his troups during mountain passages due to the "unsteadiness of the atmosphere." The first reference to mountain sickness is due to an important chinese personality, Tu-Chhin, who, around 100 A.D., dissuaded his superiors from sending ambassadors to countries with "headache mountains"—probably the Himalayas. They provoked, as he said, not only headaches but also dizziness, vomiting, and a feeling of "malaise." The first detailed description of this illness and the first knowledge of the possibilities of adaptation to high altitude are, nevertheless, owed to Father José de Agosta, who accompanied Pizzaro on his conquests in Peru around 1590. It was three centuries later (1861) that Jourdanet then Bert established the scientific evidence that mountain sickness was due to an insufficient oxygenation of the blood. Since that time, numerous researchers have become interested in altitude and hypoxia in general: de Saussure, Gay-Lussac, Boyle, Andreoli, Viault, Douglas, Barcroft, Monge, Hurtado, without forgetting Cournand, to whom cardiorespiratory physiopathology owes a lot.

II. Anatomical and Histological Changes of the Hypoxic Heart

A. Ventricular Hypertrophy

1. Right Ventricle

Hypoxia is associated with right ventricular hypertrophy (RVH) secondary to pulmonary hypertension in practically all types of hypoxic heart: neonatal or fetal heart, high-altitude heart (normal or pathological), chronic cor pulmonale, and cyanotic congenital heart disease (particularly the Eisenmenger syndrome).

RVH of the high-altitude heart has been well documented. High altitude represents an excellent model for studying the repercussions of hypoxia on the heart and on pulmonary circulation. Van Liere in 1936 already noticed that a prolonged stay at an altitude of about 5000 m provoked, in the guinea pig, an increase in heart weight, without nevertheless specifying which ventricle was hypertrophied. It was to Rotta (1955), Valdivia (1957), Hurtado (1960), Arias-Stella and Recavarren (1962), and Hultgren et al., (1963) that we owe the first exact measures. With F. Duchosal and U. Lutzen we have studied the weight variations of the heart and of the right and left ventricles, in addition to the modifications in right and left ventricular pressures and aortic and pulmonary pressures of rats placed at an altitude of 3454 m (Research Laboratory of the Jungfraujoch, Swiss alps) during periods of 3 days to 12 weeks. Each series of rats, comprised of 12–15 male Wistar rats, was compared to other series of animals of the same strain and age kept at low altitude (Geneva, 340 m), with the same dietary, light, and temperature conditions (Moret, 1971–1972; Moret and Duchosal, 1973, 1976; Moret and Lutzen, 1977a; Moret et al., 1973, 1976).

The results are shown in Fig. 1. From the third day right ventricular weight increases rapidly, as objectivated by the ratio right ventricular wet weight (RV_w)/body weight (B_w). The RV weight increase on the third day is principally due to an increase in cellular hydration. The ratio RV dry weight (RV_{dw})/RV wet weight (ww) is decreased. This tissue edema is due to important metabolic alterations with a marked decrease in high-energy phosphate compounds (see Section IVB) accompanied by disturbances of acid–base balance and electrolytes and by histological alterations. It is only after the seventeenth day that true hypertrophy is installed. The rate of development of the ventricular hypertrophy is, nevertheless, fairly rapid, taking a few weeks: 3 to 4 weeks in our experiments, 5 weeks in the experiments of Abraham et al. (1971) and of Heath et al (1973). After 12 weeks, as shown in Fig. 1, the right ventricular weight is approximately 35% greater than that of the controls kept at low altitude. The variations in ventricular weight follow fairly closely, the variations in the mean pulmonary pressure.

The existence of RVH in altitude hypoxia has been noted by numerous authors. Its importance, however, varies according to species, age, and sex. It is very marked in cattle (Brisket disease), but also present in other animals. According to Hultgren and Miller (1967), the importance of the RVH is of decreasing magnitude in the following species: rabbit, guinea pig, dog, sheep, lamb, pig, and finally man, one of the least-sensitive species. According to Vogel *et al.* (1971), the dog would, however, be more resistant than man to the development of RVH, despite the presence of more severe pulmonary hypertension. The reasons for the differences between species are not apparent. RVH in the other forms of hypoxic heart has been well

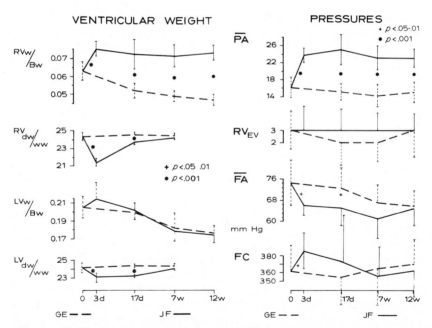

Fig. 1. Modifications in right ventricular (RV) and left ventricular (LV) weights, in mean pulmonary arterial ($\overline{PA}$) and femoral ($\overline{FA}$) pressures, in the right ventricular end-diastolic pressure (RV_{EV}), and in heart rate (FC) of rats placed at altitude (Jungfraujoch—JF) during 3 and 17 days, 7 and 12 weeks. These values are compared to those of animals kept at low altitude (Geneva—GE). RV_w/B_w or LV_w/B_w: ratio of RV or LV wet weight/body weight (B_w). $RV_{dw/ww}$ or $LV_{dw/ww}$: ratio of dry weight/wet weight for LV or RV.

documented, particularly in chronic cor pulmonale and in some cyanotic congenital heart diseases.

Providing the individual remains in a hypoxic environment, the RVH is permanently maintained. It regresses in a few months in individuals descending from a high altitude to a lower one. In the experimental animal this regression takes 5–10 weeks (Heath *et al.,* 1973; Widimsky *et al.,* 1973). In chronic cor pulmonale, the existence of this regression is known but is not always easy to detect clinically. In congenital cardiopathies it also regresses after correction of the associated anomalies (shunt or stenosis).

2. Left Ventricle

The presence of left ventricular hypertrophy (LVH) in chronic hypoxia has been the object of many controversies. In our experiments on rats at altitude (Fig. 1), we noted no development of LVH after 12 weeks of stay. On the third day the ratio of the left ventricular wet weight (LV_w) to body weight (B_W) increases slightly, but this is due, as in the right ventricle, to an increase in tissue water. This absence of development of LVH at altitude has been noted by various other authors, in both man and experimental animals (Recavarren and Arias-Stella, 1964; Wachtlova *et al.,* 1977; Widimsky *et al.,* 1973). Some authors (Burton and Smith, 1967; Van Liere *et al.,* 1965; Zhaparov and Mirrakhimov, 1977), nevertheless, have reported a LVH, but often in far from physiological conditions (very high altitude, very rapid or intermittent exposure to altitude or hypoxia). The causes of development of such a LVH are not clear; it is not impossible that important abrupt hemodynamic changes (e.g., an increase in cardiac output or heart rate) or repetitive adrenergic stimulation were of importance.

The presence of LVH in chronic cor pulmonale is debatable and has never been demonstrated with certitude (see Denolin, 1976). The prevalence of LVH in chronic cor pulmonale may vary from 0 to 85%. For some authors LVH is due to the existence of an associated pathology, such as systemic hypertension or undiagnosed coronary artery disease; for other it could be explained either by an intermittent phase of acute hypoxia favoring protein synthesis and hypertrophy of the whole heart or by acute hemodynamic or hematologic changes (e.g., an increase in cardiac output or blood volume). If the presence of LVH is disputed and rejected by many, the probability of the left ventricular function being often disturbed remains, but in our opinion, not for reasons due to hypoxia alone (see Section VA). It should be stressed that transposition of the great vessels, a frequent cyanotic congenital cardiopathy, is a good example of the small influence that pure hypoxia has on the development of LVH. The left ventricle diminishes in thickness because of its connection with the low-pressure pulmonary system, and this despite a severe hypoxemia.

B. Histological and Ultrastructural Changes

The changes in the histology and ultrastructure of the myocardium secondary to hypoxia depend on its importance, its duration (acute or chronic hypoxia), and the presence or absence of associated factors (physical effort, pressure overload).

1. Acute Hypoxia

Some experiments have been carried out under severe, short-lasting acute hypoxic conditions, particularly those conducted on the isolated heart using perfusion fluids very poor in O_2 ($P_{O_2} \leq 6$ mm Hg). These types of experiments are perhaps distant from real conditions (altitude or chronic cor pulmonale or cyanotic congenital cardiopathies), but they have served, on the one hand, to demonstrate that the myocardium is extremely resistant to hypoxia, providing the coronary perfusion is maintained, and, on the other hand, to specify the exact nature of the cellular alterations (Hearse *et al.*, 1976; Nayler and Fassold, 1977).

The ultrastructural lesions provoked by such a hypoxia consist essentially of rupture of the plasma membrane, cellular edema with mitochondrial distortion and vacuole formation, rupture of the myofilaments, development of contraction bands, aggregation of nuclear chromatin, loss of matrix density, vesiculation of the sarcoplasmic reticulum, and distortion or disintegration of the intercalated discs. According to Somogyi *et al.* (1976), these damages are preceded by alterations of the Z-bands that might form the morphological basis of the functional changes induced by hypoxia. The exact sequence of the ultrastructural changes has not been clarified. They are accompanied by important metabolic disturbances with glycogen loss, tissue edema, enzyme loss, electrolytic disturbances, and perturbation of Ca^{2+} exchange. If such hypoxias are of too long a duration, they inevitably lead to tissue necrosis. Some of these disturbances may also become of greater importance during the reoxygenation or reperfusion phase, with (again) a great variation between species (Ganote *et al.*, 1977; Hearse *et al.*, 1976).

2. Chronic Hypoxia

The different acclimatization phases at altitude have been thoroughly studied in order to analyze the effects of hypoxia on a longer-term basis (subacute and chronic). Unfortunately, the methods used are often variable. The ultrastructural modifications are apparent, particularly during the initial stage of exposure to the chronic hypoxia and may last for several weeks or months. Depending on the severity of the hypoxia or altitude, these modifications can lead to areas of necrosis, even after only a few hours exposure. According to Urbanova *et al.* (1977), histochemical techniques show minute myocardial changes in rats after four exposures of 4 hr daily at an altitude of 3000 m, and distinct changes after eight exposures at an altitude of 4500 m. Histologically, acute local necroses were evident in both ventricles after 11 exposures at an altitude of 6000 m or higher. They are of more importance if the animals are submitted to a physical effort (Eriskovskaya and Tsellarius, 1976). Scar tissue may develop with permanent fibrosis. Necrosis or ultrastructural lesions can be avoided or greatly diminished by protective myocardial agents (see Section VIIIB). It should be noted that such necrotic or scar lesions have never been described in young healthy men or animals living or born at high altitudes (e.g., the Andes or Himalayas).

After a certain duration of exposure to moderate hypoxia or altitude, an acclimatization progressively occurs, which is dependent on the species involved and its individual characteristics (e.g., genetic traits). The ultrastructural alterations will disappear. The cellular, and probably molecular, structures progressively resemble those of individuals living permanently at high altitude (Vergnes *et al.*, 1976). There is an increase in both mitochondrial mass and number. The mitochondrial internal structure is also modified in order to increase their efficiency (Meerson *et al.*, 1964; Ou and Tenney, 1970; Zhaparov and Mirrakhimov, 1976, 1977). For Eriskovskaya and Tsellarius (1976) and Kearney (1973) the ratio between mitochondrial mass and myofibrillar mass is, however, equal in subjects at low altitudes and in those acclimatized or adapted to high altitudes. For Harris (1977) the ultrastructure of the myocardium of high-altitude residents does not greatly differ from those living permanently at low altitude.

In chronic cor pulmonale, histological myocardial alterations have been noted by several authors (Samad and Noehren, 1965; Seley, 1958; Weinschenk, 1939). The lesions consist principally of small zones of necrosis with fibrosis disseminated throughout the myocardium in both the right and left ventricles. According to Samad and Noehren (1965), they are frequent, being present in up to 30% of their cases. They could be responsible for the left ventricular dysfunction reported by various authors (see Section VA), for the electrocardiographic alterations with, occasionally, images of myocardial pseudonecrosis (Moret *et al.*, 1966a), or for the disturbances in intraventricular conduction. These alterations can be compared with the earlier description concerning acclimatization to high altitude. They have been produced experimentally in animals by creating respiratory insufficiency by tracheal stenosis and development of emphysema and chronic bronchitis, or by a pulmonary resection of up to 80% (Konopinski and Zimnoch, 1976; Loiko *et al.*, 1976). In chronic cor pulmonale the lesions can be provoked by an acute phase of cardiopulmonary decompensation with marked hypoxia, acidosis, and hypercapnia. They could also be favored by the presence of undiagnosed coronary lesions. According to Mitchell *et al.* (1968), 60% of autopsied cases of obstructive bronchopneumopathies reveal a significant coronary stenosis.

In congenital cardiopathies histological and ultrastructural alterations secondary to hypoxia alone are difficult to demonstrate because of the existence of almost inevitable associated lesions. It appears that hypoxia alone of moderate severity (arterial saturation > 70%) rarely results in cellular disturbances. The additive effect of pressure or volume overload is a factor favoring cellular degeneration with the appearance of fibrosis, cellular atrophy, and lipids deposits, as recently demonstrated by Jones and Ferrans (1977). Krymsky (1965) reported, however, small infarctions of the left ventricle in cases of tetralogy of Fallot.

III. Coronary Vessels and Coronary Flow

A. Coronary Vessels

1. Coronary Arteries

The influence of chronic hypoxia on the diameter and number of large coronary arteries, on the secondary branches, and on the arterioles and capillaries is actually well known. Kerr *et al.* (1965a) have shown that the intraluminal volume of the coronary artery network in rats, excluding the capillaries, practically doubles when the rats are submitted to 2 hr a day at an altitude of 22,000 ft (6600 m) during 20 days. Arias-Stella and Topilsky (1971) have confirmed the greater myocardial vascularization of both ventricles in residents of high altitude, with also an increased number of intercoronary anastomoses. This has also been demonstrated in chronic cor pulmonale and in certain cyanotic congenital cardiopathies (Bjork, 1966; Kerr *et al.*, 1965b; Krymsky, 1965; Moffitt *et al.*, 1970; Perloff *et al.*, 1968; Zimmerman, 1952).

2. Capillaries

Like the arteries, the number and volume of capillaries also increase in all types of hypoxia (Anthony and Kreider, 1961; Diemer, 1968; Krymsky, 1965; Miller and Hale, 1970; Stere and Anthony, 1977; Tenney and Ou, 1970; Valdivia *et al.*, 1960; Zimmerman, 1952). For Eriskovskaya and Tsellarius (1976) the increase in number occurs from preexisting capillaries; for Stere and Anthony (1977) there is a formation of new capillaries. It is probable that part of the capillary network is out of use during rest but that it constitutes a greater coronary reserve, which could explain the greater resistance to anoxia or ischemia of residents at high altitude or of patients with cyanotic congenital heart diseases (see Section VIIIB).

The increase in number and volume of capillaries probably constitutes the most important phenomenon of adaptation to chronic hypoxia. It should be remembered that the number of capillaries in a given tissue does not solely depend on the O_2 consumption of the tissue but that it is directly related to the O_2 partial pressure of the perfusing blood. When this P_{O_2} diminishes, the number and the diameter of the capillaries must rise in order to decrease the diffusion distance.

B. Coronary Flow

1. Acute Hypoxia

The effects of acute hypoxia on the coronary circulation have been well documented. There is an instantaneous vasodilation and an increase in flow, which can be up to four to five times that of the basal flow rate (Berne et al., 1957; Eckenhoff et al., 1947; Moret et al., 1964). Figure 2 represents the variation of coronary flow ($\dot{Q}$ cor), and of the coronary vascular resistance when the arterial saturation in O_2 is progressively diminished by decreasing the O_2 concentration of inspired air in the dog. The $\dot{Q}$ cor increases and the O_2 saturation of the coronary sinus venous blood decreases. The percentage O_2 extraction [$\Delta(a\text{-}v)O_2/aO_2$] increases.

Once the arterial saturation attains about 35%, both the $\dot{Q}$ cor and the O_2 extraction by the myocardium have reached a maximum; the coronary venous saturation is then in the order of 15% (P_{O_2}: 10–15 mm Hg). Beyond these limits, myocardial metabolism becomes anaerobic, with release of lactate into the coronary sinus. The left ventricular end-diastolic pressure rises, cardiac insufficiency rapidly occurs, and the animal dies. These experiments, like many others, demonstrate the powerful coronary vasodilatory effect of acute hypoxia. The same does not apply to chronic hypoxia.

2. Chronic Hypoxia

In chronic hypoxia due to high altitude, to chronic cor pulmonale, or to congenital cardiopathies, the coronary flow either may remain within the normal range and comparable to that of normoxic subjects or may be inferior to the normal range.

a. HIGH-ALTITUDE HYPOXIA

The coronary flow of normal subjects born at or permanently resident at high altitude (High Plateaus of Andes) was measured for the first time in

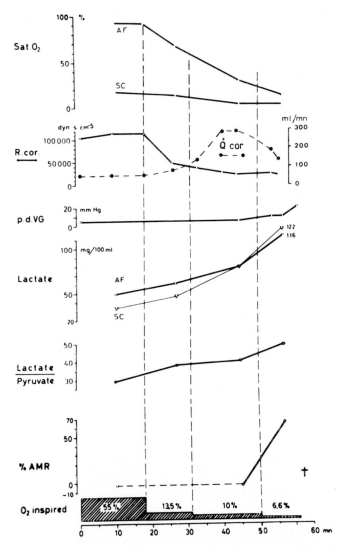

Fig. 2. Variations during acute hypoxemia in O_2 saturation (Sat O_2) of femoral arterial blood (AF) and of coronary sinus venous blood (SC), in coronary vascular resistances (R. cor.), in coronary flow (Q cor), in the left ventricular end-diastolic pressure (p.d. VG), in the lactate content of femoral arterial (AF) and coronary sinus venous (SC) blood, in the ratio lactate/pyruvate, and in the percentage of anaerobic metabolism (% AMR) according to Huckabee. At the lower part of the figure, variations in the percentage of O_2 in the inspired gaseous mixture.

1969 (Moret, 1971, 1971–1972, 1976; Moret *et al.,* 1970, 1972). During this survey, we studied, with the collaboration of Peruvian and Bolivian colleagues, three groups of healthy subjects born or permanently resident at three different altitudes: Lima, Peru (150 m or 492 ft altitude); La Paz, Bolivia (3700 m or 12,130 ft altitude); and Cerro de Pasco, Peru (4375 m, or 14,350 ft altitude). In addition to these groups of healthy subjects, six patients affected by chronic mountain sickness—or Monge disease or Soroche cronico—were studied.

i. Normal subjects. The results concerning coronary flow measured in the three groups of normal subjects, aged 18–36 (average, 23 years), are represented in Fig. 3. One notes that the coronary flow/min per 100 g of left ventricular mass ($\dot{Q}$ cor/min/100 g LV) is markedly lower at high altitude. The coronary vascular resistances, not shown on this figure, pass from approximately 112,000 dynes sec cm^{-5} at 150 m altitude to 180,000 at 4375 m. The oxygen delivery or supply (coronary flow × oxygen content of arterial blood) also diminishes with increasing altitude. The decrease in coronary flow and the drop in arterial oxygen saturation (95% at 150 m, 82% at 4375 m) at high altitude are not compensated for by the rise in the hematocrit (45% at 150 m, 52% at 4375 m). The mycardial oxygen supply remains, nevertheless, totally adequate. The percentage oxygen extraction (extraction coefficient) by the myocardium remains similar at the three

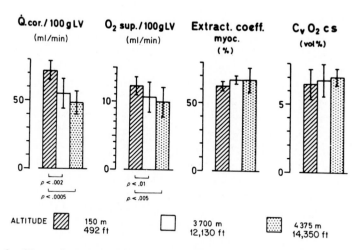

Fig. 3. Mean values with standard deviations of the coronary flow ($\dot{Q}$ cor.—ml/min/100 g LV), of the oxygen supply (O$_2$ sup.—ml/min/100 g LV), of the myocardial O$_2$ extraction coefficient (Extract. coeff. myoc.), and of the O$_2$ content of the coronary sinus blood (Cv$_{O_2}$cs—ml/100 ml of blood) in three groups of normal subjects living permanently at three different altitudes.

different altitudes (at 65% approximately). The oxygen content of the coronary sinus venous blood is also unchanged, as is the coronary venous P_{O_2}. Metabolic studies (see Section IVB) confirm the adequate oxygen supply to the myocardium and the absence of signs of anaerobic metabolism or lactate production by the myocardium. This decrease in coronary flow with altitude has been confirmed by other authors, particularly by Grover et al. (1970), who studied normal subjects transfered from sea level to an altitude of 3100 m, also by Manchanda et al. (1973) and Roy (1973) on residents of the high plateaus of the Himalayas (12,000 ft., 3500 m). All these studies used the N_2O) dilution technique to determine the coronary flow. Recently Maseri et al. (1976), using radioisotopes, also confirmed our results. It can thus be considered that permanent residents of high altitudes (over 3000 m) have a 20–30% lower coronary flow per unit of muscular mass than inhabitants of low altitudes. Similar values have also been found in animal studies (Vogel et al., 1970).

The regulation of coronary flow in high-altitude subjects is the same as that for low-altitude subjects. The coronary network is capable of dilating normally during exercise, or acute hypoxia in both man and animal (Grover et al., 1976a; Maseri et al., 1976; Moret et al., 1972). The reasons for the diminished coronary flow in normal subjects at high altitude and in a few cyanotic congenital cardiopathies will be discussed later (see Sections IV, VI,VII).

ii. Chronic mountain sickness or Monge disease or Soroche cronico. The physiopathology of Monge disease is badly known. It could be compared to a variant of chronic high-altitude cor pulmonale. It would be due to primary alveolar hypoventilation (Hurtado, 1960; Monge, 1943; Peñaloza et al., 1971). It is characterized by an important cardiorespiratory insufficiency with significant pulmonary hypertension and a high hematocrit (Hct). In the six patients we studied (Moret, 1971, 1976), the average age was 44 years—23 for the normal subjects (N) living at the same altitude; the Hct was 69% (N: 50%), the mean pulmonary arterial pressure was 35 mm Hg (N: 23), and the O_2 arterial saturation was 79% (N: 86%). Figure 4 shows the coronary flow ($\dot{Q}$ cor/min/100 g LV) and O_2 supply to be higher ($p < 0.001$). The oxygen content and saturation of the coronary venous blood are practically identical in the two groups. The study of myocardial metabolism has shown, despite the increased supply of O_2 and blood, disturbances in aerobic metabolism (see Section IVB).

b. CYANOTIC CONGENITAL HEART DISEASES.

The coronary flow in congenital cardiopathies has also been relatively little studied. Bernsmeier and Rudolph (1961), Rudolph (1971–1972), Rudolph et al. (1967), and Scheuer et al. (1970a) have shown that, as at

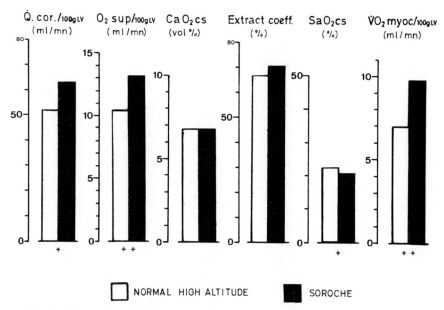

Fig. 4.   Mean values of coronary flow ($\dot{Q}$ cor.—ml/min/100 g LV), of the oxygen supply (O_2 sup.—ml/min/100 g LV), of the O_2 content of coronary sinus blood ($Ca_{O_2}cs$—ml/100 ml of blood), of the myocardial O_2 extraction coefficient (Extract. coeff.), of the O_2 saturation of coronary sinus blood ($Sa_{O_2}cs$), and of the myocardial O_2 consumption ($\dot{V}_{O_2}$ myoc.—ml/min/ 100 g LV), in patients affected by chronic mountain sickness, or Monge disease or Soroche cronico. These values are compared to those of normal subjects residing at the same altitude.

high altitude, the coronary flow per 100 g of ventricular mass is diminished when compared to that of the normal. When this low coronary flow is accompanied by an important desaturation of arterial blood (below 70% approx.), there may be associated metabolic disturbances with lactate production (see Section IVB). This lactate production during important O_2 desaturation of arterial blood has also been demonstrated by Friedli et al. (1977).

c. Chronic cor pulmonale

In chronic cor pulmonale, secondary to obstructive chronic bronchitis, the coronary flow per unit of myocardial mass is not increased. It remains practically equal to that of healthy and normoxic subjects. It was Rose and Hoffman in 1956 who produced the first results, later confirmed by Fukuda (1966), Hosono (1965), Moret et al. (1966a), and Rudolph and Fruhman (1966).

Figure 5 represents the results we obtained from a survey of 30 subjects affected by chronic cor pulmonale consecutive to obstructive chronic bron-

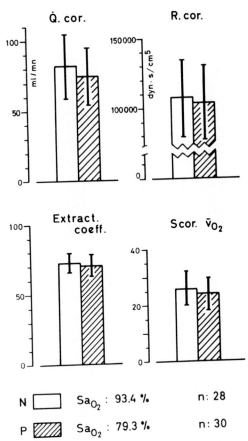

Fig. 5. Mean values, with standard deviations, of coronary flow ($\dot{Q}$ cor.—ml/min/100 g LV), of the coronary vascular resistance (R. cor.), of the myocardial O_2 extraction coefficient (Extract. coeff.), of the O_2 saturation of coronary sinus blood (S cor. $\overline{V}_{O_2}$) in 30 patients affected by chronic cor pulmonale (P). These values are compared to those of 28 normal subjects (N).

chitis (Moret, 1968). The arterial O_2 saturation in these 30 patients, with a mean age of 57, is an average 79%. The results were compared to a group of 28 normal subjects (average age 48) with an arterial saturation of 93%. One notes that the coronary flows ($\dot{Q}$ cor/min/100 g LV) are practically identical for the normal group and for the patients presenting chronic cor pulmonale. The coronary vascular resistance and the O_2 extraction coefficient are equal, as is the O_2 content of the coronary venous blood. Despite the absence of differences between the two groups there exists, at the metabolic level, evidence of perfusion insufficiencies in about 50% of our patients (see

Section IV), with disturbances of aerobic metabolism and a diminution of myocardial extraction of lactates. These metabolic alterations have been confirmed by others (Frank *et al.,* 1973; Fukuda, 1966; Hosono, 1965; Rudolph and Fruhman, 1966). Rudolph (1971–1972) occasionally found an increased coronary flow in patients with markedly diminished arterial O_2 saturation to around 60%. The regulation of coronary circulation is normal in chronic cor pulmonale and capable of increasing under stress, such as physical exercise or additional acute hypoxia (Frank *et al.,* 1973; Hosono, 1965; Moret, 1966, 1968).

IV. Myocardial Metabolism

The metabolic or biochemical processes of the myocardium are very complex; as a result it is not possible to cover all the aspects in this review. We will consider factors concerning energy-producing metabolism; O_2 consumption and mechanical efficiency, the utilization of the main substrates generally extracted by the myocardium (glucose, lactate, pyruvate, and free fatty acids), intracellular metabolites contents, and the reciprocal importance of aerobic and anaerobic metabolism. These aspects of energy metabolism concern particularly chronic hypoxia data (acclimatization and adaptation), with at first a short review on the normal energy-producing metabolism and the effects of acute hypoxia. At the end of the chapter, protein synthesis and mechanisms leading to ventricular hypertrophy are briefly discussed.

A. Normal Energy Metabolism and Effect of Acute Hypoxia

Myocardial metabolism is almost uniquely aerobic. Enzymatically, the myocardium is badly equipped for working in conditions lacking oxygen or blood supply. The principal substrates utilized by the heart are glucose, lactate, pyruvate, and free fatty acids (FFA). Glucose supplies approximately 20–30% of the total energy used by the heart; lactate, 10–20%; pyruvate, 1%; and free fatty acids, about 70%. Various conditions determine the relative percentages of each sustance used: fasting, exercise, altitude, adrenergic activity, etc. The myocardium can also use triglycerides, ketone bodies, or amino acids (see Opie, 1969).

The energy-producing pathways in conditions of normal oxygen supply are summarized in Fig. 6. Glucose is degraded to pyruvate following the classical pathway of anaerobic glycolysis (Embden-Meyerhof). Lactate, which is absorbed by the heart in conditions of normal oxygenation, is converted to pyruvate and enters the Krebs cycle. The Krebs cycle is a "melting pot" from which energy in the form of H^+ ions is produced. Direct coupling of H^+ to

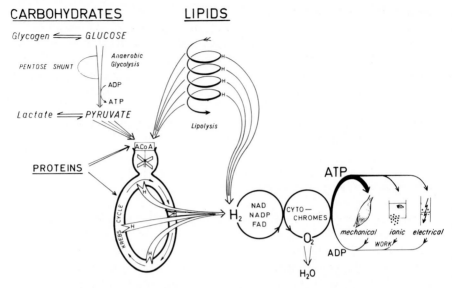

Fig. 6.   Outline of the energy-producing myocardial metabolism.

oxygen is impossible because it is too explosive. Therefore the hydrogen will progressively liberate its energy by means of the electron transport chain (NAD, NADP, FAD, cytochromes), to be finally eliminated in the form of water by binding to oxygen. The energy liberated by the hydrogen during its passage via the respiratory chain will serve to reform ATP from ADP by the process of oxidative phosphorylation. ATP will be partially stocked in the form of creatine phosphate (CrP); together they will constitute the energy reserves for the whole of the myocardial activities. About 70% of the energy produced by the heart is used in contraction, the remaining 30% being used for other functions (e.g., ionic pumps, electrical conduction, electromechanical excitation, and protein synthesis). Fatty acids follow, more or less, the same metabolic pathway, being initially split into two-carbon groups that will enter the Krebs cycle. This splitting will also be accompanied by production of H^+ ions, which will follow the electron transport chain. This is the principle of beta oxidation. Fatty acid metabolism is practically entirely intramitochondrial and O_2 dependent.

   The anaerobic glycolysis pathway alone is very little used by the normal heart for production of ATP. It offers little return from the energy aspect: one molecule of glucose produces only two molecules of ATP by this pathway, whereas in conditions of sufficient oxygenation permitting complete glucose combustion by the regular pathways of Krebs cycle and the respiratory chain, this same molecule of glucose is capable of producing 38 molecules of ATP. From the aspect of energy production, fatty acids are the greatest producers, since one molecule of palmitic acid, in the presence of oxygen, provides sufficient energy for the reconstruction of 130 ATP molecules.

A lack of oxygen supply inhibits all aerobic metabolism. In severe hypoxia the hydrogen transporting system is blocked, the Krebs cycle is incapable of functioning, and ATP synthesis is seriously impaired. Anaerobic glycolysis remains the only possibility for ATP production. Glucose is degraded, as usual, to pyruvic acid, but instead of entering the Krebs cycle, it is reduced to lactic acid, which starts accumulating. The energy return from this pathway is poor. The heart increases its glucose consumption and borrows from its glycogen reserves. Lactate extraction diminishes, and in cases of marked hypoxia, important quantities will be produced and shed into coronary venous blood. Fatty acid extraction may follow, but it is transformed into neutral fats and deposited in cells. ATP and CrP synthesis decreases, and the intracellular level of CrP and ATP diminishes and that of ADP, AMP, and P rises. Mitochondrial function and their anatomical appearance show important alterations. These disturbances of energy-producing metabolism are associated with disturbances in electrolytes and acid–base balance. The intracellular pH becomes progressively more acidic. K^+ leaves the cell to be replaced by Na^+, associated with an escape of Ca^{2+} and Mg^{2+} and an entry into the cell of water and Cl^-. These metabolic and electrolytic disturbances result in perturbations of the electrical and mechanical comportment of the heart.

B. Energy-Producing Metabolism in Chronic Hypoxia

1. Mycardial O_2 Consumption and Mechanical Efficiency

The myocardial tissue has, per unit of muscle mass, the greatest O_2 consumption of the whole organism. In chronic hypoxia, particularly of altitude, the oxygen consumption by the myocardium is less than that at lower altitudes. Figure 7 shows the values of myocardial O_2 consumption/min/100 g of left ventricular mass ($\dot{V}_{O_2}$ cor/min/100 g LV) that we determined in three population groups of young healthy subjects living permanently at three different altitudes: 150 m, 3700 m, and 4375 m. The results are compared to those we obtained in patients affected by chronic cor pulmonale and chronic mountain sickness—Monge disease or Soroche cronico (see Section IIIB).

At high altitudes the $\dot{V}_{O_2}$ cor/min/100 g LV is markedly lower than that at low altitudes. Because the cardiac output, heart rate, and mean aortic pres-

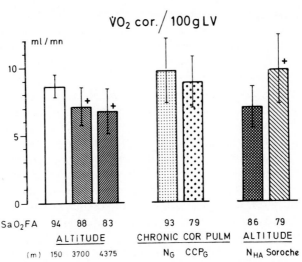

Fig. 7. Comparative values of myocardial O_2 consumption $\dot{V}_{O_2}$ cor.—ml/min/100 g LV) in different types of hypoxic heart. *On the left:* Normal subjects living permanently at different altitudes. *In the center:* Patients affected by chronic cor pulmonale (CCP_G) compared to normal subjects living at the same altitude (Geneva N_G). *On the right:* Patients affected by chronic mountain sickness or Soroche cronico, compared to normal subjects living at the same altitude (high altitude:N_{HA}). $Sa_{O_2}FA$: O_2 saturation of femoral arterial blood. +, Statistically significant.

sure are practically the same for all three groups, the external cardiac mechanical efficiency (myocardial $\dot{V}_{O_2}$/left ventricular external work) is markedly improved at high altitudes, being about 31% at 150 m, 38% at 3700 m, and 40% at 4375 m (Moret, 1971; Moret *et al.,* 1970, 1972).

In chronic cor pulmonale the $\dot{V}_{O_2}$ cor/min/100 g LV of patients with chronic cor pulmonale is practically identical to that of healthy controls residing at the same altitude (Geneva) (Moret, 1968; Moret *et al.,* 1966b).

In Soroche cronico or Monge disease, the $\dot{V}_{O_2}$ cor/min/100 g LV is greater than in the normal subjects living at the same high altitude (Moret, 1971, 1976). In the two groups of patients with chronic cor pulmonale of low altitude (Geneva, 340 m) and Monge disease of high altitude, the cardiac mechanical efficiency was not calculated.

A less important myocardial oxygen consumption in some forms of chronic hypobaric hypoxia has been found by other authors (Barbashova, 1964; Duckworth, 1961; Manchanda *et al.,* 1973; Maseri *et al.,* 1976; Roy, 1973). It has also been reported in certain cyanotic congenital cardiopathies (Bernsmeier and Rudolph, 1961; Moffitt *et al.,* 1970). However, other authors could not confirm this finding (Grover *et al.,* 1970; Rudolph,

1971–1972; Rudolph *et al.,* 1967; Scheuer *et al.,* 1970a,b). The reasons for the diminution of O_2 consumption and an improved cardiac mechanical efficiency are discussed later.

2. Substrate Utilization and Energy Supply

As stated earlier, the four principal substrates utilized by the heart as an energy source are glucose, lactate, pyruvate, and free fatty acids (FFA). Pyruvate does not play an important part in the supply of energy, but its role in the metabolic pathways is of capital importance, since it is situated at the junction between anaerobic glycolysis and the Krebs cycle. The energy supplied to the myocardium for each of these four main substrates, termed also the *O_2 extraction ratio,* can be fairly precisely calculated (Bernsmeier and Rudolph, 1961; Opie, 1969).

The arterial level, the coronary arteriovenous (a-v) difference, the myocardial consumption or extraction, and the energy supplied (O_2 extraction ratio) are compared in Table I for each of the four main substrates utilized by the heart in the different types of hypoxic heart.

a. HIGH-ALTITUDE HYPOXIA

At high altitude one notes that the arterial glucose level or content diminishes with increasing altitude; the coronary a-v difference and the myocardial consumption remain the same. The arterial level of lactate increases with altitude, as does the coronary a-v difference and myocardial consumption. The same is applicable to pyruvate. For FFA neither the arterial level nor the a-v difference vary with altitude; on the other hand, at high altitude the myocardial consumption is lower. For details of the values see Moret (1971, 1976) and Moret *et al.* (1970, 1972).

The regulations that govern the penetration of the different substrates into the myocardium are the same at both high and low altitudes. The heart performs a certain selection between the different substrates, and competition exists, for example, between carbohydrates and lipids, between lactate and glucose, and between FFA and pyruvate.

Our studies on the utilization of substrates at altitude strongly suggest that there are no signs of insufficient myocardial perfusion or oxygenation, since lactate production does not occur. On the contrary, lactate consumption is increased at altitude. The lactate/pyruvate (L/P) ratio remains constant.

The energy supplied to the heart by each of these substrates (O_2 extraction ratio) is more or less equal for glucose at both low and high altitudes (approximately 35%). Energy production from lactate, however, shows a marked increase with altitude: 9% at 150 m, 22% at 3700 m, and 25% at 4375 m ($p < 0.0005$). Energy supplied from pyruvate also increases with

TABLE I

Chronic Cor Pulmonale[a,b]

	Glucose (G)			Lactate (L)			Pyruvate (P)			L/P	FFA			O₂ extraction ratio				
	Art. cont.	A-V diff.	V or extr.	Art. cont.	A-V diff.	V or extr.	Art. cont.	A-V diff.	V or extr.	CS	Art. cont.	A-V diff.	V or extr.	G	L	P	FFA	Total
High altitude Moret et al. (1972)																		
3700 m Sa₀₂ 88% (R)	↗	=	=	↗	↗	↗	↗	↗	↗	=	=	=	↗	=	↗	↗	=	=
4375 m Sa₀₂ 83% (R)	↗↗	=	=	↗↗	↗↗	↗↗	↗	↗	↗	=	=	=	(↘)	=	↗↗	↗↗	↗	=
Chronic cor pulmonale Moret et al. (1966b)																		
Sa₀₂ 82% (R)	=	(↗)	↗	=	(↘)	↗	=	=	=	↗	(↗)	=	=	(↗)	↗	=	=	=
Rudolph (1971–1972)	=	↗	↗	=	=	=	=	=	=	—	↗	=	↗	↗	=	(↗)	=	↗
Chronic mountain sickness Moret (1971)																		
Sa₀₂ 79% (R)	=	↗↗	↗↗	=	(↘)	(↘)	=	↗	↗	(↗)	=	↗	↗	↗↗	(↘)	=	↗	↗
Congenital heart disease Scheuer et al. (1970a)																		
Sa₀₂ 83% (R)	=	=	=	=	=	=	—	—	—	=	=	=	=	(=)	(=)	(=)	(=)	(=)
Sa₀₂ 66% (S)	=	=	—	↗	=	—	—	—	—	↗	=	=	=	(=)	(=)	(=)	(=)	(=)
Rudolph (1971–1972)																		
Sa₀₂ 86% (R)	=	=	=	=	=	=	=	=	=	=	=	↗	↗↗	=	=	(=)	↗↗	=
Sa₀₂ 70% (R)	=	↗	=	↗	=	(↘)	↗	=	(↘)	(↗)	↗	↗	↗	↗	=	—	↗	↗
Friedli et al. (1977)																		
Sa₀₂ 77% (R)	—	—	—	↗	=	=	—	—	—	=	—	—	—	—	—	—	—	—
Sa₀₂ 58% (S)	—	—	—	↗	↗	↗↗	—	—	—	(↗)	—	—	—	—	—	—	—	—

[a] Comparative values of the utilization of substrates by the myocardium and the respective energy supplied (O₂ extraction ratio). Art. cont. = arterial content or level. A-V diff. = arteriovenous difference. V or extr. = consumption (V) or percentage extraction by the myocardium (Extr.). L/P CS = lactate/pyruvate ratio in coronary sinus (CS) venous blood. Sa₀₂ = O₂ saturation of arterial blood. R = values at rest. S = values during stress: exercise or atrial pacing.

[b] Sign explanation: ↗, ↘, = : increase, decrease, or no change when compared to the control values. — : values not mentioned or not measured by the authors. Values in brackets: hardly significant differences.

altitude but remains low. Free fatty acids (FFA) remain the most important energy suppliers, but a supply that does not particularly change with altitude and probably even has a tendency to diminish with increasing altitude. The energy contribution by FFA is on the order of 68% at 150 m, 65% at 3700 m, and 52% at 4375 m. These differences are nonsignificant, but this is probably due to the method of determination used (Kelley, 1965). The preceding values have been partially confirmed by Grover *et al.* (1970, 1976a). Nevertheless, to our knowledge, no other studies comparable to our own, relating to the utilization of all substrates and the energy supplied by each one, have yet been published. The absence of signs of anaerobic metabolism has not been confirmed by Roy (1973) and Manchanda *et al.* (1973). They did note an increase in arterial levels of lactate with altitude, but its extraction by the myocardium was slightly diminished, leaving one to suspect, in opposition to our observations, slight metabolic disturbances. Nevertheless, they did find, as we did, a decreased myocardial oxygen consumption and an improved cardiac mechanical efficiency at high altitude.

b. Chronic cor pulmonale

In chronic cor pulmonale we found (Table I) definite signs of insufficient oxygenation of the myocardium with an increase in glucose consumption and a decrease in consumption of lactate. For details of the values see Moret (1966, 1968) and Moret *et al.* (1966b). The utilization or consumption of pyruvate was not perturbed, but the ratio L/P in the coronary sinus was raised. These metabolic disturbances were observed in 47% of our patients. The use of free fatty acids was not modified when compared to the normal.

The metabolic alterations of the "anoxic or ischemic" kind observed in our patients with chronic cor pulmonale are not necessarily imputable, in our opinion, to hypoxemia alone. It is possible that the relatively advanced age of the patients (average: 57 years) may have played a role (undiagnosed coronary lesions), as may have other factors (see Section VD). These metabolic disturbances could be responsible for the anatomical, electrocardiographic, and hemodynamic alterations described in chronic cor pulmonale (see Section IIA, VA). These metabolic alterations have also been reported by other authors, particularly Hosono (1965) and Rudolph and Fruhman (1966). Certain disturbances in metabolism, particularly of lactate, may only become apparent during a physical effort. However, Frank *et al.* (1973), both during exercise and rest, found no metabolic disturbances of lactate or pyruvate, though the group studied involved a small number of patients, who were, in addition, very heterogeneous. Rudolph and Fruhman (1966) have shown that the hypoxia-provoked metabolic disturbances, when apparent, are reversible by the inhalation of an O_2-rich gaseous mixture.

c. CHRONIC MOUNTAIN SICKNESS—MONGE
DISEASE—SOROCHE CRONICO

The investigations performed on six patients affected by chronic mountain sickness (see Section IIIB) demonstrated that, as in severe acute hypoxia, the myocardial glucose consumption is markedly increased (Table I). Lactate consumption is little diminished, but nonsignificantly, probably because of the small number of patients examined. Pyruvate a-v difference and consumption are decreased and the ratio L/P of the sinus blood is raised. For details of values see Moret (1971, 1976).

As far as the energy supplied by each of the substrates is concerned, for glucose it passes from 35% in normal subjects living at the same altitude to 45% ($p < 0.01$). For lactate the value diminishes from 25 to 12% (NS), and for FFA there is a rise from 52 to 67% (p < 0.01). The values remain unchanged for pyruvate. The total energy supplied by the four different substrates largely exceeds 100%. This is probably due to the fact that FFA are extracted by the myocardium but are stored in the cell not being used for energy production and that part of the glucose may be utilized only through the anaerobic energy production.

From these data it can be seen that in Monge disease, despite an increased coronary flow, metabolic disturbances of the "ischemic or anoxic" type exist, which resemble the alterations described earlier in chronic cor pulmonale.

d. CONGENITAL HEART DISEASE

There are few studies on myocardial metabolism in congenital cardiopathies (Bernsmeier and Rudolph, 1961; Friedli et al., 1977; Graham et al., 1977; Greene and Talner, 1964; Moffitt et al., 1970; Rudolph, 1971–1972; Rudolph et al., 1967; Scheuer et al., 1970a). In general, one can see from Table I that, as in high-altitude subjects, there is little modification in glucose metabolism. The same applies to lactate metabolism, providing the arterial oxygen saturation is not too radically decreased either spontaneously—as in the study conducted by Rudolph (1971–1972)—or after a stress, such as exercise, isuprenaline administration, or atrial pacing (Friedli et al., 1977; Graham et al., 1977; Scheuer et al., 1970a). Generally, when the arterial saturation falls below about 70%, metabolic disturbances of the "anoxic or ischemic" type become apparent, resembling those encountered in chronic cor pulmonale or chronic mountain sickness. The a-v difference and/or consumption of FFA are either normal or lower than in the healthy normoxic subject (Moffitt et al., 1970; Rudolph, 1971–1972).

3. Intracellular Metabolic Changes

Numerous works have been devoted to the intracellular metabolic modifications in relation to energy metabolism during acute hypoxia (see

Sections IIB, IVA). In this section we will review first the intracellular changes apparent in animals after exposure to hypoxia lasting a few days to a few months—acclimatization to hypoxia—and second the small amount of data collected from biopsies of hearts (human or animal) submitted to prolonged hypoxia during several years and adapted to hypoxia.

a. ACCLIMATIZATION TO HYPOXIA

Investigations performed for several years on rats exposed to an altitude of 3454 m (Jungfraujoch Research Laboratory in the Swiss Alps, see Section IIA) will serve as an example of the different modifications involving the intracellular metabolites. These animals (male Wistar rats) stayed at this altitude for periods ranging from 3 days to 50 weeks. Each series of animals, composed of 10–12 rats, was compared to other series kept at Geneva (340 m) (Moret and Duchosal, 1973, 1976; Moret et al., 1973, 1976; Vergnes et al., 1976). Some of the results of this long-term study are represented in Figs. 8 and 9. One can distinguish two main phases during exposition to chronic hypoxia: (1) an *early* phase during 7–12 weeks characterized by intensive alterations in energy-producing metabolism and (2) a *late* phase,

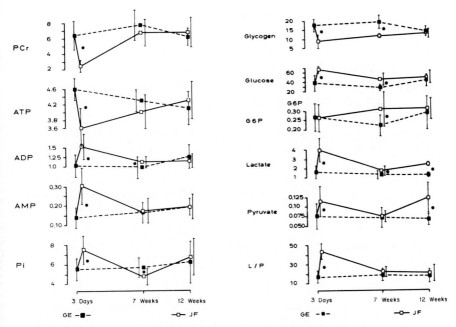

Fig. 8.   Variations in the different myocardial metabolites in the rat during stays of variable duration (3 days, 7 and 12 weeks) at high altitude: Jungfraujoch (JF). The values are compared to those of control animals kept at low altitude: Geneva (GE).

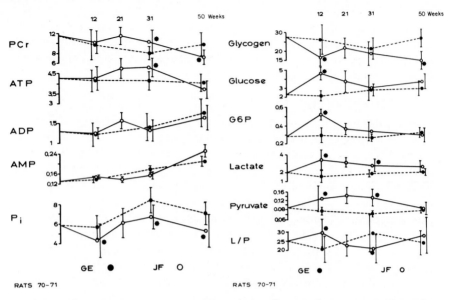

Fig. 9.   The same variation in myocardial metabolites for stays of 12, 21, 31, and 50 weeks.

starting from the twelfth to twentieth week, into which the various adaptation mechanisms fall.

i. Early Phase.   The principal modifications occurring during this period are found in Fig. 8. One remarks profound alterations in energy-rich products with a decrease in creatine phosphate (CrP) and ATP and a corresponding increase in ADP, AMP, and inorganic phosphate (P_i). These disturbances are particularly marked on the third day. By the twelfth week virtually all values have returned to normal. The principal modifications in glycolysis are manifested by an important rise in lactate (L), pyruvate (P), and the ratio L/P on the third day, where one also notes an important drop in myocardial glycogen and a rise in glucose. These metabolic alterations are slower to correct than those of CrP or ATP. By the twelfth week, disturbances of lactate and pyruvate still persist. At the blood level, there is also an increase in lactate, pyruvate, and the L/P ratio, but only on the third day, beyond which time the differences with low-altitude animals are no longer significant.

ii. Late phase.   Figure 9 illustrates the late phase, during which a new cellular equilibrium is attained. (These experiments were conducted on another group of animals, thus explaining the different results of the twelfth week on Figs. 8 and 9). At the twenty-first and thirty-first weeks, as Fig. 9

demonstrates, the CrP and ATP values are normal and even superior to those of the control animals in Geneva; the values of ADP and AMP are also comparable. The P_i, however, is below control values, whereas the glycogen, glucose, and glucose-6-phosphate values are as abnormal at the twelfth week return to the control values as at the twenty-first week. Lactate and pyruvate, on the other hand, remain high until the thirty-first week.

The effects of various so-called myocardial protective substances on metabolic alterations in the early phase—beta blockers (propranolol, practolol, alprenolol), alpha blockers (phenoxybenzamine, raubasine), and piridoxilate—have been evaluated (Moret and Duchosal, 1976; Moret and Lutzen, 1977a,b; Moret et al., 1978). Individually, none of these substances was able to prevent the alterations in CrP, ATP, or lactate noted on the third day. Only the association of propranolol and piridoxilate attenuated the drop in CrP and ATP and the rise in lactate. The propranolol had, all the same, a marked effect on ventricular edema (particularly concerning the right ventricle), pulmonary hypertension, and heart rate (see Section VIIA).

b. ADAPTATION TO HYPOXIA

Few works have been devoted to the levels of different intracellular products of energy metabolism in chronic hypoxia lasting a number of years (hearts adapted to hypoxia). Tappan et al. (1957) were the first to measure, in guinea pigs permanently living at high altitude, the intracellular content of energy-rich compounds (CrP, ATP, and ADP). They found no difference in relation to animals from low altitudes. Other metabolite levels have been determined, unfortunately very often on animals living for too short a time in a hypoxic environment. Purshottam et al. (1977) found decreased cardiac glycogen levels after 30 days of simulated altitude varying between 3660 and 7620 m. However, Zhaparov and Mirrakhimov (1976) found important glycogen deposits in the yak living permanently at altitudes over 3000 m. High intramyocardial glycogen levels are well known in the fetal heart, which, for some, is one of the reasons for the high resistance of the fetus to severe hypoxia. Mensen de Silva and Cazorla (1973) measured various Krebs cycle and glycolysis metabolites in guinea pigs living permanently at an altitude over 14,000 ft. They found no difference regarding lactate, α-glycerophosphate, fumarate, or malate from animals living at low altitudes. The values of succinate and cis-aconitate are, on the other hand, markedly raised at high altitude; citrate too is slightly raised. Later we will see the importance of these facts.

We know of no measure of intracellular metabolites taken by myocardial biopsy in man born or permanently resident at a high altitude (e.g., during cardiac surgery, as has been performed at low altitude by Sebening and Scheuer). We also have no data on chronic cor pulmonale. Sebening (1965), by means of myocardial biopsies taken during surgery, found no difference in the products of energy-producing metabolism (glycolysis or high-energy phosphate compounds) between a group of patients presenting a tetralogy of Fallot with severe arterial desaturation and another group of patients with severe pulmonary stenosis and slight arterial desaturation, except for the lactate, where the values were surprisingly lower in subjects with an important arterial desaturation. Scheuer *et al.* (1970b) remarked that in cases of patients affected by tetralogy of Fallot, the levels of myocardial glycogen were lower when the arterial saturation was below 90%.

4. Aerobic and Anaerobic Capacity of the Hypoxic Heart; Mitochondrial Function

Various reviews of these captivating problems have been published (Frisancho *et al.*, 1973; Moret, 1971–1972; Poupa, 1971–1972; Scheuer, 1975). Here we will only outline the principal characteristics.

a. ANAEROBIC METABOLISM

Several authors have supplied data favoring the increased possibilities of the chronically hypoxic heart to synthesize energy-rich compounds in the absence of O_2 (Barrie and Harris, 1976; Moret, 1971–1972; Picon Reategui, 1966; Scheuer, 1975; Simanovskij and Cotoev, 1971; Vergnes and Moret, 1976; Weissler *et al.*, 1968). As early as 1934, Evans *et al.* suggested that an increase in glycolytic flux could enhance energy formation. Scheuer (1972) and Scheuer and Stezoski (1970, 1972a) demonstrated that under severe acute hypoxia, the production of ATP by anaerobic glycolysis may greatly increase and supply 50–75% (dependent on whether glucose or glycogen is the source) of the total energy necessary for the normal functioning of the heart. Evidently this is only possible if myocardial perfusion or coronary flow is maintained, with an adequate glucose supply. In conditions of normal myocardial oxygenation and perfusion, the energy supplied by anaerobic glycolysis represents only 10–15% of the total. The increase in energy production by anaerobic glycolysis is evidently only valid for a short period of time in severe hypoxia. In moderate chronic hypoxia, the increased ATP production by anaerobic glycolysis can theoretically replace the deficient aerobic production; however, there is no definite evidence to suggest that in humans or animals living permanently at high altitudes, energy production by anaerobic glycolysis is generally accentuated. However, this appears to be accepted by numerous authors during the acclimatization phase to high altitude, or in certain other conditions (e.g., cyanotic congenital cardiopathies, chronic cor pulmonale, Monge disease, or under certain particular conditions such as superimposed acute hypoxia, ischemia, or physical exercise) (Moret, 1971, 1971–1972; Moret *et al.*,

1972, 1976; Roy, 1973; Simanovskij and Cotoev, 1971; Vergnes *et al.,* 1971, 1976).

If the high-altitude heart is capable of increasing its use of the anaerobic glycolytic pathway for energy synthesis, it has also, at its disposition, other more or less anaerobic metabolic pathways: the pentose shunt (Reynafarje, 1962)—probably playing a minimal role; the interconversion of ADP to ATP and AMP via myokinase (Vergnes *et al.,* 1971)—a badly known myocardial pathway; triglyceride catabolism—transformation of glycerol 1-phosphate to dihydroxyacetone phosphate. In addition, we will see below that mitochondria are also partially capable of functioning anaerobically. One should also not forget that the myocardial glycogen reserves also play a vital role in the possibilities of the use of anaerobic glycolysis. This is well known in the fetal or newborn heart, or in the resistance mechanisms to acute hypoxia, ischemia, or during strenuous exercise (see Section VIIIB).

b. AEROBIC METABOLISM—MITOCHONDRIAL FUNCTION

The increased capacity of aerobic metabolism in chronic hypoxia has been suggested by numerous authors. There are numerous possibilities for improving aerobic metabolism:

1. Improvement of the O_2 supply or transport to the mitochondria by an increased number of circulating red cells, by a displacement of the oxygen–hemoglobin dissociation curve to the right (2,3-DPG), by an increased number and volume of myocardial capillaries, and by an increased cellular myoglobin content (see Section IIIA,B).

2. A raised metabolic capacity of the mitochondria by an increase in number of mitochondria and/or their active surface (see Section IVC), by a greater concentration or activity of certain enzymes or cytochromes (see references in Harris, 1977, and Moret, 1971–1972), by an increased ability of the mitochondria to generate energy in the presence of a lower concentration of ADP (Reynafarje, 1971–1972), by an improvement in the efficiency of oxidative phosphorylation (ADP/O ratio), by preferential use of certain more economical or profitable substrates (carbohydrates as compared to fatty acids, for example) (Moret, 1976; Moret *et al.,* 1970; Opie, 1969; Reynafarje, 1971–1972), by a decreased activity of certain hormones (catecholamines or thyroxine) that have an uncoupling or wastage effect (see Section VIIA,B).

3. A decrease in sympathetic or adrenergic activity, which has been described by numerous authors (see Section VIIA).

4. Anaerobic energy production by the mitochondria, as suggested by Penney and Cascarano (1970) and Singer (1965). Surprisingly enough, the mitochondria might be able to produce energy in anaerobic conditions. The

anaerobic capacity is based on the possibility of ATP production via fumarate-dependent oxidation of NADH (Runeberg and Pakarinen, 1967; Sanadi and Flukarty, 1963; Wilson and Cascarano, 1970) and by the oxidation of oxylacetate and of α-ketoglutarate in the cytochrome chain (Hunter, 1949). Mensen de Silva and Cazorla (1973) have shown that in guinea pigs living at high altitudes, the fumarate pathway could be a safety mechanism for an anaerobic energy production outside ordinary glycolysis. Nevertheless, it remains to be demonstrated that this pathway is normally active in residents of high altitudes, even though Mensen de Silva and Cazorla reported raised succinate levels (supplied by the reduction of fumarate) in guinea pigs living permanently at high altitude. It is also known that succinate may stimulate heme synthesis and thus hemoglobin, myoglobin, and cytochrome c, which are particularly raised in high-altitude chronic hypoxia or in certain cyanotic congenital cardiopathies.

C. Protein Synthesis—Development of Hypertrophy

In acute hypoxia, protein synthesis is decreased principally by a diminished availability of high-energy phosphate compounds necessary for the activation of amino acids or for their translation into protein. There is an important mitochondrial deterioration, with the myosine and the cellular membrane being more resistant (Aschenbrenner et al., 1971; Klain and Hannon, 1970).

The effects of chronic hypoxia on the myocardial cell have occasionally been confused with those of pressure or volume overload. In addition, the acclimatization stage should be well differentiated from the stabilization stage or adaptation. During acclimatization to moderate hypoxia, a right ventricular hypertrophy develops (see Section IIA) because of pressure overload secondary to pulmonary hypertension. Certain authors (Meerson in particular) have also found a left ventricular hypertrophy, which we did not encounter in our experiments on the rat (see Section IIA). It is not clear if the right ventricular hypertrophy is a true hypertrophy of preexisting myofibrils (true hypertrophy) or whether there is, in parallel, a myofibrillar division (hyperplasia) (Grandtner et al., 1974; Hollenberg et al., 1976). In addition to this right ventricular hypertrophy, there is also a proliferation of the mitochondria and their contents—enzymes, coenzymes, and cytochromes (probably in both ventricles, but of more importance in the right); of the myoglobin; and of the capillaries and connective tissue in both ventricles (Grandtner et al., 1974; Hollenberg et al., 1976; Meerson, 1975; Meerson and Pomoinitsky, 1972; Stere and Anthony, 1977; Wachtlova et al., 1977). It appears that nucleic acid and protein synthesis become apparent shortly after (1–2 hr) exposition to hypoxia and are maintained during several weeks, or more than 40 days according to Meerson (1975).

The mechanisms responsible for the initiation of protein synthesis have been the object recently of numerous controversies (Gevers, 1972; Harris, 1977). According to Meerson and Pomoinitsky (1972), the stimulus to an increase in protein synthesis is a deficiency of high-energy phosphate compounds. These would stimulate the genetical apparatus of the nuclei or the mitochondria, the latter being the first to be activated. This hypothesis, agreed to by some (Fizel and Fizelova, 1971; Gibb et al., 1976), has been criticized by Gevers (1972). It should be noted that in our studies on rats exposed to an altitude of 3500 m for several weeks (see Section), we found, in both ventricles, an important decrease in high-energy phosphate compounds (CrP and ATP) with a marked increase in what Meerson termed "phosphorylation potential" (ADP × AMP/ATP) without having encountered the least weight increase or hypertrophy of the left ventricle. This does not mean that in our experiments there was no increase or activation of protein synthesis, but it was, in any case, not manifested in the form of left ventricular hypertrophy.

Rabinowitz and Zak (1972) reviewed the different hypotheses concerning the stimulus to hypertrophy in the heart. The initial stimulus would be a myocardial mechanical overload, which in the case of chronic hypoxia would be essentially localized in the right ventricle. The increased work or tension of the right ventricular wall may lead to tissue anoxia, to depletion of energy reserves, and to macromolecular breakdown, with accumulation of materials causing genetic activation. The stretching of muscle cells may also directly activate growth processes. Humoral or hormonal factors may also be involved (insulin, growth hormone).

The activity of protein synthesis in subjects or animals living permanently in a hypoxic environment remains unclear. It is probably not very different from that of those living at low altitude, being simply adapted to lower arterial P_{O_2}. The apparatus for protein synthesis is probably more developed, but its activity appears comparable. As far as protein synthesis of the development of ventricular hypertrophy in chronic cor pulmonale or cyanotic congenital heart diseases in the absence of cardiac failure is concerned, there is little difference from that of the high-altitude heart, with the exception that at high altitudes, hypoxia is not the only element to be taken into consideration. The influence of the cold should not be underestimated (Meerson, 1975), nor should the effect of dietary restriction (Krelhaus et al., 1975).

V. Cardiovascular Function

The modifications of cardiovascular function in chronic hypoxia have been the object of numerous reviews recently (Badeer, 1973; Daum, 1977;

Frisancho, 1975; Heath and Williams, 1977; Lenfant and Sullivan, 1971). Only the principal characteristics will be outlined here.

A. Myocardial Contractility—Ventricular Function

As for the variations in coronary flow or myocardial metabolism, a distinction should be made between acute hypoxia, subacute to chronic hypoxia, and long-duration chronic hypoxia. It is experiments on altitude—hypobaric hypoxia—that have led to a clarification of these conditions. The repercussions of acute hypoxia on myocardial contractility, or function, have been well documented (Little, 1976; Sonnenblick and Brutsaert, 1972). Acute or severe hypoxia provokes an important depression in the myocardial force of contraction and ventricular performance. In subacute to chronic hypoxia of moderate severity, as encountered during acclimatization at medium and high altitudes (3000–5000 m), the effects on the heart are less marked and more controversial. Most authors admit that the cardiac output at rest increases during the first days but that the stroke volume during submaximal work decreases, thus implying a diminution in myocardial function or contractility (Alexander *et al.,* 1967; Balasubramanian *et al.,* 1975; Barcroft *et al.,* 1923; Grover *et al.,* 1976a; Klausen, 1966; Maher *et al.,* 1972; McDougall *et al.,* 1976; Pugh, 1964; Tucker *et al.,* 1976). This diminution in ventricular function or contractility may persist for several months, even years. The reasons for this diminution are not clear. It appears that they are not related to modifications in pH, venous return, myocardial norepinephrine content (Maher *et al.,* 1972), or myocardial hypoxia due to insufficient O_2 supply (Grover *et al.,* 1970, 1976a). Recent studies by Grover *et al.* (1976a) have shown that hypocapnia-associated alcalosis probably plays an important part.

Like other authors (Asmussen and Consolazio, 1941; Meerson and Kapelko, 1972; Peñaloza *et al.,* 1962, 1963; Sime et al., 1963; Vogel *et al.,* 1966), we found no evidence of disturbances of myocardial function in our studies on normal subjects living permanently at high altitude (Moret *et al.,* 1970, 1972) (see Section IIIB). The stroke volume, the left ventricular ejection fraction, the mean pulmonary capillary and right atrial pressures, the right and left end-diastolic ventricular pressures, and the cardiac output or index are identical to those of people living at low altitude. Even under the effect of additional acute hypoxia no disturbances in right or left ventricular function were demonstrated.

In compensated chronic cor pulmonale, on the contrary, we found a diminished stroke volume, with the right auricular and right end-diastolic ventricular pressures often being raised (see Section IIIB). The mean pulmonary capillary pressure was increased in 25% of our patients, indicating disturbances of left ventricular function and the cardiac output decreased (mean cardiac index: 2.72 liters/min/m² in chronic cor pulmonale and 3.2 liters/min/m² in normals, $p < 0.05$ (Moret, 1966, 1968, 1976). Disturbances in right, and often left, ventricular function have been noted by other authors [see review of Denolin (1976) and Denolin et al. (1971)]. These disturbances of ventricular function are often associated with metabolic alterations. In chronic mountain sickness or Monge disease, ventricular function is often disturbed with associated metabolic perturbations. The same is applicable to congenital cardiopathies when the arterial saturation falls below 70% (see Section IVB).

B. Cardiac Output

Cardiac output rises in acute hypoxia or in transfer to high altitude. This increase is of a few days duration and then returns to normal, or even below normal, most probably due to diminished ventricular function (see above). The mechanisms responsible for this increase in cardiac output are not evident. It is probably due to a transitory rise in adrenergic activity (Grover et al., 1976b; Maher et al., 1975; Maksutov et al., 1974; Meerson and Pshennikova, 1973; Moret and Duchosal, 1976; Myles and Radomski, 1974). The altitude of the degree of arterial desaturation from which the cardiac output initially rises is badly defined. Concerning altitude, we have already noted a definite rise as from 2000 m (Weber et al., 1973). In normal subjects living permanently at high altitude, the cardiac output at rest is comparable to that of subjects at low altitude (see Section IIIB), however the maximal output during effort most probably remains inferior to that of subjects of low altitude.

In chronic cor pulmonale, the values of cardiac output have been the object of numerous controversies. It is probable that, as during acclimatization to altitude, the cardiac output increases during the initial phase of pulmonary decompensation to subsequently diminish. In the series of patients we studied, the cardiac output was slightly decreased (see Section IIIB). In Monge disease the cardiac output or index was comparable to that of normal subjects resident at the same altitude (Moret, 1971, 1976). In congenital cyanotic cardiopathies, the cardiac output is essentially dependent on the complexity of the malformations or the importance and direction of the shunts.

C. Heart Rate

During exposition to acute hypoxia there is a rise in heart rate that persists for several days or weeks, which may be hindered by administration of β blockers (Maher *et al.,* 1975; Moret and Duchosal, 1976; Richardson *et al.,* 1967) (see Section VIIA). In normal subjects living at high altitude, heart rates were comparable to those living at low altitude. It should also be noted that an additional acute hypoxia did not increase the basal frequency, as was the case in residents of low altitude (Moret *et al.,* 1970, 1972). This leaves one to suppose that in high-altitude subjects a different sympathetic regulation of the cardiovascular system exists (see Section VIIA). Monge (1942) had mentioned in his initial observations on life at high altitude that the existence of a certain degree of bradycardia was not rare. In chronic cor pulmonale, as is well known, a certain degree of tachycardia exists. In our series of patients (see Section VIIA), the average heart rate was 80/min for patients with chronic cor pulmonale and 73/min for normal subjects ($p < 0.05$). In patients with chronic mountain sickness or Monge disease, the heart rate is higher than that in normals: 82/min and 69/min in normal subjects living at the same altitude ($p < 0.02$).

D. Pulmonary Circulation

Alveolar hypoventilation or the inhalation of an O_2-poor gaseous mixture provokes, as is well known, pulmonary hypertension by increasing the pulmonary precapillary resistances. The exact location of the vasoconstriction and the mechanisms responsible have not been completely elucidated. The origin of some is local; others are dependent on the sympathetic nervous system. The reasons, or the teleological significance of the pulmonary hypertension remain debatable. It is probable that this vasoconstriction serves to adjust the perfusion/ventilation ratio in order to maintain it, particularly during physical effort, at the most efficient value. This decreases the venous admixture and ameliorates the oxygenation of arterial blood (Dawson and Grover, 1974; Fishman, 1976; Lloyd, 1968; Tucker *et al.,* 1975; Urbanova *et al.,* 1973).

It was in 1956 that Rotta *et al.* demonstrated that the pulmonary arterial pressure was increased at high altitude. This has since been confirmed by numerous authors. Some have even established a relationship between the importance of the altitude and the degree of pulmonary hypertension (Cruz-Jibana *et al.,* 1964). This does not entirely apply to our observations. It is possible that ethnic differences also play a role. This pulmonary hypertension manifested by a muscularization of the pulmonary arterioles is reversible when the subjects return to low altitude. The pulmonary hypertension provoked by high altitude, responsible for the right ventricular hypertrophy, has been found in numerous experimental animals either transfered to or living permanently at high altitudes (see Section IIA). It varies according to age, sex, and species. The increase in pulmonary pressure may appear very early after arrival at high altitude, reaching a maximum after 3–7 days.

Pulmonary hypertension in cor pulmonale is well known. Hypoxia is not the only cause; many other factors are also of importance—acidosis, hypercapnia, vascular lesions, etc. The same is also applicable to congenital cardiopathies or Monge disease.

E. Systemic Circulation

Various studies on the populations of the Andean, Himalayan, or Ethiopian high plateaus have shown that their systolic and diastolic pressures are lower when compared to those of populations of low altitudes (for references, see Moret *et al.*, 1978). In the studies we performed on three population groups living permanently at three different altitudes, no significant difference was observed between the three groups (Moret *et al.*, 1970, 1972). It appears, however, according to Cruz-Coke *et al.* (1973), Marticorena *et al.* (1969), Page (1976), Peñaloza (1966), and Ruiz *et al.* (1969), that the prevalence of arterial hypertension is very low in the populations resident at high altitude and that, contrary to what is found at low altitude, the systolic and diastolic pressures do not have a tendency to rise with age. The reasons for these differences are not evident, but it is possible that a greater tissue vascularization (greater number of capillaries per unit mass of tissue), a different distribution of the cardiac output toward various organs (see below), a less important sympathetic activity, and a decrease in aldosterone secretion (see Section VIIB) are at the origin of these differences.

In the acclimatization phase at high altitude, the systemic arterial pressures generally increase during the first days with a decrease in arterial resistance (increase in cardiac output). In hypertensive subjects the fluctuations in arterial pressure are very variable and unpredictable from one individual to another and may appear at moderate altitudes (1500 m) (Weber *et al.*, 1973; Weidemann, 1972).

In compensated chronic cor pulmonale or in chronic mountain sickness—Monge disease—we did not find any difference in systolic, diastolic, or mean pressures or in systemic vascular resistances when compared to control healthy subjects residing at the same altitude. Some authors, however, have found certain "coexistences" of systemic arterial hypertension with pulmonary arterial hypertension in patients with chronic cor pulmonale, which for them would be one of the principal reasons for the left ventricular hypertrophy occasionally encountered in chronic cor pulmonale (see Section IIA).

F. Regional Blood Flow

The exposition to chronic hypoxia results in modifications in the distribution of the systemic blood flow to the organs. Figure 10 compares regional flow in two groups of normal subjects, one resident at low altitude and the other at high altitude. At high altitude the cerebral, muscular, and coronary blood flows are distinctly lower than at low altitude (Bidart *et al.*, 1975; Durand *et al.*, 1969; Marc-Vergnes *et al.*, 1974; Martineaud *et al.*, 1972; Moret *et al.*, 1970; Sørensen *et al.*, 1974). The retinal flow is also diminished (Frayser *et al.*, 1974). The renal blood flow has been found to be lower, unchanged, or even slightly increased. According to Ramsøe *et al.* (1970), the hepatic circulation appears to be greatly increased (+33%). The values for the splanchnic circulation have not been fully elucidated, but they appear also to be increased (Zelter *et al.*, 1976).

The reasons for this different redistribution of the systemic circulation at high altitude have not been clarified. The global cardiac output being practically identical at high and low altitude, a decrease in certain regional blood flows must necessarily be compensated for by an increase in flow in other

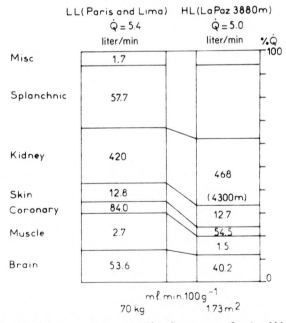

Fig. 10. The distribution, as a percentage of cardiac output, of regional blood flows at low altitude (Paris, Lima) and at high altitude (La Paz). The values apparent in each box indicate the regional blood flow in ml/min/100 g. (From Zelter *et al.*, 1976, by permission of the authors and Editions, INSERM, Paris).

territories—for example, splanchnic. The hematocrit and the hemoglobin concentrations being higher at altitude, Zelter *et al.* (1976) have calculated from data obtained from the literature, the plasma flow ($\dot{Q}_p$) and the red blood cell or globular flow ($\dot{Q}_g$) of certain regional circulation (Table II). Among the least decreased $\dot{Q}_g$, one finds two territories where the O_2 consumption is critical (coronary and cerebral) and in the comparable $\dot{Q}_p$ one finds the splanchnic and renal blood flows whose role is predominantly that of epuration of the plasma. Little, if anything, is known of the distribution of systemic flow in compensated chronic cor pulmonale. It is known that in cardiac insufficiency a redistribution of regional flow is produced in order to safeguard vital organs such as the heart and brain.

VI. Oxygen Transport: Pulmonary, Hematologic, and Tissue Adaptations

Because the arterial P_{O_2} is by definition diminished in all forms of chronic hypoxia, the organism must make all possible efforts to assure an adequate O_2 supply to all cells by the most effective and rapid means. Structural and functional modifications affect the pulmonary ventilation and the alveolo-capillary diffusion, the O_2 transport by the blood, the diffusion and O_2 transport at the tissue level, and finally, the utilization of the O_2 in the tissues.

TABLE II

Systemic Circulation at High Altitude [a,b]

	Sea level		3750 m − 12,130 ft		4375 m − 14,350 ft	
Organ	$\dot{Q}_p$	$\dot{Q}_g$	$\dot{Q}_p$	$\dot{Q}_g$	$\dot{Q}_p$	$\dot{Q}_g$
Heart	39.5	31.2	27.4	27.1	22.7	26.5
Brain	28.1*	22.0*	20.1	20.0		
Skin	0.84	0.66	0.5	0.5		
Muscle	1.13	0.89	0.76	0.74		
Kidney	721.1	568.9	646		461.0	539.0
Splanchnic circulation	855.3*	674.7*	860.1	849.9		

[a] Plasma flow ($\dot{Q}_p$) and globular or red blood cell flow ($\dot{Q}_g$) at sea-level and at altitude. Values calculated from those of Fig. 10. The flows are expressed in ml/min/100 g or ml/min depending on the method used. * = values for caucasian subjects.

[b] From Zelter *et al.,* 1976, by permission of the authors and Editions, INSERM, Paris.

A. Pulmonary Adaptation

The modifications, relative to the O_2 load at the pulmonary level, have been the subject of numerous studies concerning both altitude hypoxia and chronic cor pulmonale (Eckes, 1976; Frisancho, 1975; Konietzko and Matthys, 1976; Lenfant and Sullivan, 1971). Only the main characteristics will be recapitulated here, and particularly those relevant to residents of high altitudes. In the latter or in those transfered to high altitudes several months or years beforehand, one notes an increase in pulmonary ventilation. The obvious purpose of this is to increase the alveolar P_{O_2} (PA_{O_2}) and as a consequence, the arterial $P_{O_2}(Pa_{O_2})$. In order to maximize the chances of the highest Pa_{O_2} possible, subjects of high altitudes have greater pulmonary volumes with a greater surface for gaseous exchange and a greater diffusion capacity. The ventilation/perfusion ratio appears also to be constantly adapting in order to maximize its efficiency. The consequence of the slight pulmonary hypertension noted at high altitude has the effect, for some authors at least, of an adaptation of the pulmonary perfusion to the alveolar ventilation, which is particularly true during exercise (see Section VIIIA). The sensitivity of the respiratory centers to the hypoxia and hypercapnia of residents of high altitude is lower than that of subjects resident at low altitude. It is not really known if this constitutes an adaptation mechanism that is favorable or unfavorable because of a deterioration of the mechanisms governing the regulation of ventilation. The hypertrophy of the carotid bodies at high altitude is fascinating (Arias-Stella and Valcarcel, 1973). Since the works of Heymans *et al.* (1930), it is admitted that the carotid bodies monitor the oxygen saturation of systemic arterial blood. This hypertrophy of the carotid bodies has also been described in other forms of hypoxemia (see "Carotid Bodies in Heath," 1977). It usually appears (but not always) to be associated with a diminution of the ventilatory response to hypoxemia.

B. Hematologic Adaptation

During the chronic phase of hypoxia, the cardiac output and heart rate are practically comparable to those of normoxic subjects (see Section VB,C). The evident aim of this is to economize on useless energy expenditure for O_2 transport. The improvement of O_2 transport is achieved by an increase in the number of red blood cells, thus hemoglobin, and by an increase in blood volume or globular volume. The erythrocytosis of altitude, like that of congenital cardiopathies or chronic cor pulmonale, is well known. Viault in 1891 was the first to demonstrate an erythrocytosis in animals living at high altitude. The mechanisms responsible for the erythrocytosis are a stimulation of erythropoietin production by the kidney (Faura *et al.*, 1969; Siri *et al.*, 1966). A more or less close relationship exists between the degree of hypoxemia and the erythrocytosis, hematocrit (Hct), and hemoglobin (Hb) values.

In our studies on three populations resident at three different altitudes (see Section IIIB), we noted at 150 m altitude a Hct of 45%, a Hb level of 15 g/100 ml; at 3700 m, Hct is 51% and Hb is 18 g/100 mg; and at 4375 m, Hct is 53% and Hb is 19 g/100 ml. The increase in Hb constitutes an important mechanism for the improvement of O_2 transport, the limitations of its effectiveness being defined by the severity of the hypoxemia and the increase in blood viscosity (Hussan and Otis, 1957; Lenfant and Sullivan, 1971; Murray *et al.*, 1963; Stone *et al.*, 1968). Because of the rise in Hb levels, the capacity for O_2 transport increases until an arterial desaturation of the order of 70% and/or a Hct of 70% is reached; beyond these values the capacity decreases again. It is interesting to note that, concerning the congenital cardiopathies, for example, this represents the limit beyond which metabolic disturbances of the "anoxic or ischemic" type become apparent (see Section IVB). These values also represent the altitude at which the well-acclimatized man may reside permanently (about 5000 m). This erythrocytosis is accompanied by a rise in total blood volume with, in residents of high altitude, a slight decrease in plasma volume (Sanchez *et al.*, 1970). The rise in Hct, Hb, and blood volume is associated with modifications in the O_2–Hb dissociation curve, which becomes displaced to the right (because of an increase in intraerythrocytic 2,3-diphosphoglycerate (2,3-DPG) (Keys *et al.*, 1936; Lenfant *et al.*, 1968). This does not constitute a true improvement in the O_2 transport capacity of the blood, but it has the advantage of facilitating the release of oxygen into the tissues. The pulmonary adaptation facilitates the oxygen loading of the erythrocytes, and the increase in 2,3-DPG facilitates the oxygen unloading to the tissues. The importance of this adaptation mechanism is debated by certain authors. It has not been ascertained that this mechanism plays a preponderant role above 3500 m (Lenfant *et al.*, 1971; Torrance *et al.*, 1970–1971). It is interesting to note that the camelids (llamas, alpacas, and vicunas) that live at very high altitudes have a particular form of hemoglobin dissociation curve (Reynafarje *et al.*, 1975), which permits, on the one hand, a greater affinity of Hb for O_2 at the pulmonary level (which is not the case when the curve is displaced to the right) and, on the other hand, facilitates the release of O_2 into the tissues. This is probably a result of the presence in the erythrocytes of a greater quantity of fetal Hb. It is of interest to add that the Hb level of these animals is only 13–15 g/100 ml, their Hct is 35–38%, and their erythrocytes are smaller and elliptical.

C. Tissue Adaptation

The tissue adaptations to an impoverished O_2 content of capillary blood are multiple. We have already seen (see Section IIIA) that in practically all forms of hypoxia there exists an increase in capillary number and surface per unit of tissue mass. The purpose of this is to facilitate O_2 diffusion toward the mitochondria by diminishing the distance traveled. This increase, by the opening of preexisting and new capillaries, may reach 35–50% (Hultgren *et al.*, 1963; Rotta *et al.*, 1956). The O_2 diffusion at the tissue level is also greatly enhanced by the myoglobin that numerous authors have shown to be distinctly raised at altitude, and in congenital cardiopathies (Hurtado *et al.*, 1937; Poupa *et al.*, 1966; Reynafarje, 1962; Ward, 1975; Wittenberg, 1965). In addition, as previously noted, the specific shape of the dissociation curve permits a facilitated and rapid transfer of O_2 from the erythrocyte to the mitochondria. Moreover, there are at the cellular and mitochondrial level (see Section IVB) a large number of modifications that facilitate the utilization of oxygen: increase in number and active surface of the mitochondria, increased content or activity of the mitochondrial enzymes, increase in cytochrome and cytochrome oxidase concentration (Barbashova, 1964; Korecky and Rakusan, 1967; Tappan *et al.*, 1957; Tenney and Ou, 1969). The total result is an enhancement of the possibilities of O_2 finding the most rapid and shortest path to the enzyme site.

VII. Adrenergic and Other Hormonal Activities

A. Sympathetic Activity and Catecholamines

Exposure to chronic hypoxia leads to important modifications in adrenergic activity. There is initially an increase in sympathetic activity, thus explaining the rise in cardiac output and heart rate during the first days of exposure, which is often not in proportion to the degree of hypoxemia. This increase in sympathetic activity is accompanied by a rise in the renal elimination and the plasma concentrations of catecholamines—in particular, norepinephrine (Cunningham *et al.*, 1965; Grover *et al.*, 1976a; Maher *et al.*, 1973; Maksutov *et al.*, 1974; Myles and Radomsky, 1974; Pace *et al.*, 1964; Surks, 1967). These plasmatic and urinary modifications are, for many authors, accompanied by a diminution in myocardial catecholamine and particularly norepinephrine levels (Davis and Carlsson, 1973; Hurwitz *et al.*, 1971; Maksutov *et al.*, 1974; Meerson and Pshennikova, 1973; Rapin *et al.*, 1977; Stupfel and Roffi, 1961). This drop in myocardial catecholamines is generally of several days duration and may be of variable importance. According to Meerson and Pshennikova (1973), the decrease in myocardial norepinephrine may reach 70% after 10 days in rats exposed to an altitude of 7000 m and may last for 7–8 weeks. It is associated with energy-producing metabolic disturbances, as we demonstrated in rats exposed to altitude (see Section IVB). This could also explain the diminished contractility or ventricular performance reported by several authors in both man and animals transfered to altitude (see Section VA).

The variations in myocardial, plasmatic, and urinary catecholamines are not always in direct relationship to the chronotropic and perhaps inotropic cardiac regulation as demonstrated by Maher *et al.* (1975). Figure 11 reports some of their results. One notes in the upper part of the figure that the plasmatic norepinephrine levels progressively rise during exposure to hypoxia, but after 10 days (chronic hypoxia) the heart rate diminishes while the norepinephrine rises. Figure 11 shows also (lower part) that the cumula-

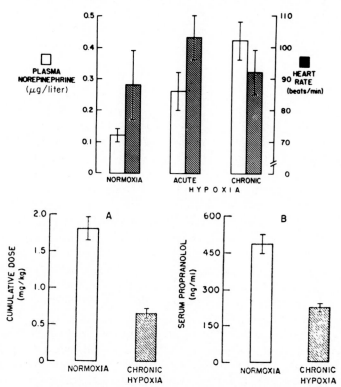

Fig. 11. (*Above*) Variations in the rat (mean ± SE) of plasma norepinephrine levels and heart rates during normoxia and after acute (24 h) and chronic (10 days) hypoxia. (*Below*) Cumulative dose of propranolol required to achieve maximal beta blockade (A); serum propranolol concentration on attainment of maximal β blockade (B). (From Maher *et al.*, 1975, and the American Physiological Society, by permission.)

tive propranolol dose necessary to block the β adrenergic activity is much lower in rats exposed to chronic hypoxia for 10 days than in the controls. This is confirmed by the serum level of propranolol, which is lower, thus demonstrating that despite high plasmatic levels of norepinephrine the response of the vascular system is different and that after 10 days there exists a relative refractoriness of the β receptors of the sinoatrial node.

The response of the sympathetic system of subjects or animals living permanently at high altitude and the myocardial or plasmatic catecholamine content is badly known. It appears that the latter is little modified (Moncloa *et al.,* 1965). In our studies on populations resident on the high Andean plateaus, we tested the sympathetic regulation by inhalation of an O_2-poor gaseous mixture (Moret *et al.,* 1970, 1972). We noted that an acute hypoxia superimposed on the effect of altitude provokes an increase in cardiac output, as at low altitude, but no increase in heart rate (see Section VC). It appears as though the inotropic receptors were as sensitive as at low altitude but that the chronotropic receptors were inhibited. This is in accordance with the experiments of Maher *et al.,* (1975), reported earlier.

α and β Blockades

Several authors have demonstrated that β blockers can partially diminish the metabolic alterations or the hemodynamic modifications during acute hypoxia (Maher *et al.,* 1975; Nayler *et al.,* 1977; Richardson *et al.,* 1967). In our experiments on rats placed at high altitude (Jungfraujoch, 3454 m; see Section IIA), we tested the effects of α and β blockers (Moret and Duchosal, 1976; Moret and Lutzen, 1977a,b; Moret *et al.,* 1976). Alpha blockers (phenoxybenzamine and raubasine) had no effect on the metabolic disturbances or on the hemodynamic modifications. Among the β blockers (propranolol, practolol, and alprenolol), the propranolol (4 mg/kg/day administered before and during the stay of high altitude) had, during the initial stay at high altitude, the effect of inhibiting the rise in mean pulmonary pressure ($\overline{P}A$) (see Fig. 12), probably by preventing the increase in cardiac output usually present during the early phase of acclimatization. After 12 weeks, however, the animals under propranolol had a higher pulmonary pressure than those without propranolol.

Propranolol also has the effect of preventing the rise in heart rate during the first weeks, but it provokes, on the other hand, at least initially, a slight rise in right ventricular end-diastolic pressure (RV_{ED}). The right ventricular edema (tissue water) is, however, less important under propranolol, probably due to a minimal rise in pulmonary pressure. There was, however, no effect on metabolic disturbances (see Section IVB) unless the propranolol was associated with piridoxilate, a protective myocardial substance analogous to dichloroacetate (Moret and Lutzen, 1977a,b,c).

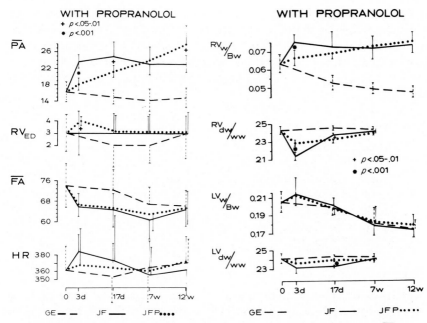

Fig. 12. Effects of propranolol or mean pulmonary arterial ($\overline{PA}$) and femoral ($\overline{FA}$) pressures, on the right ventricular end-diastolic pressure (RV_{ED}), on the heart rate (HR), and on the ventricular weights (see Fig. 1). Control animals kept at low altitude: Geneva—GE. Animals placed at high altitude (Jungfraujoch), not treated: JF, treated by proprapronol: JFP.

The effect of propranolol on heart rate is comparable to that noted by Maher *et al.* (1975). The effect on pulmonary pressure has not been noted by others. We believe that this is an indirect effect resulting from a decrease in cardiac output. This effect, even secondary, may all the same be of clinical interest for short stays at high altitude, despite the only slight rise in right ventricular end-diastolic pressure. The late rise in pulmonary arterial pressure under propranolol confirms the role of the autonomic nervous system in the regulation of the pulmonary circulation during hypoxia (Buss and Bisgard, 1976; Fishman, 1976).

B. Other Hormonal Activities

1. Thyroid

The studies concerning the activity of the thyroid gland are contradictory. Some have demonstrated high thyroxine levels during the initial exposure to altitude (Kotchen *et al.,* 1973; Surks *et al.,* 1967). In chronic hypoxia of long duration thyroid activity is, for the majority of authors, diminished (see "Endocrines in Heath," 1977). This would be of capital importance to define, since it could contribute to the explanation of the low myocardial oxygen consumption we noted in residents of high altitude. Despite the iodide lack, the prevalence of goiters at high altitude is lower that at low altitude.

2. Adrenals

The exposure to chronic hypoxia as for catecholamines provokes a rise in 17-hydroxycorticosteroids during several weeks. It appears that the secretion of aldosterone is diminished at high altitude (Hogan *et al.*, 1973). Changes in intravascular volume could be of importance in its regulation. This decrease in aldosterone secretion would play, for some, a protective role against hypertension, the low prevalence of which is known at high altitude (see Section VE).

3. Insulin

Despite the importance of insulin in glucose metabolism, particularly in chronic hypoxia, its variations are little known. The glucose blood level is lower at high altitude (see Section IVB). A faster rate of disappearance of blood glucose has been reported at high altitude (Picon Reategui, 1966). It should also be remembered that insulin is necessary to ensure correct protein synthesis, which is important during exposition to hypoxia and severe hypoxia in particular.

VIII. Exercise Tolerance—Myocardial Resistance to Ischemia or Necrosis

A. Maximum Oxygen Consumption ($\dot{V}_{O_2\ max}$—Aerobic Capacity)—Endurance to Exercise

The influence of altitude chronic hypoxia on the maximum oxygen consumption ($\dot{V}_{O_2\ max}$, or maximum aerobic capacity) has been, and continues to be, the object of numerous controversies, particularly since the Mexico Olympic games in 1969, where the athletes from high altitudes dominated the endurance events (i.e., those events requiring concurrent oxygen intake).

Various studies have demonstrated that transfer to high altitude of subjects born or resident at low altitude is accompanied by a decrease in the maximal aerobic capacity. The importance of this decrease is dependent on the altitude and the age of the subject (Burkirk *et al.*, 1967; Consolazio *et al.*, 1967; Faulkner *et al.*, 1968; Hansen *et al.*, 1967; Pugh *et al.*, 1964; Saltin *et al.*, 1968; Sen Gupta *et al.*, 1975; Sime *et al.*, 1974; Vogel *et al.*, 1974b). In the person nonacclimatized to altitude, there is a 3% decrease in $\dot{V}_{O_2\,max}$ for each 1000 ft or 300 m altitude difference. This decrease amounts to only 2% for those who are partially acclimatized. The diminished $\dot{V}_{O_2\,max}$ is in relation to the degree of hypoxemia and probably originates from a decrease in myocardial contractility or left ventricular function (see Section VA) and from an increase in pulmonary pressure. The decrease in $\dot{V}_{O_2\,max}$ progressively diminishes, returning after several months to values comparable to those of subjects permanently resident at high altitudes. This acclimatization is more efficient and rapid when the transfer to high altitude is accomplished during the earlier years of life—preferably during the growth period (Frisancho *et al.*, 1973).

The $\dot{V}_{O_2\,max}$ of subjects living permanently at altitude would be, for many authors, equal to that of subjects residing at low altitude or, for some, would be even greater (Buskirk *et al.*, 1967; Hansen *et al.*, 1967; Kollias *et al.*, 1967; Mazess, 1969; Velasquez, 1964). It increases by approximately 10% when these residents are transferred to low altitude (Vogel *et al.*, 1974a), hence the still discussed interest or benefit of training athletes at high altitude. In addition, it should be noted that maximal physical effort in those born or resident at high altitude is accompanied by a less important increase in blood lactate, leading one to suppose a higher rate of disappearance or a reduced production of lactate (Reynafarje and Velasquez, 1966; Lahiri and Milledge, 1966).

The preceding values concerning $\dot{V}_{O_2\,max}$, lactate production during exercise, or endurance to effort can evidently not be found in chronic cor pulmonale, since the cardiac and pulmonary functions are seriously restricted. There are relatively few studies on cyanotic congenital cardiopathies. As opposed to that observed at high altitude, Scheuer *et al.* (1970a) have shown that during exercise, arterial lactate rises to a greater extent in cyanosed patients than in those who are noncyanosed. Moffitt *et al.* (1970) have, however, demonstrated that cyanosed patients are more tolerant to aortic clamping, with arrest of the coronary circulation during open-heart surgery, than noncyanosed patients. After aortic declamping and coronary reperfusion, the myocardium of cyanosed patients not only did not produce lactate but continued to consume it, as opposed to the noncyanosed patients, whose myocardium eliminated large quantities of lactate during reperfusion. These observations approach those noted in high-altitude subjects at the peripheral and myocardial level.

B. Resistance of the Chronic Hypoxic Heart to Ischemia or Necrosis

The rarity of ischemic cardiopathies (angina and infarction) in high-altitude residents was already noted by Hurtado in 1960. This has been reaffirmed by Arias-Stella and Topilsky (1971), Mirrakhimov (1972), and Ruiz *et al.* (1969). Mortimer *et al.* (1977) recently reported a reduction in mortality from coronary heart disease in men residing at high altitudes. Similar observations have also been reported in chronic cor pulmonale. Samad and Noehren (1965) noted that in autopsy controls the presence of infarction is much less frequent in chronic cor pulmonale than in a control series of the same age, despite comparable arteriosclerotic coronary lesions in the two groups. This has been confirmed by Schoenmackers and Schoene (1972). For Bhargava and Woolf (1971) and Karpick *et al.* (1970), it appears that, on the contrary, there is no difference between the two groups.

The resistance to total anoxia, ischemia, or necrosis of the heart adapted to high altitude has been reported by numerous authors on different animal species (Kopecky and Daum, 1958; McGrath and Bullart, 1968; McGrath *et al.*, 1973; Poupa, 1971–1972; Poupa *et al.*, 1965a,b, 1966; Meerson *et al.*, 1973). With Opie we have ourselves (Moret *et al.*, 1976; Opie *et al.*, 1978) studied, on the isolated rat heart adapted to altitude during several weeks (16–28 weeks), the resistance to necrosis provoked by ligature of the main left anterior coronary artery. Figure 13 represents the metabolic modifications. The altitude-adapted animals (Jungfraujoch, 3454 m altitude) had a greater ability to maintain tissue contents of glycogen, creatine phosphate (CP), and adenosine triphosphate (ATP), and the lactate content is lower. The hemodynamic values are not modified and remain as deteriorated as in the control animals.

The reasons for this improved resistance to anoxia, ischemia, or necrosis of animals adapted to chronic hypoxia (altitude or hypobaric chamber), as well as for the low incidence of ischemic heart disease and mortality by cardiovascular disease in high-altitude residents, can be found in the preceding chapters. The high-altitude heart is endowed with a greater arterial coronary, capillary, and anastomotic network than the low-altitude heart. There is an improved O_2 transport by the blood and the diffusion of O_2 into the tissues to the mitochondria is ameliorated. The aerobic and anaerobic metabolic capacities are greater and more efficient. The myocardial O_2 demands are probably less important, thus constituting a form of protective factor. The adrenergic, and probably also thyroid, activity is lower. These various properties of the high-altitude heart result in a protection against anoxia or ischemia. This protection probably does not stem uniquely from hypoxia; it is possible that physical activity submitted by those living at high

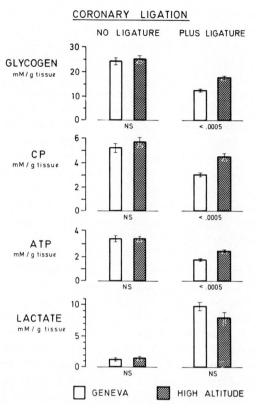

Fig. 13. Protective effect of altitude chronic hypoxia on myocardial necrosis provoked by coronary ligation.

altitude also plays a role. However, as previously noted, a part of these properties is also found in chronic cor pulmonale, in certain cyanotic congenital cardiopathies and in the fetal or newborn heart. In the latter the role of physical activity is evidently not relevant. It appears as though the high-altitude heart retained some of the properties that enabled it to develop and live during its intrauterine life in a very hypoxic environment. This might provide ischemia-resistant properties that, unfortunately, are lost after birth in the low-altitude heart.

IX. Conclusions

The hypoxic heart secondary to moderate chronic hypoxemia demonstrates a different comportment to the ischemic heart. After several months or years of "adaptation," compensation mechanisms appear that, excluding the right ventricular hypertrophy, may even result in various advantages over the normoxic heart. Among these advantages one notes a more developed coronary vascular network with a capillary–mitochondria O_2 diffusion distance reduced to a minimum, an increased capacity in the O_2 transport system, an improved aerobic and anaerobic metabolism that are able to function during more pronounced decreases in blood O_2 saturation or decreases in blood flow. In addition, there is reduced adrenergic and probably thyroid activity. The overall result is an increased protection of the chronically hypoxic heart to ischemia or necrosis. However, the disadvantages are an associated pulmonary hypertension which, in certain situations as for example chronic mountain sickness or Monge disease, chronic cor pulmonale, or the Eisenmenger syndrome in congenital cardiopathies, will greatly complicate the clinical evolution and lead the patient toward severe right heart insufficiency and an increasingly severe hypoxemia. Below an arterial desaturation of about 70%, or a hematocrit greater than 70–75%, the compensatory mechanisms are no longer functional and one enters a vicious circle. The myocardium suffers to a continually greater extent from a lack in O_2 supply and metabolic alterations of the "anoxic or ischemic" type become apparent with the associated repercussions on the anatomical structure, and electrical and mechanical comportment. Some of the above pathological conditions are partially reversible providing the arterial saturation, the P_{CO_2} disturbances and acid/base disequilibrium often accompanying severe decompensation states, can be sufficiently and durably corrected. Monge disease, for example, is, to a large extent, reversible if the patients are transferred to low altitude.

The study of the hypoxic heart is not only of clinical interest. The numerous works both in man and animal, and particularly those concerning altitude hypoxia, have supplied many new facts related to physiology, pathophysiology, and biochemistry and have contributed to an improved understanding of the normal and pathological heart and to ameliorated therapeutic possibilities. The present review has attempted to demonstrate this.

Acknowledgment

The personal studies reported in this review were supported by the University and Cantonal Hospital of Geneva, the Fonds National Suisse for Scientific Research, the Swiss Foundation of Cardiology, the World Health Organization, the Foundation S. I. Patino, Geneva. It was accomplished in collaboration with the Instituto de Investigaciones de la Altura, Universidad Peruana Cayetano Heredia, Lima, Peru, the Instituto de Biologia de la Altura, Instituto del

Torax, La Paz, Bolivia, the Research Laboratory of the Jungfraujoch (Swiss Alps), and the Centre of Hemotypology of Toulouse, France.

We would like to thank all our past and present collaborators, and particularly Mrs. S. Sheehey, who helped in the preparation of the English text, and Miss M. Turrian for her secretarial assistance.

References

Abraham, A. S., Kay, J. M., Cole, R. B., and Pincock, A. C. (1971). *Cardiovasc. Res.* 5, 95.

Alexander, J. K., Hartley, L. H., Modelski, M., and Grover, R. F. (1967). *J. Appl. Physiol.* 23, 849–858.

Anthony, A., and Kreider, J. (1961). *Am. J. Physiol.* 200, 523–525.

Arias-Stella, J., and Recavarren, S. (1962). *Am. J. Pathol.* 41, 55–64.

Arias-Stella, J., and Topilsky, M. (1971). *In* "High Altitude Physiology—Cardiac and Respiratory Aspects" (R. Porter and J. Knight, eds.), pp. 149–157. Churchill-Livingstone, Edinburgh and London.

Arias-Stella, J., and Valcarcel, J. (1973). *Pathol. Microbiol.* 39, 292–297.

Aschenbrenner, V., Zak, R., Cutilletta, A. F., and Rabinowitz, M. (1971). *Am. J. Physiol.* 221, 1418–1425.

Asmussen, E., and Consolazio, F. C. (1941). *Am. J. Physiol.* 132, 555–563.

Badeer, H. S. (1973). *Aerosp. Med.* 44, 1173–1179.

Balasubramanian, V., Kaushik, V. S., Manchanda, S. C., and Roy, S. B. (1975). *Br. Heart J.* 37, 272–276.

Barbashova, Z. I. (1964). *In* "Handbook of Physiology" (D. B. Dill, ed.), Sect. 4, Vol. I, pp. 37–54, Williams & Wilkins, Baltimore, Maryland.

Barcroft, J., Binger, C. A., Boch, A. V., Doggart, J. H., Forbes, H. S., Harrop, G., Meakins, J. C., and Redfield, A. C. (1923). "Observations Upon the Effect of High Altitude on the Physiological Processes of the Human Body Carried Out in Peruvian Andes, Chiefly at Cerro de Pasco," pp. 351–480. Philos. Trans. R. Soc., London.

Barrie, S. E., and Harris, P. (1976). *Am. J. Physiol.* 231, 1308–1313.

Berne, R. M., Blackmon, J. R., and Gardner, T. A. (1957). *J. Clin. Invest.* 36, 1101–1106.

Bernsmeier, A., and Rudolph, W. (1961). *Verh. Dtsch. Ges. Kreislauf. forsch.* 27, 59–76.

Bhargava, R. K., and Woolf, C. R. (1971). *Chest* 59, 254–261.

Bidart, J., Drouet, L., and Durand, J. (1975). *J. Physiol. (Paris)* 70, 333–337.

Bjork, L. (1966). *Radiology* 87, 33–34.

Burton, R. R., and Smith, A. H. (1967). *J. Appl. Physiol.* 22, 782–785.

Buskirk, E. R., Kollias, J., Akers, R. F., Prokop, E. K., and Picon Reategui, E. (1967). *J. Appl. Physiol.* 23, 259–266.

Buss, D. D., and Bisgard, G. E. (1976). *Basic Res. Cardiol.* 71, 456–468.

Consolazio, C. F., Johnson, H. G., Matausch, L. O., Nelson, R. A., and Isaac, G. C. (1967). *U.S. Army Med. Res. Nutr. Lab. Rep.* No. 300.

Cruz-Coke, R., Donoso, H., and Barrera, R. (1973). *Clin. Sci. Mol. Med.* 45, 55.

Cruz-Jibana, J., Banchero, N., Sime, F., Peñaloza, D., Gamboa, R., and Marticorena, E. (1964). *Dis. Chest* 46, 446–451.

Cunningham, W. L., Becker, E. J., and Kreuzer, F. (1965). *J. Appl. Physiol.* 20, 607–610.

Daum, S. (1977). "Cor Pulmonale Chronicum." Eur. Soc. Clin. Respir. Physiol. and Eur. Soc. Cardiol., München.

Davis, J. N., and Carlsson, A. (1973). *J. Neurochem.* 21, 783–790.

Dawson, A., and Grover, R. F. (1974). *J. Appl. Physiol.* **36**, 294–298.

Denolin, H. (1976). *Bull. Eur. Physiopathol. Respir.* **12**, 407–413.

Denolin, H., de Coster, A., and Bernard, R. (1971). *Prog. Respir.* **6**, 147–161.

Diemer, K. (1968). "Capillarization and Oxygen Supply of the Brain. Oxygen Transport in Blood and Tissue," p. 118. Thieme, Stuttgart.

Dill, D. B. (1968). *J. Am. Med. Assoc.* **205**, 747–753.

Duckworth, M. W. (1961). *J. Physiol. (London)* **156**, 603–610.

Durand, J., Verpillal, J. M., Pradel, M., and Martineaud, J. P. (1969). *Fed. Proc., Fed. Am. Soc. Exp. Biol.* **28**, 1124–1128.

Eckenhoff, J. E., Hafkenskiel, J. H., and Landmesser, C. M. (1947). *Am. J. Physiol.* **148**, 582–596.

Eckes, L. (1976). *Gegenbaurs Morphol. Jahrb. (Leipzig)* **122**, 826–863.

Elsner, R. W., Bolstad, A., and Forno, C. (1964). *In* "The Physiological Effects of High Altitude" (W. H. Weihe, ed.), pp. 217–223. Macmillan, New York.

Eriskovskaya, N. K., and Tsellarius, Y. G. (1976). *Bull. Exp. Biol. Med. (Engl. Transl.)* **82**, 1727–1729.

Evans, C. L., De Graff, A. L., Kosaka, T., McKenzie, K., Murphy, G. E., Vacek, T., Williams, D. H., and Young, F. G. (1934). *J. Physiol. (London)* **80**, 21–40.

Faulkner, J. A., Kollias, J., Favour, C. B., Buskirk, E. R., and Balke, B. (1968). *J. Appl. Physiol.* **24**, 685–691.

Faura, J., Ramos, J., and Reynafarje, C. (1969). *Blood* **33**, 668–676.

Fishman, A. P. (1976). *Circ. Res.* **38**, 221–231.

Fizel, A., and Fizelova, A. (1971). *J. Mol. Cell. Cardiol.* **2**, 187–192.

Frank, M. J., Weisse, A. B., Moschos, C. B., and Levinson, G. E. (1973). *Circulation* **47**, 798–806.

Frayser, R., Gray, G. W., and Houston, C. (1974). *J. Appl. Physiol.* **37**, 302–304.

Friedli, B., Haenni, B., Moret, P. R., and Opie, L. H. (1977). *Circulation* **55**, 647–652.

Frisancho, A. R. (1975). *Science* **187**, 313–319.

Frisancho, A. R., Martinez, C., Velasquez, T., Sanchez, J., and Montoye, H. (1973). *J. Appl. Physiol.* **34**, 176–180.

Fukuda, M. (1966). *Jpn. Circ. J.* **30**, 693–702.

Ganote, C. E., Worstell, J., Ianotti, J. P., and Kaltenbach, J. P. (1977). *Am. J. Pathol.* **88**, 95–118.

Gevers, W. (1972). *J. Mol. Cell. Cardiol.* **4**, 537–541.

Gibb, L., Bishop, S. P., Nesher, R., Robinson, W. F., Berry, A. J., and Kruger, F. A. (1976). *J. Mol. Cell. Cardiol.* **8**, 419–429.

Graham, T. P., Buckspan, G. S., and Fisher, R. D. (1977). *Pediatr. Res.* **11/4**, No. 124.

Grandtner, M., Turek, Z., and Kreuzer, F. (1974). *Pfluegers Arch.* **350**, 241–248.

Greene, N. M., and Talner, N. S. (1964). *N. Engl. J. Med.* **270**, 1331–1336.

Grover, R. F., Lufschanowski, R., and Alexander, J. K. (1970). *Adv. Cardiol.* **5**, 72–79.

Grover, R. F., Lufschanowski, R., and Alexander, J. K. (1976a). *J. Appl. Physiol.* **41**, 832–838.

Grover, R. F., Reeves, J. T., Maher, J. T., McCullough, E., Cruz, J. C., Denniston, J. C., and Cymerman, A. (1976b). *Circ. Res.* **38**, 391–396.

Hansen, J. E., Vogel, J. A., Stelter, G. P., and Consolazio, C. F. (1967). *J. Appl. Physiol.* **23**, 511–522.

Harris, P. (1977). *In* "Man at High Altitude" (D. Heath and D. R. Williams, eds.), pp. 174–190. Churchill-Livingstone, Edinburgh.

Hearse, D. J., Humphrey, S. M., and Garlick, P. B. (1976). *J. Mol. Cell. Cardiol.* **8**, 329–339.

Heath, D., and Williams, D. R., eds. (1977). "Man at High Altitude." Churchill-Livingstone, Edinburgh and London.

Heath, D., Edwards, C., Winson, M., and Smith, P. (1973). *Thorax* **28**, 24.

Heymans, C., Bouckaert, J. J., and Dautrebande, L. (1930). *Arch. Int. Pharmacodyn. Ther.* **39**, 400–450.

Hogan, R. P., III, Kotchen, T. A., Boyd, A. E., III, and Hartley, L. H. (1973). *J. Appl. Physiol.* **35**, 385–390.

Hollenberg, M., Honbo, N., and Samorodin, A. J. (1976). *Am. J. Physiol.* **231**, 1445–1450.

Hosono, K. (1965). *Jpn. Heart J.* **6**, 318–324.

Hultgren, H. N., and Miller, H. (1967). *Circulation* **35**, 207–218.

Hultgren, H. N., Marticorena, E., and Miller, H. (1963). *J. Appl. Physiol.* **18**, 913–918.

Hunter, F. E. (1949). *J. Biol. Chem.* **177**, 361–372.

Hurtado, A. (1960). *Ann. Intern. Med.* **53**, 247–258.

Hurtado, A., Rotta, A., Merino, C., and Pons, J. (1937). *Am. J. Med. Sci.* **194**, 708.

Hurwitz, D. A., Robinson, S. M., and Barofsky, J. (1971). *Psychopharmacologia* **19**, 26.

Hussan, G., and Otis, A. B. (1957). *J. Clin. Invest.* **36**, 270–278.

Jones, M., and Ferrans, V. J. (1977). *Am. J. Cardiol.* **39**, 1051–1063.

Karpick, R. J., Pratt, P. C., and Asmundsson, T. (1970). *Ann. Intern. Med.* **72**, 267–279.

Kearney, M. S. (1973). *Pathol. Microbiol.* **39**, 258–265.

Kelley, T. (1965). *Anal. Chem.* **37**, 1078.

Kerr, A., Jr., Diasio, R. B., and Bommer, W. J. (1965a). *Am. Heart J.* **69**, 841.

Kerr, A., Jr., Pilato, S., and Foster, E. J. (1965b). *Proc. Soc. Exp. Biol. Med.* **119**, 717.

Keys, A., Hall, F. G., and Barrón, E. S. G. (1936). *Am. J. Physiol.* **115**, 292–307.

Klain, G. J., and Hannon, J. P. (1970). *Proc. Soc. Exp. Biol. Med.* **134**, 1000–1004.

Klausen, K. (1966). *J. Appl. Physiol.* **21**, 609–616.

Kollias, J., Buskirk, E. R., Akers, R. F., Prokop, E. K., Baker, P. T., and Picon Reategui, E. (1967). *J. Appl. Physiol.* **24**, 792–799.

Konietzko, N., and Matthys, H. (1976). *Klin. Wochenschr.* **54**, 1161–1167.

Konopinski, M., and Zimnoch, L. (1976). *Anaesth. Resusc. Intensive Ther.* **4**, 95–103.

Kopecky, M., and Daum, S. (1958). *Cesk. Fysiol.* **7**, 518.

Korecky, B., and Rakusan, K. (1967). *Physiol. Bohemoslov.* **16**, 33.

Kotchen, T. A., Mougey, E. H., Hogan, R. P., Boyd, A. E., Pennington, L. L., and Mason, J. W. (1973). *J. Appl. Physiol.* **34**, 165–168.

Krelhaus, W., Gibson, K., and Harris, P. (1975). *J. Mol. Cell. Cardiol.* **7**, 63–69.

Krymsky, L. D. (1965). *Circulation* **32**, 814–827.

Lahiri, S., and Milledge, J. S. (1966). *Fed. Proc., Fed. Am. Soc. Exp. Biol.* **25**, 1392–1396.

Lenfant, C., and Sullivan, K. (1971). *N. Engl. J. Med.* **284**, 1298–1309.

Lenfant, C., Torrance, J., English, E., Finck, C. A., Reynafarje, C., Ramos. J., and Faura, J. (1968). *J. Clin. Invest.* **47**, 2652–2656.

Lenfant, C., Torrance, J. D., and Reynafarje, C. (1971). *J. Appl. Physiol.* **30**, 625–631.

Little, R. C. (1976). *Am. Heart J.* **92**, 609–614.

Lloyd, T. C., Jr. (1968). *J. Appl. Physiol.* **25**, 560–565.

Loiko, I. K., Gaziuk, A. P., and Loiko, V. V. (1976). *Arch. Anat. Histol. Embryol.* **71**, 60–67.

McDougall, J. D., Reddan, W. G., Dempsey, J. A., and Forster, H. (1976). *J. Hum. Ergol.* **5**, 103–11.

McGrath, J. J., and Bullart, R. W. (1968). *J. Appl. Physiol.* **25**, 761–764.

McGrath, J. J., Prochazka, J., Pelouch, V., and Ostadal. B. (1973). *J. Appl. Physiol.* **34**, 289–293.

Maher, J. T., Goodman, A. L., Bowers, W. D., Hartley, L. H., and Angelakos, E. T. (1972). *Am. J. Physiol.* **223**, 1029–1033.

Maher, J. T., Jones, L. G., and Hartley, L. H. (1973). *Fed. Proc. Fed. Am. Soc. Exp. Biol.* **32**, 435.

Maher, J. T., Manchanda, S. C., and Cymerman, A. (1975). *Am. J. Physiol.* **228**, 477–481.

Maksutov, K. M., Kirianova, R. I., and Shapovalova, S. S. (1974). *Sechenov Physiol. J. USSR* **60**, 733–739.

Manchanda, S. C., Shrivastava, L. M., Tandon, R., and Roy, S. B. (1973). *Indian J. Physiol. Pharmacol.* **17**, 79–82.

Marc-Vergnes, J. P., Antezana, G., Coudert, J., Gourdin, D., and Durand, J. (1974). *J. Physiol. (Paris)* **68**, 633–654.

Marticorena, E., Ruiz, L., Severino, J., Galvez, J., and Peñaloza, D. (1969). *Am. J. Cardiol.* **23**, 364–368.

Martineaud, J. P., Tillous, M. C., Le Moel, J. F., and Durand, J. (1972). *J. Physiol. (Paris)* **65**, 272A.

Maseri, A., L'Abbate, A., Coudert, J., Biagini, A., Michelassi, C., and Distanta, A. (1976). *In* "Anthropologie des populations andines," pp. 363–370. INSERM, Paris.

Mazess, R. B. (1969). *Hum. Biol.* **41**, 494.

Meerson, F. Z. (1975). *Physiol. Rev.* **55**, 79–123.

Meerson, F. Z., and Kapelko, V. I. (1972). *Cardiology* **57**, 183–199.

Meerson, F. Z., and Pomoinitsky, V. D. (1972). *J. Mol. Cell. Cardiol.* **4**, 571–597.

Meerson, F. Z., and Pshennikova, M. G. (1973). *Int. J. Biometeorol.* **17**, 83–93.

Meerson, F. Z., Zaletaeva, T. A., Lagutchov, S. S., and Pshennikova, M. G. (1964). *Exp. Cell Res.* **36**, 568–578.

Meerson, F. Z., Gomzakov, O. A., and Shimkovich, M. V. (1973). *Am. J. Cardiol.* **31**, 30–34.

Mensen de Silva, E., and Cazorla, A. (1973). *Am. J. Physiol.* **224**, 669–672.

Miller, A. T., and Hale, D. M. (1970). *Am. J. Physiol.* **219**, 702–704.

Mirrakhimov, M. M. (1972). *Klin. Med. (Moscow)* **50**, 104–109.

Mitchell, R. S., Walker, S. H., and Maisel, J. C. (1968). *Am. Rev. Respir. Dis.* **98**, 611–612.

Moffitt, E. A., Rosevear, J. W., and McGoon, D. C. (1970). *J. Am. Med. Assoc.* **211**, 1518–1524.

Moncloa, F., Gomez, M., and Hurtado, A. (1965). *J. Appl. Physiol.* **20**, 1329–1331.

Monge, M. C. (1942). *Science* **95**, 79.

Monge, M. C. (1943). *Physiol. Rev.* **23**, 166–184.

Moret, P. R. (1966). *Proc. World Congr. Cardiol., 5th, 1900* pp. 158–171.

Moret, P. R. (1968). *In* "Le poumon et le coeur," pp. 421–439. Vigot Frères, Paris.

Moret, P. R. (1971). *In* "High Altitude Physiology: Cardiac and Respiratory Aspects" (R. Porter and J. Knight, eds.), pp. 131–148. Churchill-Livingstone, Edinburgh and London.

Moret, P. R. (1971–1972). *Cardiology* **56**, 161–172.

Moret, P. R. (1976). *In* "Anthropologie des populations Andines," pp. 371–380. INSERM, Paris.

Moret, P. R., and Duchosal, F. (1973). *Schweiz. Med. Wochenschr.* **103**, 1796–1797.

Moret, P. R., and Duchosal, F. (1976). *Schweiz. Med. Wochenschr.* **106**, 1564–1566.

Moret, P. R., and Lutzen, U. (1977a). *Ann. Cardiol. Angeiol.* **26**, 85–94.

Moret, P. R., and Lutzen, U. (1977b). *Schweiz. Med. Wochenschr.* **107**, 1585–1586.

Moret, P. R., and Lutzen, U. (1977c). *J. Mol. Cell. Cardiol.* **9**, Suppl. No. 53.

Moret, P. R., Mégevand, R., Pattay, J., Infante, F., and Bopp, P. (1964). *Cardiologia* **44**, 208–217.

Moret, P. R., Bopp, P., Grosgurin, J., Hatam, K., Ahmadi, N., and Odier, J. (1966a). *Cardiologia* **48**, 182–202.

Moret, P. R., Fournet, P. C., Bopp, P., and Infante, F. (1966b). *Helv. Med. Acta* **33**, 468–478.

Moret, P. R., Covarrubias, E., Coudert, J., and Duchosal, F. (1970). *Schweiz. Med. Wochenschr.* **100**, 2186–2189.

Moret, P. R., Covarrubias, E., Coudert, J., and Duchosal, F. (1972). *Acta Cardiol.* **27**, 285–305, 483–503, and 596–619.

Moret, P. R., Vergnes, H., and Duchosal, F. (1973). *Schweiz. Med. Wochenschr.* 103, 293–294.

Moret, P. R., Duchosal, F., and Opie, L. (1976). *In* "Anthropologie des populations andines," pp. 523–530. INSERM, Paris.

Moret, P. R., Duchosal, F., Weber, J., and Lutzen, U. (1978). *Coeur Med. Interne* 17, 75–85.

Mortimer, E. A., Jr., Monson, R. R., and McMahon, B. (1977). *N. Engl. J. Med.* 296, 581–585.

Murray, J. F., Gold, P., and Johnson, B. L., Jr. (1963). *J. Clin. Invest.* 42, 1150–1159.

Myles, W. S., and Radomski, M. W. (1974). *Aerosp. Med.* 45, 422–424.

Nayler, W. G., and Fassold, E. (1977). *J. Mol. Med.* 2, 299–308.

Nayler, W. G., Grau, A., and Yepez, C. (1977). *Cardiovasc. Res.* 11, 344–352.

Opie, L. H. (1969). *Am. Heart J.* 77, 100–122.

Opie, L. H., Duchosal, F., and Moret, P. R. (1978). *Eur. J. Clin. Invest.* 8, 309–315.

Ou, L. C., and Tenney, S. M. (1970). *Respir. Physiol.* 8, 151.

Pace, N., Griswold, R. L., and Grunbaum, B. W. (1964). *Fed. Proc., Fed. Am. Soc. Exp. Biol.* 23, 521.

Page, L. B. (1976). *Am. Heart J.* 91, 527–534.

Peñaloza, D. (1966). *Sci. Publ., Pan Am. Health Organ.* 140, 27.

Peñaloza, D., Sime, F., Banchero, N., and Gamboa, R. (1962). *Med. Thorac.* 19, 449–460.

Peñaloza, D., Sime, F., Banchero, N., Gamboa, R., Cruz, J., and Marticorena, E. (1963). *Am. J. Cardiol.* 11, 150–157.

Peñaloza, D., Sime, F., and Ruiz, L. (1971). *In* "High Altitude Physiology: Cardiac and Respiratory Aspects" (R. Porter and J. Knight, eds.), pp. 41–60. Churchill-Livingstone, Edinburgh and London.

Penney, D. G., and Cascarano, J. (1970). *Biochem. J.* 118, 221–227.

Perloff, J. K., Urschell, C. W., Roberts, W. C., and Caulfield, W. H. (1968). *Am. J. Med.* 45, 802–810.

Picon Reategui, E. (1966). *Arch. Inst. Biol. Andina* 1, 255–285.

Poupa, O. (1971–1972). *Cardiology* 56, 188–196.

Poupa, O., Krofta, K., Prochazka, J., and Chvapil, M. (1965a). *Physiol. Bohemoslov.* 14, 233–257.

Poupa, O., Turek, Z., Kalus, M., and Krofta, K. (1965b). *Physiol. Bohemoslov.* 14, 542–545.

Poupa, O., Krofta, K., Prochazka, J., and Turek, Z. (1966). *Fed. Proc., Fed. Am. Soc. Exp. Biol.* 25, 1243–1246.

Pugh, L. G. C. E. (1964). *J. Appl. Physiol.* 19, 441–447.

Pugh, L. G. C. E., Gill, M. B., Lahiri, S., Milledge, J. S., Ward, M. P., and West. J. B. (1964). *J. Appl. Physiol.* 19, 431–440.

Purshottam, T., Kaveeshwar, U., and Brahmachari, H. D. (1977). *Aviat. Space Environ. Med.* 48, 351–355.

Rabinowitz, M., and Zak, R. (1972). *Annu. Rev. Med.* 23, 245–262.

Ramsφe, K., Jarnum, S., Preisig, R., Tauber, J., Tygstrap, N., and Westergaard, H. (1970). *J. Appl. Physiol.* 28, 725–727.

Rapin, J. R., Coudert, J., Drouet, L., Durand, J., and Cohen, Y. (1977). *Experientia* 33, 739–740.

Recavarren, S., and Arias-Stella, J. (1964). *Br. Heart J.* 26, 806–812.

Reynafarje, B. (1962). *J. Appl. Physiol.* 17, 301–305.

Reynafarje, B. (1971–1972). *Cardiology* 56, 206–208.

Reynafarje, B. and Velasquez, T. (1966). *Fed. Proc., Fed. Am. Soc. Exp. Biol.* 25, 1397–1399.

Reynafarje, C., Faura, J., Villavivencio, D., Curaca, A., Reynafarje, B., Oyola, L., Contreras, L., Vallenas, E., and Faura, A. (1975). *J. Appl. Physiol.* 38, 806–810.

Richardson, D. W., Kontos, H. A., Raper, A. J., and Patterson, J. L., Jr. (1967). *J. Clin. Invest.* 46, 77–85.

Rose, L. B., and Hoffman, D. L. (1956). *Circ. Res.* **4**, 130–132.

Rotta, A. (1955). *Rev. Peru. Cardiol.* **4**, 71.

Rotta, A., Canepa, A., Hurtado, A., Velasquez, T., and Chavez, R. (1956). *J. Appl. Physiol.* **9**, 328–336.

Roy, S. B. (1973). "Circulatory and Ventilatory Effects of High Altitude-Acclimatization and Deacclimatization of Indian Soldiers. A Prospective Study. 1964–1972." Indian Counc. Med. Res., New Delhi.

Rudolph, W. (1971–1972). *Cardiology* **56**, 209–215.

Rudolph, W., and Fruhman, G. (1966). *Verh. Dtsch. Ges. Inn. Med.* **72**, 560–573.

Rudolph, W. Meister, W., and Kriener, J. (1967). *Verh. Dtsch. Ges. Inn. Med.* **73**, 751–755.

Ruiz, L., Figueroa, M., Horna, C., and Peñaloza, D. (1969). *Arch. Inst. Cardiol. Mex.* **39**, 474.

Runeberg, L., and Pakarinen, A. (1967). *Ann. Med. Exp. Biol. Fenn.* **45**, 428–433.

Saltin, B., Grover, R. F., Blomqvist, C. G., Hartley, L. H., and Johnson, R. L., Jr. (1968). *J. Appl. Physiol.* **25**, 400–409.

Samad, I. A., and Noehren, T. N. (1965). *Dis. Chest* **48**, 376–379.

Sanadi, D. R., and Flukarty, A. I. (1963). *Biochemistry* **2**, 523–528.

Sanchez, C., Merino, C., and Figallo, M. (1970). *J. Appl. Physiol.* **28**, 775–778.

Scheuer, J. (1972). *J. Mol. Cell. Cardiol.* **4**, 689–692.

Scheuer, J. (1975). *Recent Adv. Stud. Card. Struct. Metab.* **10**, 195–207.

Scheuer, J., and Stezoski, S. W. (1970). *Circ. Res.* **27**, 835–849.

Scheuer, J., and Stezoski, S. W. (1972a). *Circ. Res.* **30**, 418–429.

Scheuer, J., and Stezoski, S. W. (1972b). *J. Mol. Cell. Cardiol.* **4**, 599–610.

Scheuer, J., Shavers, J. A., Kroetz, F. W., and Leonard, J. J. (1970a). *Cardiology* **55**, 193–210.

Scheuer, J., Shavers, J. A., Kroetz, F. W., and Leonard, J. J. (1970b). *Abstr. World Congr. Cardiol., 6th, 1900* p. 278.

Schoenmackers, J., and Schoene, D. (1972). *Z. Kardiol.* **62**, 555–567.

Sebening, F. (1965). Uber klinische und experimentelle Untersuchungen des Myokardstoffwechsels während der Operation Korrektur von Herzfehlern. Habilitations schrift, München.

Seley, H. (1958). "The Chemical Prevention of Cardiac Necrosis." Ronald Press, New York.

Sen Gupta, J., Dua, G. L., Srinivasulu, N., and Malhotra, M. S. (1975). *Aviat. Space Environ. Med.* **40**, 907–910.

Simanovskij, L.N., and Cotoev, Z. A. (1971). *Bull Exp. Biol. Med. (Leningrad)* **5**, 65–66.

Sime, F., Banchero, N., Peñaloza, D., Gamboa, R., Cruz, J., and Marticorena, E. (1963). *Am. J. Cardiol.* **11**, 143–149.

Sime, F., Peñaloza, D., Ruiz, L., Gonzalez, M., Covarrubias, E., and Postigo, R. (1974). *J. Appl. Physiol.* **36**, 561–565.

Singer, T. P. (1965). *In* "Oxidases and Related Redox System" (T. E. King, H. S. Manson, and M. Morrison, eds.). Wiley, New York.

Siri, W. E., Van Dyke, D. C., Winckell, H. S., Pollycove, M., Parker, H. G., and Cleveland, A. S. (1966). *J. Appl. Physiol.* **21**, 73–80.

Somogyi, E., Balogh, I., and Sotonyi, P. (1976). *Acta Morphol. Acad. Sci. Hung.* **24**, 35–45.

Sonnenblick, E. H., and Brutsaert, D. L. (1972). *Cardiology* **57**, 11–15.

Sørensen, S. C., Lassen, N. A., Severinghaus, J. W., Coudert, J., and Zamora, M. P. (1974). *J. Appl. Physiol.* **37**, 305–310.

Stere, A. J., and Anthony, A. (1977). *J. Appl. Physiol.* **42**, 501–507.

Stone, H. O., Thompson, H. K., Jr., and Schmidt-Nielsen, K. (1968). *Am. J. Physiol.* **214**, 913–918.

Stupfel, M., and Roffi, J. (1961). *C. R. Seances Soc. Biol. Ses Fil.* **155**, 237.

Surks, M. I. (1967). *In* "Biomedicine Problems of High Terrestrial Elevations" (A. H. Hegnauer, ed.), pp. 186–203. US Army Res. Inst. Environ. Med., Washington, D.C.

Surks, M. I., Beckwill, H. J., and Chidsea, C. A. (1967). *J. Clin. Endocrinol. Metab.* 27, 789–799.

Tappan, D. V., and Reynafarje, B. (1957). *Am. J. Physiol.* 190, 99–103.

Tappan, D. V., Reynafarje, B., Van Potter, R., and Hurtado, A. (1957). *Am. J. Physiol.* 190, 93–98.

Tenney, S. M., and Ou, L. C. (1969). *In* "Biomedicine Problems of High Terrestrial Elevations" (A. H. Hegnauer, ed.), p. 160. US Army Res. Inst. Environ. Med., Washington, D.C.

Tenney, S. M., and Ou, L. C. (1970). *Respir. Physiol.* 8, 134–150.

Torrance, J. D., Lenfant, C., and Cruz, J. (1970–1971). *Respir. Physiol.* 11, 1–15.

Tucker, A., McMurtry, I. F., Reeves, J. T., Alexander, A. F., Will, D. H., and Grover, R. F. (1975). *Am. J. Physiol.* 228, 762–767.

Tucker, C. E., James, W. E., Berry, M. A., Johnstone, C. J., and Grover, R. F. (1976). *J. Appl. Physiol.* 41, 356–361.

Urbanova, D., Ressl, J., Widimsky, J., Ostadal, B., Pelouch, V., and Prochazka, J. (1973). *Beitr. Pathol.* 150, 389–399.

Urbanova, D., Pelouch, V., and Ostadal, B. (1977). *Cor Vasa* 19, 246–250.

Valdivia, E. (1957). *Circ. Res.* 5, 612–616.

Valdivia, E., Watson, M., and Dass, C. M. (1960). *Arch. Pathol.* 69, 199–208.

Van Liere, E. J. (1936). *Am. J. Physiol.* 116, 290–294.

Van Liere, E. J., Krames, B. B., and Northrup, D. W. (1965). *Circ. Res.* 16, 244–248.

Velasquez, T. M. (1964). *In* "The Physiological Effects of High Altitude" (W. H. Weihe, ed.), p. 289. Macmillan, New York.

Velasquez, T. M. (1966). *Arch. Inst. Biol. Andina* 1, 189–212.

Vergnes, H., and Moret, P. R. (1976). *Enzyme* 21, 516–523.

Vergnes, H., Moret, P., and Duchosal, F. (1971). *In* "Extractive Colloque de Préadaptation génétique," pp. 81–102. INSERM, Paris.

Vergnes, H., Moret, P. R., and Duchosal, F. (1976). *Enzyme* 21, 66–75.

Vogel, J. A., Hansen, J. E., and Harris, C. W. (1966). *U.S. Army Med. Res. Nutr. Lab. Rep.* 294.

Vogel, J. A., Genovese, R. L., Powell, T. L., Bishop, G. W., Bucci, T. J., and Harris, C. W. (1971). *Am. J. Vet. Res.* 32, 2059.

Vogel, J. A., Hartley, H., Cruz, J. C., and Hogan, R. (1974a). *J. Appl. Physiol.* 36, 169–172.

Vogel, J. A., Hartley, L. H., and Cruz, J. C. (1974b). *J. Appl. Physiol.* 36, 173–176.

Vogel, J. H. K., Jamieson, G., Delivoria-Papadopoulos, M., Lueker, R. D., Brammell, H. L., and Brake, D. (1970). *Adv. Cardiol.* 5, 80–85.

Wachtlova, M., Mares, V., and Ostadal, B. (1977). *Virchows Arch. B* 24, 335–342.

Ward, M. (1975). "Mountain Medicine. A Clinical Study of Cold and High Altitude." Crosby Lockwood Staples, London.

Weber, J., Clara, F. R., Horvat, L., Cougn, R., and Moret, P. R. (1973). *Schweiz. Med. Wochenschr.* 103, 295–297.

Weidemann, H. (1972). *Fortschr. Med.* 90, 381–384.

Weinschenk, V. K. (1939). *Beitr. Pathol. Anat. Allg. Pathol.* 102, 477–484.

Weissler, A. M., Kruger, F. A., Baba, N., Scarpelli, D. G., Leighton, R. F., and Gallimore, J. K. (1968). *J. Clin. Invest.* 47, 403–416.

Widimsky, J., Urbanova, D., Ressl, J., Ostadal, B., Pelouch, V., and Prochazka, J. (1973). *Cardiovasc. Res.* 7, 798–808.

Wilson, M. A., and Cascarano, J. (1970). *Biochim. Biophys. Acta* 216, 54–62.

Wittenberg, J. B. (1965). *J. Gen. Physiol.* **49**, 57–74.

Zelter, M., Capderou, A., Poliansky, J., and Mensch-Dechene, J. (1976). *In* "Anthropologie des populations andines," pp. 383–402. INSERM, Paris.

Zhaparov, B., and Mirrakhimov, M. M. (1976). *Bull. Exp. Biol. Med. (Engl. Transl.)* **81**, 906–908.

Zhaparov, B., and Mirrakhimov, M. M. (1977). *Bull. Exp. Biol. Med. (Engl. Transl.),* 109–112.

Zimmerman, H. A. (1952). *Dis. Chest* **22**, 269–273.

8

The Heart and Exercise Training

H. Lowell Stone

I. Introduction

Exercise training has been shown to result in metabolic changes in skeletal muscle and changes in the cardiovascular system (Scheuer and Tipton, 1977; Clausen, 1977). The cardiovascular changes that have been most noticeable are (1) a decrease in resting heart rate, (2) an increase in resting stroke volume, (3) a reduced heart rate at submaximal workload, and (4) an increase of the cardiac size at rest. The classical definition of a training effect has long been the resting cardiac bradycardia and the increase in maximal oxygen consumption. Associated with these training effects has been the ability, particularly in experimental animals, to demonstrate the metabolic changes in skeletal muscle, i.e., an increase in the aerobic capacity. Using these criteria in both experimental animals and human subjects, this chapter will endeavor to delineate the present state of our knowledge in terms of the changes that occur in the heart during training and the possible mechanism that might be involved. For the sake of presentation of material, the chapter will begin with changes occurring in the cardiac muscle cell, the intact heart, and the intact animal. Included within this discussion will be the changes that may occur in the coronary vascular bed of the heart and the role of the autonomic nervous system in the overall response of the heart to exercise training. The material covered will deal mainly with *dynamic* exercise and not *static* exercise. The primary reason for this is the lack of any good experimental data on the mechanism of the effect of repetitive static exercise on the heart.

II. Effects of Training on the Cardiac Muscle Cell

A. Structure

Repetitive exercise has been found to result in either no change in heart weight or an increase in heart weight, depending on the type of exercise used. In studies (Dowell *et al.,* 1976; Tomanek, 1969) using treadmill exercise in rats, no significant difference has been found in heart weights, whereas using swimming as the exercise stress, an increase in heart weight has been reported (Leon and Bloor, 1968, 1976). *Fiber diameter* in the treadmill-trained rats did not change, whereas in the swimming-trained rats, the increase in heart weight was associated with both a hyperplasia of the cardiac muscle cell and an increase in sarcoplasmic volume. In dogs trained by treadmill running, no significant increase in heart weight (Stone, 1977a) or cell size (McGill and Stone, 1977) has been observed.

The preceding studies raise the question of the difference in the response of the heart to training by treadmill or swimming exercise. It should be noted at this point that many differences will appear at the cellular level between these two methods of producing the physiological changes associated with training. Despite these differences, there are apparently two responses of the heart to repetitive intermittent regular exercise. This should be kept in mind as the various cellular changes are discussed. Emphasis will be placed on the similarities that exist but the differences will be pointed out.

Other membrane systems of the myocardial cell have been found to change with training accomplished by swimming. The intercalated disc (Sohal *et al.,* 1968) and mitochondria (Arcos *et al.,* 1968; Aldinger and Rajindar, 1970) appear to be altered, with the effects being related to the duration of the training program. In rats trained by treadmill running, the mitochondria appeared to be smaller (Edington and Cosmas, 1972), but in subsequent studies, no difference in cellular membranes or mitochondria were found. Morphometric analysis of the data utilizing the determination of mitochondrial volumes and surface area in the trained dog shows no significant difference from studies conducted on hearts from sedentary animals (McGill and Stone, 1977).

The effect of repetitive exercise on the mass of the heart has varied from none to a significant increase in myocardial mass. There appears to be no relationship of the heart mass to the type of exercise used to obtain the training but rather more of an effect of the intensity and possibly the duration of the training program. In rats trained by treadmill running, many investigators do not find any change in heart weight (DeSchryver et al., 1969; Oscai et al., 1971), whereas others using a more intensive training program have found an increase in heart weight (Spear et al., 1978; Tipton, 1965; Siguardsson et al., 1977; Ostman and Sjöstrand, 1971). Rats trained by swimming exercise generally have been reported to have an increased heart weight as compared to sedentary controls (Leon and Bloor, 1968; Crews and Aldinger, 1967). Cats trained by treadmill running (Williams and Potter, 1976) and dogs trained in a similar manner (Stone, 1977a; Wyatt and Mitchell, 1974) do not increase their heart weight with the training program. In these latter two cases (i.e., cat and dog) a slight increase of 8–10% was found, which is much less than that found in swimming-trained rats. In the unanesthetized dog undergoing a training program, angiographic studies (Stone, 1977b) demonstrated that there was an increase in left ventricular end-diastolic volume prior to achieving the criteria for training and this was followed in time by an increase in wall thickness. In these experiments, when training was achieved, both an increase in end-diastolic volume and wall thickness was found.

The classical finding in highly trained human subjects is the increase in heart shadow size when a roentgenogram is taken of the chest. The question has been whether this represented an increase in heart chamber volume, wall thickness, or both. Alluding to the preceding study in unanesthetized dogs (Stone, 1977b), it could be concluded that the increase in heart shadow size represents an increase in both heart chamber volume and wall thickness. In two recent studies (DeMaria et al., 1978; Gilbert et al., 1977), the left ventricular chamber volume and wall thickness have been measured by echocardiography. In one study (DeMaria et al., 1978), pre- and post-training echocardiographic measurements were obtained in a group of subjects, whereas in the second study (Gilbert et al., 1977) using similar methodology, trained and untrained subjects were compared. In subjects compared before and after training (DeMaria et al., 1978) the ultrasonic left ventricular end-diastolic dimension increased from 4.8 ± 0.1 to 5.0 ± 0.1 cm and wall thickness increased from 9.1 ± 1.3 to 10.1 ± 1.2 mm. These dimensions are taken with the subjects at rest. Calculated left ventricular mass was augmented by 12%. In the study (Gilbert *et al.*, 1977) using two separate populations, similar results were obtained. The increase in the heart shadow on roentgenograph examination of athletes is a result of an increase in both left ventricular volume and mass of the heart.

B. Mitochondria and Sarcoplasmic Reticulum

The primary subcellular particle to be described here is the mitochondria. In all mammalian tissues, the mitochondria are the sole energy-producing sources for cellular function. The oxidative capacity of these organelles seems to be governed chiefly by the content of an electron transport chain located on their internal cristae. The inner mitochondrial membrane contains many transporter molecules and enzyme systems that shuttle substrate into the mitochondria and also subserves ion transport functions. In skeletal muscle the major adaptation found is an increase in the aerobic capacity associated with the mitochondria (Holloszy and Booth, 1976). The increase in skeletal muscle aerobic capacity is directly correlated with a pronounced increase in respiratory enzyme activity of the mitochondria. In the heart, similar studies have failed to find any changes in the respiratory activity (Oscai *et al.*, 1971; Scheuer *et al.*, 1974; Sordahl *et al.*, 1977) of isolated mitochondria. This implies that any mitochondrial adaptation in the heart does not involve a change in respiratory enzyme content and that heart and skeletal muscle adaptation are clearly different. No difference has been found in heart mitochondria for the phosphorylating efficiency (ADP:O) or the tightness of respiratory coupling (Scheuer *et al.*, 1974; Sordahl *et al.*, 1977). However, in the rat trained by swimming (Scheuer *et al.*, 1974) a decrease in the active mitochondrial respiratory component (state 3) has been found, which would indicate either an uncoupling of mitochondrial phosphorylating function or a different population of mitochondria in this study. A distinction between these two possibilities cannot be made at the present time.

Another functional aspect of the mitochondria is the energy-linked calcium ion transport, which either may have physiological significance in intracellular ionic homeostasis or under certain conditions may play a role in excitation–contraction coupling. The latter function of mitochondria has been suggested by Lehninger (1974), but definitive proof for this role is lacking. Mitochondria will take up calcium ion from a medium when supplied with a substrate and oxygen. When the system becomes anaerobic the mitochondria will release calcium ion back into the medium. This effect in mitochondria isolated from control dog hearts can be seen in Fig. 1. With the addition of substrate (succinate) and in the presence of 150 μm calcium there is a rapid uptake of calcium that is held in the mitochondria until release occurs in the absence of oxygen. The second curve in Fig. 1 was obtained from mitochondria isolated from a heart taken from an exercise-trained dog. There are two noticeable differences between the curves: (1) not as much calcium is actively transported by the mitochondria from the exercise-trained dog heart and (2) there is an early release of calcium from the mitochondria prior to the point of the system being anaerobic. This difference in mitochondrial function implied the possibility that a new type of mitochondria existed with different kinetic behavior for calcium transport. This possibility was probed by exposing the mitochondria to an agent (ruthenium red) that specifically blocks the calcium transport sites on the inner mitochondrial membrane. The results of such a study are shown in Fig. 2. It is clear from the data presented by Sordahl and associates (1977) that the number of calcium transportation sites on the inner mitochondrial membrane observed from trained dog hearts has decreased to approximately 50% of that in control mitochondria. Less calcium sequestration by the mitochondria would imply either that there is more free intracellular calcium at any time or that if the mitochondria are buffering the intracellular calcium over several minutes, the degree of buffering has diminished. In a subsequent study (Penpargkul *et al.*, 1978) on hearts taken from rats trained by swimming, mitochondrial calcium uptake and retention was not different from that of control mitochondria using similar substrates, as discussed in

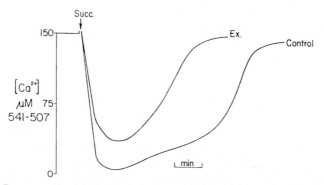

Fig. 1. Representative dual-beam spectrophotometric tracings of calcium uptake by mitochondria from control and exercised-trained (Ex) dog hearts. Addition of respiratory substrate succinate (Succ) produces a rapid energy-dependent uptake of calcium by mitochondrial preparations (downward deflection of traces). Preparations from exercise-trained hearts (Ex) exhibited incomplete uptake and rapid, premature release of calcium (upward deflection of trace) compared with control mitochondria. (Sordahl *et al.*, 1977, by permission.)

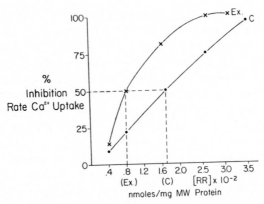

Fig. 2.   Effects of increasing concentration of ruthenium red (RR) on rates of calcium up-take by mitochondria isolated from control (c, circles) and exercise-trained (Ex, x's) dog hearts. Ruthenium red at a concentration of 0.8×10^{-2} nmoles/mg mitochondrial protein produces 50% inhibition of the rate of calcium uptake in exercised-trained preparations (Ex, dashed lines), whereas a concentration of 1.7×10^{-2} nmoles ruthenium red per mg mitochondrial protein was necessary to produce a similar degree of inhibition in control (c, dashed line) mitochondrial preparations. (Sordahl *et al.*, 1977, by permission.)

the previous study (Sordahl *et al.*, 1977). However, it was found (Penpargkul *et al.*, 1978) that in the presence of physiological concentration of adenosine triphosphate, calcium uptake in the mitochondria taken from hearts of trained rats was reduced compared with the control mitochondria.

A membrane system that has been implicated in excitation contraction coupling in the heart is the sarcoplasmic reticulum (Fozzard, 1977). This membrane system is less plentiful in heart muscle than in skeletal muscle (Katz, 1970) but has similar properties. The sarcoplasmic reticulum binds calcium and releases this ion into the cell cytoplasm following the depolarization of the sarcolemmal membrane. An active potassium plus calcium ATPase located in the sarcoplasmic reticulum actively removes calcium ion from the surrounding medium, apparently during the relaxation phase of the muscle cell (Jones *et al.*, 1977). Changes in the amount of calcium bound, released, and taken up and the rates of the release or uptake would influence the cytoplasmic calcium ion concentration and thus the behavior of the contractile proteins. Two studies have reported on the sarcoplasmic reticulum from exercise-trained animals. The model used in one study was the rat trained by swimming (Penpargkul *et al.*, 1977); the other study used the treadmill-trained dog (Sordahl *et al.*, 1977). In the study using swimming-trained rats, an increased transport of calcium was found, whereas in the study using treadmill-trained dogs, no difference in calcium transport was observed. Both studies used similar techniques for isolation of the sarcoplasmic reticulum and the reason for the difference is not readily apparent. It would be easy to say the difference was due to species of animals or type of training program, but there is a great deal of uncertainty in this area of cardiac biochemistry at the current time (Jones *et al.*, 1977).

In summary, the oxidative phosphorylation function of the mitochondria is not altered by training but the calcium transport function does appear to be changed. The sarcoplasmic reticulum may or may not be altered following training. The importance of the calcium transport function resides in the excitation–contraction scheme of the myocardium. There have been no measurements made of the sarcolemmal calcium transport in hearts from trained animals which serves a major portion of the calcium transport in the heart. This membrane system may hold the key to the relationship between calcium transport and change in cardiac function following exercise training.

C. Contractile Proteins

The cellular system that might most logically be affected by repetitive exercise leading to training would be the contractile protein of the muscle cell. In skeletal muscle the contractile function of various types of muscle has been shown to be related to the enzymatic activity (ATPase) of the contractile proteins (Close, 1972). Evidence has been accumulating that suggests this same relationship in cardiac muscle (Dowell, 1976; Shiverick *et al.*, 1976; Yazaki and Raben, 1974). An increase in myofibrillar enzymatic activity would imply an increase in contractile properties and could explain the potential increase in contractile function observed with exercise training in the heart.

The studies of contractile proteins in exercise-trained animals have been conducted on the swimming-trained rat and treadmill-trained rat and dog. The results obtained in the swimming-trained rat versus the treadmill-trained rat and dog are different and this difference may be the result of the mode of training or the stress involved in the training. The data will be discussed therefore first for the swimming-trained rat and then for the treadmill-trained animals, and little attempt will be made to reconcile the measurements.

The hearts from swimming-trained rats may or may not be hypertrophied, meaning that the actual mass of heart may or may not be increased. This is a critical question, since contractile protein changes associated with overt hypertrophy (Katz, 1970) may not have any relationship to exercise training. Actomyosin ATPase activity has been determined in swimming-trained rats (Bhan and Scheuer, 1972). There are two types of ATPase activity that can be activated in either myofibrillar or actomyosin preparations. One ATPase can be activated by the addition of calcium and is felt to be associated with the myosin molecule, while a second ATPase can be activated by magnesium and is associated with the actomyosin complex. Magnesium-activated ATPase in the myofibrillar preparation and in actomyosin preparation is felt to be the physiological representative of a change in contractile behavior of the intact muscle cell. An increase in actomyosin magnesium-ATPase occurred in the rats following 60 hours (8 weeks) of swimming with no increase in heart weight compared to the sedentary control group (see Fig. 3). The calcium-activated ATPase also increased in the actomyosin preparation from the trained-rat hearts. Figure 3 demonstrates these results and would indicate an increase in contractile behavior of the heart, and the increase in the calcium-ATPase suggests that the myosin molecule may have changed in these animals hearts. In subsequent studies (Bhan and Scheuer, 1975; Bhan *et al.,* 1975; Scheuer *et al.,* 1974), the Ca–ATPase activity of a purified myosin preparation was found to increase with training and this change was related to a structural change of the molecule in the region of the active site. These changes were used to explain the increase in intrinsic cardiac function, discussed later in this chapter, observed in isolated hearts from swimming-trained rats.

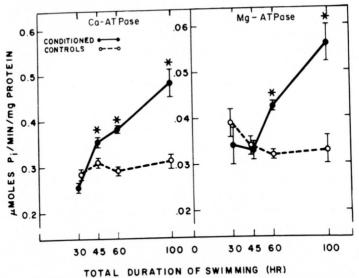

Fig. 3. The effect of total duration of swimming on Ca^{2+} and Mg^{2+}-stimulated ATPase activities of cardiac actomyosin. Results are mean ± SE. Asterisk indicates $P < 0.01$ when comparing hearts from control and conditioned animals. Thirty, 45, and 60 hr represent swimming 90 min/day for 4, 6, and 8 weeks. One hundred hours represent swimming 150 min/day for 8 weeks. Swimming was conducted 5 days/week. (Bhan and Scheuer, 1972, by permission.)

In the treadmill-trained rat and dog, the cardiac myofibrillar ATPase or actomyosin ATPase activity does not change as compared with control measurements (Dowell *et al.*, 1977; Baldwin *et al.*, 1975; Tibbits *et al.*, 1978). Values for these measurements can be found in Table I, taken from the references cited. It can be seen that the rat with a higher heart rate and index of contractility (*dP-dt*) has a higher Mg^{2+}-activated ATPase activity than the dog, which exactly fits the trend of data from skeletal muscle (Close, 1972). Thus any adaptation of intrinsic contractile function in this case must be derived from mechanisms other than changes in the contractile proteins. The sensitivity to increasing concentration of potassium was used to determine if there were any changes in the actomyosin molecule (Dowell *et al.*, 1977) and there was no difference found between sedentary and trained animals.

In summary, the contractile proteins of the heart in rats trained by swimming have an increased contractile ability that is evidenced by an increase in the ATPase activity of actomyosin and myosin. The behavior of the contractile proteins from treadmill-trained rats and dogs is no different before or after a training program. This fundamental difference may reside in the intensity of the training program and the stress imposed on the animals during the training. Both rats and dogs have been reported to increase or decrease the contractile protein function in states such as hyperthyroidism, pressure overload hypertrophy, cardiac failure, and catecholamine-induced hypertrophy. All of these states are recognized not to be physiologically normal. Whether the rat trained by swimming is responding solely to the repetitive exercise or some other stresses is not clear at this time.

D. Cellular Metabolism

Holloszy and Booth (1976) have reviewed the metabolic alterations that take place in skeletal muscle with training, but similar changes have not been found to be as prominent in the heart.

Glycogen content of rat hearts trained by swimming has been shown to be increased (Scheuer *et al.*, 1970; Shelley *et al.*, 1942), whereas the glycogen content of hearts from treadmill-trained rats does not change (Segel and Mason, 1978). Glycogen synthase activity did not increase in the same animals (Segel and Mason, 1978), which would indicate that in this study at least the glycogenolytic pathways have not changed with training. The glycolytic pathway has not been studied extensively in the heart from trained animals. The few studies that have been done indicate that there are no major changes in glucose metabolism or glycolytic enzymes with the exception of pyruvate kinase (York *et al.*, 1975).

In the rat myocardium, lower triglyceride stores and an increased turn-

TABLE I

Mg^{2+}-Activated Myofibrillar ATPase Activity from Untrained (UT) and Trained (T) Animals

Species	HR[a]	Myofibrillar ATPase[b]		dP/dt[c]		Ref.
		UT	T	UT	T	
Rat	403 ± 9	0.324 ± 0.006	0.308 ± 0.012	6550 ± 350	6392 ± 374	Dowell et al. (1976)
						Tibbits et al. (1978)
Dog	132 ± 8	0.199 ± 0.012	0.194 ± 0.012	2620 ± 450	2969 ± 423	Dowell et al. (1977)

[a] Heart rate in beats per minute. All values are ± 1 standard error of the mean.
[b] Mg-activated expressed in μmol P$_i$/mg min^{-1}.
[c] Maximum rate of rise of left ventricular pressure at rest expressed in mm Hg/sec.

over of fatty acids through the triglyceride pool have been found (Fröberg, 1971). Lipoprotein lipase activity in heart following training did not increase as found in skeletal muscle (Borensztajn *et al.,* 1975). Other studies of the palmatylcarnitene transferase system of the inner mitochondrial membranes have not been done in hearts from trained animals to determine if the use of free fatty acid residues has changed in the heart from trained animals.

The adaptation of the metabolic pathways found in skeletal muscle with training is not evident in cardiac muscle under similar conditions.

III. Effects of Training on Papillary Muscle and Isolated Heart

A. Papillary Muscle

Muscle mechanics have been studied extensively in skeletal muscle taking advantage of the parallel organization of the skeletal muscle fibers. In the heart a parallel arrangement of fibers does not occur very often but can be found in the papillary muscle. The force–velocity relationship of cardiac papillary muscles has been well described (Sonnenblick, 1962; Jewell, 1977; Abbott and Gordon, 1975; Julian and Sollins, 1975), and this preparation should reflect any intrinsic changes in the muscle that results from an experimental procedure. Thus in the previous section we found some changes suggested in exercise-trained animals that should be reflected in various parameters of tension, rate of tension development, and time of contraction in the papillary muscle.

Table II summarizes the results from the animal preparation that have been used to study papillary muscle mechanics following some form of exercise training. It should be noted that no changes have been found in any study of passive characteristics in papillary muscle from trained animals. The results are very contradictory even with the same animal species (rat), but in the cat there is some agreement that no change in papillary muscle from heart of trained animals has been found. Thus at least in the papillary muscle preparation the cellular effects of exercise training observed by some authors (Bhan and Scheuer, 1972) have not been manifested. The reasons for this are unclear at the present time.

B. Isolated Heart

The isolated heart preparation has been used to study the effect of exercise training on the pump function of the heart and on some aspects of

TABLE II

Effect of Training on Papillary Muscle Mechanics[a]

| | | | Mechanics | | |
Animal	Training	Hypertrophy	Isotonic	Isometric	Ref.
Rat	Swimming	15%↑	↑	↑	Mole (1978)
Rat	Swimming	↑	N.C.	↑	Steil *et al.* (1975)
Rat	Running	↑	N.C.	↓	Grimm *et al.* (1962)
Rat	Running	↑	—	↓	Nutter and Fuller (1977)
Rat	Running	—	—	↑	Tibbits *et al.* (1978)
Cat	Running	N.C.	N.C.	N.C.	Williams and Potter (1976)
Cat	Swimming	N.C.	—	N.C.	Wyatt *et al.* (1978)

[a] (—) Not measured, (↑) increase, (↓) decrease, (NC) no change in parameter.

cardiac metabolism (Scheuer, 1977). This type of preparation has been primarily used in trained rats, where the hearts are smaller than other animals and can be maintained for several hours in a perfusion apparatus. The heart is removed from the animal and placed in a chamber that permits the investigator to control many parameters simultaneously, but this preparation is devoid of any nervous system influence. The contractile properties of the intact isolated heart can be studied under a variety of conditions such as hypoxia, ischemia, or elevation of filling pressure. Such studies have been accomplished and tend to indicate that the hearts from the trained animals have improved pump function and are more resistant to hypoxia and possibly ischemia (Penpargkul and Scheuer, 1970; Scheuer and Stezoski, 1972; Bersohn and Scheuer, 1977; Schaible and Scheuer, 1980). Many of these studies have been accomplished on the swimming-trained rat.

In a recent study (Bersohn and Scheuer, 1977), pump function was studied by varying the left atrial filling pressure in the isolated heart preparation. Aortic flow, end-diastolic ventricular volume, and left ventricular pressure was measured during the variation in left atrial filling pressure in hearts from swimming-trained rats and control rats. End-diastolic volume was found to be the same in the hearts from the two groups of animals (see Fig. 4) as filling pressure was varied. This was a very important finding, since some of the previous observations could have been explained on the basis of an increase in end-diastolic volume in the hearts from the trained animals. At the initial filling pressure used (10 mm Hg) stroke volume of the hearts from trained animals was larger than in the control group and the ejected fraction was larger. When filling pressure was increased (20 mm Hg) the differences in stroke volume and ejected fraction became larger, with the hearts from trained animals increasing stroke volume, whereas in the hearts from control animals stroke volume changed very little. Calculation of the contractile element velocity and total contractile fiber shortening again showed that these calculated values were higher under similar conditions in trained hearts as compared with the control hearts. These latter data were obtained in the absence of any apparent change in diastolic ventricular compliance. The authors concluded from these studies that the hearts from the trained animals showed an enhanced performance that did not depend on an increase in diastolic fiber length (Starling effect) and that the increase in ejected fraction and fiber shortening were indicative of an increase in

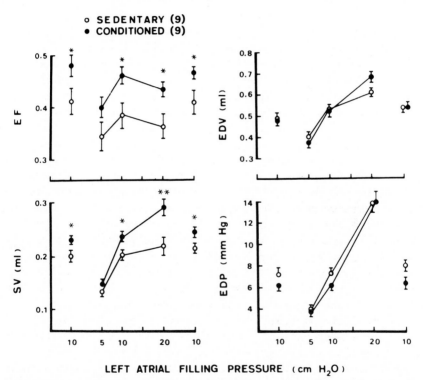

Fig. 4. Ejection fraction (EF), end-diastolic volume (EDV), stroke volume, (SV), and end-diastolic pressure (EDP) of hearts from conditioned and sedentary rats. Data for three different atrial filling pressures are shown. Data for each heart were recorded with 5-minute intervals between successive conditions, proceeding from left to right in each panel. Each point is the mean value for that atrial pressure. Vertical lines indicate ±1 SE. The number of hearts are shown in parenthesis. Asterisks indicate significance of the difference between groups at a particular atrial pressure. *P, 0.05; **P, 0.01. (Bersohn and Scheuer, 1977, by permission of the American Heart Association, Inc.)

contractility. Thus these data substantiate in the intact heart the findings at the subcellular level in the swimming-trained rat—namely, the increase in contractile protein function and calcium handling discussed previously.

A subsequent report (Schaible and Scheuer, 1979) has compared the response of the isolated hearts from treadmill-trained and swimming-trained rats in the same system. The experiments used a change in filling pressure as the stimulus with which to test the hearts from the trained animals. This study was particularly interesting, since it was the first comparison of the two types of programs to produce the cardiac changes synonymous with exercise training. The heart rate was measured in a group of animals in both the treadmill- and swimming-trained groups at the end of the training program. Resting heart rates were similar in the two trained groups and significantly lower than in a group of sedentary control animals. During either treadmill or swimming exercise, however, the treadmill-trained group had a significantly higher heart rate than the swimming group in the last 15–20 min of exercise. In general, the heart rate during treadmill running tended to be higher during the entire exercise period than the heart rate during swimming exercise. In the isolated heart preparation, the hearts from animals trained by swimming or treadmill exercise responded almost identically to changes in filling pressure, as discussed previously and as shown in Fig. 4. Both of the exercise-trained groups had a significantly higher stroke work, maximum power, and ejected fraction at the same end-diastolic volume as compared with the sedentary control group. The major difference found in this isolated heart study was that the hearts from swimming-trained animals had a larger negative rate of fall of left ventricular pressure (relaxation) than either the sedentary control or the treadmill-trained group. In neither trained group was there evidence of left ventricular hypertrophy. The authors concluded that the two types of training protocols were similar with the exception that the swimming exercise may have been more strenuous than the treadmill exercise in this study. If this were the case, it might explain the exercise heart rate and the negative rate of fall of left ventricular pressure difference between the two groups. In any event both groups of exercise-trained rats showed improved pump performance of the heart.

In summary, in the isolated working heart preparation a consistent improvement in pump function has been found, which supports some of the data obtained from isolated papillary muscle and at the cellular level. The improvement in pump function was found to be independent of the autonomic nervous system in this preparation and may be the result of changes at the cellular level in calcium handling or the contractile proteins.

As stated earlier, the hallmark of exercise training has been the resting bradycardia and the reduction in heart rate at submaximal workloads. The question arises whether the change in heart rate is intrinsic to the heart as a result of a new balance in the autonomic nervous system control of heart rate. Using an isolated heart preparation, Tipton *et al.* (1977) examined the question of intrinsic changes in heart rate produced by exercise training. In a group of trained rats, these investigators found a resting bradycardia in the intact animal, but in the isolated heart preparation this difference disappeared. In the resting animal, an intraperitoneal injection of isoproterenol (50 μg/kg) increased heart rate for the first 4 min following injections in both the trained and untrained groups. The heart rate increase in the trained group was larger than in the untrained group. This same increase in sensitivity to isoproterenol was found in the isolated heart preparation. Other investigators have found differences in the intrinsic rate of isolated sinoatrial tissue taken from exercise-trained rats (Bolter *et al.*, 1973; Hughson *et al.*, 1975, 1977). These investigators found that the intrinsic rate was 146 bpm (beats per minute) in control atria and 128 bpm in atria from trained animals. The difference between the two groups was significant. The reason for the different conclusions in these studies is not readily apparent at the present time.

A change in the intrinsic rate of the sinoatrial node in the trained rat would imply that the diastolic potential of these cells was different in hearts from trained as compared with untrained rats (Fozzard, 1977). This difference would implicate some change in the potassium channel of the sarcolemmal membrane such that the conductance of potassium was increased. The change in potassium conductance may be independent of any type of change observed in tissue neurotransmitters or enzymes in the synthetic pathway for the neurotransmitters as has been measured in many instances. Herrlich *et al.* (1960) and DeSchryver and Mertens-Strythagen (1975) have found significant increases in acetylcholine in the myocardium of trained rats when compared with untrained control animals. A 94% and 44% increase in acetylcholine was found in the two studies. Ekström (1974) has found that the level of choline acetyltransferase in the hearts from trained rats was increased. This enzyme is a key enzyme in the synthetic pathway for acetylcholine. Stone (1977a) has reported a decrease in the atrial content of acetylcholinesterase in trained dog hearts. This enzyme is the major enzyme responsible for the degradation of acetylcholine released from parasympathetic nerve terminals. All of these data indicate some possible change in either the synthesis or degradation of acetylcholine that would tend to reduce the resting heart rate in trained animals. Conversely, data on changes in the sympathetic nervous system are conflicting. Myocardial catecholamine levels have been reported to be increased, decreased, or unchanged (DeSchryver *et al.*, 1969; Leon *et al.*, 1975; Ostman and Sjöstrand, 1971; Ostman *et al.*, 1972) following exercise training.

In summary the intrinsic heart rate changes found in the isolated heart preparation may be due to changes in the diastolic potential of the sinoatrial nodal cells of the exercise trained heart. Additionally, the quantity of the parasympathetic nervous system neurotransmitter released may be changed and/or the degradation of this neurotransmitter may be altered.

C. Coronary Flow in the Isolated Heart Preparation

In the isolated heart preparation coronary flow has been measured during conditions of elevated filling pressure (Penpargkul and Scheuer, 1970; Schaible and Scheuer, 1980), hypoxia (Scheuer and Stezoski, 1972), and ischemia (Bersohn and Scheuer, 1977). When filling pressure was changed in one study to increase cardiac work, coronary flow was found to increase in both the sedentary control and swimming-trained rat hearts. The coronary blood flow in the hearts from the swimming-trained group increased more than in the sedentary group. Since there was more work being done by the hearts from the swimming-trained animals, coronary flow may have been increased to support this increased workload. In a subsequent study (Schaible and Scheuer, 1980) using a similar preparation, the coronary flow response to changes in filling pressure was found to be similar in hearts from sedentary controls and animals trained by either swimming or treadmill exercise. Hypoxia was used as another means to determine if the hearts from trained and sedentary animals were different. The coronary flow response to a combination of hypoxia and elevation of filling pressure was not different between the two groups of animals. As with the elevation of filling pressure alone, the work output by the hearts from trained animals was higher when compared with the hearts from sedentary control animals. Thus in this study the coronary flow response was not matched to the increase in work performed by the trained hearts. Ischemia was produced in the isolated heart preparation by restricting the total diastolic coronary flow. When this was done, there was no difference between the coronary flow in hearts from trained or sedentary animals. Upon reestablishment of normal coronary flow, the hearts from trained animals had a larger coronary flow, which might imply a larger coronary vascular bed in these animals.

In summary, the coronary flow changes in the isolated heart preparation do not directly indicate any specific difference as compared with hearts from sedentary control animals. It must be emphasized that these experiments were performed in isolated hearts that were deprived of any neural innervation. More will be said about coronary flow in a subsequent section.

IV. Effects of Training in the Intact Animal and Human

A. The Autonomic Nervous System—Heart Rate

The control of heart rate is through the autonomic nervous system effect on the intrinsic firing rate of the specialized cells of the sinoatrial node. In cardiac transplant patients the intrinsic rate seems to be approximately 100 bpm (Orlick *et al.*, 1978) and in cardiac denervated dogs approximately 100 bpm (Donald and Shepherd, 1963) also. An increase in vagal activity and the release of acetylcholine will reduce the rate of spontaneous discharge of the sinoatrial nodal cells and reduce heart rate. Conversely, an increase in the level of sympathetic activity to this region of the heart will increase the rate of discharge and increase heart rate. Clearly, there is an overlap in the effect of these two parts of the autonomic nervous system on heart rate. An increase in heart rate can be brought about by a decrease in vagal activity or an increase in sympathetic activity. As discussed previously, evidence has been obtained in both rats and dogs indicating that both the synthesis and degradation of acetylcholine may be affected by exercise training. There has been no direct measure of the neural activity traveling in the efferent vagal fibers to indicate whether an increase in vagal efferent activity also occurs with exercise training. A major difference has been found in the various species relating to the dominant portion of the autonomic nervous system that controls heart rate at rest. In the rat this seems to be primarily accomplished by the sympathetic nerves, whereas in the human and dog this appears to be accomplished by the vagus nerve.

As stated earlier, the major hallmark of world class athletes has been resting heart rates 15–20 bpm lower than those found in sedentary individuals (Branwell and Ellis, 1929). Numerous other studies in humans and animals have also found that the bradycardia is an adaptation to chronic exercise (Frick, 1967; Marsland, 1968; Tipton *et al.*, 1974; Tipton, 1965; Saltin *et al.*, 1968). The exact mechanisms responsible for the reduction in resting heart rate and submaximal exercise heart rate are not completely clear. It does seem evident that some change in the parasympathetic efferent fibers to the heart occurs such that there is an increase in vagal efferent neural signals, in increase in acetylcholine released, or a reduction in degradation of acetylcholine at the effector site. Any or all of these mechanisms may explain the results obtained in experimental studies to date.

Atropine, a cholinergic receptor blocking agent, has been used in trained and sedentary animals to demonstrate the probable role of the parasympathetic nervous system in the bradycardia (Lin and Horvath, 1972; Tipton and Taylor, 1965). Using submaximal doses of atropine, the heart rates of trained animals were found to be lower than those in sedentary controls. This would indicate that either there was an increase in acetylcholine in the trained hearts or there was a decrease in sensitivity to atropine. From what has been presented previously, there could also be a reduction in sympathetic activity to the heart resulting in a reduction in heart rate. The evidence to support this possibility is conflicting and again no direct measurements have been made of neural activity.

Another important question concerns the underlying changes in the circulatory system that lead to the bradycardia whether this be caused by a change in the efferent vagal or sympathetic nervous system activity. Clausen (1977) has presented the idea that in human subjects there are two possible components to the reduction in heart rate. One component may be an intrinsic change in the heart or parasympathetic nervous system component, which may primarily affect the resting heart rate and possibly the exercise heart rate also. Using subjects in which either both arms or both legs were used in training program, submaximal work with the trained muscle groups (legs or arms) resulted in a reduction in heart rate while a reduction was also found with submaximal work with the nontrained muscle groups. However, when the fact that a resting heart rate change had occurred with the training program was considered, exercise with the trained muscle groups resulted in a significant reduction in heart rate change from resting conditions as compared with the pretrained values. On the contrary, exercise with the nontrained muscle groups resulted in the same heart rate change as observed prior to training. These studies lead to the second component of the reduction in heart rate with training, which is the possible influence of the trained muscles on the sympathetic nervous system activity going to the heart. This component would be confined to the period of exercise. Afferent nerve fibers arising from skeletal muscle have been shown to influence both heart rate and blood pressure (Foreman *et al.,* 1979; Sato and Schmidt, 1973; Coote *et al.,* 1971; McCloskey and Mitchell, 1972; Coote and Sato, 1978). The working skeletal muscle component of the heart rate response to exercise would appear to travel over these same afferent fibers. It is fairly clear that the cardiac sympathetic nerves will increase their discharge frequency when the muscle afferents are activated. An adaptation in this reflex pathway could occur at any level of the nervous system (afferent receptors, spinal cord, or brain) with repetitive exercise leading to training. This proven reflex pathway would explain the possibility advanced by Clausen (1977) of the relationship between the exercising-trained muscle groups and the influence on heart rate. However, another possibility must also be considered, namely, the role of cardiac afferent receptors in the genesis of the exercise bradycardia (Linden, 1972). The sympathetic efferent fibers reaching the heart from the right stellate ganglion control heart rate more than the sympathetic efferent fibers from the left stellate ganglion (Norris *et al.*, 1974). In dogs with the left stellate ganglion removed (Schwartz and Stone, 1979) the heart rate response to submaximal exercise was greater at the higher workloads as compared with the same animals prior to the removal of the ganglion. When animals with the left stellate ganglion removed were trained, the bradycardia during submaximal exercise was not present, even though all other criteria for training were found (Stone, 1978a). This later evidence implicates the sympathetic afferent fibers traveling through the left stellate ganglion as being very important to the exercise-training resultant exercise bradycardia. Resting bradycardia was not examined in this study, but it would seem that this would also have been affected by the removal of the left stellate ganglion.

In summary (see Fig. 5), the bradycardia of exercise training may result from (1) adaptations at the effector organ such as changes in acetylcholine, choline acetyltransferase, or acetylcholinesterase; (2) an increase in vagal efferent nerve activity; and/or (3) a reduction in sympathetic efferent nerve

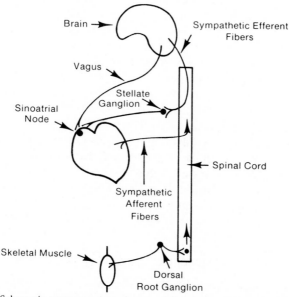

Fig. 5. Schematic representation of some of the autonomic innervation of the heart and afferent innervation of skeletal muscle. Afferent fibers reach the brain from the vagus nerve, sympathetic nerves, and muscle afferent nerves. The afferent nerves of the sympathetic system and muscle system have cell bodies located in the dorsal root ganglion of the spinal cord. The afferent information is integrated in the brain and the efferent vagal and/or sympathetic nerves are activated to change heart rate or other target tissues of the cardiovascular system. See text for more detail.

activity. It seems clear that afferent fibers from both the exercising muscle groups and the heart play a key role in the bradycardia response.

B. Ventricular Function

As discussed previously, an improved ventricular function was found in the isolated heart preparation from trained rats. In human subjects (Clausen, 1977) an improved ventricular function has not been measured directly following training but has been implied from the ability to increase maximum cardiac output.

A direct measurement of ventricular function has been accomplished in trained dogs (Stone, 1977a). Ventricular function was measured by rapidly loading the heart and increasing filling pressure. Previous studies (Bishop *et al.*, 1964; Stone *et al.*, 1967) have shown that when filling pressure was elevated in the conscious dog, heart rate, stroke volume, and cardiac output would all increase to a plateau level. The plateau of cardiac output was dependent on the level of heart rate achieved with the volume loading. In animals with both vagus nerves blocked the heart rate was very high and the maximum plateau of the cardiac output curve was obtained. This would correspond to a condition where no vagal activity existed and some high level of sympathetic activity was acting on the heart. The cardiac reserve would be the difference between any level of cardiac output and this maximum level when filling pressure is raised.

In the exercise-trained dog the cardiac reserve is increased (Fig. 6) by a reduction in the plateau of the cardiac output curve with volume loading. There is a greater difference between the cardiac output curve obtained in the trained animals and that obtained in animals during elimination of any vagal effect on the heart. Referring to Fig. 6, the cardiac reserve of the untrained animal has been labeled with the number 1 and that of the trained animal has been labeled with the number 2. The increase in cardiac reserve in this study directly demonstrates that ventricular pump function has been improved by exercise training.

C. Coronary Flow and Myocardial Oxygen Consumption

Change in coronary blood flow or in the coronary vasculature has long been cited by many exercise physiologists as a result of exercise training. This has been particularly true since the advent of major efforts to increase the physical conditioning of large segments of the public to reduce the effect or incidence of coronary artery disease. It must be said from the beginning of this section that there is no evidence to date that proves that any change in the coronary vasculature produced by exercise training pro-

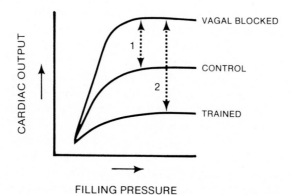

FILLING PRESSURE

Fig. 6. Schematic drawing of three ventricular junction curves showing the change in cardiac output resulting from an increase in filling pressure. As filling pressure is increased cardiac output reaches a plateau value in the conscious dog, which is highly reproducible for each animal. With a high level of sympathetic activity (vagal blocked) the maximum cardiac output plateau has been found to be considerably above the control value. Cardiac reserve in these two conditions would be the difference between the curves labeled control and vagal blocked at the plateau (number 1). Training increases the cardiac reserve (number 2).

vides protection against coronary artery disease or induces the growth of collateral vessels in the normal heart.

Exercise training has been shown by several methods to either increase or not affect the size or number of coronary vessels or capillaries. The coronary vessels of hearts from sedentary and trained rats have been injected with materials that harden within them, and the heart tissue can then be digested away. This method has been termed "corrosion casting." Using this method, studies have shown that exercise training increases the ratio of vascular space to myocardial mass in rats (Denenberg, 1972; Stevenson *et al.,* 1964; Tepperman and Perlman, 1961). Using a microscopic approach, Tomanek (1969) found an increase in capillary density in the absence of myocardial hypertrophy in exercise-trained rats. This finding of an increase in the capillary/fiber ratio was independent of age and appeared to depend only on the training. In another study (Leon and Bloor, 1968), rats trained by swimming had a significant increase in extracoronary collateral vessels and capillary/fiber ratio in the presence of cardiac hypertrophy (14%). The capillaries were identified in this light microscopic study by the presence of a red blood cell in the lumen of the capillary. It is entirely possible that with the cardiac hypertrophy in the trained animals more capillaries were open at the time of death of the animal, which would produce a high capillary/fiber ratio as compared with normal hearts. Maximal dilation prior to fixation would have precluded this problem. Radioactive thymidine was used in swimming-trained rats to label mitotically active endothelial cells of capillaries (Ljungqvist and Unge, 1977). In this study an increase in the heart weight/body weight ratio was found. There was a fivefold increase in labeling of the capillary walls in the hypertrophied heart indicative of the formation of new capillaries. More specifically, this increased labeling indicates an increase in DNA synthesis, which can lead to cell division. In treadmill-trained dogs (Wyatt and Mitchell, 1978), an increase in the diameter of the left circumflex coronary artery was found by angiographic techniques. This increase in diameter translated into a 20% increase in cross-sectional area of the vessel. In this same study on treadmill-trained dogs, biopsy material was taken from the right ventricular endocardium and examined under the electromicroscope for capillary density. A small but insignificant increase was found. The capillary was examined in yet another manner in exercise-trained dogs by determining the permeability–surface area product (Laughlin and Diana, 1975). This measurement is a functional measurement of the transport characteristics of the capillary. If the permeability of the capillary to a certain molecular size tracer has not changed with training, then any change in the permeability–surface area product would reflect a change in the surface area of the capillary network. In this study in the presence of an increase in heart weight/body weight ratio there was no difference in the permeability–surface area product compared with the control animals. This would indicate no change in the number of capillaries. The major drawback of this study was similar to that stated previously, namely, the coronary vascular bed was not intentionally maximally dilated. From these studies the capillary density of the rat heart may increase with training, but in the exercise-trained dog heart no increase in capillaries has been found. In both the dog and rat, the large coronary arteries appear to increase in diameter with exercise training. This may be the major specific adaptation of the coronary system to exercise training.

Coronary blood flow in the intact animal has been measured following exercise training in only a few studies (Spear et al., 1978; Laughlin et al., 1978; Bove et al., 1979; Stone, 1978b; von Restorff et al., 1977; Sanders et al., 1978; Heiss et al., 1976). In these studies rats (Spear et al., 1978), dogs (Laughlin et al., 1978; Bove et al., 1979; Stone, 1978b; von Restorff et al., 1977; Sanders et al., 1978), and human volunteers (Heiss et al., 1976) were used as the experimental subjects. In the rat study (Spear et al., 1978), coronary blood flow was measured by the injection of microspheres (15 ± 5 μm in diameter) into the left ventricle of the anesthetized animal. Maximal coronary vasodilation was achieved by respiring the animal on 12% oxygen while infusing a vasoactive drug to maintain aortic pressure near control levels. The ventricular weight of the trained animals was increased by 17% over matched sedentary control animals. When the animals were exposed to both a low oxygen breathing mixture and the infusion of the vasoactive drug, near maximal coronary vasodilation should have been achieved. Under these conditions a 60% increase in coronary conductance (flow/pressure) was found in the trained animals whereas in the sedentary control group no change in conductance was observed. The effect of the hypertrophy of the trained heart was accounted for by using sedentary control animals with similar-sized hearts. These authors (Spear *et al.*, 1978) concluded that the vascularity of the trained rat heart was greater than that found in sedentary control animals and represented a direct effect of exercise training. Contrary to this conclusion, a study in anesthetized trained dogs (Bove *et al.*, 1979) found that the coronary flow response to increasing afterload and filling pressure was not different when compared to sedentary control animals. The reason for the difference between the two studies is not clear unless it is simply a species difference.

In anesthetized trained dogs, the coronary flow response to a brief occlusion was measured (Laughlin *et al.*, 1978). The coronary blood flow response to the release of a brief total occlusion is termed the "reactive hyperemic response" and is always very large in the resting condition in the heart. There are two features of this response that have been used to determine the characteristics of the coronary vascular bed distal to the occlusion (Olsson and Gregg, 1965). The first feature is the peak of the flow response on release of the occlusion, which should be the maximum flow through the dilated vascular bed. The second feature is the total reactive hyperemic response in comparison to the lost occluded flow, which should be influenced by the washout of vasoactive metabolites that accumulated during the period of occlusion. It was found in the anesthetized trained dog (Olsson and Gregg, 1965) that the peak coronary flow following the release of the occlusion was greater in the trained dogs as compared with controls but that the reactive hyperemic response was not different. This would indicate that the coronary vascular bed had increased in size so that the washout of metabolites was the same. In similar studies using unanesthetized dogs (Stone, 1978b), the peak flow response to a brief occlusion was not found to change over time during a training program, but the reactive hyperemic response was significantly reduced. Since these two studies used the same duration of occlusion and the same animal species, we will discuss the possible reasons for these differences. Two major differences are the use of anesthesia in one study and the use of the same animal population through the other study. The peak hyperemic flow will be determined by the size of large conducting arteries and the size of the capillary bed as well as the resting flow. As stated previously, in the dog evidence has been presented to indicate that the size of the coronary arteries was greater in trained animals, and additional evidence was presented that capillary bed size may not have changed in the trained animals. The difference in the two studies cannot be the severity of the training program since the same program was used in both studies. The difference in the peak flow response could be the result of removal of a tonic vasoconstrictor tone from the coronary vessels by the anesthesia, thus simulating the increase in coronary vessel size. A tonic vasoconstrictor tone on coronary vessels has been clearly demonstrated by several investigators (Schwartz and Stone, 1977; Feigl, 1967; Gwirtz and Stone, 1979; Gwirtz et al., 1979). The difference in the reactive hyperemic responses may reside in the fact again that anesthesia and a high heart rate influence response. The reduction in the hyperemic response found in the one study (Stone, 1978b) could be explained by (1) a change in metabolism such that less vasoactive metabolites are produced; (2) a decrease in the distal area of myocardium being perfused, signifying a possible increase in collateral flow; or (3) a decrease in flow through epicardial vessels relative to endocardial vessels. At the present time, it is impossible to distinguish between these mechanisms but it should be appreciated that all would lead to an increase in coronary reserve capacity or improvement in coronary flow. In the end, both studies indicate that there is a change in the coronary vasculature of the trained dog that implies an improvement in the coronary vascular perfusion of the heart.

Direct measurement of coronary blood flow in a major coronary vessel has been made in two studies (von Restorff et al., 1977; Stone, 1979) in trained animals during exercise and coronary blood flow in untrained and trained human volunteers has been measured by a radioactive gas washout technique (Heiss et al., 1976). In the one study (von Restorff et al., 1977), two groups of dogs were used that were littermates. One group was maintained as a sedentary control group and the second group was trained for 8 weeks. The training regimen used in this study produced a reduction in exercise heart rate, but no other evidence was given for a training effect of the exercise program. At rest, blood flow through the left circumflex coronary artery was reduced compared to the littermate control group and the coronary sinus oxygen content was lower than that found in the sedentary control group. Myocardial oxygen consumption was similar in the two groups. On exercising the increase in coronary blood flow and myocardial oxygen consumption was less in the trained animals than in the controls. Cardiac output and arterial blood pressure were also reduced in the trained animals. The three major determinants of myocardial oxygen consumption are the heart rate, contractility, and tension developed by the heart. In this study, arterial pressure was reduced as well as heart rate, which would contribute to a reduction in myocardial oxygen consumption. No measure was made of the contractile state of the myocardium so the effect of this variable on myocardial oxygen consumption in the study is not known.

Using data presented in this study, mean coronary resistance was calculated and found to be the same at rest and at the highest level of exercise studies. This would indicate that the decrease in flow may have been the result of the decrease in driving pressure. One very interesting facet of this study was the decrease in coronary sinus oxygen saturation at rest and during exercise in the trained group of dogs.

In the second study (Stone, 1979), different results were found in trained dogs. Resting coronary blood flow and exercise coronary blood flow velocity were not different in the same group of dogs before and after training (i.e., untrained 19 ± 4 cm/sec versus trained 22 ± 4 cm/sec at rest). Myocardial oxygen consumption was also found to be the same before and after training at rest and during exercise (5.05 ± 0.85 ml O_2/min untrained versus 4.13 ± 1.49 ml O_2/min trained at rest). This result is not surprising, since in a previous study (Stone, 1978b) there was a small decrease in resting heart rate and contractility and arterial pressure were similar under the two conditions. The increase in volume and wall thickness of the left ventricle would result in an increase in coronary blood flow and myocardial oxygen consumption, whereas the decrease in heart rate at rest would result in a reduced flow and oxygen consumption (Stone, 1977c). These two types of changes apparently result in no changes in the resting values. During submaximal exercise the trained dog had a reduced heart rate but the contractility of the left ventricle was found to be increased above untrained values during the same level of exercise (Stone, 1977a). The increased contractility and the increased end-diastolic volume during exercise may again affect the decrease in heart rate as these factors influence myocardial oxygen consumption. However, an important finding in this study was a decrease in coronary blood flow velocity during submaximal exercise when the dogs were not fully trained (i.e., no reduction in submaximal heart rate). The reduction in coronary blood flow velocity occurred at a time during the training program when no other changes resulting from exercise could be observed except the reduction in the reactive hyperemic response discussed previously. The reduction in coronary flow was accompanied by a decrease in coronary sinus oxygen saturation and a slight increase in the arteriovenous oxygen content difference. The extraction of oxygen was increased by approximately 10%. Myocardial oxygen consumption was unchanged. These results taken together indicate that there may have been a change in the coronary vascular bed such that an improved perfusion of the myocardium resulted. Clearly the reduction in coronary blood flow during exercise would imply an increase in coronary flow reserve, but the mechanisms underlying this change in coronary blood flow are unknown at the present time.

One study (Heiss *et al.*, 1976) measuring coronary sinus blood flow in human volunteers has been reported. Two groups of college students were used, one group being trained and the other group sedentary. Coronary sinus blood flow was the same at rest, but much lower in the trained group during exercise. The level of training in the trained group was not given except that this group had a lower resting heart rate. The tension-time index was measured in this study and this variable has been shown to be a relative index of myocardial oxygen consumption. During exercise the tension-time index was lower in the trained group and was the same as the reduced myocardial oxygen consumption. From this study it appears that the reduction in myocardial oxygen consumption was related to the decrease in all major determinants of oxygen consumption. No indication was given whether the studies were accomplished at the same level of maximal whole body oxygen consumption so that a realistic comparison could be made. Nonetheless, potential changes in human subjects have been reported, but clearly more studies in normal human volunteers should be done.

A major unresolved question is the role of exercise training in the development of coronary collateral vessels, which would influence the myocardial response to ischemia. Several studies have addressed this problem but with varying results (Eckstein, 1957; Burt and Jackson, 1965; Sanders et al., 1978; Cohen et al., 1978; Heaton et al., 1978). In an early study by Eckstein (1957), the coronary artery was initially narrowed and then the animals were subjected to repetitive exercise. Later, the same coronary vessel was completely occluded and the retrograde flow measured. Retrograde flow was greater in the exercised animals compared to nonexercised animals. This would indicate an increase in collateral vessel development produced by the repetitive exercise program. In three other studies (Burt and Jackson, 1965; Sanders et al., 1978; Cohen et al., 1978), using different methods to measure collateral flow and imposing the occlusion of the coronary vessel after the animals were trained, no difference in collateral vessel flow was found. One study (Heaton et al., 1978) performed following a total ligation of one coronary vessel followed by repetitive exercise demonstrated an improvement in collateral vessel development into the underperfused myocardial region. The difference in these studies may be the relationship between the timing of the occlusive event with the training program. Training followed by occlusion of a major coronary vessel does not seem to demonstrate an immediate change in the collateral vessels. However, the degree of vessel occlusion prior to training does seem to result in improvement of collateral vessel function.

In summary, coronary blood flow has been found to be either unchanged or decreased during submaximal exercise following training. The current studies in human volunteers or animals directly indicate a decrease in the coronary sinus oxygen content during exercise after some degree of training. This could indicate an improvement in myocardial blood flow distribution toward the endocardial surface. The increase in coronary flow with volume loading in the isolated rat heart, the increase in coronary vessel size, and the change in the reactive hyperemic response all tend to indicate some type of change in the coronary vascular perfusion. Whether this change is completely anatomical or can involve a neurogenic component is unknown at the present time.

V. Conclusion

The changes in the heart following a program of exercise training are varied and probably small in each system under investigation. The only real test for a change in the heart following training is to force the heart to increase its performance by some means such as exercise, volume loading, or hypoxia. Resting values are of little interest from a physiological viewpoint. In this context, exercise training by treadmill running in rats and dogs does not result in any detectable changes in the contractile protein system of the heart, but other cellular systems may change to increase intracellular free calcium during contraction. Muscle function in hearts from trained animals also does not appear to be affected by training when the muscle is viewed in the classical ways. Efforts were made in these studies to detect small differences but little has been found to date. The pumping function of the heart has been shown to be improved in both trained rats and dogs. Data from human studies imply that pump function has also improved with training. The improvement in pump function does not appear to be related to cardiac hypertrophy but may be related to the summation of small changes in intrinsic mechanisms and, more likely, to changes in the autonomic nervous system activity to the heart.

Coronary blood flow may well change in the trained heart to improve the distribution across the myocardial wall or to increase the total conductance of the vascular bed. This change in the coronary vascular bed may or may not reflect the formation of new vessels or the opening of collateral vessels; yet the functional changes observed in several studies must be accounted for by one of these two mechanisms. It seems fairly clear at present that collateral coronary vessel growth can be stimulated by training following an ischemic episode. This effect may be explained by the effect of hypoxia in underperfused regions on the growth of collateral vessels. Further studies are needed to define the changes in collateral vessels in the trained heart and in hearts with partial stenosis of coronary vessels.

Acknowledgment

This work was supported in part by NIH Grant HL22154.

References

Abbott, B. C., and Gordon, D. G. (1975). *Circ. Res.* 36, 1–7.

Aldinger, F. E., and Rajindar, S. S. (1970). *Am. J. Cardiol.* 26, 369–374.

Arcos, J. C., Sohal, R. S., Sun, S. C., Argus, M. F., and Burch, G. E. (1968). *Exp. Mol. Pathol.* 8, 49–65.

Baldwin, K. M., Winder, W. W., and Holloszy, J. O. (1975). *Am. J. Physiol.* 229, 422–426.

Bersohn, M. M., and Scheuer, J. (1977). *Circ. Res.* 40, 510–516.

Bhan, A. K., and Scheuer, J. (1972). *Am. J. Physiol.* 223, 1486–1490.

Bhan, A. K., and Scheuer, J. (1975). *Am. J. Physiol.* 228, 1178–1182.

Bhan, A. K., Malhotra, A., and Scheuer, J. (1975). *J. Mol. Cell. Cardiol.* 7, 435–442.

Bishop, V. S., Stone, H. L., and Guyton, A. C. (1964). *Am. J. Physiol.* 207, 677–782.

Bolter, C. P., Hughson, R. L., and Critz, J. B. (1973). *Proc. Soc. Exp. Biol. Med.* 144, 364–367.

Borensztajn, J., Rone, M. S., Babirak, S. P., McGarr, J. A., and Oscai, L. B. (1975). *Am. J. Physiol.* 229 394–397.

Bove, A. A., Hultgren, P. B., Ritzer, T. F., and Carey, R. A. (1979). *J. Appl. Physiol.* 46, 571–578.

Branwell, C., and Ellis, R. (1929). *Arbeitsphysiologie* 2, 51–60.

Burt, J. J., and Jackson, R. (1965). *J. Sports Med. Phys. Fitness* 4, 203–206.

Clausen, J. P. (1977). *Physiol. Rev.* 57, 779–815.

Close, R. I. (1972). *Physiol. Rev.* 52, 129–197.

Cohen, M. V., Yipintsoi, T., Malhotra, A., Penpargkul, S., and Scheuer, J. (1978). *J. Appl. Physiol.* 45, 797–805.

Coote, J. H., and Sato, A. (1978). *Brain Res.* 142, 425–437.

Coote, J. H., Hilton, S. M., and Perez-Gonzales, S. F. (1971). *J. Physiol. (London)* 215, 780–804.

Crews, J., and Aldinger, E. E. (1967) *Am. Heart J.* 74, 536–542.

DeMaria, A. N., Neumann, A., Lee G., Fowler, W., and Mason, D. T. (1978). *Circulation* 57, 237–244.

Denenberg, D. L. (1972). *J. Sports Med. Phys. Fitness* 18, 76–81.

DeSchryver, C., and Mertens-Stythagen, J. (1975). *Experientia* 31, 316–318.

DeSchryver, C., Mertens-Strythagen, J., Becsei, I., and Lammerant, J. (1969). *Am. J. Physiol.* 217, 1589–1592.

Donald, D. E., and Shepherd, J. T. (1963). *Am. J. Physiol.* 205, 393–400.

Dowell, R. T. (1976). *Circ. Res.* 39, 683–689.

Dowell, R. T., Tipton, C. M., and Tomanek, R. J. (1976). *J. Mol. Cell. Cardiol.* 8, 407–418.

Dowell, R. T., Stone, H. L., Sordahl, L. A., and Asimakis, G. K. (1977). *J. Appl. Physiol.* 43, 977–982.

Eckstein, R. W. (1957). *Circ. Res.* 5, 230–235.

Edington, D. W., and Cosmas, A. C. (1972). *J. Appl. Physiol.* 33, 715–718.

Ekström, J. (1974). *Q. J. Exp. Physiol. Cogn. Med. Sci.* 59, 73–80.

Feigl, E. O. (1967). *Circ. Res.* 20, 262–271.

Foreman, R. D., Schmidt, R. F., and Willis, W. D. (1979). *J. Physiol. (London)* 286, 215–231.

Fozzard, H. A. (1977). *Annu. Rev. Physiol.* **39**, 201–220.

Frick, M. H. (1967). *In* "Physical Activity and the Heart" (M. J. Karvonen and A. J. Barry, eds.), pp. 33–41. Thomas, Springfield, Illinois.

Fröberg, S. O. (1971). *Metab. Clin. Exp.* **20**, 1044–1051.

Gilbert, C. A., Nutter, D. O., Felner, J. M., Perkins, J. V., Heymsfield, S. B., and Schlant, R. C. (1977). *Am. J. Cardiol.* **40**, 528–533.

Grimm, A. R., Kubota, R., and Whitehorn, W. V. (1963). *Circ. Res.* **12**, 118–124.

Gwirtz, P. A., and Stone, H. L. (1979). *Am. J. Cardiol.* **43**, 392.

Gwirtz, P. A., Laughlin, M. H., Stone, H. L., and Yipintsoi, T. (1979). *Fed. Proc, Fed. Am. Soc. Exp. Biol.* **38**, 3569.

Heaton, W. H., Marr, K. C., Capuno, N. L., Goldstein, R. E., and Epstein, S. E. (1978). *Circulation* **57**, 575–581.

Heiss, H. W., Barmeyer, J., Winks, K., Hell, G., Cerney, F. J., Keul, J., and Reindell, H. (1976). *Cardiology* **71**, 658–675.

Herrlich, H. C., Raab, W., and Gigee, W. (1960). *Arch. Int. Pharmacodyn. Ther.* **129**, 201–215.

Holloszy, J. O., and Booth, F. W. (1976). *Annu. Rev. Physiol.* **38**, 273–291.

Hughson, R. L., Sutton, J. R., Fitzgerald, J. D., Cadle, J. F., and Jones, N. L. (1975). *Med. Sci. Sports* **7**, 69–70.

Hughson, R. L., Sutton, J. R., and Jones, N. L. (1977). *Med. Sci. Sports* **9**, 70.

Jewell, B. R. (1977). *Circ. Res.* **40**, 221–230.

Jones, L. R., Besch, H. R., Jr., and Watanabe, A. M. (1977). *J. Biol. Chem.* **252**, 3315–3323.

Julian, F. J., and Sollins, M. R. (1975). *Circ. Res.* **37**, 299–308.

Katz, A. M. (1970). *Physiol. Rev.* **50**, 63–158.

Laughlin, M. H., and Diana, J. N. (1975). *Am. J. Physiol.* **229**, 838–846.

Laughlin, M. H., Diana, J. N., and Tipton, C. M. (1978). *J. Appl. Physiol.* **45**, 604–610.

Lehninger, A. L. (1974). *Circ. Res.* **34/35**, III-83–III-90.

Leon, A. S., and Bloor, C. M. (1968). *J. Appl. Physiol.* **24**, 485–490.

Leon, A. S., and Bloor, C. M. (1976). *Adv. Cardiol.* **18**, 81–92.

Leon, A. S., Horst, W. D., Spirit, O. N., Wiggan, E. B., and Womelsday, A. H. (1975). *Chest* **67**, 341–343.

Lin, Y., and Horvath, S. M. (1972). *J. Appl. Physiol.* **33**, 796–799.

Linden, R. J. (1972). *Cardiovasc. Res.* **6**, 605–626.

Ljungqvist, A., and Unge, G. (1977). *J. Appl. Physiol.* **43**, 306–307.

McCloskey, D. I., and Mitchell, J. H. (1972). *J. Physiol (London)* **224**, 173–186.

McGill, M., and Stone, H. L. (1977) *Circulation* **56**, 478.

Marsland, W. P. (1968). *J. Appl. Physiol.* **24**, 98–101.

Mole, P. A. (1978). *Am. J. Physiol.* **234**, H421–H425.

Norris, J. E., Foreman, R. D., and Wurster, R. D. (1974). *Am. J. Physiol.* **227**, 9–12.

Nutter, D. O., and Fuller, E. O. (1977). *Med. Sci. Sports* **9**, 239–245.

Olsson, R. A., and Gregg, D. E. (1965). *Am. J. Physiol.* **208**, 231–236.

Orlick, A. E., Ricci, D. R., Alderman, E. L., Stimson, E. B., and Harrison, D. C. (1978). *J. Clin. Invest.* **62**, 459–467.

Oscai, L. B., Mole, P. A., Brei, B., and Holloszy, J. O. (1971). *Am. J. Physiol.* **220**, 1238–1241.

Ostman, I., and Sjöstrand, N. O. (1971). *Acta Physiol. Scand.* **82**, 202–208.

Ostman, J., Sjöstrand, N. O., and Sividin, G. (1972). *Acta Physiol. Scand.* **86**, 299–308.

Penpargkul, S., and Scheuer, J. (1970). *J. Clin. Invest.* **49**, 1859–1868.

Penpargkul, S., Repke, D. I., Katz, A. M., and Scheuer, J. (1977). *Circ. Res.* **40**, 134–138.

Penpargkul, S., Schwartz, A., and Scheuer, J. (1978). *J. Appl. Physiol.* **45**, 978–986.

Saltin, B., Blomqvist, G., Mitchell, J. H., Johnson, R. L., Wildenthal, K., and Chapman, C. B. (1968). *Circ.* **32**, Suppl. 7, VII-1–VII-55.

Sanders, M., White, F. C., Peterson, T. M., and Bloor, C. M. (1978). *Am. J. Physiol.* **234**, H614–H619.
Sato, A., and Schmidt, R. F. (1973). *Physiol. Rev.* **53**, 916–947.
Schaible, T. F., and Scheuer, J. (1979). *Am. J. Physiol.* **46**, 854–860.
Scheuer, J. (1977). *Med. Sci Sports* **9**, 231–238.
Scheuer, J., and Stezoski, S. W. (1972). *Circ. Res.* **30**, 418–429.
Scheuer, J., and Tipton, C. M. (1977). *Annu. Rev. Physiol.* **39**, 221–251.
Scheuer, J., Kapner, L., Stringfellow, C. A., Armstrong, C. L., and Penpargkul, S. (1970). *J. Lab. Clin. Med.* **75**, 924–929.
Scheuer, J., Penpargkal, S., and Bhan, A. F. (1974). *Am. J. Cardiol.* **33**, 744–751.
Schwartz, P. J., and Stone, H. L. (1977). *Circ. Res.* **41**, 51–58.
Schwartz, P. J., and Stone, H. L. (1979). *Circ. Res.* **44**, 637–645.
Segel, L. D., and Mason, D. T. (1978). *J. Appl. Physiol.* **44**, 183–189.
Shelley, W. B., Code, C. F., and Visscher, M. B. (1942). *Am. J. Physiol.* **138**, 652–658.
Shiverick, K. T., Hamrell, B. B., and Alpert, N. R. (1976). *J. Mol. Cell. Cardiol.* **8**, 837–851.
Siguardsson, K., Suanfeldt, E., and Kilbom, A. (1977). *Acta Physiol. Scand.* **101**, 481–488.
Sohal, R. S., Sun, S. C., Calcolough, H. L., and Burch, G. E. (1968). *Lab. Invest.* **18**, 49–53.
Sonnenblick, E. H. (1962). *Am. J. Physiol.* **202**, 931–939.
Sordahl, L. A., Asimakis, G. K., Dowell, R. T., and Stone, H. L. (1977). *J. Appl. Physiol.* **42**, 426–431.
Spear, K. L., Koerner, J. E., and Terjung, R. L. (1978). *Cardiovasc. Res.* **12**, 135–143.
Steil, E., Hansis, M., Hepp, A., Kissling, G., and Jacob, R. (1975). *Recent Adv. Stud. Card. Struct. Metab.* **5**, 491–496.
Stevenson, J. A., Feleki, V., Rechnitzer, P., and Beaton, J. R. (1964). *Circ. Res.* **15**, 265–269.
Stone, H. L. (1977a). *J. Appl. Physiol.* **42**, 824–832.
Stone, H. L. (1977b). *Med. Sci. Sports* **9**, 253–261.
Stone, H. L. (1977c). *Fed. Proc., Fed. Am. Soc. Exp. Biol.* **36**, 449.
Stone, H. L. (1978a). *Physiologist* **21**, 117.
Stone, H. L. (1978b). *Fed. Proc., Fed. Am. Soc. Exp. Biol.* **37**, 1161.
Stone, H. L., (1979). *Fed. Proc., Fed. Am. Soc. Exp. Biol.* **38**, Pt. II, 4348.
Stone, H. L., Bishop, V. S., and Dong, E., Jr. (1967). *Circ. Res.* **20**, 587–593.
Tepperman, J., and Perlman, D. (1961). *Circ. Res.* **11**, 576–584.
Tibbits, G., Koziol, B. J., Roberts, N. K., Baldwin, K. M., and Barnard, R. J. (1978). *J. Appl. Physiol.* **44**, 85–89.
Tipton, C. M. (1965). *Am. J. Physiol.* **209**, 1089–1094.
Tipton, C. M., and Taylor, B. (1965). *Am. J. Physiol.* **208**, 480–484.
Tipton, C. M., Carey, R. A., Eastin, W. C., and Erickson, H. H. (1974). *J. Appl. Physiol.* **37**, 271–275.
Tipton, C. M., Matthews, R. D., Tcheng, T. K., Dowell, R. T., and Vailas, V. C. (1977). *Med. Sci. Sports* **9**, 220–230.
Tomanek, R. J. (1969). *Anat. Rec.* **167**, 55–62.
von Restorff, W., Holtz, J., and Bassenge, E. (1977). *Pfluegers Arch.* **372**, 181–185.
Williams, J. F., Jr., and Potter, R. D. (1976). *Circ. Res.* **39**, 425–428.
Wyatt, H. L., and Mitchell, J. H. (1974). *Circ. Res.* **35**, 883–889.
Wyatt, H. L., and Mitchell, J. H. (1978). *J. Appl. Physiol.* **45**, 619–625.
Wyatt, H. L., Chuck, L., Rabinowitz, B., Tybert, J. V., and Parmley, W. W. (1978). *Am. J. Physiol.* **234**, H608–H613.
Yazaki, Y., and Raben, M. S. (1974). *Circ. Res.* **35**, 15–23.
York, S. W., Penny, D. G., and Oscai, L. B. (1975). *Biochim. Biophys Acta* **381**, 22–27.

Cardiac Hypertrophy

Russell T. Dowell

I. Introduction

Historical Perspective and Methodology

The ability of the mammalian heart to undergo adaptive changes has been the subject of investigation for many years. Particularly fascinating among the capabilities of the heart is its remarkable ability to increase myocardial mass. An enlarged heart is characteristically observed when the work requirements of the heart are increased and remain elevated for somewhat extended periods of time (days–weeks). Experimental methods have been developed and used in animal models to simulate pathological conditions resulting in elevated cardiac work and heart enlargement. Studies have been conducted using these experimental models in an effort to elucidate the control and mechanisms of adaptive heart growth.

Two methods have been used extensively for producing cardiac enlargement, namely, volume loading or pressure loading of the heart. Volume loading conditions can be produced experimentally (1) treating the animal with a salt retaining substance such as deoxycorticosterone acetate (DOCA), (2) developing nutritional anemia, or (3) surgically creating valvular insufficiency or arteriovenous fistula. Pressure loading conditions can be produced by constricting one of the major vessels leading from the heart. Right ventricular enlargement results from pulmonary artery constriction. Either ascending or subdiaphragmatic aortic constriction have been utilized to create enlargement of the left ventricle. Of the preceding experimental methods for producing cardiac enlargement, most investigations have employed subdiaphragmatic aortic constriction to establish left ventricular enlargement. Furthermore, the enlarged rat left ventricle resulting from pressure overload has been most extensively characterized, beginning with the detailed description by Dr. Margaret Beznak (1955) of a method for creating subdiaphragmatic aortic constriction in the rat. The popularity and utility of this procedure over the last 20–25 years is perhaps best illustrated by the fact that Beznak's paper has undergone "citation annihilation" to such a degree that a method for subdiaphragmatic aortic constriction in the rat was "rediscovered" by Malik et al. in 1974. Ascending aortic constriction has also been employed to produce left ventricular enlargement in the rat; however, the required surgical procedures (Nair et al., 1968; Fanburg and Posner, 1968) are technically difficult and the resulting cardiac enlargement mechanisms, insofar as they have been studied, do not differ substantially, regardless of the method for inducing left ventricular pressure overload. In fact, most cardiac enlargement responses seem to be quite similar, irrespective of the enlarging stimulus (volume overload or pressure overload). Therefore subsequent discussion in this chapter will relate to cardiac enlargement responses that have been shown or will be assumed to occur irrespective of the enlarging stimulus. Exceptions to the preceding general assumption will be noted.

II. Biochemical Aspects of Cardiac Enlargement

A. Protein Synthesis

Much attention has been devoted to the biochemical aspects of cardiac enlargement. Because cardiac enlargement involves the net accumulation of mycardial tissue, protein synthetic mechanisms have received particular emphasis. Ribonucleic acid synthesis (Koide and Rabinowitz, 1969; Posner and Fanburg, 1968; Schreiber et al., 1968) and synthesis and degradation of contractile proteins (Morkin et al., 1972; Zak et al., 1976) have been extensively characterized. Review articles (Fanburg, 1970; Rabinowitz and Zak, 1972) containing general descriptive aspects of protein synthesis in cardiac enlargement have been published previously. Information dealing with cardiac enlargement in terms of specific molecular mechanisms is contained in the review by Zak and Rabinowitz (1979).

B. Mitochondrial Synthesis

In order for cardiac enlargement to be an effective adaptive response, cardiac muscle cells and their various components should accumulate in proportion to the increase in heart mass. The large quantities of ATP required for heart muscle contraction are normally supplied almost exclusively by aerobic metabolism via mitochondrial oxidative reactions. Since sustained pressure or volume overload conditions elevate myocardial energy requirements, it might be expected that concomitant synthesis of mitochondria would be initiated. An extensive biochemical description (Dart and Holloszy, 1969) of enlarged, nonfailing, adult rat heart indicated that the respiratory capacity of cardiac muscle increased in proportion to heart mass when cardiac enlargement was induced by volume overload (arteriovenous fistula). However, it is now clear that during "stable" pressure-induced cardiac enlargement in the adult heart the accumulated myofibrillar mass outstrips mitochondrial mass. During the very early stages of pressure overload (hours–days), mitochondria may be preferentially accumulated (Albin *et al.,* 1973; Page *et al.,* 1972). At later time periods (days–weeks), however, mitochondrial cytochrome content per gram tissue (Albin *et al.,* 1973) and the relative cardiac muscle cell volume occupied by mitochondria (Page and McCallister, 1973; Page *et al.,* 1974) are substantially reduced. Information concerning the synthesis and degradation of mitochondrial components during cardiac enlargement has been reviewed (Rabinowitz and Zak, 1975).

C. Contractile Protein Synthesis

Considerable quantities of myofibrillar protein are synthesized and accumulated during cardiac enlargement. In contrast to mitochondria, myofibrillar protein accumulates approximately in proportion to the overall increase in heart mass. This adaptive response would be appropriate provided that the additional contractile protein synthesized is functionally normal with regard to its enzymatic (ATPase) properties. In skeletal muscle a direct relationship exists between muscle contractile properties and the ATPase activity of contractile proteins (Bárány, 1967; Close, 1972). Evidence is accumulating that suggests a similar relationship in cardiac muscle. Thus knowledge of contractile protein enzymatic properties in the enlarged heart could be related to the functional status of the myocardium. Unfortunately, investigations of the ATPase activity of myofibrillar, actomyosin, and myosin preparations from hyperthrophied hearts have yielded conflicting results, with normal (Nebel and Bing, 1963), reduced (Chandler *et al.,* 1967; Alpert *et al.,* 1974; Wikman-Coffelt *et al.,* 1976), or enhanced (Wikman-Coffelt *et al.,* 1975) enzymatic activity having been reported. These divergent results may be related to (1) the overload stimulus applied, (2) the stage of cardiac enlargement at which the measurements were taken, and (3) the relative magnitude of the enlargement achieved. Studies related to contractile protein turnover (Zak *et al.,* 1976) and the enzymatic properties of contractile proteins (Swynghedauw *et al.,* 1976) in the enlarged heart have been reviewed recently.

III. Cellular Responses During Heart Growth

A. Adaptive Responses in Adult and Neonatal Heart

Although cardiac enlargement is an end result common to a variety of experimental models, there has been controversy as to whether cardiac enlargement results from growth of preexisting cells, increased cell numbers resulting from mitotic division, or a combination of both processes. In the adult heart it is generally agreed that an elevated workload elicits an increased myocardial mass due primarily to growth of preexisting cardiac muscle cells (hypertrophy) (Zak, 1973, 1974). Cellular proliferation does occur in the enlarging adult rat heart, as evidenced by an increased DNA content; however, radioautographic analysis of labeled nuclei indicates nonmuscle cell proliferation (hyperplasia) with essentially no DNA synthesis within cardiac muscle cells (Zak, 1973, 1974). Increased proline incorporation into collagen hydroxyproline during developing cardiac enlargement (Skosey *et al.,* 1972) also supports the conclusion that nonmuscle cells respond quite actively.

Other investigators dealing with cardiac adaptation have suggested that the animal's age at the time an elevated workload is imposed on the heart may be a major factor determining the heart's cellular response to overload, i.e., hypertrophy or hyperplasia. When nutritional anemia was created in neonatal rats (21 days of age) to induce a heart volume overload, cardiac muscle cells as well as nonmuscle cells were stimulated to undergo active mitotic division (Neffgen and Korecky, 1972). Nutritional anemia produced considerable cardiac enlargement in mature rats (70 days of age), but no evidence of muscle cell division was found (Neffgen and Korecky, 1972). Mitotic division of cardiac muscle cells has also been reported in puppy ventricle after aortic constriction (Bishop, 1971) and in hypertensive neonatal rats (Sasaki *et al.,* 1970). Nevertheless, it was not completely clear from the preceding experiments whether any stimulus that increased the work requirements of the neonatal heart would elicit muscle cell proliferation. To answer this question, pressure overload was created in neonatal rats by subdiaphragmatic aortic constriction (Dowell and McManus, 1978). A left ventricular pressure overload of approximately 40 mm Hg was in effect 2 weeks following aortic constriction and was maintained throughout the 5-week experimental period. Left ventricular mass was elevated by approximately 50% in aortic constricted animals at all time points studied (Fig. 1). Biochemical results indicated that left ventricular total DNA content was elevated in aortic constricted animals, suggesting mitotic division of some cellular population(s) (Fig. 2). Radioautographic studies demonstrated a marked elevation in [³H]thymidine-labeled nuclei in *both* cardiac muscle and nonmuscle cells in aortic constricted animals (Table I). Since neither ascending nor subdiaphragmatic aortic constriction in adult rats results in cardiac muscle cell division (Morkin and Ashford, 1968; Grove *et al.,* 1969), it would appear that age-related factors dictate in some way the heart's response to overload insofar as the cardiac muscle cell is concerned. Selective activation of cell division must also occur, since nonmuscle cell DNA synthesis is observed in hearts of both neonatal and adult animals during overload stress.

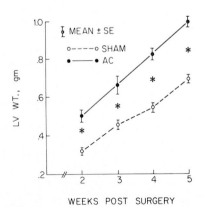

WEEKS POST SURGERY

Fig. 1. Left ventricular weights of sham-operated and aortic-constricted neonatal rats. LV = left ventricle; AC = aortic constricted. *$P < 0.05$ compared to sham. (From Dowell and McManus, 1978. By permission of the American Heart Association, Inc.)

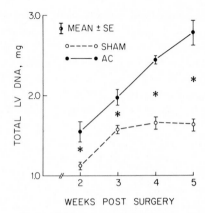

Fig. 2. Total left ventricular DNA content of sham-operated and aortic-constricted neonatal rats. Total DNA content was calculated as the product of left ventricular wet weight and left ventricular DNA concentration. LV = left ventricle; AC = aortic constricted. *P < 0.05 compared to sham. (From Dowell and McManus, 1978. By permission of the American Heart Association, Inc.)

B. Normal Developmental Responses

Recent studies of normal development and DNA synthesis in the mammalian heart provide important information regarding factors that may regulate cardiac cell differentiation and cell division. Spontaneous cell division, as indicated by [³H]thymidine incorporation into nuclear DNA, occurs frequently in the rat heart at birth, but declines rapidly during the early neonatal period. Radioautographic data of Neffgen and Korecky (1972) and Klinge and Stocker (1960) indicated that [³H]thymidine incorporation

TABLE I

Nuclear Incorporation of [³H]Thymidine in Sham-Operated and Aortic-Constricted Neonatal Rat Left Ventricle[a,b]

Group	n	Muscle cells	Nonmuscle cells
SHAM	6	9 ± 2	23 ± 4
AC	6	73 ± 15*	104 ± 23*

[a] Values are mean ±SE-labeled nuclei index (labeled nuclei/1000), n = number of rats, *P < 0.05 compared to sham. Radioautographic determination of relative numbers of labeled muscle and nonmuscle cell nuclei was performed 1–2 weeks after surgery.

[b] Data taken from Dowell and McManus, 1978. By permission of The American Heart Association, Inc.

reaches a minimum at 32–34 days and 4 months of age, respectively. A more recent study (Claycomb, 1975) shows that [³H]thymidine incorporation into DNA extracted from rat heart essentially ceases 17 days after birth. The progressive reduction and eventual cessation of heart DNA synthesis correlate with the gradual decline in cytoplasmic DNA polymerase activity (Claycomb, 1975) (Fig. 3). Thymidine kinase is another key enzyme involved in DNA synthesis via the so-called salvage pathway. Gillette and Claycomb (1974) reported that thymidine kinase activity in heart tissue declined progressively from birth to 17 days after birth. Temporal similarities in the change of activity of several key enzymes (Gillette and Claycomb, 1974; Claycomb, 1975; Limas, 1978) and of cell constituents (Claycomb, 1976a) associated with DNA synthesis indicate that differentiation of cardiac muscle may be controlled by a single, unified mechanism. Although it has not been established whether this mechanism initiates events leading to the irreversible loss or simply an inhibition of DNA synthetic activity in the fully differentiated cardiac muscle cell, the latter view appears more likely (Zak, 1973). It is clear, however, that spontaneous cessation of heart DNA synthesis is initiated by the loss of replicative DNA polymerase activity (Claycomb, 1978).

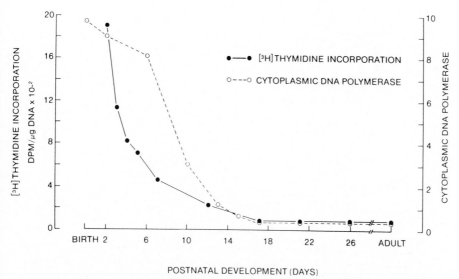

Fig. 3. Incorporation of [³H]thymidine into DNA and cytoplasmic DNA polymerase activity in heart during postnatal development. (Adapted from Claycomb, 1975, by permission.)

C. Potential Role of Cyclic Nucleotides

The involvement of cyclic AMP in cell differentiation and cell division in tissues other than heart presents the possibility that adenylate cyclase and cyclic AMP could be associated with the mechanism responsible for terminal cell differentiation in heart muscle. Adenylate cyclase activity increases progressively in the heart during neonatal development (Brus and Hess, 1973; Yount and Clark, 1976). The progressive development of the enzyme system responsible for cyclic AMP synthesis correlates positively with the cyclic AMP levels in heart tissue. Cyclic AMP levels in the rat heart are relatively low at birth but increase progressively during neonatal development (Novak *et al.*, 1972) (Fig. 4). The similarities between the time course of adenylate cyclase activity, cyclic AMP level, and arrested spontaneous mitotic activity suggested that cyclic AMP levels may regulate cardiac muscle differentiation. Subsequently, experiments by Claycomb (1976b) clearly demonstrated that mitotic activity in the neonatal heart can be prematurely arrested either by dibutyryl cyclic AMP or compounds that are known to elevate cyclic AMP levels (Fig. 5). Inhibition of [³H]thymidine incorpora-

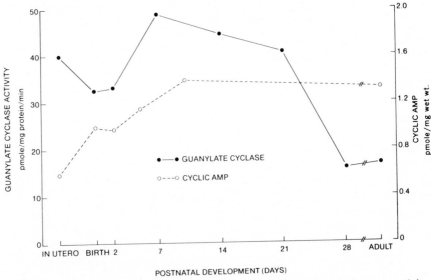

Fig. 4. Cyclic AMP level and guanylate cyclase activity in rat heart during postnatal development. Adult levels of cyclic AMP and, presumably, adenylate cyclase are reached approximately 10–14 days after birth. In contrast, guanylate cyclase activity at 21 days after birth is nearly 2.5-fold higher than adult levels. Thus quite different intracellular conditions exist in the heart when pressure overload is created in neonatal (21 days of age) or adult (>28 days of age) rats. (Adapted from Novak *et al.*, 1972, and Vesely *et al.*, 1976, by permission.)

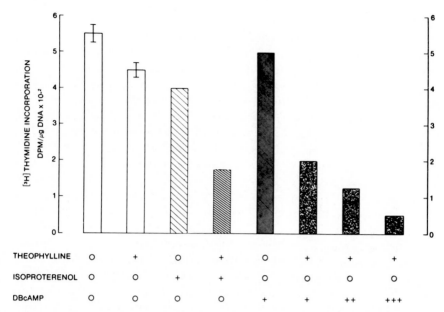

Fig. 5. Effect of theophylline, isoproterenol, and dibutyryl cyclic AMP (DBcAMP) on the incorporation of [³H]thymidine into DNA of differentiating heart. Rats were injected on the fifth or sixth day of postnatal development with: theophylline (50 mg/kg), isoproterenol (5 mg/kg), and dibutyryl cyclic AMP (25 mg/kg, [+]; 50 mg/kg, [++]; and 75 mg/kg [+++] either singly or in combination as indicated. Controls received saline injections. Fifteen hours later, animals were injected with [³H]thymidine and incorporation into DNA was measured. Standard error is indicated for control and theophylline response. Note dose-dependent response to DBcAMP. (Adapted from Claycomb, 1976b, by permission.)

tion into DNA was demonstrated both *in vivo* and *in vitro*. Although cyclic AMP inhibited heart thymidine kinase activity *in vivo,* enzyme activity was not influenced when cyclic AMP was added to neonatal heart tissue slices (Gillete and Claycomb, 1974). The preceding experimental results led Claycomb (1976b, 1977) to propose that, "cell proliferation and cell differentiation in cardiac muscle may be controlled by adrenergic innervation with norepinephrine and cyclic AMP serving as chemical mediators."

The intracellular level of a second cyclic nucleotide, cyclic GMP, is also related to DNA synthesis and cell division in a variety of tissues and cells. A recent study (Vesely *et al.,* 1976) provides evidence that the heart enzyme system that catalyzes the conversion of guanosine triphosphate to cyclic GMP exhibits developmental changes. Guanylate cyclase activity was determined at selected time periods in the developing rat heart (Fig. 4). Enzyme activity levels were relatively high *in utero* and remained elevated until approximately 3 weeks after birth. At that time enzyme activity began to decline until the characteristically low adult myocardial levels were achieved at 4 weeks after birth. The progressive decline in heart cyclic GMP levels reported during postnatal development (Kim and Silverstein, 1975) apparently occurs as the result of alterations in the heart guanylate cyclase enzyme system. It is of interest that the intracellular level of cyclic AMP increases progressively as the cyclic GMP level declines during postnatal myocardial development. A reciprocal relationship between cyclic AMP and cyclic GMP appears to play a role in several biologic processes, including cell division. However, the relationship between these cyclic nucleotides and the control of heart muscle differentiation is not completely clear, since cyclic GMP or compounds that elevate cyclic GMP levels do not further enhance [^{3}H]thymidine incorporation into DNA of neonatal rat heart (Gillette and Claycomb, 1974; Claycomb, 1976b).

Cyclic nucleotide regulation of cell differentiation and cell division is rapidly becoming an accepted principle in many mammalian cells. Burk (1968) was among the first to advocate a regulatory role for cyclic AMP in cell division. Cyclic AMP inhibited cell division in proliferating hamster cells and cells transformed by polyoma virus were found to have reduced adenylate cyclase activity. Subsequent experiments in a wide variety of cultured cells (Chlapowski *et al.*, 1975; Friedman *et al.*, 1976; Goldberg *et al.*, 1974) demonstrated that cyclic AMP, when added to the extracellular medium, inhibited cell division in both normal and transformed cell lines. Inhibition of cell division by exogenous cyclic AMP suggested an inverse relationship between cyclic AMP levels and cell growth rate. It was anticipated that low levels of this cyclic nucleotide would be found in rapidly dividing cells and high levels in nondividing cells. Furthermore, if cyclic AMP levels were the signal for the cell either to remain in an arrested state or to divide, then intracellular levels of cyclic AMP would be expected to fluctuate appropriately through the cell cycle.

The predicted results have been documented in a number of cell populations (Chlapowski *et al.*, 1975; Friedman *et al.*, 1976; Goldberg *et al.*, 1974). Intracellular levels of cyclic AMP are lowest (1) in differentiating tissue, (2) in rapidly dividing cells, and (3) during the mitotic phase of the cell cycle in synchronized cells. Conversely, cyclic AMP levels are highest (1) in fully differentiated tissue, (2) in nondividing cells, and (3) during the quiescent phase of the cell cycle in synchronized cells. Although elevated cyclic AMP levels were clearly shown to inhibit or limit cell division, a number of studies failed to demonstrate the initiation of cell division when cyclic AMP levels were reduced. This discrepancy led to the proposal that a second cyclic nucleotide, cyclic GMP, was required to mediate the mitogenic signal (Hadden *et al.,* 1972; Goldberg *et al.,* 1974; Goldberg and Haddox, 1977).

During phytohemagglutinin and concanavalin A-induced cell division in human and rat lymphocytes, intracellular cyclic GMP levels were dramatically increased, whereas cyclic AMP levels were unchanged. Similar results were obtained in cultured fibroblasts. Rapidly dividing fibroblasts exhibited markedly higher levels of cyclic GMP than fibroblasts that had undergone contact inhibition. Elevated cyclic GMP levels have also been implicated in the excessive epidermal cell division associated with psoriasis (Voorhees and Duell, 1975). Moreover, cyclic GMP has been shown to stimulate the degradation of cyclic AMP in cell-free systems by activating cyclic AMP phosphodiesterase (Beavo *et al.,* 1971; Appleman and Terasaki, 1975). If these mechanisms operate *in vivo,* then elevated cyclic GMP levels could serve concomitantly to reduce cyclic AMP levels and, in this way, ensure optimum conditions for the initiation of cell division.

The antagonistic, inverse relationship between the intracellular levels of cyclic AMP and cyclic GMP was proposed by Goldberg *et al.* (1974) as the "yin–yang" or "dualism" concept of biological regulation. This concept has been extended to involve monodirectional and bidirectional regulation by cyclic nucleotides. In a monodirectionally regulated cell population, control is exercised by an on–off principle. When an elevated cyclic nucleotide level is present, the cellular response is activated until the stimulus abates. Activation occurs irrespective of the cyclic nucleotide involved. In a bidirectionally regulated cell population, stimulation and recovery are mediated by reciprocal cyclic nucleotide stimuli, Cellular activity in bidirectionally regulated cells is determined by a balance between the two opposing cyclic nucleotide levels. Examples of bidirectional control by cyclic nucleotides have been documented in heart tissue. Catecholamine stimulation of cardiac contractile function is associated with elevated cyclic AMP levels (Kukovetz and Poch, 1972; Morkin and LaRaia, 1974) and a concomitant decrease in cyclic GMP (George *et al.,* 1973). Conversely, contractile function is suppressed when intracellular cyclic GMP levels are elevated by acetylcholine (George *et al.,* 1973, 1976). Brooker (1975) and Wollenberger *et al.* (1973) have described marked oscillations in the intracellular level of cyclic nucleotides during heart muscle contraction. Prior to the onset of contraction, cyclic AMP levels rise and cyclic GMP levels are dramatically lowered. During relaxation the cyclic nucleotide levels return to the original control value. A developmentally related reciprocal relationship has been noted between the activities of cyclic AMP-dependent and cyclic GMP-dependent protein kinase in guinea pig heart (Kuo, 1975). A recent study (Nesher *et al.,* 1977a) indicates that hypoxia results in a marked elevation in heart cyclic AMP levels and a reduced tissue level of cyclic GMP.

With regard to cellular division, it appears likely that the relative level of cyclic nucleotides is involved in regulating normal heart growth. In addition, the dualism concept of Goldberg when combined with the monodirectional and bidirectional concepts provides an attractive explanation for the DNA synthetic responses observed during adaptive heart growth. A limited number of studies have been conducted to determine adenylate cyclase activity and cyclic AMP levels in the hearts of adult animals undergoing cardiac enlargement. Schreiber *et al.* (1971) demonstrated elevated adenylate cyclase activity in isolated perfused guinea pig heart after a relatively brief (10 min) period of pressure overload. Nair *et al.* (1973) have reported elevated cyclic AMP levels in enlarged hearts from cardiomyopathic hamsters. Similar elevations in cyclic AMP were noted by Kleitke *et al.* (1976) in enlarged hearts from aortic-constricted animals. The preceding studies suggest that increased adenylate cyclase activity leads to elevated cyclic AMP levels, which, in turn, are associated in some way with the early events leading to the development of cardiac enlargement. Nuclear RNA polymerase activation is among the earliest events detectable following the imposition of a given heart overload (Nair *et al.*, 1968, 1973). Exogenous cyclic AMP has been shown to activate RNA polymerase in a heterogeneous population of cell nuclei isolated from rat heart (Nesher *et al.*, 1977b). Thus experimental data exist that implicate elevated cyclic AMP levels as a potential mechanism leading to the activation of myocardial protein synthesis. The possibility exists that DNA synthesis and cell division during cardiac enlargement may also be regulated by intracellular levels of cyclic AMP and/or cyclic GMP.

IV. Future Directions and Considerations

Adaptive cardiac enlargement in the adult heart results from growth of preexisting muscle cells that is accompanied by mitotic division of nonmuscle cells. In contrast, volume overload and pressure overload created in neonatal animals elicit adaptive heart growth that is accompanied by DNA synthesis and mitotic activity in both cardiac muscle and nonmuscle cells. The preceding responses identify a significant qualitative difference between cardiac enlargement mechanisms; however, the factors responsible for these divergent cellular responses are unknown. In fact, no information currently exists to explain the apparent selective activation of cellular division within the adult heart during adaptive growth.

Any significant advancement of our understanding of how cellular division is controlled during adaptive heart growth requires consideration of homogeneous heart cell populations. Techniques have recently been developed that allow the separation and isolation of muscle and nonmuscle cell populations from heart tissue (Cutilletta *et al.*, 1977). Homogeneous cell populations can be obtained that have essentially no cross-contamination. Isolated homogeneous cells retain good viability and enzymatic activity. Subcellular systems (i.e., nuclei) can be isolated from homogeneous cells for further detailed analysis and initial studies of homogeneous cell responses to left ventricular pressure overload have been reported (Cutilletta *et al.*, 1978). Therefore experimental models and techniques are available that can be utilized to define the cellular control mechanisms regulating adaptive heart growth.

Acknowledgment

This work was supported, in part, by NIH grants HL 23025 and HL 23206. The expert technical assistance of Judith Haithcoat and Kathe Whitten is gratefully acknowledged.

References

Albin, R., Dowell, R. T., Zak, R., and Rabinowitz, M. (1973). *Biochem. J.* **136**, 629–637.
Alpert, N. R., Hamrell, B. B., and Halpern, W. (1974). *Circ. Res.* **34–35**, Suppl. II, 71–81.
Appleman, M. M., and Terasaki, W. L. (1975). *Adv. Cyclic Nucleotide Res.* **5**, 153–162.
Bárány, M. (1967). *J. Gen. Physiol.* **50**, 197–218,
Beavo, J. A., Hardman, J. G., and Sutherland, E. W. (1971). *J. Biol. Chem.* **246**, 3841–3846.
Beznak, M. (1955). *Can. J. Biochem. Physiol.* **33**, 985–1002.
Bishop, S. P. (1971). *Circulation* **44**, Suppl. 2, 142.
Brooker, G. (1975). *Adv. Cyclic Nucleotide Res.* **5**, 435–452.
Brus, R., and Hess, M. E. (1973). *Endocrinology* **93**, 982–985.
Burk, R. R. (1968). *Nature (London)* **219**, 1272–1275.
Chandler, B. M., Sonnenblick, E. H., Spann, J. F., and Pool, P. E. (1967). *Circ. Res.* **21**, 717–725.
Chlapowski, F. J., Kelly, L. A., and Butcher, R. W. (1975). *Adv. Cyclic Nucleotide Res.* **6**, 245–338.
Claycomb, W. C. (1975). *J. Biol. Chem.* **250**, 3229–3235.
Claycomb, W. C. (1976a). *Biochem. J.* **154**, 387–393.
Claycomb, W. C. (1976b). *J. Biol. Chem.* **251**, 6082–6089.
Claycomb, W. C. (1977). *Biochem. J.* **168**, 599–601.
Claycomb, W. C. (1978). *Biochem. J.* **171**, 289–298.
Close, R. I. (1972). *Physiol. Rev.* **52**, 129–197.
Cutilletta, A. F., Aumont, M. C., Nag, A. C., and Zak, R. (1977). *J. Mol. Cell. Cardiol.* **9**, 399–407.
Cutilletta, A. F., Rudnik, M., and Zak, R. (1978). *J. Mol. Cell. Cardiol.* **10**, 677–687.
Dart, C. H., Jr., and Holloszy, J. O. (1969). *Circ. Res.* **25**, 245–263.

Dowell, R. T. and McManus, R. E. (1978). *Circ. Res.* **42,** 303–310.

Fanburg, B. L. (1970). *N. Engl. J. Med.* **282,** 723–732.

Fanburg, B. L., and Posner, E. I. (1978). *Circ. Res.* **23,** 123–135.

Friedman, D. L., Johnson, R. A., and Zeilig, C. E. (1976). *Adv. Cyclic Nucleotide Res.* **7,** 69–114.

George, W. J., Wilkerson, R. D., and Kadowitz, P. J. (1973). *J. Pharmacol. Exp. Ther.* **184,** 228–235.

George, W. J., Polson, J. B., O'Toole, A. G., and Goldberg, N. D. (1976). *Proc. Natl. Acad. Sci. U.S.A.* **66,** 398–403.

Gillette, P. C., and Claycomb, W. C. (1974). *Biochem. J.* **142,** 685–690.

Goldberg, N. D., and Haddoz, M. K. (1977). *Annu. Rev. Biochem.* **46,** 823–896.

Goldberg, N. D., Haddox, M. K., Dunham, E., Lopez, C., and Hadden, J. W. (1974). *In* "The Regulation of Proliferation in Animal Cells" (B. Clarkson and R. Baserga, eds.), pp. 609–625. Cold Spring Harbor Lab., Cold Spring Harbor, New York.

Grove, D., Zak, R., Nair, K. G., and Aschenbrenner, V. (1969). *Circ. Res.* **25,** 473–485.

Hadden, J. W., Hadden, E. M., Haddox, M. K. and Goldberg, N. D. (1972). *Proc. Natl. Acad. Sci. U.S.A.* **69,** 3024–3027.

Kim, G., and Silverstein, E. (1975). *Fed. Proc., Fed. Am. Soc. Exp. Biol.* **34,** 231.

Kleitke, B., Wollenberger, A., Krause, E. G., Will-Shahab, L., and Bartel, S. (1976). *Adv. Cardiol.* **18,** 27–40.

Klinge, O., and Stocker, E. (1960). *Experientia* **24,** 167–168.

Koide, T., and Rabinowitz, M. (1969). *Circ. Res.* **24,** 9–18.

Kukovetz, W. R., and Poch, G. (1972). *Adv. Cyclic Nucleotide Res.* **1,** 261–290.

Kuo, J. F. (1975). *Proc. Natl. Acad. Sci. U.S.A.* **72,** 2256–2259.

Limas, K. J. (1978). *Am. J. Physiol.* **235,** H338–H344.

Malik, A. B., Shapiro, J., Yanics, J., Rojales, A., and Geha, A. S. (1974). *Cardiovasc. Res.* **8,** 801–805.

Morkin, E., and Ashford, T. P. (1968). *Am. J. Physiol.* **215,** 1409–1413.

Morkin, E., and LaRaia, P. J. (1974). *N. Engl. J. Med.* **290,** 445–451.

Morkin, E., Kimata, S., and Skillman, J. J. (1972). *Circ. Res.* **30,** 690–702.

Nair, K. G., Cutilletta, A. F., Zak, R., Koide, T., and Rabinowitz, M. (1968). *Circ. Res.* **23,** 451–462.

Nair, K. G., Umali, T., and Potts, J. (1973). *Am. J. Cardiol.* **32,** 423–426.

Nebel, M. L., and Bing, R. J. (1963). *Arch. Intern. Med.* **111,** 190–195.

Neffgen, J. F., and Korecky, B. (1972). *Circ. Res.* **30,** 104–113.

Nesher, R., Robinson, W. F., Gibb, L., Bishop, S. P., and Kruger, F. A. (1977a). *Experientia* **33,** 215–217.

Nesher, R., Robinson, W. F., Gibb, L., Bishop, S. P., and Kruger, F. A. (1977b). *J. Mol. Cell. Cardiol.* **9,** 579–593.

Novak, E., Drummond, G. I., Skala, J., and Hahn, P. (1972). *Arch. Biochem. Biophys.* **150,** 511–518.

Page, E., and McCallister, L. P. (1973). *Am J. Cardiol.* **31,** 172–181.

Page, E., Polimeni, P. I., Zak, R., Earley, J., and Johnson, M. (1972). *Circ. Res.* **30,** 430–439.

Page, E., Earley, J., and Power, B. (1974). *Circ. Res.* **34–35,** Suppl. II, 12–16.

Posner, B. I., and Fanburg, B. L. (1968). *Circ. Res.* **23,** 137–145.

Rabinowitz, M., and Zak, R. (1972). *Annu. Rev. Med.* **23,** 245–261.

Rabinowitz, M., and Zak, R. (1975). *Circ. Res.* **36,** 367–376.

Sasaki, R., Morishita, T., Ichikawa, S., and Yamagata, S. (1970). *Tohoku J. Exp. Med.* **102,** 159–167.

Schreiber, S. S., Oratz, M., Evans, C. D., Silver, E., and Rothschild, M. A. (1968). *Am. J. Physiol.* **215,** 1250–1259.

Schreiber, S. S., Klein, I. L., Oratz, M., and Rothschild, M. A. (1971). *J. Mol. Cell. Cardiol.* **2**, 55–65.

Skosey, J. L., Zak, R., Aschenberger, V., and Rabinowitz, M. (1972). *Circ. Res.* **31**, 145–157.

Swynghedauw, B., Leger, J. J., and Schwartz, K. (1976). *J. Mol. Cell. Cardiol.* **8**, 915–924.

Vesely, D. L., Chown, J., and Levey, G. S. (1976). *J. Mol. Cell. Cardiol.* **8**, 903–913.

Voorhees, J. J., and Duell, E. A. (1975). *Adv. Cyclic Nucleotide Res.* **5**, 735–758.

Wikman-Coffelt, J., Fenner, C., Coffelt, R. J., Salel, A., Kamiyama, T., and Mason, D. T. (1975). *J. Mol. Cell. Cardiol.* **7**, 219–224.

Wikman-Coffelt, J., Walsh, R., Fenner, C., Kamiyama, T., Salel, A., and Mason, D. T. (1976). *J. Mol. Cell. Cardiol.* **8**, 263–270.

Wollenberger, A., Babskii, E., Krause, E., Blohm, D., and Bagdanova, E. (1973). *Biochem. Biophys. Res. Commun.* **55**, 446–452.

Yount, E. A., and Clark, C. M., Jr. (1976). *Fed. Proc., Fed. Am. Soc. Exp. Biol.* **35**, 423.

Zak, R. (1973). *Am. J. Cardiol.* **31**, 211–219.

Zak, R. (1974). *Circ. Res.* **34–35**, Suppl. II, 17–26.

Zak, R., and Rabinowitz, M. (1979). *Annu. Rev. Physiol.* **41**, 539–552.

Zak, R., Martin, A. F., Reddy, M. K., and Rabinowitz, M. (1976). *Circ. Res.* **38**, Suppl. I, 145–150.

10

Effects of Bedrest and Weightlessness on the Heart

H. Sandler

I. Introduction

Significant changes occur in the cardiovascular systems of both men and animals during and after exposure to weightlessness. During space flight the body adapts to weightlessness, and changes in the cardiovascular system during this period are manifested only with provocative testing. On return to earth, however, many physiological systems evidence difficulty in readapting to terrestrial gravity. Both American and Russian investigators have observed this problem (Berry *et al.,* 1966; Hoffler and Johnson, 1975; R. L. Johnson *et al.,* 1977; Kolenchenko *et al.,* 1976) and have noted that the condition persists for several hours to almost a week (Berry *et al.,* 1966; Gazenko *et al.,* 1976; Vorob'yev *et al.,* 1976).

Cardiovascular deconditioning following exposure to weightlessness is manifested principally by orthostatic intolerance, which includes tachycardia, narrowed pulse pressure, and an inability to control blood pressure

HEARTS AND HEART-LIKE ORGANS, VOL. 2

adequately when in the vertical position (including presyncope and frank syncope). The exact changes that occur during adaptation to weightlessness, which are probably responsible for the inability to readapt to earth gravity, are still unclear. Some investigators believe that a change in the distribution of fluid in the body is the primary biological reaction of the body to the force of gravity (Graveline, 1962). It is hypothesized that in the absence of gravity, there is a loss of the normal pressure force that acts to displace fluid (primarily blood) downward to the lower half of the body. The result is a loss of periodic distention of blood vessel walls and body fluid compartments in the lower half of the body. With the lack of gravity, changes may occur in the vessel walls themselves or in the central nervous system mechanisms that are responsible for their control.

The conditions of weightlessness have been simulated in the laboratory environment by the use of bedrest, chair rest, and immersion in humans and immobilization in animals (Dorchak and Greenleaf, 1976; Greenleaf et al., 1976; Kollias et al., 1976). These simulation studies, together with the data from both American and Russian space flights, have contributed heavily to the knowledge of cardiovascular responses to weightlessness. But much still remains to be determined concerning the mechanisms and course of cardiovascular deconditioning. The relevant information will come from the experience of future space flights and ground-based studies.

This review is concerned with (1) discussing representative previous studies that have provided pertinent information on cardiovascular changes that occur during weightlessness and (2) indicating areas that require further investigation using ground-based studies.

II. Mission Experience

A. Manned Flight

Cardiovascular changes have been observed both during and after each manned space flight to date (Berry et al., 1966; Dietlein, 1977; Gazenko et al., 1976; Hoffler and Johnson, 1975; Sandler, 1976). In the American space program cardiovascular deconditioning was first noted following the Mercury flights. The conditions manifested were a drop in systolic pressure, narrowing of or a drop in pulse pressure, and substantially increased heart rate. Russian investigators have observed the same responses in returning cosmonauts and have noted that the conditions persisted for as long as 6 days after recovery (Gazenko et al., 1976). The Gemini flight experience also showed the persistence of orthostatic intolerance following flight. In addition to the symptoms observed previously, the Gemini astronauts experienced a moderate loss of red blood cells, increased heart rate both at rest and when stressed, and a loss of exercise capacity on return to earth (Berry et al., 1966). No significant changes were observed, however, in blood pressure, electrocardiograms, or systolic time intervals. All Apollo astronauts following reentry exhibited orthostatic intolerance, decreases in the mass and volume of red blood cells, and reduced exercise capacity (Hoffler and Johnson, 1975; Rummel et al., 1975). Furthermore, in the Apollo 15 flight, bigeminy and bradycardia were observed as well as the previously documented responses. These additional changes were felt to have resulted from the astronauts' having had to work in severe heat (with consequent mineral loss) prior to lift-off. Identical or similar changes have been reported by Russian investigators (Gazenko et al., 1976; Sandler, 1976).

Postflight measurements of oxygen uptake in both astronauts and cosmonauts have shown a substantial decrease. Following the Apollo missions, crews exhibited a 25% decrease in submaximal oxygen uptake (Rummel et al., 1975). The experience of the three Skylab missions was similar. Using the single-breath CO_2 method, tests indicated that without exercise the body's oxygen needs can be readily satisfied by the increased cardiac output that occurs in weightlessness (Buderer et al., 1976). Oxygen consumption increased with exercise on a bicycle ergometer because the arms play a more active role in the zero-G environment than they do on earth. In all three Skylab missions, the oxygen uptake of the astronauts during submaximal exercise did not indicate that pulmonary efficiency was degraded, perhaps because of their exercise regimens. Following flight, however, all Skylab crewmen exhibited decreased oxygen pulse (Michel et al., 1977).

The Skylab missions were the first American flights in which cardiovascular changes were documented during flight (Johnson, et al., 1977). These flights lasted far longer than had previous manned missions—a duration of 28 days for Skylab 2, 59 days for Skylab 3, and 84 days for Skylab 3. The crews of all three missions exhibited elevated mean systolic and pulse pressures and depressed mean diastolic and mean arterial pressures at rest as compared with their preflight levels. In the crewmen of both Skylab 3 and Skylab 4, mean resting heart rates were also elevated, but they were lower than preflight levels in the Skylab 2 crewmen. This group also exhibited cardiac dysrhythmias during exercise (Smith et al., 1977). In all Skylab missions, heart rate during stress was consistently higher than preflight levels.

Lower body negative pressure (LBNP) measurements were made by the fifth day of each Skylab flight. Substantially greater increases in calf volume were noted during LBNP as compared with preflight measurements. The Skylab experience confirmed that LBNP in the weightless environment creates a more severe stress on the cardiovascular system than it does at earth gravity. This situation may be explained in part by the changes that weightlessness causes in relationships in the anatomical distribution of blood volume and extravascular fluids, as well as concomitant alterations in blood flow patterns and decrease in total circulating blood volume. In the Skylab 4 crewmen, the severity of responses to LBNP were found to subside after 30–50 days in flight (Johnson *et al.*, 1977). The responses of all three crews to LBNP postflight were similar to those of most previous crews of manned space flights in that recovery was rapid.

During reentry all Skylab crewmen wore cardiovascular pressure garments, which were controlled manually with air pressure bulbs. The garments were designed to provide counterpressure to the lower extremities to reduce postural hypotension after landing and while standing upright in earth gravity. The suits succeeded, in most cases, in decreasing heart rate and maintaining blood pressure at close to supine levels during standing. Despite these procedures, however, the science pilot of Skylab 2 experienced postural hypotension.

In December 1977, the Soviets launched two cosmonauts aboard Soyuz 26 to spend 96 days in their Salyut space laboratory. Soviet investigators have not yet published their findings concerning the experience of these crewmen. Preliminary reports, however, have stated that both crewmen tolerated weightlessness for a prolonged period without ill effects. But, as in previous manned flights, cardiovascular deconditioning again occurred despite the use of LBNP suits periodically during flight, regular exercise on a specially designed treadmill, and ingestion of fluids to replace plasma volume (Pestov *et al.*, 1974).

Both American and Russian crewmen have been assigned regimens of moderate exercise in space to counteract cardiovascular deconditioning resulting from weightlessness. But, to date, exercise has not proved to be a useful countermeasure. Investigations are continuing in this area, however, because exercise has improved the mental well-being of the crewmen and because, to this point, maximum exercise loads have not been imposed in space. The cardiovascular responses of the astronauts to weightlessness are shown in Table I; those for the cosmonauts appear in Table II.

B. Animal Flights

Animals have consistently preceded man into space in both the U.S. and Soviet space programs. United States animal flights have used nonhuman primates primarily, whereas the animal of choice by Soviet investigators has been the dog (Sandler, 1977). The more important flights launched by the two countries and their results are shown in Table III.

1. United States Animal Flights

United States investigators began sending animals into space as early as 1948, when Air Force investigators initiated a series of eight vertical V-2 rocket flights with animal payloads to obtain physiological information on the effects of suborbital flight (Henry *et al.*, 1962). During these flights, seven anesthetized rhesus, *Cebus,* and *Cynomolgus* monkeys and 14 unanesthetized mice served as animal subjects. The monkeys were used to observe changes in pulse and respiration rates and arterial and central venous pressure during flight; the mice were photographed to study performance in weightlessness.

The early American animal flights were an exercise in failure; the animals were not recovered alive because of failure of either the parachute system or the life support system. These failures were offset, however, by increased technical knowledge gained with each flight that made future successful flights possible. Technical advances included improvements in the nose cone and life support system, development in instrumentation for telemetering physiological data to earth, and improvements in the parachute recovery system.

The first successful animal rocket flight was accomplished by U.S. investigators in September 1951. The flight was made in a newly developed, high-altitude Aerobee sounding rocket. The rocket, Aerobee 2, carried an unanesthetized rhesus monkey and 11 unanesthetized mice and returned safely to earth. The monkey was instrumented to record electrocardiograms, as well as arterial and central venous pressure; the mice were again used to study performance in weightlessness. Although the animals returned safely, the monkey died after recovery from exposure to the hot desert environment where they touched down.

In May 1952, Aerobee 3 was launched carrying two *Cebus* monkeys (Mike and Patricia) and two mice. Mike was placed in a seated position to receive acceleration forces in the $+G_z$ mode while Patricia was in the supine position to receive stress in the $+G_x$ mode. ECGs were obtained from both monkeys, but arterial and venous pressure could not be measured. The mice again were studied for performance. All animals survived the flight.

The first suborbital flight, which was made possible by improvements in rocket design, was launched in April 1958. The flight carried a mouse to an altitude of 870 km. In this and two subsequent flights carrying mice, the biologic capsules were not recovered, although the mice survived reentry into the atmosphere and physiological data were telemetered to earth.

Bioflight I was launched on December 13, 1958, and carried a 0.5-kg

TABLE I

Summary of U.S. Manned Space Flight Experience

Orbiter Designation	Launch Date	Length of Flight	Astronauts	Comments	Cardiovascular Responses Encountered
Mercury MA-6	20 February 1962	4 hr, 55 min	Glenn	81,000-mile flight; difficulty encountered with autopilot.	Two short bursts (9 and 17 beats) of nodal tachycardia observed in astronaut during postponed MA-6 launch.
Mercury MA-7	24 May 1962	4 hr, 56 min	Carpenter	81,200-mile flight; 200-mile over-shoot on landing.	No cardiovascular deconditioning observed.
Mercury MA-8	3 October 1962	9 hr, 13 min	Schirra	160,000-mile flight.	First incidence of orthostatic intolerance.
Mercury MA-9	15 May 1963	34 hr, 20 min	Cooper	Last and longest Mercury flight.	Astronaut suffered dizziness and orthostatic intolerance on standing, dehydration, and hemoconcentration.
Gemini GT-3	23 March 1965	4 hr, 53 min	Grissom Young	Objective: to achieve altitude and orbital plane changes.	During all Gemini flights, the astronauts were subjected to the following measurements: 2-lead ECG, blood pressure, respiration, and body temperature. Peak heart rates were observed at launch and re-entry; the only abnormalities noted were very rare, premature auricular and
Gemini GT-4	3 June 1965	97 hr, 48 min	McDivitt White	First extravehicular activity in which astronauts maneuvered with hand-held reaction device.	ventricular contractions; no significant changes were observed in the duration of specific segments of the ECGs. Blood
Gemini GT-5	21 August 1965	190 hr, 59 min	Cooper Conrad	Cooper was the first U.S. astronaut to make a second flight.	pressure measurements during Gemini 7 showed that systolic and diastolic values remained within the range of normalcy
Gemini GT-6	15 December 1965	25 hr, 51 min	Schirra Stafford	First rendezvous flight; rendezvous successfully performed.	throughout the 14-day flight (including reentry). Orthostatic intolerance as
Gemini GT-7	4 December 1965	13 days, 18 hr, 35 min	Borman Lovell	First long-duration flight.	measured with a tilt table was noted for some 50 hours postflight; reduction in red-
Gemini GT-8	16 March 1966	10 hr, 42 min	Armstrong Scott	First docking maneuver successfully performed (with unmanned Agena target satellite); vehicles went into roll. Gemini 8 quickly separated	cell mass of 5 to 20 per cent.

Mission	Date	Duration	Crew	Description	Notes
				and slowly regained altitude. Mission aborted.	See above.
Gemini GT-9	3 June 1966	72 hr, 22 min	Stafford, Cernan	New rendezvous techniques demonstrated, but Gemini vehicle failed to dock because of problem with nose cover on target vehicle. Cernan left space craft for 2-hour, 7-minute walk in space.	See above.
Gemini GT-10	18 July 1966	70 hr, 46 min	Young, Collins	Rendezvous docking with two targets; change of altitude using the propulsion system of one of the target vehicles; mission included an extended EVA.	See above.
Gemini GT-11	12 September 1966	71 hr, 17 min	Conrad, Gordon	Successful rendezvous and docking. EVA successful although tiring for Gordon.	See above.
Gemini GT-12	11 November 1966	94 hr, 34½ min	Lovell, Aldrin	Multiple rendezvous, docking; extensive EVA including astronauts working with tools.	See above.
Apollo 204			Grissom, White, Chaffee	Orbiter destroyed by fire and astronauts killed, 27 January 1967.	
Apollo 7	11 October 1968	260 hr, 9 min	Cunningham, Shirra, Eisele	First manned Apollo flight; test in earth orbit; rendezvoused with burnt-out final stage, using sextant and telescope for direction finding.	The following information on cardiovascular responses during the Apollo program applies to all Apollo missions except Apollo 15. This mission is considered separately because cardiovascular findings differed substantially from responses observed in all of the other flights.
Apollo 8	21 December 1968	147 hr	Borman, Lovell, Anders	First manned orbit of the moon.	
Apollo 9	3 March 1969	241 hr, 1 min	McDivitt, Scott, Schweickart	Docking operation with lunar module.	Heart rate was elevated during launch and reentry but tended to stabilize at lower-than-preflight levels during weightlessness.

(*Continued*)

TABLE I—*Continued*

Orbiter Designation	Launch Date	Length of Flight	Astronauts	Comments	Cardiovascular Responses Encountered
Apollo 10	18 May 1969	192 hr, 3 min	Stafford Cernan Young	Descended to within 9 miles of the moon.	Postflight, resting heart rates were elevated, but returned to preflight levels within 30 to 50 hours. Orthostatic intolerance was evidenced by elevated heart rates during the application of lower-body negative pressure. ECG measurements during flight revealed no dramatic changes. Vectorcardiograms were significantly altered postflight. Heart size also decreased in most crewmen. Labile blood pressure observed for up to 3 days postflight. In 18 of 27 crewmen, a significant decrease in work capacity and oxygen uptake was observed postflight. All cardiovascular changes were reversed within 2 to 3 days postflight.
Apollo 11	16 July 1969	195 hr, 18 min	Armstrong Aldrin Collins	First lunar landing. Armstrong and Aldrin land in Sea of Tranquility.	
Apollo 12	14 November 1969	244 hr, 36 min	Conrad Bean Gordon	Conrad and Bean land in Sea of Storms; collected and labeled 108 pounds of rock.	
Apollo 13	11 April 1970	142 hr, 52 min	Lovell Haise Swigert	Pressure vessel explosion in service module caused orbiter to return to earth after a partial lunar orbit.	
Apollo 14	2 February 1971	216 hr, 1 min	Shepard Roosa Mitchell	Shepard and Mitchell landed in lunar module in the Fra Mauro area of the moon.	
Apollo 15	26 July 1971	295 hr, 12 min	Scott Worden Irwin	Scott and Irwin in lunar module landed in the Hadley Rille area of the moon and explored the region in a land rover. Worden, in the command module, performed lunar orbital experiments and the first deep space walk—200,000 miles from earth.	Cardiac arrhythmias and extrasystoles observed during flight. Crewmen exhibited all cardiovascular changes noted in other Apollo missions; the notable difference was that the Apollo 15 crew took a much longer time to return to preflight levels and reached complete recovery only after 2 weeks.
Apollo 16	16 April 1972	254 hr, 51 min	Duke Mattingly Young	Duke and Young spent 71 hours, 2 minutes on the moon; returned with 214 pounds of lunar rock and soil.	

Mission	Date	Duration	Crew	Description	Findings
Apollo 17	7 December 1972	301 hr, 51 min	Cernan Evan Schmitt	Cernan and Schmit spent a record 74 hours, 59 minutes on the moon and returned with 250 pounds of lunar material.	Single episode of significant cardiac arrhythmias in one crewman during exercise early in mission. Cardiac deconditioning observed during flight; crew returned to preflight cardiovascular status on 21st day postflight.
Skylab 2	25 May 1973	672 hr, 49 min	Conrad Kerwin Weitz	First manned flight to Skylab space station and longest space flight to date. First comprehensive medical studies performed in flight.	Cardiovascular deconditioning noted during flight and decreased cardiac output and exercise capacity postflight. Crew members returned to preflight cardiovascular status by the fourth day postflight. Increased exercise regimen thought to be a factor in the improved recovery rate.
Skylab 3	28 July 1973	59 days	Bean Garriott Lousma	Continuation of extensive medical studies utilizing specially designed equipment.	Cardiovascular deconditioning noted during flight; decreased cardiac output and lowered exercise capacity observed postflight. Crew members returned to preflight cardiovascular status on 5th day postflight. Stepped-up exercise regimen believed to be responsible for improved recovery rate.
Skylab 4	16 November 1973	84 days	Carr Gibson Pogue	Astronauts remained in space for the longest period to date; continued with scientific and biomedical experiments.	No significant cardiovascular problems during flight. Accidental release of nitrogen tetroxide into environmental control system on reentry exposing all three crew members. Postflight evidence of chemical pneumonitis. Postflight examination on Slayton revealed pulmonary nodule. Surgery four weeks after flight revealed benign lesion.
Apollo-Soyuz	15 July 1975	9 days	Stafford Brand Slayton	Joint Russian-American space flight experiment. Transfer of Russian and American astronauts from their respective spacecrafts.	

TABLE II

Summary of Soviet Manned Space Flight Experience

Orbiter Designation	Launch Date	Length of Flight	Cosmonaut(s)	Comments	Cardiovascular Responses Encountered
Vostok 1	12 April 1961	1 hr, 48 min	Gagarin	World's first manned orbital flight.	Pulse rate and respiration normal during flight.
Vostok 2	6 August 1961	25 hr, 18 min	Titov	Distance covered: 435,000 miles.	Pulse rate ranged from 80 to 100 per minute, which was within limits of preflight level; respiration rate was 18–22. Pulse rate dropped to 54–56 during sleep, in line with preflight responses. Form and intervals of ECG tracings did not undergo substantial changes.
Vostok 3	11 August 1962	94 hr, 22 min	Nikolayev	With Vostok 4, which was launched the following day, objectives were to (1) obtain data on the possibility of establishing close contact between two ships, (2) coordinate the actions of the cosmonauts, and (3) check the influence of identical conditions of space flight on human organs.	Cosmonauts felt well throughout flight; no cardiovascular problems encountered. A-V conduction time slightly prolonged.
Vostok 4	12 August 1962	70 hr, 57 min	Popovich	Coordinated with Vostok 3 to fulfill the above objectives.	Cosmonauts felt well throughout flight; no significant cardiovascular problems encountered. A-V conduction time slightly prolonged.
Vostok 5	14 June 1963	119 hr, 6 min	Bykovsky	Dual flight with Vostok 6.	Cosmonauts felt well during flight; no cardiovascular problems encountered. A-V conduction time slightly shortened.

Mission	Date	Crew	Mission notes	Cardiovascular notes
Vostok 6	16 June 1963	Tereshkova	70 hr, 50 min	First flight of a woman into space. During first orbit, Vostok 5 and Vostok 6 came within three miles of one another.	No cardiovascular problems encountered. A-V conduction time slightly shortened.
Voskhod 1	12 October 1964	Komarov Feoktistov Yegorov	24 hr, 17 min	First multiman flight into space; first flight with cosmonauts in "shirtsleeve" condition.	No cardiovascular problems encountered. Pilots wore no pressure suits. Inversion illusion present during flight. Yegorov showed marked bradycardia (46 beats/min) while asleep. Blood samples taken during flight.
Vokshod 2	18 March 1965	Belyaev Leonov	26 hr, 2 min	For first time, cosmonaut left orbiter and walked in space.	No cardiovascular problems observed although cosmonaut stated that he felt tired after reentering the orbiter following his space walk.
Soyuz 1	23 April 1967	Komarov	27 hr	Test flight of Soyuz vehicle. Mission halted prematurely because of communications and stabilization problems. Recovery system failed on reentry, resulting in death of cosmonaut and destruction of vehicle.	No information available on cardiovascular function during flight.
Soyuz 3	26 October 1968	Beregovoy	94 hr, 51 min	Radar lock-on with unmanned Soyuz 2 achieved but docking not accomplished.	Cosmonaut's pulse and respiration rate increased to 109 and 36 cycles per minute, respectively, during launch and reached maximum on insertion into orbit. Pulse rate variability exceeded preflight levels throughout the entire flight, but mean respiration rate did not differ from preflight level. ECG and seismocardiogram did not reveal any change in form.

(Continued)

445

TABLE II—*Continued*

Orbiter Designation	Launch Date	Length of Flight	Cosmonaut(s)	Comments	Cardiovascular Responses Encountered
Soyuz 4	14 January 1969	71 hr, 14 min	Shatalov	Docking operation with passive Soyuz 5; automatic docking maneuver to within 350 feet; docking accomplished manually.	During active phase of launch, pulse rate increased to 94 and respiration rate to 25 cycles per minute. Pulse rate variability in revolutions 33–34 substantially exceeded preflight level, but remained within the limits of the initial values during the rest of the orbital flight. However, the cosmonaut's mean respiration rate exceeded the preflight level during the entire orbital flight.
Soyuz 5	15 January 1969	72 hr, 46 min	Volynov Khrunov Yeliseyev	Soyuz 5 joined to Soyuz 4 for about four hours at perigee-apogee altitude of 131–156 miles; Khrunov and Yeliseyev transferred to Soyuz 4.	Pulse and respiration rates did not accelerate as markedly as those of cosmonauts on Soyuz 3 and 4; pulse rate ranged from 88–106 and respiration rate from 24–28. During transfer, respiration rates of both cosmonauts increased sharply but returned to the initial level during the 38th revolution. During preparation for transfer and entry into orbit, systolic time intervals were appreciably shortened, particularly so during transfer operations.
Soyuz 6	11 October 1969	118 hr, 42 min	Shonin Kubasov	Welding of metals in space.	Heart rate and respiration increased prior to launch. During flight, cardiac contractions became more frequent and the main phases of the cardiac cycle were appreciably shortened. Variations in pulse rate during orbital flight were greater for all crew members than during the preflight period. Performance of complex work tasks resulted in accelerated heart rates and respira-

Flight	Date	Duration	Crew	Description	Cardiovascular responses
Soyuz 7	12 October 1969	118 hr, 41 min	Filipichenko Volkov Gorbatko	Tests for building an orbiting space laboratory.	tions. Prior to descent the frequency of cardiac contractions again increased. No significant changes were noted in ECGs or SCG wave-forms except that Kubasov exhibited a brief displacement of the S-T segment below the isoelectric line during the 20th flight revolution.
Soyuz 8	13 October 1969	118 hr, 41 min	Shatalov Yeliseyev	Further tests for building an orbiting space laboratory.	Same responses observed in Soyuz 6 except that Filipichenko exhibited S-T segment depression during the 49th revolution. Same responses as those exhibited in Soyuz 6 and 7.
Soyuz 9	1 June 1970	424 hr, 59 min	Nikolayev Sevastyanov	Longest space flight to date; extensive scientific experiments and biomedical observations, such as prolonged weightlessness responses.	Cardiac reaction to standard physical loads did not exhibit significant changes and remained virtually unchanged from preflight levels. After flight, cosmonauts exhibited weakness, dizziness, and increased heart rate while standing or tilted. Orthostatic tests were tolerated with difficulty by both cosmonauts. By Day 11 postflight, the conditions of both were close to preflight level.
Soyuz 10	22 April 1971	48 hr	Shatalov Yeliseyev Rukavishnikov	Docked with Salyut 1 for 5½ hours while crew checked out space station systems, including a new docking device.	No information available on cardiovascular responses.
Soyuz 11	6 June 1971	276 hr	Dobrovolsky Volkov Patsayev	Spacecraft docked with Salyut 1 space station; cosmonauts orbited in space station for 23 days. During return to earth, pressure leak in Soyuz vehicle resulted in death of all three cosmonauts.	No unusual cardiovascular responses observed during Salyut segment of mission.

(Continued)

TABLE II—*Continued*

Orbiter Designation	Launch Date	Length of Flight	Cosmonaut(s)	Comments	Cardiovascular Responses Encountered
Soyuz 12	27 September 1973	2 days	Lazarev Makarov	Test of redesigned version of spacecraft; modified to hold two crewmen in space suits rather than three in coveralls. Reached record altitude for Soyuz of 214 miles.	Definite feeling of chest fullness and uneasiness when breathing. Weight loss pilot and engineer: 2.8 kg and 1.7 kg respectively.
Soyuz 13	19 December 1973	8 days	Klimuk Lebedev	Astronomical and earth observations stressed in mission; studies of brain circulation during weightlessness; observation of on-board greenhouse.	No alteration of cardiovascular responses during flight. Postflight orthostatis and exercise decrements present.
Soyuz 14	4 July 1974	16 days	Popovich Artyukhin	First Salyut docking since Soyuz 11. Photographed earth, studied atmosphere and performed a variety of scientific tasks in the space station.	Lung efficiency and cardiovascular changes tested in flight; cosmonauts appeared to adapt to weightlessness in 3–4 days. Postflight orthostasis exercise degradation.
Soyuz 15	26 August 1974	3 days	Sarafanov Dyemin	Rendezvous achieved with Salyut 3 space station; failed to dock. Returned to earth because of limited battery power of Soyuz vehicle.	Cardiovascular responses as with previous flights. Main findings after flight.
Soyuz 16	2 December 1974	7 days	Filipichenko Rukavishnikov	Warm-up flight for the Soviet portion of Apollo-Soyuz Program; evaluation of a variety of equipment for the two-nation program.	No significant changes in cardiovascular responses. Findings during and after flight similar to those on previous flights.
Soyuz 17	9 January 1975	30 days	Gubarev Grechko	Docked to Salyut 4 space station; cosmonauts lived and worked in	Regimen of 2 hours a day exercising on bicycle ergometer and treadmill; test of

Flight	Date	Duration	Crew	Description	Medical findings
				space station. Numerous biological and physiological observations made as well as earth and astronomical studies. New Russian record of 30 days in orbit.	negative pressure suits. Cosmonauts suffered fatigue at first, but were reported to have "withstood well the long space flight." Specific studies were conducted to monitor cerebral blood flow during flight using rheo-encephalography.
Soyuz 18A	5 April 1975	Aborted	Lazarev, Makarov	First manned space vehicle to abort during launch when third stage rocket moved off course. Soyuz vehicle jettisoned automatically and made soft landing in Siberia. Both cosmonauts safe.	No significant medical findings.
Soyuz 18	25 May 1975	63 days	Klimok, Sevastyanov	Docking accomplished with Salyut 4 space laboratory placed in orbit December 26, 1974; cosmonauts transferred safely to Salyut.	Longest Russian manned flight to date. Provocative tests done weekly in order to develop prognostic indices for continuing flight which were positive. Early adaptation occurred. Heart rate and blood pressure changes as on previous flights. Specific countermeasures evaluated during flight: Anti-G suits, bicycle ergometer, in-flight treadmill, water loading, and LBNP suits.
Soyuz 19	15 July 1975	6 days	Kubasov, Leonov	ASTP flight, docked with American Apollo vehicle.	No significant cardiovascular or biomedical findings.
Soyuz 21	6 July 1976	49 days	Volynov, Zholobov	Vehicle docked with Salyut 5 space laboratory and cosmonauts transferred to Salyut.	No significant cardiovascular or biomedical findings.
Soyuz 22	15 September 1976	7 days+	Bykovskiy, Aksenor		No significant cardiovascular changes; cosmonauts subjective findings were that they felt fine.

(Continued)

TABLE II—*Continued*

Orbiter Designation	Launch Date	Length of Flight	Cosmonaut(s)	Comments	Cardiovascular Responses Encountered
Soyuz 23	14 October 1976	48 hours	Zudov Razhdestvenskiy	Failed to dock with Salyut 5 space laboratory.	No significant cardiovascular findings.
Soyuz 24	7 February 1977	17+ days	Gorbatko Glazkov	Docked with Salyut 5 space laboratory and cosmonauts transferred to Salyut.	No significant cardiovascular findings.
Soyuz 25	9 October 1977	48 hours	Kavalenak Ryumin	Failed to dock with Salyut 6 space laboratory.	No significant cardiovascular findings.
Soyuz 26	10 December 1977	96 days	Romanenko Grechko	Docked and transferred to Salyut 6; longest period spent aboard space laboratory.	Heavy use of exercise. Decreased exercise and orthostatic tolerances for 1 month postflight.
Soyuz 27	10 January 1978	6 days	Dzhanibekow Makarov	Docked with Salyut 6 and Soyuz 26.	No significant cardiovascular changes.
Soyuz 28	2 March 1978	7+ days	Gubarev Remek	Docked with Salyut 6 and Soyuz 27.	No significant cardiovascular changes.
Soyuz 29	15 June 1978	139 days+	Kovalenok Ivanchenko	docked and transferred to Salyut 6; longest stay in space to date.	Findings similar to Soyuz 26. Less postflight exercise intolerance.
Soyuz 30	27 June 1978	8 days	Plimick Hermaszewski	Docked with Salyut 6 and Soyuz 29.	No significant cardiovascular changes.
Soyuz ?	25 February 1979	175 days	Lyakhov Ryumin	Cosmonauts docked with and transferred to Salyut 6 space laboratory.	Cosmonauts carried from spacecraft. Findings similar to Soyuz 29.

unanesthetized squirrel monkey to an altitude of 186 km. Although data were telemetered to earth for 13.3 min, the animal was not recovered. The life support system functioned satisfactorily, as did all biosensors except for respiration, which was lost early in flight. Heart rate, heart sounds, and body temperature were monitored (Graybiel *et al.,* 1959).

Bioflight II, which followed in May 1959, carried two monkeys—a 3.2-kg rhesus and a 0.5-kg squirrel—into weightlessness. All measurements made during Bioflight I were repeated, except that colonic temperature replaced axillary measurements and electromyograms were added. Performance monitoring was included, with the rhesus monkey trained to perform a task in weightlessness; however, data transmission on the performance testing ceased just before takeoff. Both animals were recovered unharmed.

The first American attempt to place a biologic payload in orbit occurred on June 3, 1959. A Discoverer 3 satellite carrying two mice was successfully launched but failed to go into orbit, so that the animals were lost.

In December 1959, a 3.6-kg rhesus monkey was sent into weightlessness on a Little Joe solid-fuel launch vehicle. He was followed in January 1960 by a 2.7-kg female rhesus. Both animal flights were used to verify the adequacy of the flight equipment to be used in Project Mercury. They were monitored for biologic reactions to acceleration, as well as performance. Both animals were recovered, and neither exhibited findings of note.

Three mice were launched to an altitude of 400 km in October 1960. The flight was boosted by an Atlas RZX-2A missle but did not go into orbit. Nevertheless, it provided important information because the vehicle passed through the Van Allen radiation belt. The animals were recovered and exhibited no effects from radiation exposure either individually or in their subsequent offspring.

On January 31, 1961, a 16.7-kg male chimpanzee preceded Alan Shepard into ballistic space flight (Clamann, 1961). The vehicle was a Mercury capsule powered by a Red Stone booster (MR-2). The animal was monitored for lead I and lead III of the ECG, respiratory waveform, and rectal temperature, and was required to perform two psychomotor tests (discrete and continuous avoidance tasks). The animal survived the flight with no ill effects.

A second male chimpanzee (18.9 kg) next preceded astronaut John Glenn in flight, spending 183 min in weightlessness and reaching an altitude of 90 km (Henry and Mosely, 1963). The flight was made in a Mercury capsule powered by an Atlas missile (MA-5). The animal was monitored for ECG, respiration, and body temperature; he was also required to perform psychomotor tasks. Arterial and venous pressure were recorded from intravascular cathethers. The blood pressure recording system was similar to that used in the Aerobee flights. Blood pressure readings in the animal were

TABLE III

Significant American and Russian Animal Flights

Vehicle Designation	Origin	Launch Date	Flight Duration	Animal Description	Physiological Measurements	Comments
Sputnik 2	USSR	3 Nov. 1957	25 hours	Dog, Laika	Pulse rate, blood pressure, chest ECG leads	No ill effects from ascent and injection into orbit; in orbit, took food from automatic dispenser, barked, and moved about. Animals not recovered.
Bioflight I	US	13 Dec. 1958		Unanesthetized squirrel monkey (0.5 kg) named Old Reliable	Heart rate, heart sounds, body temperature	Suborbital flight; animal not recovered.
Bioflight II	US	28 May 1959		Two unanesthetized monkeys: Able (3.2 kg Rhesus) and Baker (0.5 kg squirrel monkey)	Heart rate, heart sounds, body temperature, colonic temperature, electromyograms. Performance tests attempted.	Suborbital flight; animals recovered. Heart sounds and performance not recorded, no significant changes in other measurements from preflight values.
Bioflight III	US	4 Dec. 1959		Unanesthetized monkey, Sam (3.6 kg Rhesus)	Biological effects of acceleration; performance testing.	No significant cardiovascular changes; animal recovered; testing for Project Mercury.
Bioflight IV	US	21 Jan. 1960		Unanesthetized female monkey, Miss Sam (2.7 kg Rhesus)	Biological effects of acceleration; performance testing.	No significant cardiovascular changes; animal recovered. Preliminary to Project Mercury. Animal did not perform as well as Sam.
Sputnik 4	USSR	19 Aug. 1960	25 hours	Dogs: Belka (5.5 kg) and Strelka (4.5 kg); 40 mice; 2 rats	Pulse rate, chest ECG leads, blood pressure, phonocardiograms.	First successful recovery of animals from orbital flight.
Sputnik 5	USSR	1 Dec. 1960	25 hours	Dogs: Pchelka and Mushka; mice; insects	Pulse rate, ECG, phonocardiograms, seismocardiograms.	Vehicle destroyed on re-entry.
Mercury/Red Stone	US	31 Jan. 1961		Chimpanzee, Ham (16.7 kg)	ECG recordings (Lead I and	Suborbital flight; all biological data

					Lead III); performance testing.	successfully transmitted; no significant cardiovascular changes.
Sputnik 6	USSR	9 Mar. 1961	65 minutes	Dog, Chernushka (5.9 kg); guinea pigs; mice; other living organisms.	Pulse rate, ECG, sphygmogram.	Space craft completed only one orbit.
Sputnik 7	USSR	25 Mar. 1961	65 minutes	Dog, Zvezdochka	Pulse rate, ECG, sphygmogram.	Preceded Yuri Gagarin into orbit; animal successfully recovered.
Mercury/MA-5	US	29 Nov. 1961	183 minutes	Chimpanzee, Enos (18.9 kg)	ECG, arterial and venous pressure, body temperature, performance testing.	Blood pressure high; extra systoles recorded occasionally during flight.
Kosmos 110	USSR	22 Feb. 1966	22 days	Dogs: Veterok (7.6 kg) and Ugolek (8.3 kg)	ECG, pulse rate, blood pressure, respiration rate, seismocardiograms, hematology.	30% loss in body weight, primarily fluid. No ECG changes. Altered STIs indicating a decrease in stroke volume.
Biosatellite III	US	28 June 1969	8.8 days	Monkey, Bonnie (5.5 kg pigtail)	ECG, EMG, EOG, body temperature, direct measurement of arterial and venous pressure by catheters.	Animal died shortly after recovery; weighed only 4.4 kg; exhibited marked dehydration. Slight but significant increase in central venous pressure during flight.
Kosmos 605	USSR	31 Oct. 1973	22 days	Rats, tortoises	Pathophysiological studies before and after flight.	No significant cardiovascular changes.
Kosmos 690	USSR	22 Oct. 1974	20.5 days	Rats (200 gm)	Same as Kosmos 605, plus radiation testing.	No significant cardiovascular changes.
Kosmos 782	USSR	25 Nov. 1975	19.5 days	Rats (200 gm)	Same as Kosmos 605.	U.S. investigators participated in experimentation; no significant cardiovascular changes.
Kosmos 936	USSR	3 Aug. 1977	18.5 days	Rats (200 gm)	Same as Kosmos 605, plus centrifugation of 10 rats at 1 G during flight; no centrifugation of other 9 rats.	No significant cardiovascular changes.

high, probably because of the stress of the instrumentation and flight procedures. Peak systolic values were not obtained because of the limits set for galvanometer deflection. Extra systoles were recorded occasionally in flight and were believed to result from the presence of the venous catheter in the right ventricular chamber. The animal was recovered and showed no adverse physiological effects.

With the advent of man into space, less emphasis has been placed on animal payloads. Biologic payloads have continued to be sent into space, however, to investigate further the long-term effects of weightlessness. Some of these payloads have flown aboard manned space flights and in bioscience satellites. They have included such biologic systems as human serum, rabbit antiserums, frog eggs and frog otiliths, seeds, viruses, bacteria, tissue culture cells, and various insects.

The last flight using a nonhuman primate was launched on June 28, 1969 (Adey and Hahn, 1971). The subect was a 5.5-kg pig-tailed monkey. The flight lasted only 8.8 days of a planned 30 days and had to be terminated because the animal demonstrated physiological deterioration during flight. The capsule was recovered, but the animal died shortly after recovery. He weighed only 4.4 kg at the time of death and was markedly dehydrated. There has been considerable controversy over the cause of death. But most likely, death resulted from a combination of heavy instrumentation in the animal and the stress of space flight.

Animal flights prior to man's entry into space demonstrated that the organism could adapt to weightlessness and withstand the stresses of flight without serious or long-term effects on the body. With the outlook for increasingly longer stays in space, questions arise about the long-term effects of weightlessness on the cardiovascular system. Prolonged animal flights in the future offer the only reliable means of obtaining further knowledge on these effects.

2. Soviet Animal Flights

As indicated earlier, Soviet investigators have preferred dogs over primates for their animal flights. In 1949 the Soviets began a systematic program of animal flights, with vehicles that progressed from small rockets to increasingly larger boosters that could achieve an altitude of 450 km. Between 1949 and 1960, 40 animal flights were made, all of which carried dogs. Most of the animals made more than one flight, some as many as five flights; others were killed on their first or second flight. These flights were directed toward determining the effects of acceleration forces, developing a retrieval system, and recording physiological functions during flight. The animals were monitored for ECG, blood pressure, and respiratory frequency; motion pictures were also taken occasionally.

Between 1949 and 1952, nine dogs were sent in hermetically sealed cabins to altitudes of about 100 km (Galkin *et al.*, 1962). The animals were monitored for heart rate, blood pressure, and respiration rate. From 1953 to 1956, 12 additional dogs were launched (Bugrov *et al.*, 1962). In this group of flights, the cabins were not sealed; instead, the animals wore ventilated space suits.

In 1957 a series of five dogs was launched in hermetically sealed cabins to altitudes between 200 and 212 km (Galkin *et al.*, 1962). Results of these flights showed that the dogs responded to the acceleration, noise, and vibration by exhibiting increases in blood pressure, pulse frequency, and respiration rate.

The dog Laika, who preceded Yuri Gagarin into space, was launched November 3, 1957 (Gurovskiy and Kieslev, 1973). Laika's flight was a pioneer in space because it was the first biologic payload to be placed in orbit. The animal died during flight because of limitations in the environmental control system; the capsule disintegrated on reentry.

Following the flight of Laika, four ballistic flights were conducted to acquire additional information for the development of more effective orbital recovery systems. In August 1958, two dogs were launched in hermetically sealed cabins to an altitude of 450 km; both were recovered. In July 1959, two dogs and a rabbit were launched to an altitude of 160 km and were successfully recovered. The outcome of additional animal flights during this period is not known.

On May 15, 1960, Sputnik IV was launched containing one dog. The vehicle was placed in orbit to test orbital recovery systems. Although the animal was not recovered, the mission marked the first successful telemetry of biologic information to earth, including data on respiratory frequency, arterial blood pressure, and ECG.

Sputnik V was launched on August 20, 1960, and recovered 24 hr later. The flight vehicle contained two dogs, 21 black mice, 21 white mice, and several rats, as well as scores of fruit flies, seeds, and cellular organisms.

Two more dogs were launched in Sputnik VI on December 1, 1960. The biologic payload also included insects and plants. The satellite orbited for two days, during which biologic data were telemetered to earth. Heart performance of one dog was measured by a seismocardiographic (vibration-sensing) transducer and on the other dog by phonocardiograms. ECGs, and EMGs, and deep-body temperature were also obtained for each dog. Television was successfully transmitted from the satellite. The vehicle was destroyed on reentry because of a faulty recovery system.

The last dog flight was launched on February 22, 1966, and marked the first of the Kosmos series of biologic flights. The satellite vehicle remained in space 22 days and was successfully recovered. It contained two dogs, as well as mice, fruit flies, seeds, and cellular systems. The dogs were monitored by ECGs, phonocardiograms, and carotid arterial tracings to determine systolic time intervals. The findings were later used to assess cardiovascular status during flight. Both dogs showed a decrease in cardiac output and stroke volume. Attempts to withdraw blood and measure intravascular arterial pressure failed.

Four more Kosmos flights were launched between 1973 and 1977. All contained rats and consisted of pathophysiological studies before and after flight. The satellites spent from 18 to 22 days in orbit, and all were successfully recovered.

Physiological responses during the first of these flights (Kosmos 605) were reported by Portugalov and co-workers (1976). The 27 rats who made this flight were sacrificed on days 1 and 2 and 26 and 27 after landing. Perceptible morphological and biochemical shifts were observed postflight in the musculoskeletal, hemo- and lymphopoiesis, and hypothalmic–hypophyseal–adrenal systems, as well as in the juxtaglomerular apparatus of the kidney. The observed changes were nonspecific and reversible; such changes had been observed previously during both ground-based hypokinesia and other forms of stress. Significant changes could not be detected in any of the heart chambers or major blood vessels. Gayevskaya and co-workers (1976) also reported on electron microscopic studies of the myocardium and anlaysis of its protein fractions and enzymatic activity. They concluded that the animals showed no significant alterations in the content of sarcoplasmatic and myofibrillar proteins. Such changes as were noted (decrease in ATPase activity of the myocardial myosin) were considered by the authors to be an adaptive reaction to the weightless state.

The animals in the remaining three flights also have evidenced no significant cardiovascular changes as a result of their prolonged exposure to weightlessness.

III. Physiological Responses Associated with Postural Changes

The circulatory effects of gravity and weightlessness (including simulated weightlessness) can be better understood from a discussion of the physiological changes that occur with a change in body position. When an individual is standing, the body must adjust for gravitational pull by making significant compensatory adjustments so that the blood flow will be maintained to the head and blood volume will be distributed adequately. If the compensatory mechanisms are insufficient or retarded, the individual experiences orthostatic intolerance or hypotension. Orthostatic responses are complex and involve physical, hormonal, and central nervous system changes (Rushmer, 1970). Figure 1 shows the circulatory events that accompany a change in body position; Fig. 2 indicates the measureable hemodynamic results.

Gauer and Thron (1963), as well as others, have pointed out that the normal functional condition of circulation is in the upright position, since man spends at least two-thirds of his time in this position. In the vertical position the long axis of the body is oriented parallel to the pull of gravity. In this position there is a shift of blood from the head and chest toward the feet. When the body is changed to the horizontal position, blood that has accumulated in the lower limbs shifts immediately back to the rest of the body because of the loss of hydrostatic distending pressure in the peripheral veins and other vascular structures (Sjöstrand, 1955). When this occurs, an average of 640 ml of blood (or 11% of the average blood volume) shifts, with approximately 80% moving to the thorax (McCally and Graveline, 1963; Sjöstrand, 1955).

This same change very probably occurs in weightlessness, with the blood volume redistributions being of equal or greater magnitude, although definitive measurements have not yet been made. This conclusion has been supported by flight experience—neck vein distention and facial puffiness have occurred consistently in both astronauts and cosmonauts (Thornton *et al.*, 1977). These changes also occur as the result of simulated weightlessness (bedrest, immersion, and immobilization). The redistribution of the blood produces an immediate increase in cardiac output through the Frank–Starling's mechanism; long-term effects, however, have not yet been adequately studied.

Despite the increase in cardiac output and stroke volume (Fig. 2), with supine posture arterial blood pressure does not change significantly; the heart rate slows, and arterial flow resistance decreases. The depressor signals for these changes result from the stimulation of the baroreceptors in the central and peripheral circulations and in the heart itself (Pelletier and Shepherd, 1972). In the intact unanesthetized animal and in man, the latter reflex adjustments may overshadow changes resulting from increased venous return or an increase in cardiac size (Rushmer, 1970, pp. 148–150).

Adjustments in mean arterial pressure and the factors that change it—such as blood flow, nervous influences, vessel elasticity, and contained volume—are more readily understood by applying the concepts of hydraulics to the systems. In its simplest form the concept of hydraulics allows mean arterial pressure to be related to the product of cardiac output and peripheral vascular resistance (Rushmer, 1970, pp. 192–220). The manner in which these principles operate physiologically is shown in Fig. 2; as the figure illustrates, mean arterial pressure drops slightly, but insignificantly,

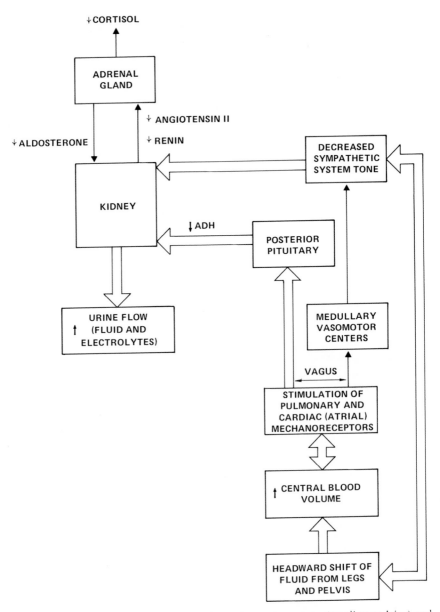

Fig. 1. Circulatory events accompanying a change in posture (standing to lying) and possibly weightlessness.

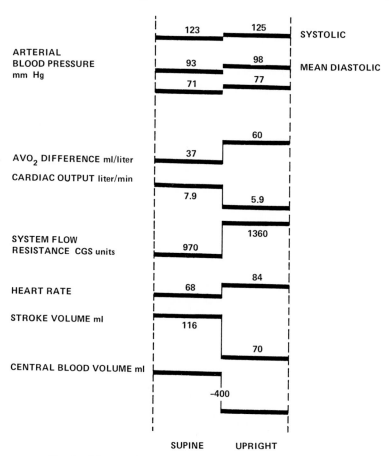

Fig. 2.   Measurable hemodynamic effects. (From Gauer, 1971.)

when the individual is in the supine position despite a significant increase in blood flow resulting from the concomitant decrease in flow resistance.

Mean arterial blood pressure measurements show little change as the blood passes down the aorta and larger arteries. Mean pressure drops only as the blood enters the small arteries and capillary beds of each organ. As the blood passes down the larger arteries, the systolic pressure rises slightly while the diastolic pressure falls because of reflected waves that amplify the systolic pressure somewhat and depress the trailing portion of the diastolic segment of the pulse pressure curve (Remington and Wood, 1956).

Measured pressure, therefore, may vary significantly at various sites in the body and during changes in body position or exposure to aerospace-induced stresses. Examples of such changes are shown in Table IV and the

TABLE IV

Comparison of Systolic Blood Pressure Values in mmHg under Space Environmental Conditions

Organ	Vertical +1 G	Recumbent	Any Position During Orbit	Moon Vertical +1/6 G	Mars Vertical +1/3 G	Seated +3 G_z
Eye	80	104	104	100	96	32
Brain	100	124	124	120	116	52
Heart	124	124	124	124	124	115
Ankle	210	140	140	152	162	350

pressures are idealized for the hemodynamic values given in Fig. 2. Systolic pressures are compared at the level of the heart, brain, and eye (30 cm above the heart) and at the ankle. It is interesting to note that when the individual is recumbent or in null gravity, the heart-to-ankle gradient is markedly decreased from that when he is standing upright (or tilted) or during +G_z acceleration. The ability to compensate or adjust physiologically depends on a multitude of factors related to the force of contraction of the heart, the level of aortic pressure, the compliance of the aortic wall, the magnitude of the intravascular volume, and the responsivness of the peripheral vascular bed.

When vascular resistance increases and the heart is called on to work against a greater pressure load, it undergoes a sequence of adaptive changes. Systolic ejection is less complete, causing, first, an increase in end-systolic volume and, then, an increase in end-diastolic volume. This change improves ventricular emptying by the mechanism of heterometric autoregulation. The decreased load secondarily induces the true inotropic changes referred to as homometric autoregulation. By these two adaptive mechanisms, the heart through autoregulation is able to maintain a normal output during large changes in vascular resistance.

The influence of the neurotransmitter substance norepinephrine on the mechanical and electrical properties of the myocardium in accomplishing these purposes has long been recognized (Rushmer and Smith, 1959; Wurtman, 1965). The response of the intact heart to augmented adrenergic influences has been defined during exercise and the Starling response. In the intact animal, these adrenergic effects are evidenced by tachycardia, a reduction in cardiac dimensions, increased velocity of ejections, and an increased rate of force development (Rushmer, 1959).

The development of cardiac-denervated animals and the techniques of heart transplant have contributed importantly to an understanding of the adrenergic regulation of the heart. The denervated heart appears capable of meeting the demands of muscular exercise. The mechanisms used by the denervated heart to increase cardiac output to compensate for postural changes differ from those used by the intact heart (Donald *et al.*, 1964; Donald and Shepherd, 1963). Tachycardia is less marked in the denervated heart, and the Frank–Starling mechanism is utilized to increase stroke volume and cardiac output.

Changes in peripheral circulation during postural changes occur in the following circuits: (1) windkessel vessels, (2) peripheral resistance vessels, (3) precapillary sphincters, (4) exchange vessels, (5) postcapillary resistance vessels, (6) capacitance vessels, (7) shunt vessels. The pre- and postcapillary sphincters and the capacitance vessels are the areas of greatest importance in assessing physiological responses during weightlessness and simulated weightlessness. The sum of the pre- and postcapillary resistances determines the blood flow to any region, and the ratio of the two determines blood volume. The reactivity of the capacitance vessels determines ventricular filling, which has a direct bearing on cardiac performance in producing modifications of heart rate and, particularly, stroke volume (Shepherd, 1966).

Maximal vascular dilation is reached only in exceptional circumstances (Saltin and Steinberg, 1964). Normally, the flow capacity to the various tissues is adjusted by the functioning of the vascular smooth muscle to meet physiological requirements. The vascular smooth muscle is controlled by its own intrinsic activity, which is facilitated, to some extent, by the distention resulting from the normal fluctuation of the pulsatile flow. This intrinsic muscle activity, on the other hand, receives a powerful negative feedback from the steadily produced muscle metabolites. This system accounts for the autoregulation of blood flow and for the automatic adjustments in the perfused capillary surface area that occur with changes in posture. Negative feedback control stems from the combined action of a series of tissue-produced vasodilator metabolites. The importance of the individual components varies from tissue to tissue: CO_2 appears to be the most important for brain tissue; potassium ion for activated skeletal muscle; adenosine and possibly prostaglandin for coronary vessels; and bradykinin for sweat glands, salivary glands, and pancreas (Zelis, 1975).

Control of the cardiovascular changes by means of sympathetic vasoconstrictor discharge, mediated through the central nervous system, is superimposed on the local regulation of the precapillary vessels (Folkow, 1955, 1960). The discharge in itself may not be as important as the rate of discharge. Constrictor activation increases the precapillary/postcapillary resistance ratio and increases total resistance to flow. "Depot" blood within the capacitance vessels is also mobilized. These mechanisms operate particularly in skeletal muscle and skin and cause an autotransfusion of interstitial fluid to the vascular bed as the result of a consequent capillary pressure decrease resulting from the disturbance of the Starling filtration–absorption equilibrium across the capillary walls. An identical type of mechanism can be expected to operate during the initial phases of space flight and immobilization in the laboratory environment because of the loss of hydrostatic gradients.

Sympathetic tone emerges from the bulbar vasomotor center and is continuously adjusted by different sets of highly sensitive cardiovascular proprioreceptors, which create both inhibitory and excitatory effects on the center. Depending on their location and design, the inhibitory mechanoreceptors (baroreceptors) are able to sense (1) the filling of the system, (2) the wall tension in various cardiac sections, and (3) the pulse and mean pressures in the pulmonary and systemic arteries. The excitatory chemoreceptors, on the other hand, sense the composition of the arterial tree.

Normally, cardiovascular hemostatic mechanisms do not disturb cutaneous and renal mechanisms (Vatner, 1975). These circuits are involved only when there is intense alteration of the vasomotor center—that is, during a considerable loss of blood, pain, fear, and the like. Usually, centrally induced autonomic discharge is linked to specific somatomotor–hormonal adjustments that condition the entire organism to a new situation, such as feeding or exercise. Man's adjustment to weightlessness and simulated weightlessness occurs because of these reactions.

Reflex nervous influence on the capacitance vessels can be considered to be the first line of defense against the effects of postural changes because it occurs so rapidly after the onset. This influence on fluid partition at the level of the pre- and postcapillary sphincters can be considered to be a second line of defense. The latter mechanism is probably more important than the influence on the capacitance vessels because it increases the absolute volume of the cardiovascular system rather than redistributing its contents. The mechanisms concerned with maintaining proper blood volume through neurohumoral functions are the third line of defense against the physiological effects of weightlessness and immobilization.

The presence of low-pressure mechanoreceptors has been known for a considerable time, but their effects on cardiovascular function have been studied only recently (Gauer *et al.,* 1970; Goetz *et al.,* 1975; Linden, 1973; Pelletier and Shepherd, 1973). These sensors consist of complex, unencapsulated nerve endings that are situated primarily in the wall of the cardiac atria—in the left atrium, in the vicinity of its junction with the pulmonary veins, and in the right atrium, near the caval entrances. The nerve endings appear to be of two types—one that is activated by distention and another that is activated by atrial contraction. To date, no clear differences have been noted in the action of either type.

Traffic is carried in medullated afferents, which, on stimulation, result in an increase in heart rate, a decrease in sympathetic activity to the kidney, and a water diuresis that is probably caused by the inhibition of antidiuretic hormone secretion (or increased secretion of such elements as natiuretic hormone) (Chapman and Henry, 1973; Gauer et al., 1970; Goetz et al., 1975).

A significant early diuresis producing a dilute urine regularly occurs with human bedrest and water immersion experiments (Cardus et al., 1965; Epstein, 1978; Lynch et al., 1967; McCally and Graveline, 1963; Stevens and Lynch, 1965). Clinical experiments with normal individuals have indirectly supported the foregoing conclusions by showing compensatory events, the opposite of those just described, when central venous volume is lowered as the result of positive pressure breathing or LBNP (Hunt, 1967; Lamb and Stevens, 1965; McCally et al., 1968; Stevens, 1966). Changes in body fluid content, especially intravascular volume, mediated through the stimulation of the central low-pressure mechanoreceptors, are considered to be one of the most significant features of the adaptive process to the recumbent state.

Whenever the cardiovascular system is unable to compensate for the erect posture, syncope or fainting results. Its incidence and the rate of onset in man can be measured during standing or tilting by blood withdrawal, the use of vasodilator drugs, immobilization, prior exercise, or the use of venous occlusive tourniquets or cuffs. The cause appears to be an increased vagal discharge superimposed on the already basic sympathetic response to tilt or change in body position and, therefore, has been termed "vasodepressor or vasovagal syncope" (Lamb et al., 1964a; Weissler et al., 1957).

The exact trigger mechanism for the vagotonic discharge remains unknown, but the work of Epstein et al., (1968a,b) strongly supports a primary role for the cardiovascular system, depending on minimal cardiac volume. Such a possibility in bedrested subjects is supported by recent work of Sandler and co-workers (1977).

Vasovagal syncope during tilt is characterized by the sudden onset of bradycardia, nausea, pallor, sweating, dizziness, and a sudden drop in blood pressure. In general, such syncopal reactions can occur in any clinical state that reduces heart rate, stroke volume, or peripheral resistance (Sandler, 1976). Severe postural hypotension may also occur with such clinical states as diabetes or Addison's disease or with other uncommon states that disturb the sympathetic innervation—for example, idiopathic chronic orthostatic hypotension. With regard to the latter, investigators (Bevegard et al., 1962; Ibrahim et al., 1975; Ziegler et al., 1977) have shown that the subjects do not pool more blood in dependent regions than normal individuals, but such pooling nevertheless causes a marked fall in blood pressure because of an absence or deficiency in reflex arteriolar and venous constriction. These findings are the opposite of changes occurring during a vasovagal faint.

Prolonged bedrest is associated with distinct changes in body fluid volumes (intra- and extravascular) and volume distribution, as well as deterioration of the normal reflex mechanisms that are responsible for peripheral vascular tone. These changes are clinically manifested primarily when bedrested individuals stand up suddenly or are stressed by upright tilting or LBNP. The resulting postural hypotension is regularly accompanied by decreased pulse pressure and tachycardia. In more susceptible individuals, when orthostatic stress is continued, vasodepressor syncope occurs.

During the period when an individual is bedrested, these cardiovascular changes do not appear to constitute a serious health hazard. Periods of bedrest lasting from several weeks to 120 days have been tolerated without evidence of harm, as is shown in Table V. Longer studies (1–2 years), which are usually concerned with orthopedic or neurological illnesses and conducted in a hospital environment, have also been reported in the literature with no indication of cardiac problems (Browse, 1965; Buhr, 1963; Stevenson, 1952). In fact, several studies have used bedrest for periods of 1–2½ years to treat chronic cardiac disease with beneficial effects (McDonald *et al.*, 1971, 1972).

IV. Changes in Resting Hemodynamic Parameters Resulting from Bedrest, Immersion, and Immobilization

With the advent of the space age, scientists began seeking an environment on earth that could be used to study physiological reactions to weightlessness. Brief periods of weightlessness could be achieved using Keplerian trajectory, but they lasted only about 1 min and, of course, did not provide a suitable environment for studying the long-term effects of exposure to zero gravity. Bedrest and fluid immersion, as well as immobilization of animals, were found to be suitable simulations. None of the methods, however, duplicates the weightless condition precisely because they do not reproduce the complete removal of the hydrostatic pressure gradient on the body or the removal of the constant action of gravity on the vestibular organs (semicircular canals and otoliths). Nonetheless, studies using all methods for simulating weightlessness have resulted in expanding man's knowledge of the physiological responses related to weightlessness.

Bedrest has been used more extensively in studying man's responses than immersion has, although the physiological mechanisms respond more rapidly during immersion. The preference for the bedrest regimen probably stems from the methodological difficulties related to immersion—that is, the necessity for precise thermal regulation of the immersion medium, maceration of the skin resulting from prolonged contact with water, and the complexity of carrying out hygienic procedures. Immobilization studies of small animals have also been used to a considerable extent in learning how weightlessness affects the heart.

A. Animal Experimentation

In assessing the effects of weightlessness, both American and Russian investigators have utilized animals not only in space flights but also in immobilization studies in the laboratory to simulate a null-gravity environment. Through immobilization studies, data have been accumulated on a small, but reasonably diverse, group of animals, including dogs, rabbits, rats, and monkeys. The physiological responses of the animals have varied in many cases, but, following prolonged immobilization, most have exhibited orthostatic intolerance and shifts in body fluids—both of which conditions have also been observed in man following space flight or bedrest.

Dogs have been immobilized to study the effects of simulated weightlessness (Asyamolov and Voskresenskiy, 1968; Kolpakhov *et al.,* 1970; Korol'kov, *et al.,* 1977; Novikov and Vlasov, 1976). Kolpakhov and co-workers (1970) documented significant decreases in resting cardiac output and blood pressure in dogs who had been immobilized for 2 weeks in body casts. Asyamolov and Voskresenskiy (1968), on the other hand, could not find consistent evidence of orthostatic intolerance or significant decrements in acceleration tolerance in dogs that were similarly treated. Animals kept immobilized for 6 months (Novikov and Vlasov, 1976) exhibited distinct changes in microvascular structure in most tissues, indicating a loss of vascular tonus, as well as a loss of muscle mass. Following 1 month of recovery, small vessel changes in the structure of the hind extremities (hard and soft bone tissue and bone marrow) were still present in the dogs. In addition, a number of investigators have found that bone metabolism is disordered in these animals as the result of immobilization (Katkovskiy and Pometov, 1976; Kolpakhov *et al.,* 1970; Kovalenko, 1976).

Rabbits subjected to hypokinesia for from 1 to $7\frac{1}{2}$ months showed a weight loss of 15–35%, depending on the length of immobilization (Karapu and Ferents, 1978). When exposed to a single treadmill run to capacity (at 1.27 km/hr) following immobilization, the animals exhibited complete fatigue in half the time of unrestricted controls. During hypokinesia, heart rate in-

TABLE V

Summary of Major Bedrest Studies Emphasizing Cardiovascular Changes

Investigator(s)	Publication Year	No. of Subjects	Duration	Study Emphasis
Tenney	1959	24	30 minutes	Fluid volume redistribution
Widdowson and McChance	1950	10 (5 f, f m)	2 hours-3 days	Plasma volume
Torphy	1966b	5	6 hours	Water immersion versus bedrest
McCally et al.	1966a	6	6 hours	Effect of LBNP on tolerance
McCally et al.	1968	9	6 hours	Venous cuffs/leotard/ADH injection/cold immersion
Reck et al.	1975	10	10 hours	Control of plasma aldosterone during upright posture
Lubin et al.	1976	40	10 hours	Effects of exercise, bedrest, and napping on performance
Vogt	1967a,b	9	12 hours	Water immersion/chair rest/bedrest/occlusive cuffs
Pestov and Asyamolov	1972	8	18 hours and 30 days	Water immersion/bedrest/LBNP as countermeasure
Spealman	1948	4	24 hours	Tilt versus stand tests
Birkhead et al.	1964	4	24 hours	16 hours bedrest/4 hours chair rest
Nixon et al.	1979	8	24 hours	5° head down/central venous pressure/heart dimensions
Leverett et al.	1971	9	24 hours	Experienced centrifuge subjects—Shuttle re-entry
Sokolkov	1971	24	24 hours	Basal metabolism
Leach et al.	1972	9	24 hours-7 days	Centrifugation/serum thyroid function tests
Volicier et al.[1]	1977	9	27 hours	5° head-down tilt
Vanyushina et al.	1966	21	1.5–11.5 days	Chair rest/water immersion/physiological changes
DiGiovanni and Birkhead	1964	1	2 days	Heat and restriction of fluid
Zhdanova	1965	18	2–10 days	Bedrest/water immersion
Chazov and Ananchenko	1963	12	2–20 days	Anticoagulation studies

Duration	Author	n	Description	Year
3 days	Cardus et al.[2,3]	6	Plasma levels; 17 OHC at rest; isometric exercise/Valsalva	1965
3 and 20 days	Kotovskaya et al.	2	$+G_x$ acceleration tolerance	1965
3 days	Pestov	16	Bedrest/water immersion/countermeasures	1968
3 days	Shurygin et al.	7	Chair rest/adrenal responses	1976
3 days	McCutcheon and Sandler[4]	3	Acceleration tolerance/LBNP/body composition	1975
3 days	Chavarri et al.	5	Circadian rhythms of hormones	1977
4 days	Lamb	6	Chair rest	1964
4–10 days	Lamb et al.	23	Chair rest	1965
4 days	Galle et al.	6	Reactions to low-intensity $+G_z$	1976
5–20 days	Panferova et al.	16	Chair rest/bedrest/arterial tone	1967
5 days	Olree et al.	20	Effects of physical training	1973
5–15 days	Melada et al.	6	Evans blue cardiac output and F-E changes	1975
5 days	Kakurin et al.	8	Antiorthostatic bedrest ($-4°$, $-8°$, $-12°$)	1976
6 days	Stevens and Lynch	4	9-alphafluorohydrocortisone as countermeasure	1965
6 days	Cherepakhin	12	Reduced diet/hypokinesia/tolerance to static load	1970
6 days	Vyazitskiy and Kumanichkin	8	Chair rest at various altitudes	1970
6 days	Johnson et al.	9	Fluid and electrolyte changes	1971b
6 days	Ivanov	10	Tissue oxygen metabolism	1972
6 days	Ivanov and Orlov	21	Oxygen metabolism in elderly and senile subjects	1973
7–21 days	Lurwak and Whedon	10	Effects of physical conditioning on glucose tolerance	1959
7 and 30 days	Birkhead et al.	8	Bicycle ergometer exercise as countermeasure	1964
7 days	Lamb and Stevens	4	LBNP as countermeasure	1965
7 days	Yegorov et al.	4	Effects of diet	1966
7 days	Udalov et al.	6	Effects of diet on metabolic function	1967

(Continued)

TABLE V—*Continued*

Duration	No. of Subjects	Investigator(s)	Publication Year	Study Emphasis
7–20 days	42	Kotovskaya *et al.*	1969	+G_z acceleration
7 days	9	Zubek	1968	Urinary excretion of steroids
7 days		Leverett *et al.*	1971	Shuttle re-entry/LBNP using experienced subjects
7 days	14	Friman and Hamrin	1976	Reactive hyperemia in forearm and calf muscle
7 days	8	Hyatt and West	1976	Horizontal versus 5° head down
7 days	3	McCutcheon and Sandler	1975	Acceleration tolerance
7 days (2)	6	Hyatt and West	1977	LBNP and fluid ingestion as countermeasures
8–15 and 20 days	21	Vasil'yev and Kotovskaya	1965	Physiological reactions to acceleration
8, 10, and 12 days	19	Syzrantsev	1967	Bedrest/water immersion/nitrogen metabolism/exercise
9 days	8	Bartok *et al.*	1968	Leg negative pressure
9 days	7	Goldwater *et al.*	1977	Shuttle re-entry profiles/LBNP; males 35–45 years
9 days	10	Sandler *et al.*	1978	Shuttle re-entry profiles/LBNP; females 35–45 years
9½ days	8	Bernauer *et al.*	1968	Renal function/blood and urine composition/metabolism
10 days		Ioffe *et al.*	1966	Noninvasive measurement of central and peripheral circulatory function
10 days	8	White *et al.*	1966	Repeated acceleration as countermeasure
10 days	11	Cardus[5,6]	1966	O_2 alveolar-arterial tension changes
10–12 days	13	Buyanov *et al.*	1967	Limb compression and exercise as countermeasures

Duration	Author	Year	n	Study
10 days	Zav'yalov et al.	1967	6	Bedrest in isolation chamber/scanning ability
10 days	Bohnn et al.	1970	8	Effect of 9-alphafluorohydro-cortisone on orthostatism
10 days	Vaysfel'd and Il'icheva	1972	6	Diurnal rhythms of steroid hormones
10 and 24 days	Isabayeva and Ponomareva[7,8]	1973	12	Adaptation to high altitude conditions as countermeasure
10 days	Korol'kov	1973	10	Hyperoxic & hypercapnic gas mixture as countermeasure
10 days	Chambers and Vykukal	1972	8	Jet pilots ($+G_z$/G suits)
10 days	de Marees et al.	1974	10	Endurance training/orthostatic regulation
12 days	McCally et al.	1971	4	Leg volume changes with tilt; forearm vessel responses
12 days	Hyatt et al.	1973	2	Potassium balance/Apollo 15 simulation
13 days	Epstein[96]	1970	8	Renal diluting capacity
14 days	Schønheyder and Christensen	1957	1	Creatinuria during bedrest
14–28 days	Miller and Leverett	1963	22	Tolerance to $+G_z$
14 days	Katz	1964	11	Fluid and electrolyte changes/plasma 17-OHCS
14 days	Miller et al.	1964a	72	Venous cuffs/head-up tilt/isotonic exercise
14 days	Cardus et al.[9–11]	1965	6	Respiratory measurement/isotonic & isometric exercise/Valsalva
14 days	Stevens et al.	1966c	18	LBNP as countermeasure
14 and 21 days	Umapathy	1967	8	Creatine and creatinine excretion
14 days	Vogt and Johnson[12]	1967	6	Arm cuffs/arm-leg cuffs/radioisotope measurements of blood volume changes
14 days	Schmid et al.	1968	4	Forearm venous response to norepinephrine & tyramine

(Continued)

TABLE V—*Continued*

Duration	No. of Subjects	Investigator(s)	Publication Year	Study Emphasis
14 days	2	Menninger et al.	1969	Leg volume changes with LBNP
14 days	20	Hyatt[13-16]	1971	Electrolyte balance/tyramine/9-AFHC/cardiac catheterization
14 days	8	Greenleaf et al.[17-21]	1973a,b	+G_z/oral hydration/exercise/hematocrit & plasma volume
14-21 days	6	Chobanian et al.	1974	Infusion of NE and angiotensin/NE turnover
14 days	7,8	Dolkas and Sandler[22,23]	1974	Exercise and reverse gradient garment as countermeasures
14 days	5	Ellis et al.	1974	Forearm amino acid metabolites
14 days	6	Jacobson et al.[33]	1974	Low-level +G_z tolerance/effect of G suits
14 days (3)	7	Greenleaf et al.[24-28]	1975	+G_z tolerance/LBNP/isotonic and isometric exercise
14 days	5	Hyatt et al.	1975	Comparison of tilt, LBNP, and passive standing tests
14 days	6	Buderer et al.[29]	1976	Cardiovascular evaluation/exercise stress testing
14 days	8	Hyatt and West	1977	Horizontal/antiorthostatic bedrest (−5°)
14, 49 days	24	Kakurin et al.	1978b	Head-down bedrest (−4°)
15 days	12	Chase et al.	1966	Supine ergometer exercise/trampoline as countermeasures
15 days	12	Anashkin	1969	Blood coagulation studies
15 days	18	Smirnova[30]	1971	Bedrest/acceleration/oxygen consumption/restricted diet
15 days	3	Ellis et al.	1972	Confinement in small, airtight environmental chamber
17 days	8	Sandler and Winter[31-33]	1978	First female bedrest study; +G_z/LBNP/F-E balance
18-32 days	5	Birkhead et al.	1966	Bicycle exercise

Duration	Reference	N	Description	Year
20 days	Kakurin et al.[34-37]	4	Motor, circulatory, and respiratory systems/exercise testing	1963
20 and 62 days	Katkovsky[38]	6	Basal metabolism/centrifugation effects	1967
20 days	Panferova et al.	15	Chair rest/cardiac contractions/isometric exercise	1967
20 days	Blomquist et al.[39]	5	Heart rate and cardiac output at rest and with exercise	1971
21 days	Taylor et al.	5	Cardiac output/acetylene breathing/plasma volume/treadmill	1945
21–28 days	Taylor et al.	6	Cardiac size and function	1949
21 days	Vogt et al.[40]	5	Gravitation acceleration simulation suit as countermeasure	1967a
	McCutcheon and Sandler	3	LBNP	1975
21 days	Birkhead et al.[41]	4	Supine, sitting, and bicycle exercise	1963
24 days	Lynch et al.	44	Metabolic effects of bedrest	1959
28 days	Miller et al.[42]	12	Cardiac catheterization/anti-G suits/F-E changes/treadmill	1964b
28 days	Miller and Leverett	11	$+G_x$ and $+G_z$ tolerance	1965
28 days	Speckman et al.	12	Basal metabolic rate/isotonic exercise	1965
28 days	Meehan et al.	14	$+G_x$/blood volume/tilt	1966
28 days	Stevens et al.[43]	22	Simulated altitude/RBC changes/LBNP as countermeasure	1966d
28 days	Stevens et al.	12	LBNP, 8 hours a day	1966c
28–78 days	Stevens et al.	9	9-AFHC/venous occlusive cuffs as countermeasures	1966b
28 days+	Oberfield et al.	10 m, 1 f	Blood volume measured by sodium radiochromate	1968
28 days	Hyatt et al.[44-47]	24	Hemodynamics/body fluid changes/apexcardiography	1969
28 days	Hoffler et al.[45-49]	6	Fluid volume changes/muscle atrophy/LBNP/hematology and biostereometric measurement	1977
30 days	Birkhead et al.	4	Ergometer exercises	1964

(Continued)

TABLE V—_Continued_

Duration	No. of Subjects	Investigator(s)	Publication Year	Study Emphasis
30 days	8	Chase et al.	1966	Five weeks of physical training before bedrest
30 days	4	Chung	1966	Creatine, creatinine, and nitrogen excretion
30 days	5	Vogt	1966	Plasma volume/tilt response
30 days	15	Voskresenskiy et al.[50–67]	1972	Horizontal/−4° bedrest/remedial procedures
30 days, 100 days	27	Bokhov et al.[68–70]	1975	Orthostatic bedrest (+6°) with physical load and LBNP; anti-orthostatic (−2°, −4°, −6°) with electrical stimulation
30 days	8	Kakurin	1976	Antiorthostatic body positions (0, −4°, −8°, −12°)
30, 49, 120 days	33	Krotov et al.[71–82]	1976	Orthostatic vs. antiorthostatic/hemodynamics/renal functon
35 days	13	Morse	1967	RBC kinetics
35 days	8	Triebwasser et al.	1970	Total body exercise/RBC kinetics
40 days	10	Ioffe et al.	1968	Adjustment of cardiovascular system to physical work
42 days	4	Deitrick et al.	1948	Metabolic and physiologic functions
42 days	4	Birkhead et al.	1963a	Exercise
42 days	6	Mikhaylovskiy et al.	1967	+G_x tolerance (12 to 14 G) before and after bedrest
49 days	4	Stevens et al.	1966b	Venous occlusive duffs/9-AFHC
49 days	12,9	Kakurin et al.[83–84]	1976	Physical work capacity/exercise electrostimulation
56 days	12	Vernikos-Danellis et al.[85–87]	1972	Ambulatory controls/hormonal activity/exercise
60 days	30	Brannon et al.	1963	Exercise
62–84 days	5	Stevens et al.	1966b	9-AFHC
62 days	6	Yegorov et al.[88–95]	1967	Physiological effects/acceleration/exercise

70–75 days	Gurvich et al.[96-102]	16	1967	Cardiac activity/CNS/vector analysis/drugs/exercise
84 and 210 days	Texas Woman's University	8	1970	Bone density/potassium phosphate supplement/exercise
90–94 days	Zvonarev[103]	6	1971	Cardiac output by acetylene method
120 days	Parin et al.[104-110]	10	1971	Physiological responses/hormonal drugs
168–560 days	Leach et al.[111,112]	8	1973	Exercise/potassium phosphate as countermeasure

ADDITIONAL PUBLICATIONS

1. Nixon et al., 1979
2. Vallbona et al., 1965
3. Vogt, 1965
4. Pace et al., 1974
5. Vogt, 1966
6. Vogt and Johnson, 1967
7. Korol'kov and Mirakhimov, 1976
8. Korol'kov et al., 1976
9. Mack et al., 1965
10. Vallbona et al., 1965
11. Vogt et al., 1965
12. Vogt, 1967b
13. Smith et al., 1966
14. Hyatt et al., 1969
15. Hyatt, 1971
16. Hyatt et al., 1973
17. Van Beaumont et al., 1972
18. William and Resse, 1972
19. Haines, 1973c
20. Haines, 1973a
21. Haines, 1973b
22. Dolkas and Greenleaf, 1977
23. McDonald et al., 1974
24. Sandler et al., 1973
25. Stremel et al., 1976
26. Greenleaf et al., 1977d
27. Hoffler et al., 1977
28. Katkovskiy et al., 1971
29. Hoffler, 1976
30. Pace et al., 1974
31. Van Beaumont et al., 1974a
32. Myasnikov et al., 1963
33. Jacobson et al., 1973
34. Katkovskiy, 1966
35. Iseyev and Katkovskiy, 1968b
36. Georgievskiy and Mikhaylov, 1968
37. Saltin et al., 1968
38. Birkhead et al., 1964
39. Miller et al., 1965
40. Gatts and Beard, 1967
41. Hyatt, 1970
42. Hyatt, 1971
43. Lynch et al., 1967
44. Spears et al., 1973
45. Herron and Keys, 1977
46. Homick et al., 1977
47. Johnson and Driscoll, 1977
48. LaFevers et al., 1977
49. Rinks, 1977
50. Balakhoviskiy et al., 1972
51. Drozdova and Grishin, 1972
52. Genin and Kakurin, 1972
53. Pometov and Katkovskiy, 1972
54. Stepantsov et al., 1972
55. Yakoleva, 1972
56. Asyamolov et al., 1973
57. Dlusskaya et al., 1973
58. Georgievskiy et al., 1973
59. Aleksandrov and Kochetov, 1974
60. Beregovkin and Kaliminchenko, 1974
61. Katkovskiy et al., 1974
62. Krasnykh, 1974
63. Suvorov, 1974
64. Belaya et al., 1975
65. Kiselev et al., 1975
66. Krotov and Romanskaya, 1975
67. Fedorov, 1976
68. Maksimov and Domracheva, 1976
69. Krupina and Fedorov, 1977
70. Grigor'yev, 1978
71. Mikhaylov and Georgievskiy, 1976
72. Kovalenko and Krotov, 1975
73. Krupina et al., 1976
74. Krotov et al., 1977
75. Maksimov et al., 1978
76. Kakurin et al., 1978b
77. Gayevskaya et al., 1976
78. Shurygin et al., 1976
79. Tkachev and Kul'kov, 1975
80. Bychkov and Markaryan, 1976
81. Ushakov and Vlasova, 1976
82. Ushakov et al., 1977
83. Balakhovsky et al., 1972
84. Vlasova et al., 1978
85. Rambaut et al., 1973
86. Vernikos-Danellis et al., 1972
87. Vernikos-Danellis et al., 1974
88. Benevolenskaya et al., 1967
89. Georgievskiy and Mikhaylov, 1968
90. Kakurin, 1968
91. Maslov, 1968
92. Kakurin et al., 1970
93. Korolev, 1968a,b
94. Korolev, 1969
95. Sorokin et al., 1969
96. Epstein, 1971
97. Gurvich and Yefimenko, 1967
98. Yefimenko, 1969
99. Panov and Lobzin, 1968
100. Buznik and Kamforina, 1973
101. Bobkova and Grinio, 1971
102. Boldov, 1971
103. Grigor'yev, 1971
104. Krupina et al., 1971
105. Yakoleva, 1971
106. Panferova, 1972
107. Purakhin et al., 1972
108. Kuz'min, 1973
109. Pak et al., 1973
110. Grigor'yev et al., 1976
111. Schneider et al., 1974
112. Donaldson et al., 1970

creased even when the animals were at rest, with a further significant increase when they were exposed to a static load. The major disorders observed after immobilization were a decrease in myocardial contractility and an encroachment on functional cardiac reserves. In the immobilized animals, the subsequent treadmill load resulted in changes similar to those reported in rats (Baranski *et al.*, 1975).

Medionecrotic changes in the aorta, with subsequent mediocalcinosis and the formation of aneurysms of various sizes, were found in rabbits after 19–30 days of immobilization (Vikhert *et al.*, 1972). The myocardium exhibited areas of increased fatty deposits and the development of protein dystrophy, necrobiosis, and necrosis of small groups of muscle fibers, with evidence of fine-focal fibrosis. The investigators were unable to determine the etiology of these changes.

Fedorova in 1973 summarized the Soviet experience with rabbits immobilized for up to 6 weeks (Fedorova and Shurova, 1973). The studies emphasized changes occurring for the myocardium. Included was work conducted by Krupina and co-workers (1971) with 60 animals to assess changes in T waves that had been noted in bedrested subjects. They recorded ECGs and analyzed the adrenals for catechol content. By days 12–14 of immobilization, myocardial content of norepinephrine (micrograms per gram of tissue) was reduced by more than half (from $0.8 \pm 0.06 \mu g/g$ to $0.37 \pm 0.06 \mu g/g$); after 30 days, it continued to be reduced ($0.33 \pm 0.05 \mu g/g$). A considerable decrease was also observed in norepinephrine content in hypothalamic tissues (from $0.16 \mu g/g$ in the control period to $0.08 \mu g/g$ on day 30 of immobilization). Adrenal function was also observed to decrease. On day 12, norepinephrine content was $202 \pm 18 \mu g/g$ (control $243 \pm 22 \mu g/g$); by day 30, the value was $90 \pm 8 \mu g/g$. Plasma 11-oxycorticosteroids also decreased significantly ($P < 0.01$) from $10 \mu g\%$ in the control period to $4.7 \mu g\%$ on day 12 and $3.9 \mu g\%$ on day 30. Electron microscopic studies of the animals conducted on days 12, 14, and 30 revealed changes in the mitochondria (edema, lysis, and formation of lipid granules in sarcoplasm, and a decrease in the number of cristae and myofibrils), as well as changes in the capillaries (plethors and lamination of basement membranes). Federova concluded that changes in the catechol content of the central nervous system indicated primary changes in neural regulatory mechanisms, which imply possible loss of sympathetic nervous system tone. This conclusion was borne out by distinct changes (increase) observed in the threshold to electrostimulation and the prolonged time for recovery. It was felt that these changes occur as the body attempts to compensate for depression in the myocardium and changes in vessel tone. Changes in hormonal metabolism were manifested by a decrease in functional activity and hormone content of the adrenal cortex, adrenal medulla, and thyroid glands.

The mechanisms or reasons for the myocardial changes were not determined.

Rats subjected to 30–40 days of immobilization (Prozkhazka *et al.,* 1973) also exhibited a sharp decrease in body weight and heart weight, especially for the right ventricle. The investigators also observed that the animals showed a decrease in myocardial contractility and a lowering of cardiovascular resistance to hypoxic stress. During hypoxia the anaerobic metabolism rate in the ventricles decreased—with a decrease in glycolysis and glycogenolysis in the right ventricle and glycogenolysis in the left ventricle. The glycogen content of the heart muscles of the animals was unchanged after 30–40 days of immobilization. As with the rabbit studies, the findings indicated that specific cardiac changes occurred with immobilization, implicating a degradation of function.

Baranski and co-workers (1975) kept male Wistar rats under restraint for 6–7 months and used unrestrained animals as controls. Following hypokinesia, ECGs were made of the animals before and after a 1- to 2-hr swimming test. Resting ECGs showed no change, but the animals exhibited an accelerated heart rate during the swimming test. In the hypokinetic animals, changes were also present in the S–T segment and the T wave, indicating hypoxia of the heart muscle. Succinic acid dehydrogenase activity of heart muscle sections were noted to be slightly decreased in the immobilized animals at rest, but accentuated after exertion. Electron microscopic examination of the heart muscle of both the control and immobilized animals revealed no abnormalities except that occasional hypokinetic animals exhibited vacuolization of mitochondria. After exertion, the hypokinetic animals exhibited enlargement of the mitochondria, vacuolization, and loss of internal structure. The mitochondria remained unchanged, however, in the vicinity of the blood vessels. No alterations in the ultrastructure of the myofibrils were noted.

Restraint of male rats for up to 120 days (Romanov, 1976) also resulted in changes in myocardial mitochondria similar to those observed by Baranski above. Quantitative analysis of electron microscopic data demonstrated that, by day 14 of immobilization, the number of mitochondria had increased but their size had decreased. By day 30, the number had decreased slightly as their size increased. By days 45–60, both size and number returned to normal, and by day 120, both were higher than control values. The changes that had occurred by the fourth month of immobilization were interpreted to indicate that a new level of cardiac activity had been reached. Quantitative changes in the organelles were more significant in the left ventricle than in the right. The reason for these changes remains unexplained. The investigators hypothesized, however, that the changes indicated that the animals had adjusted to the hypokinetic state.

In an earlier study of mature male rats restricted for up to 60 days, Pruss and Kuznetsov (1972) found that the contractile function of the myocardium during hypokinesia is characterized by temporal changes. During the first 5 days of immobilization (first phase), contractile function was reduced. By day 15 (beginning of the second phase), changes did not differ significantly between the control animals (unrestrained) and the hypokinetic animals. By days 45 to 60, the rate of myocardial contraction and the strength of cardiac contractions increased. It was felt that these compensations were brought about by a decrease in the functional reserve of the heart, which, if continued, would later lead to the development of cardiac failure. Such an extrapolation is highly speculative, since myocardial failure has not been a factor in the longer-duration animal studies cited earlier or during longer-duration human space flights. There have been some indications, however, of myocardial muscle deterioration occurring during human bedrest studies (Saltin *et al.,* 1968) and immobilization of nonhuman primates (Bourne, 1977).

Immobilized rats have also been used to study microhemodynamics. Shtykhno and Udovichenko (1978) restrained rats for 30 days and found a decrease in the number of true capillaries, the appearance of nonfunctioning empty vessels, and an opening of arteriovenular shunts. Changes were also found in the rheological properties of the blood, including increased viscosity, adhesiveness, hematocrit, and erythrocyte sedimentation rate. These changes were interpreted to indicate reduced blood flow and decreased nutrition of the tissues, which could lead to primary changes or reflect adaptation to the hypodynamic state.

Nonhuman primates have been used successfully in both space flights and immobilization studies. This species was chosen because, like man, they spend more time in the upright position. Histopathological examinations of rhesus monkeys immobilized in body casts in the horizontal position for between 2 and 6 months showed progressive changes in the myocardium, which were significant after 3 months of restraint (Golarz and Bourne, 1972; Golarz *et al.,* 1973, 1974). In these experiments initial myocardial changes were exhibited by the accumulation of fat droplets within the cells. Some fibers exhibited excessive thinning whereas others showed vascular degeneration, which varied in extent between different animals. There was also some round cell infiltration and a significant increase in intercellular connective tissue as the duration of immobilization progressed. Figure 3 shows a typical electron micrograph of the myocardium from one such animal. At the top right portion of the photograph is an abnormal aggregation of mitochondria between the myofibrils; more normal-appearing fibers are seen at the lower left. At the right middle border, one of the myofibrils can be seen to be fragmented and degenerating; another torn or similarly

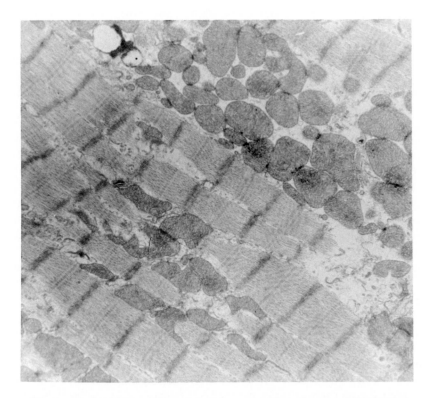

Fig. 3. Typical electron micrograph of the myocardium of an immobilized animal.

degenerating fiber is seen at the upper left. Other studies have shown fibrotic infiltration when animals have been immobilized for up to 6 months (Bourne, 1977).

Biochemical studies of bedrested animals have revealed elevated levels of hydroxyproline in both the right and left ventricles, confirming an increase in fibrous tissue seen by electron and light microscopy. Both total and free lysosomal enzyme activities were also elevated in both the right and left ventricle, suggesting increased net accumulation of lysosomes, coupled with enhanced active degradation. Ribonucleic acid was reduced, indicating reduced protein synthesis. Deoxyribonucleic acid changes were ambiguous, but the lower levels observed could indicate a loss of cellular populations or dilution of nuclear material by increased accumulation of other heart components. Magnesium-stimulated ATPase activity for the right ventricle was also measured and showed a pronounced reduction, indicating that contractility in the right ventricle was depressed.

The changes in the cardiovascular system that have been observed in hypokinetic primates have occurred in the absence of abnormal ECGs. Golarz and co-workers (1977) demonstrated that even more extensive but localized changes can occur in the myocardium without producing changes in the ECG. Data were obtained from monkeys in whom pressure sensors were chronically implanted in the left ventricle by surgical incision through the apex. Careful microscopic studies were conducted of the ventricles of the animals from 1 month to a year after surgery. Their findings showed considerable fibrotic reaction in the myocardium in the area where the transducer was implanted and extending at least ½ cm distally into the ventricles from the apex.

Male rhesus monkeys placed in a reduced gravitational stand for up to 26 days in some cases exhibited orthostatic hypotension and collapse after immobilization (Belkaniya *et al.*, 1973). Rokotova and co-workers (1962), on the other hand, concluded that three rhesus monkeys immobilized for 10 days showed no adverse effects. But two animals immobilized for more than 100 days exhibited a significant weight loss and loss of skeletal muscle in the lower extremities. However, cardiovascular responses were not tested in these animals.

On the basis of animal findings to date, it appears that significant cardiovascular changes occur in all animal species with immobilization—the most striking have been in rabbits and the most resistant has been the rat. Studies following space flights have also indicated that few or no significant cardiovascular changes occur in the rat (Belkaniya, 1978). The most promising animal model appears to be the monkey, because of his similarity to man phylogenetically and because of recent findings of significant cardiovascular changes in the animals with immobilization. Final verification of the similarity of changes and findings in men and animals during immobilization must await definitive measurements made during space flight. Flights that would accomplish such measurements are planned by both U.S. and Soviet investigators over the next several years.

B. Human Experimentation

1. Bedrest Studies

A summary of the major bedrest studies emphasizing cardiovascular changes is given in Table V. A total of 120 days of bedrest, 7 days of complete immersion, and 3 months of weightlessness have shown that diastolic pressures remain within normal limits even in the face of marked physical inactivity (Berry *et al.*, 1966; Birkhead *et al.*, 1963a; Deitrick *et al.*, 1948; Graveline and Jackson, 1962; Miller *et al.*, 1964a,b; Purakhin *et al.*,

1972; Sandler, 1976; Stevens, 1966; Vallbona et al., 1965; Vogt, 1967a). Changes in pulse rate and cardiac electrical activity have been more variable, with heart rate usually showing slight increases over time as bedrest exposure progresses (Birkhead et al., 1963a,b; Cardus et al., 1965; Georgiyevskiy and Mikhaylov, 1968; Miller et al., 1964a,b; Taylor et al., 1945). The relationship of an increase in heart rate of 0.5 bpm per day of bedrest, which was first pointed out by Taylor and co-workers (1949), has generally been the rule. Korolev (1968a,b, 1969) has also demonstrated slight, but significant, T wave changes in standard limb leads and by vector electrocardiography. In 16 bedrested subjects studied weekly during a 10-week bedrest period, increasing T wave amplitude could be detected in most subjects using standard limb leads; U waves of increasing amplitude appeared in precordial leads. Significant U wave changes are detected in most subjects by the second to third week of bedrest; they were registered in the standard limb leads by the fifth to sixth week. Korolev and co-workers felt that these changes were associated with altered blood and cellular (K^+ and Ca^{2++}) content induced by bedrest, but data supporting such a conclusion were not presented, although it is known that changes in these electrolytes do occur with bedrest (Donaldson, 1970; Hyatt et al., 1973). Vector electrocardiographic tracings confirmed the standard lead findings.

Similar T wave findings have been reported in various manned space flights (Sandler, 1976). Hyatt and co-workers (1973), however, did not observe significant ECG changes during a 2-week bedrest study that was devoted to assessing the effect of altered potassium ingestion. During the Skylab missions, slight but significant changes were noted in vector electrocardiograms in QRS and T wave magnitude (Smith et al., 1977). Tkachev and Kul'kov (1975) also reported significant changes in ECG during venipuncture in a 49-day bedrest study. As the duration of bedrest progressed in the latter study, the subjects showed significant increases in heart rate and decreases in registered T wave either in anticipation of or during venipuncture. The investigators concluded that these changes resulted from emotional or electrolyte factors. They might also be explained by the known decreases that occur in heart size with bedrest (Saltin et al., 1968) and space flight (Nicogossian, 1977), since changes in ECG waveforms could result from an altered position of the heart within the chest.

Under conditions of bedrest and particularly with water immersion, subjects have consistently exhibited a decrease in plasma volume accompanied by a diuresis (Deitrick et al., 1948; Graveline, 1962; Hyatt, 1971; Miller, 1965; Miller et al., 1965; Stevens, 1966; Stevens and Lynch, 1965; Vogt, 1967a,c; Vogt and Johnson, 1967). Most of the blood volume contraction has occurred during the first 48 hr of exposure (Hyatt, 1971; Lancaster and Triebwasser, 1971). Maximal plasma volume increases have usually been in the range of 500 ml or about 10% of body weight (Chobanian *et al.*, 1974; Hyatt, 1971; Johnson *et al.*, 1971a,b; Miller *et al.*, 1964b; Pace *et al.* 1975; Stevens, 1966; Stevens and Lynch, 1965; Van Beaumont *et al.*, 1972, 1974a,b; Vogt and Johnson, 1967). Various studies have demonstrated that, after the typical initial decrease, both blood volume and plasma volume tend to remain constant or even to begin to return toward preexposure values (Deitrick *et al.*, 1948; Hyatt, 1971; Lancaster, and Triebwasser, 1971; Vogt, 1966).

To learn more about the mechanisms underlying the preceding changes, two bedrest studies of 2 and 3 weeks duration were devoted to assessing red blood cell changes (Kiselev *et al.*, 1975; Morse, 1967). In each study the decrease in plasma volume observed was associated with an increase in hematocrit, indicating hemoconcentration and a decrease in red blood cell mass with evidence of slight but significant red cell destruction indicated by reticulocytosis. These findings are shown in Fig. 4. After the initial shifts of blood and plasma volume, values have remained reasonably constant over the period of study. The mechanisms of the physiological changes observed have not as yet been explained and require further investigation.

The changes in red blood cells and blood volume noted during bedrest and immersion studies have been reinforced by findings from other immobilization studies. Results from chair rest and confinement studies have shown that red blood cell mass and plasma volume decrease even though intravascular hydrostatic pressure gradients resulting from gravity remain unaltered (Birkhead *et al.*, 1964; Lamb, 1964, 1965; Lamb *et al.*, 1964b). Both plasma volume contractions and hematologic changes have occurred during chair rest and confinement. This finding strongly suggests that inactivity may be as important as weightlessness in enhancing plasma volume contraction during immobilization. This conclusion is partially supported by a comparison of bedrest findings with chair rest and confinement results (Iseyev and Nefedov, 1968; Lamb, 1964; Panferova *et al.*, 1967). Although changes brought about by the two regimens are similar, the magnitude of the changes is greater with bedrest.

Plasma volume also decreases when dehydration occurs, probably because of an inadequate intake of fluids or excess body fluid loss through urine excretion and sweating (Gauer *et al.*, 1970). The possibility that excess body fluid may be lost through sweating during bedrest has been reinforced by Williams and Resse (1972), who demonstrated that sweating occurred at a lower mean temperature in male subjects during a 2-week bedrest study than was experienced during the control and recovery periods. In stressful situations it is also possible that thirst can be markedly suppressed and sweating increased (Greenleaf *et al.*, 1976). Finally, antidiuretic hormone secretion is known to be controlled by the central ner-

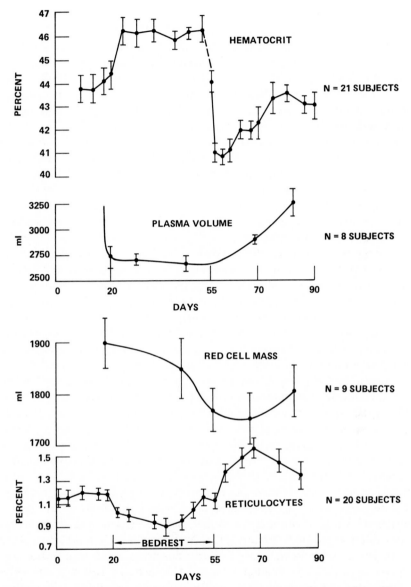

Fig. 4. Serial determination of red blood cell dynamics during bedrest. (From Morse, 1967.)

vous system so that emotional stress, as well as physical stimuli, can result in suppression of its release (Gauer *et al.,* 1970; Verney, 1946).

Changes in body fluid compartments and hormonal and electrolyte contents at rest have been reported by various investigators (Chavarri *et al.,* 1977; Chobanian *et al.,* 1974; Hyatt, 1971; Leach *et al.,* 1973; Melada *et al.,* 1975; Pace *et al.,* 1974; Vernikos-Danellis *et al.,* 1974). Most of the reported changes have been associated with the initial salt and water diuresis accompanying bedrest and immersion. During bedrest lasting longer than 2 weeks, subjects have regularly exhibited changes in adrenal hormones, serum, and urine or body content of potassium and calcium. These changes appear to be related to the known stresses of prolonged immobilization and losses of muscle mass and bone content (Birkhead *et al.,* 1964. 1966; Donaldson *et al.,* 1970; Oganov, 1977). During bedrest, resting plasma levels of most variables (electrolytes and hormones) have shown little change or only slight decreases (Greenleaf *et al.,* 1977a–d). Notable exceptions have been cortisol, which showed a slight increase during the first 3 weeks of an 8-week study and then a significant two- to threefold increase by the end of bedrest (Vernikos-Danellis *et al.,* 1974), and plasma renin activity. Figure 5 shows the ACTH and cortisol changes. Others (Chavarri *et al.,* 1977; Chobanian *et al.,* 1974) have found no changes. In contrast, urinary cortisol has increased throughout bedrest periods, urinary norepinephrine has increased, and urinary epinephrine has remained unchanged (Sandler and Winter, 1978; Zubek, 1968).

Resting cardiac output and stroke volume during bedrest have been found variously to increase, to remain normal, or more usually to decrease (Hyatt, 1971; Kakurin, 1978; Katkovskiy and Pometov, 1971a,b; Pometov and Katkovskiy, 1972; Saltin *et al.,* 1968; Sandler *et al.,* 1977; Stevens, 1966). A slight decrease in cardiac output is consistent with the diuresis and decrease in heart size and end-diastolic volume with bedrest (Hyatt, 1971; Krasnykh, 1973; Melada *et al.,* 1975; Sandler *et al.,* 1977; Taylor *et al.,* 1949; Vetter *et al.,* 1971). Some of the inconsistencies in findings may have resulted from the methodologies used, which have varied from measurements made at the time of cardiac catheterization using Fick or indicator dilution methods (Hyatt, 1971; Melada *et al.,* 1975; Pekshev, 1969; Saltin *et al.,* 1968; Stevens, 1966) to measurements using echocardiography (Nixon *et al.,* 1979; Sandler *et al.,* 1977; Sandler and Winter, 1978), vibrocardiography (Simonenko, 1969), and single breath CO_2 detection or CO_2 or acetylene rebreathing methodologies (Fahri *et al.,* 1976; Katkovskiy and Pometov, 1971a,b; Michel *et al.,* 1977; Triebwasser *et al.,* 1977; Zvonarev, 1971). Teleroentgenokyograms were also used by Krasnykh (1973) in one study. Clinical experience has shown that catheterization and echocardiography are the most reliable of the methods. To date, these two

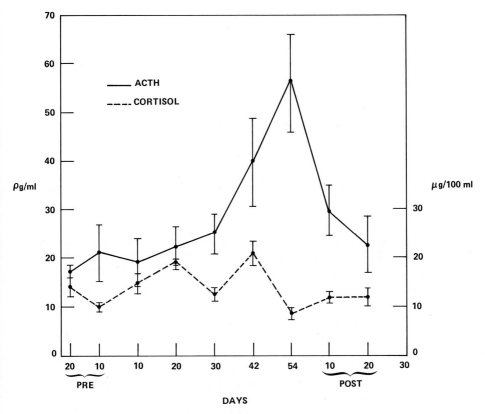

Fig. 5. Mean plasma ACTH and cortisol.

methods have indicated either no change in or a slight suppression of resting cardiac output and stroke volume during bed rest.

Since losses in skeletal muscle mass occur with bed rest, questions have
arisen as to whether vascular smooth muscle might undergo similar changes,
resulting in an inability to respond properly during tilt or LBNP. If such
changes occur, they would be expected to affect both arterial vessels (particularly arterioles) and veins, especially in the lower extremities. However,
measurements using primarily plethysmographic techniques have failed to
demonstrate significant impairment of the mechanisms controlling
peripheral resistance vessels (McCally *et al.,* 1971; Montgomery *et al.,*
1977; Musgrave *et al.,* 1969; Sandler and Winter, 1978; Schmid *et al.,*
1971; Stevens *et al.,* 1966a–d). In addition, responsiveness of vascular smooth
muscle to norepinephrine has been tested by direct infusion (Chobanian *et
al.,* 1974; Schmid *et al.,* 1971), and release of endogenous norepinephrine

has been tested by the infusion of tyramine (Hyatt, 1971; Schmid *et al.*, 1971). Forearm vascular resistance and venous tone increased appreciably during both types of provocation. Following bedrest, seven times more tyramine was required to achieve the same level of vascular resistance and three times more to increase venous tone compared with the control and recovery periods. In contrast, dose response to norepinephrine did not change during any of the three test periods. These findings have been interpreted as strongly suggesting a change in the functional state of the peripheral sympathetic nervous system. The conclusion that a distinct change occurs is supported by the finding that urinary norepinephrine excretion decreases significantly and regularly during bedrest (Leach *et al.*, 1973; Schmid *et al.*, 1971; Vernikos-Danellis *et al.*, 1974; Zubek, 1968). The magnitude of the decrease has been correlated with the ability to tolerate tilt or bedrest or both (Zubek, 1968).

Chobanian and co-workers (1974) confirmed the preceding findings but failed to provide evidence that the changes resulted from a depressed capacity for norepinephrine synthesis. During a 3-week bedrest study, labeled norepinephrine was used to detect circulating blood levels of hormone and its disappearance rates from plasma. Plasma catecholamines became slightly lower during bedrest and slightly exaggerated with tilting, as shown in Fig. 6, but changes were not significant for the group as a whole. Plasma disappearance rates remained unchanged from control levels. From these findings it appears that norepinephrine release, or uptake into granules, may be impaired, but the mechanisms underlying this change remain unknown and will require further careful study.

a. Response to Lower Body Negative Pressure

Definite symptoms of orthostatic intolerance have occurred consistently after as little as 3 days of bedrest and 6–12 hr of water immersion (Birkhead *et al.*, 1963a; Deitrick *et al.*, 1948; Graveline, 1962; Hyatt, 1971; McCally and Graveline, 1963; McCutcheon and Sandler, 1975; Miller *et al.*, 1964b; Taylor *et al.*, 1949). Failure of the body to compensate under these circumstances has led to vasopressor syncope (Lamb, 1964; McCally and Graveline, 1963; Stevens *et al.*, 1966b,d) aggravated by the known early losses of intravascular volume. This altered state after bedrest and space flight has been termed "cardiovascular deconditioning."

The earliest, most sensitive, and most consistent finding of deconditioning has been an increase in registered heart rate during provocation—that is, passive standing (Hyatt *et al.*, 1975), tilt, or LBNP (Hyatt, 1971; McCally *et al.*, 1966a; Miller *et al.*, 1964b; Stevens *et al.*, 1966a,c,d). Changes in heart rate have been gauged according to prebedrest or preflight responses, and most individuals have exhibited 30–50% increases as a result of the decon-

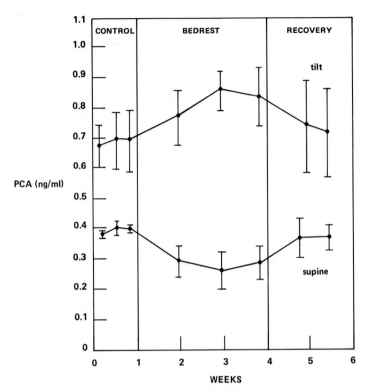

Fig. 6. Serial changes in plasma catecholamine activity with passive tilting and recumbency. *Note:* Plasma catecholamine activity (PCA) values with passive tilting are plotted above, and with recumbency, below. Each point represents ±SE for five subjects.

ditioning process (Asyamolov *et al.*, 1973; Hyatt, 1971; Korobkov *et al.*, 1968; Stevens *et al.*, 1966a). The reasons for these responses remain obscure. Some insight into their cause, however, has been gained from comparing male and female responses (Sandler and Winter, 1978). Typically, heart rate responses during LBNP following bedrest, as shown in Fig. 7, have been significantly greater in females ($P < 0.001$). These changes may best be correlated with alterations in heart volume. Hemodynamic measurements (Sandler *et al.*, 1977) determined noninvasively using single-crystal echocardiography, as shown in Table VI, have indicated lower end-diastolic volumes at rest for both males and females, with marked decreases occurring during lower body suction. Losses in ventricular volume at rest of 10–12% are consistent with previous changes in total heart volume as determined by plain films of the chest (Krasnykh, 1973; Nicogossian, 1977; Saltin *et al.*, 1968; Taylor *et al.*, 1949). Such losses in heart volume at rest

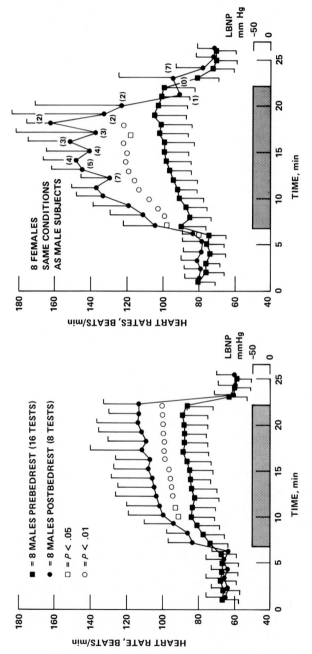

Fig. 7. Male and female LBNP heart rate responses following 2 weeks of bedrest.

are undoubtedly associated with the diuresis of recumbency, which results in a change in central nervous system responsiveness (inhibition of vagal tone or increased sympathetic discharge or both) (Epstein *et al.,* 1968a). These changes are exaggerated by decreases in end-diastolic volume resulting from peripheral volume displacement during suction. The magnitude of the changes in females appears to be correlated with the significantly lower ventricular volumes demonstrated to be present at all stages of testing (Table VI).

Echocardiographic studies of bedrest-induced changes at rest have demonstrated significant findings (Sandler *et al.,* 1977), as shown in Table VII. In females at rest after 14 days of bedrest, stroke volume decreased by 25% (prebedrest, 68 ± 10 ml), cardiac output decreased by 21%, (prebedrest, 5.2 ± 0.8 L/min), and end-diastolic volume decreased by 12% (prebedrest, 99 ± 8 ml). In a matched group of male subjects, bedrest induced a significant 14% decrease in cardiac output (prebedrest, 5.4 ± 1.1 L/min) and a 10% decrease in end-diastolic volume (prebedrest, 119 ± 18 ml). All males (N = 7) were able to complete 15 min of −50 mm Hg LBNP both before and after bedrest. All females (N = 12) were able to do so before bedrest, but none could tolerate the exposure afterward.

Analysis of end-diastolic volume data during LBNP to determine minimal values reached during tests revealed significantly lower values ($P < 0.001$) in females than in males. End-diastolic volume in the females was 40 ± 7 ml before bedrest and 28 ± 9 ml after; in the males, prebedrest and postbedrest values were 68 ± 13 ml and 54 ± 8 ml, respectively. The smaller female end-diastolic volumes regularly seen during LBNP after bedrest also occurred with marked increases in heart rate, which would account for most of this finding. As discussed previously, the female end-diastolic volumes following bedrest were associated with syncope or presyncope in all cases; the male values, however, were not. Cardiac output during these LBNP studies was maintained principally by an increase in heart rate; as much as 30–60% of resting end-diastolic volume was shifted to the periphery during suction in both males and females (Sandler *et al.,* 1977). The magnitude of this shift was not affected by bedrest. In more recent female tests LBNP was performed after exposure to $+G_z$ acceleration rather than before, as it had been in previous studies. With this approach marked changes in cardiac output and end-diastolic volume were not observed. However, postbedrest syncope or presyncope was seen in 6 out of 10 subjects. The fact that syncope was not seen in all subjects could stem from a reconditioning caused by the acceleration exposure and associated increases in plasma volume.

Reports of increased blood pooling in the legs during tilt or LBNP after bedrest have varied considerably, with most investigators reporting either

TABLE VI

Hemodynamic Changes During LBNP

	Control		Peak LBNP			
	HR beats/min	EDV ml	HR beats/min	EDV ml	ΔEDV ml	%Δ ml
FEMALE n = 7 LBNP −50 mmHg						
PRE BR	76 ± 8	99 ± 8	98 ± 18	40 ± 7	59 ± 12	59 ± 8
POST BR	80 ± 9	87 ± 7	139 ± 25	28 ± 9	59 ± 9	66 ± 7
		$p < .001$	$p < .001$	$p < .001$		
MALE n = 7 LBNP −50 mmHg						
PRE BR	70 ± 10	119 ± 14	87 ± 9	68 ± 13	52 ± 14	43 ± 10
POST BR	62 ± 8	112 ± 16	108 ± 16	54 ± 8	54 ± 10	48 ± 4
	$p < .02$	$p < .001$	$p < .001$	$p < .05$		
MALE n = 7 LBNP −20, −30, −40 mmHg						
PRE BR	59 ± 4	141 ± 20	71 ± 10	101 ± 19	40 ± 13	29 ± 9
POST BR	58 ± 8	125 ± 18	94 ± 15	63 ± 14	62 ± 24	49 ± 14
		$p < .02$	$p < .02$	$p < .001$	$p < .05$	$p < .01$

TABLE VII

Resting Hemodynamic Data

	HR beats/min	CO L/min	EDV ml	ESV ml	SV ml/beat	MEAN BP mm Hg
FEMALES CONTINUOUS LBNP −50 mmHg n = 7						
PRE BR	76 ± 8	5.2 ± 0.8	99 ± 8	31 ± 6	68 ± 10	79 ± 5.8
POST BR	80 ± 8	4.1 ± 0.8	87 ± 7	36 ± 9	51 ± 9	85 ± 6.1
MALES CONTINUOUS LBNP −50 mmHg n = 7						
PRE BR	70 ± 9	5.4 ± 1.1	119 ± 18	42 ± 9	77 ± 13	90 ± 7.9
POST BR	62 ± 8	4.7 ± 0.9	112 ± 15	38 ± 6	75 ± 11	87 ± 9.1
INCREMENTAL LBNP −20, −30, −40 mmHg						
PRE BR	57 ± 6	5.2 ± 0.6	140 ± 18	47 ± 12	93 ± 14	82 ± 7.6
POST BR	59 ± 9	4.9 ± 0.7	125 ± 19	39 ± 10	85 ± 12	85 ± 5.2

no change or a decrease in leg volume (Bartok *et al.*, 1968; McCally *et al.*, 1971; Menninger *et al.*, 1969; Sandler and Winter, 1978). These findings are diametrically opposed to reports of significant increases in leg volume during LBNP tests in all of the Skylab missions (Johnson *et al.*, 1977). The findings may be more apparent than real because of the methods of measurement and the known marked decreases in leg girth, which are significantly greater during space flight as compared with ground-based conditions. During space flight leg volume changes were determined using a capacitance leg band (Gowen *et al.*, 1977; Johnson *et al.*, 1977). A Whitney gauge has been used during tilt or LBNP studies (Bartok *et al.*, 1968; McCally *et al.*, 1971). These devices are capable of accurately detecting only the percentage change from resting leg dimensions. If the resting leg dimensions were to decrease significantly for any reason (as was the case during the Skylab mission because of cephalad shift of blood *and* disuse atrophy of muscles) and if the same amount of blood is displaced into the leg by tilt or LBNP, the apparent or measured leg girth percentage would change significantly, but absolute volume or blood displacement to the measured limb would be the same under both conditions.

Limb girth decreased dramatically during the Skylab missions (Johnson *et al.*. 1977). Correction for such changes markedly decreases the apparent significance that more blood is displaced to the lower extremities during LBNP. These findings also point out the need for positioning the measurement gauges accurately (particularly the Whitney transducers) if quantitative results are to be obtained during repeated measurements of the lower extremities, which have such highly variable cross-sectional areas. In an attempt to remedy these shortcomings, Musgrave and co-workers (1969) developed a water plethysmograph for leg measurement during LBNP. It has been used extensively by McCutcheon during bedrest studies (Sandler and Winter, 1978). With this method it was found that leg volume increases occur with exposure to LBNP. However, the increase was less in the majority of subjects with this technique after bedrest. This difference in pooling after bedrest has also been noted by several investigators who used Whitney strain gauges (McCally and Wunder, 1971; Stevens *et al.*, 1966a). Montgomery and co-workers (1977) also applied impedance plethysmographic methods to the study of leg volume changes during tilt and LBNP; these investigators also found no change or less pooling during LBNP after bedrest. Females measured by impedance plethysmography during bedrest studies exhibited a significantly smaller increase in leg volume than did males during passive tilt, but the females suffered a higher incidence of syncope. Much less is known about the accuracy of the impedance plethysmographic approach than is known about the methods discussed previously. A recent finding of a close correlation between the results of impedance plethysmographic and findings with the use of capacitance leg bands (as used in Skylab) during LBNP before and after bedrest is encouraging.

In female subjects tested to date, leg volume increases have been less during LBNP after bedrest despite vasopressor syncope. This finding lessens the feasibility of the hypothesis that a significant loss of blood to the legs is a key factor or contributor to syncope in these cases. Epstein and co-workers (1968a,b) came to a similar conclusion regarding venous pooling during studies of vasovagal syncope in normal subjects. They hypothesized that the magnitude of cardiac volume or size (filling) may be important in these instances, initiating reflex bradycardia when a minimal or critical right or left heart volume is reached, which increases intramyocardial (wall) pressure. Female echocardiographic findings before and after bedrest (Tables VI and VII) support such a possibility. Before bedrest both male and female subjects were able to tolerate a 15-min exposure to -50 mm Hg suction. After bedrest none of the female subjects could tolerate this exposure because of the onset of presyncope or syncope. None of the male subjects experienced syncope before or after bedrest. End-diastolic volume in the females just prior to the onset of vasodepressor syncope was 28 ± 4 ml, which was significantly lower than that of the males and may indicate the level of end-diastolic volume required to trigger the myocardial component of the fainting response.

b. DIMINISHED WORK CAPACITY

Decreased work capacity has been observed consistently in bedrest and immersion studies. It has been manifested as an impaired capacity to accomplish treadmill or bicycle exercises, either maximal or submaximal (Cardus, 1966; Chase et al., 1966; Convertino et al., 1975; Georgiyevskiy et al., 1966; Iseyev and Katkovskiy, 1968a,b; Kakurin, 1976; Katkovskiy et al., 1974; Saltin et al., 1968; Stepantsov et al., 1972). Identical responses have been observed after space flight (Gazenko et al., 1974, 1976; Michel et al., 1977).

Changes measured before and after bedrest and immersion have usually demonstrated decreases in oxygen uptake, cardiac output, and stroke volume; ventilatory volumes; and maximal heart rate, with anteriovenous oxygen (AVO_2) showing only minor variations or no change (Saltin et al., 1968). Decreases in maximal oxygen uptake following bedrest have ranged from 17% to 28% (Cherepakhin, 1968; Graveline et al., 1961; Miller et al., 1964a; Saltin et al., 1968; Taylor et al., 1949). Chase and co-workers (1966), on the other hand, found no changes. Saltin's finding (Saltin et al., 1968) of a 28% decrease following 20 days of bedrest was based on measurements in both the upright and supine positions; the decrease, therefore, could not be attributed to impairment of venous return during upright exercise. Blomquist and co-workers (1971) concluded that a primary decrease in myocardial function may play a role in these findings.

The use of various exercise programs to counteract these events has had highly variable results and has failed to fully reverse decrements in cardiovascular performance (Birkhead *et al.*, 1963a,b, 1964, 1966; Buznik and Kamforina, 1973; Cardus *et al.*, 1965; Cherepakhin, 1968; Greenleaf *et al.*, 1975; McCally *et al.*, 1968; Miller and Leverett, 1965; Stepantsov *et al.*, 1972). Circulatory findings during maximal work have shown that decreases in maximal oxygen uptake resulted primarily from a decrease in stroke volume and cardiac output, with anteriovenous oxygen difference not changing significantly (Convertino *et al.*, 1975; 1978; Georgiyevskiy *et al.*, 1966; Kakurin *et al.*, 1966; Katkovskiy *et al.*, 1969; Katkovskiy and Pomotov, 1976; Saltin *et al.*, 1968). Postbedrest, maximal heart rate has usually increased by 14–19%, maximal decline in cardiac output has been 14–16%, and stroke volume has decreased by 24–25%. Exercise at submaximal levels, both in the upright and supine positions, has resulted in changes that are consistent with those occurring during maximal exercise (Birkhead *et al.*, 1963a; Cardus, 1966; Convertino *et al.*, 1975, 1978; Katkovskiy and Pomotov, 1976).

Physical inactivity—failure to maintain skeletal muscle strength and tone as well as loss of pumping effectiveness of muscle contraction—may contribute to the observed findings. Miller and Leverett (1965) found that the dependent cyanosis associated with bedrest could be reduced with exercise. As pointed out previously, however, periodic exercise generally has failed to be an effective countermeasure for the orthostatic intolerance seen after bedrest and space flight. Nonetheless, following the last Skylab flight and its heavy use of in-flight exercise, the postflight recovery period appeared to be markedly shortened compared with those of previous flights.

A large portion of the changes noted with regard to diminished work capacity may be explained by changes in intravascular volume and shifts of fluid (including redistribution of blood flow). Data from exercise studies indicate that a reduction in stroke volume may also play a role. In this regard the reduction in stroke volume when exercising in the supine position (24%) has been almost as large as that occurring during upright exercise (27–30%) Katkovskiy and Pomotov, 1971a,b; Saltin *et al.*, 1968).

c. Changes Associated with Acceleration

Responses to $+G_x$ acceleration have usually shown slight or no degradation following bedrest (Kotovskaya *et al.*, 1965, 1969; Krupina *et al.*, 1967; Miller and Leverett, 1965). In contrast, numerous studies have shown that significant decrements occur in $+G_z$ tolerance following hypokinesia.

Leverett and co-workers (1971) studied nine male subjects (ages 20–36 years) after sequential bedrest periods of 24 hr and 7 days. Acceleration exposures consisted of consecutive $+G_z$ profiles at $+2.5$, $+3.0$, $+3.5$, and $+4.0$ G_z, with onset rates of 1 G/min and the peak held for 270 sec. Cardiovascular deconditioning was noted after only 24 hr of bedrest; 20% of the group developed visual symptoms or blackout at $+2.5$ G_z, and 40% showed similar responses at $+3.0$ G_z. The subjects in this study were experienced centrifuge riders; less experienced individuals could be expected to have even greater degrees of intolerance. The investigators suggested that G-suits be used to improve the observed decrements in tolerance. Subsequent studies by Jacobson and co-workers (1974) and Chambers and Vykukal (1972) have provided evidence that G-suits afford subjective and objective physiological benefits for acceleration tolerance up to $+4.0$ G_z after bedrest.

Various other countermeasures have not improved acceleration tolerance. In 1973 Greenleaf and co-workers (1973a,b) studied the effects of rehydration as a countermeasure. Eight male subjects (ages 21–23 years) underwent two 14-day periods of bedrest with a 2-week period in between. The first bedrest period served as the control. One hour before exposure to $+G_z$ acceleration, the subjects were given a saline-grapefruit juice drink to test the effects of rehydration on tolerance. They were then centrifuged at $+2.0$ G_z for 11 min, at $+3.0$ G_z for 3.5 min, and at $+4.0$ G_z for 3 min. None of the subjects were experienced centrifuge riders. Bedrest induced a 36% decrease in tolerance at $+2.0$ G_z, a 30% decrease at $+3.0$ G_z, and a 44% decrease at $+4.0$ G_z. Rehydration was effective only at $+2.0$ G_z and even then did not restore the subjects to prebedrest levels. The study did demonstrate, however, that bedrest deconditions the majority of unprotected, inexperienced, younger individuals to the point where their acceleration tolerance is below the maximal levels projected for Space Shuttle reentry ($+2.0$ G_z), particularly if off-nominal $+G_z$ levels occur (Sandler *et al.*, 1976).

In another study conducted by Greenleaf and co-workers (1975), the investigators sought to determine the effect of isometric and isotonic exercise on $+G_z$ tolerance. Seven male subjects were bedrested for three 2-week periods. The findings indicated that neither type of exercise had a remedial effect on bedrest deconditioning as measured by $+G_z$ tolerance, maximal oxygen uptake, and LBNP.

Finally, in 1976, Sandler and co-workers studied the responses of eight male subjects (ages 19–22 years) to determine whether deliberate intermittent venous pooling in the extremities could reverse bedrest-induced cardiovascular changes (Annis, 1974). No improvement from venous pooling could be determined. After bedrest, $+G_z$ tolerance compared with control values decreased by 75% at $+2.5$ G_z (average control value 10.5 min) and by 87% at $+3.0$ G_z (average control value 8.6 min).

In contrast to the preceding findings, two early investigations failed to demonstrate markedly significant decrements in $+G_z$ tolerance following bedrest. The reasons remain obscure. In the first study, Meehan and Jacobs (1959) exposed six subjects to a 15-sec $+G_z$ tolerance test following 30 days of bedrest. The onset of G was rapid at 1 G/sec. The effects on the ability to withstand this stress were observed in terms of blood pressure, blood volume, and physical condition. The subjects were retested after one month of physical training. Although they experienced a 28.4% decrease in total blood volume after bedrest, no statistically significant changes were noted in $+G_z$ tolerance. In the second study, Miller and Leverett (1965) observed the responses of 22 male subjects (ages 17–23 years) to $+G_x$ and $+G_z$ acceleration after prolonged bedrest. Half of the group was subjected to 4 weeks of complete bedrest and the other half to 2 weeks of modified bedrest (allowed to sit and dangle their feet but not to walk). Both groups were exposed to $+G_z$ until grayout or blackout under two conditions of acceleration—rapid onset of acceleration (ROR) at 1 G/sec and gradual onset of acceleration (GOR) at 0.1 G/sec. The subjects who had undergone strict bedrest were less able to tolerate GOR and ROR. The modified bedrest group also had a slight decrease in $+G_z$ tolerance.

There is little information in the literature concerning the effects of age, sex, or the presence of disease states on tolerance to $+G_z$ acceleration. Although a large literature (beginning in 1929) has been accumulated on $+G_z$ tolerance in males (Gauer, 1950; Gauer and Zuidema, 1961; Howard, 1965; Roth et al., 1968), all of the subjects studied have been below the age of 45 years. In addition, tolerance data in these cases were collected for the purpose of monitoring pilot performance in military aircraft, where acceleration exposures are of high magnitude ($+8.0$ and $+10$ G_z) and short duration (no longer than several minutes) (Clarke and Leverett, 1976; Howard, 1965). Here again, the flyers were all of a younger age.

Most astronauts and cosmonauts selected for flight have been in the 35–45-year age group (Sandler, 1976). One older astronaut did fly during the ASTP in July 1975. He had no difficulties before or during flight. His postflight responses were complicated, however, by exposure to toxic gas fumes (nitrogen tetroxide) during reentry, requiring hospitalization and treatment (Nicogossian, 1977). He tolerated all procedures without adverse effects and has had no subsequent complications.

Data on female responses to $+G_z$ acceleration became available recently (Newsom et al., 1977; Sandler and Winter, 1978). Twelve flight nurses (age 24–35 years) who were experienced centrifuge riders were studied before and after bedrest. GOR of 0.03 G/sec was used to determine physiological responses to low-level, prolonged acceleration such as might occur with Space Shuttle flights. Each subject was exposed twice to levels of $+2.5$,

$+3.0$, $+3.5$, and $+4.0$ G_z before bedrest. Length of tolerance varied widely at $+2.5$ G_z: three subjects tolerated 2.3–5.4 min; six subjects, 9.1–13.4 min; and three subjects, 15.1–20 min. There was considerably less variation at $+3.0$ G_z; four subjects tolerated 1.2–1.8 min; four subjects, 3.1–4.6 min; and four subjects, 6–6.8 min. At $+3.5$ G_z, one subject could not complete the ramp (117 sec) to peak G, whereas seven subjects completed 0.4–1.4 min and four subjects completed 2.8–4.7 min. At $+4.0$ G_z, three subjects could not complete the ramp and one barely did; the remaining eight subjects tolerated peak G for 10–117 sec. Following bedrest, tolerance times at $+3.0$ G_z were decreased by an average of 66% (mean prebedrest, 288 sec). This finding compared favorably with an 87% decrease in male tolerance during similar studies (Sandler *et al.*, in preparation).

More recently, 10 females (ages 35–44 years) were studied before and after 7 days of bedrest, using the more realistic Shuttle reentry profiles of $+1.5$, $+2.0$, and $+3.0$ G_z (Goldwater *et al.*, 1977). All subjects were able to complete the $+1.5$ G_z runs. Six subjects were unable to complete the $+2.0$ G_z exposures; two had grayout on the ramp up and two at peak G, and two during the ramp down. There was a 57% decrease in tolerance to $+3.0$ G_z after bedrest (mean prebedrest, 266 sec), which was compatible with the previous female bedrest study (Newsom *et al.*, 1977) and with a 50% decrease in similarly aged male subjects (Goldwater *et al.*, 1977). Prebedrest tolerance to $+3.0$ G_z among the females, however, was significantly lower than that of their male counterparts (266 sec vs. 749 sec).

d. HEAD-DOWN VERSUS HORIZONTAL BEDREST

American and Russian investigators have been attempting to determine whether a different body position during bedrest would induce physiological responses that would be closer to those observed after exposure to weightlessness (Bokhov *et al.*, 1975; Hyatt and West, 1976; Kakurin, 1976, 1976a; Krotov *et al.*, 1976; Nixon *et al.*, 1979; Volicier *et al.*, 1977; Voskresenskiy *et al.*, 1972). Head-down bedrest studies (varying in body position from $-2°$ to $-12°$) were first introduced by Soviet investigators because the cosmonauts had expressed a feeling that the head-down position best reproduced the conditions of head fullness and awareness felt during flight. The first study (Genin *et al.*, 1969) consisted of a 30-day comparison of horizontal (0°) and head-down tilt ($-4°$). Subsequent studies have consisted of multiple 5-day bedrest exposures at 0°, $-4°$, $-8°$ and $-12°$ (Kakurin, 1976) and 30 days using body positions of $+6°$, and $-2°$, and $-6°$ (Bokhov *et al.*, 1975). Results have indicated an increase in subjective and objective physiological findings because of headward fluid movement with increasing severity of downward head inclination. The most significant subjective findings have been complaints of blood rushing to the head, heaviness of the head, and vessel pulsations in the temple area. Objectively, findings have shown neck vein engorgement and increased venous distention of the retinal veins. Most signs and symptoms reached maximum intensity within 3 hr after beginning the experiment. In general, investigators have not observed any increase in illness or clinically significant changes of biochemical parameters in blood or urine samples.

During bedrest in the head-down position, Soviet investigators have noted no significant changes in heart rate, but repeatedly have observed increases in cardiac output and, therefore, stroke volume as well. Changes were usually most prominent by the sixth to ninth day of bedrest and returned to baseline levels by the fifteenth to twentieth day. Such changes have occured in both horizontal and head-down positions, but the changes occurred earlier and were more pronounced in subjects in the head-down position. The accuracy of such measurements must be questioned, however, since they were determined noninvasively using CO_2 rebreathing techniques. Tests for orthostatic tolerance failed to demonstrate increased losses resulting from a change in body position. Changes in blood redistribution have been measured using radioactive iodinated serum albumin (RISA) (Kakurin, 1976, 1978); the results are shown in Table VIII. Significantly greater headward shifts of volume were documented in the head-down body position; these shifts persisted throughout the bedrest period. However, the accuracy of this method has been questioned, since it is determined from the number of counts obtained by scanning a given area of the body using a scintillation crystal (Wolthuis *et al.*, 1975).

Two American bedrest studies, each lasting 24 hr, have compared the horizontal and −5° head-down body positions. The first, which was conducted by Volicier and co-workers (1977), studied fluid and electrolyte balance and found that the change in body position induced a sodium diuresis and stimulated the renin–angiotensin, aldosterone system. Plasma renin activity and plasma aldosterone levels were not significantly different from findings in the horizontal position during the first 6 hr, but were significantly increased by the end of the 24-hr period. Nixon and co-workers (1979) measured cardiovascular changes in eight subjects under conditions of horizontal and −5° head-down tilt. Changes in central venous pressure (CVP) are shown in Fig. 8. CVP rose transiently and significantly by 40 min after placement in the head-down position and returned to control levels (pretilt) by 90 min. Arterial pressure, cardiac output, and left ventricular contractile state did not change. Blood volume decreased significantly by 0.6 liter. Contrary to the findings of Volicier, plasma renin activity and aldosterone tended to be depressed over the first 12 hr and returned to baseline by the end of the study. The reasons for the differences in the two studies are unclear and will require attention during subsequent inves-

TABLE VIII

Comparison of Blood Distribution in Orthostatic and Antiorthostatic Bedrest Positions[a,b]

Positions	Head	Chest	Abdomen	Pelvic Area	Lower Extremities
Horizontal before bedrest	665.7	1263.4	819.4	624.0	1099.0
Antiorthostatic (−4°) before bedrest	735.4	1400.7	924.7	678.1	799.0
antiorthostatic (−4°) after 45 days of bedrest	727.6	1574.8	814.8	713.7	626.3

[a] From Kakurin, 1976.
[b] In ml.

tigations. Hyatt and West (1976) exposed eight healthy males to 1 week of horizontal (0°) and 1 week of −5° head-down bedrest. Heart rate, blood pressure, LBNP tolerance, fluid and electrolyte balance, and echocardiographic parameters were measured. The investigators failed to find qualitative or quantitative differences in cardiovascular or metabolic effects.

From the data collected to date, it appears that head-down bedrest shows promise of quantitatively simulating cardiovascular changes that occur early in space flight. The accuracy of such changes must await definitive human measurements during flight, which appear to be possible in the upcoming Space Shuttle flights.

2. Water Immersion Studies

Fluid immersion duplicates zero gravity in two ways. First, within a few hours after immersion, there is a prompt, involuntary diuresis and a loss of body and plasma fluid (Epstein, 1978; McCally and Wunder, 1971; Kollias et al., 1976). Second, prolonged immersion produces physiological deconditioning and orthostatic intolerance similar to what is experienced with exposure to weightlessness. Immersion for up to 56 days has been tolerated without ill effects (Shulzenko et al., 1976). Immersion differs from true weightlessness, however, in that (1) hydrostatic forces exerted on the body create a state of negative pressure breathing that, in itself, shifts blood into the intrathoracic circulation, (2) the influence of gravity is still present, although bodily movement requires less muscular effort, and (3) the high specific heat of water results in an abnormal heat exchange with the environment. The advantages of immersion for simulating weightlessness are that physiological mechanisms respond rapidly and closely duplicate those associated with the zero-gravity state. Considerable immersion studies have been directed toward assessing the effects of this simulator on the cardiovascular system.

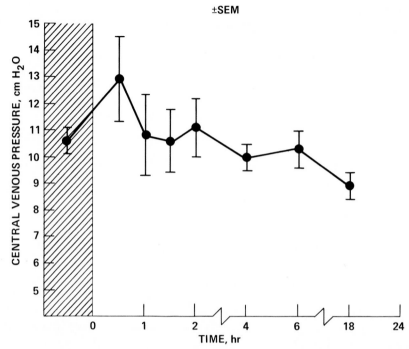

Fig. 8. Central venous pressure after 24 hr of antiorthostatic hypodynamia ($-5°$). (From Nixon *et al.*, 1979.)

Orthostatic intolerance, a key indicator of cardiovascular deconditioning, has been observed consistently following immersion (Epstein, 1978; Gauer, 1971; Arborelius *et al.*, 1972; Graveline *et al.*, 1961; Graybiel and Clark, 1961; Kaiser *et al.*, 1963; McCally *et al.*, 1966a; McCally and Wunder, 1971; Stegemann *et al.*, 1969). With a relatively short time, diuresis occurs, followed by a decrease in plasma volume (Behn *et al.*, 1969; Gauer, 1971; Kaiser *et al.*, 1963, 1969; McCally and Wunder, 1971; Torphy, 1965; Vogt, 1967a). Heart rate and pulse rate can increase, and systolic and diastolic blood pressure have been found to drop even with a constant pulse rate (Kaiser *et al.*, 1963). Most investigators have found significant symptoms of cardiovascular deconditioning during immersion studies.

These effects are believed to be caused by excitation of the central cardiac mechanoreceptors (Arborelius *et al.*, 1972; Behn *et al.*, 1969; Epstein, 1978; Gauer *et al.*, 1970). During immersion the hydrostatic pressure effects on the body surface shift approximately 700 ml of blood into the intrathoracic space—an amount greater than that which occurs when changing from a standing to recumbent body position (Gauer, 1971; Lange *et al.*,

1974). Using biplane plane films of the chest, Lange and co-workers (1974) demonstrated a mean increase in heart volume of 180 ± 62 ml with initiation of immersion in upright normal subjects. Study of the X-ray plates shows that a major component of the heart volume increase is localized to the atria.

As discussed earlier, these alterations can cause reflex and humoral changes to decrease plasma volume and alter renal handling of fluid and electrolytes (Epstein, 1978). The principal mechanism responsible for these changes has been shown to be an inhibition of the release of antidiuretic hormone (ADH), resulting in a persistent diuresis and a condition like diabetes insipidus (Gauer, 1971). Kaiser and co-workers (1963) found that the diuresis was 3.5 times greater in the immersed subjects than in the controls. In a later study (1969), when these investigators immersed 20 subjects for 8 hr, plasma volume was noted to decrease by 494 ml (14%) and body weight to decrease by 6.4 kg. Similar changes have been found by a number of other investigators (Gauer, 1971). McCally and co-workers (1971) were able to show that 80% of the expected change occurred during the first 25 min of immersion. However, Behn and co-workers (1969) pointed out that the amount and nature of the diuresis depended on the state of hydration of the subjects: normally hydrated subjects showed a rise in free water clearance, whereas hydropenic subjects exhibited an increased osmolar clearance.

Epstein (1978) recently completed an extensive review of the renal mechanisms involved in volume homeostasis during immersion. Aside from the inhibition of ADH, he pointed out that important roles were also played by renal prostaglandins (Berl and Schrier, 1973) and sympathetic nervous system activity (DiBona, 1978). Epstein (1978) also stressed the importance of the temporal dissociation between renal salt and water excretion. In most cases (90% of subjects), a naturesis and kaliuresis occur subsequent to the large water diuresis as a result of the preceding factors, either alone or in combination with aldosterone suppression or release of a naturietic factor (Epstein et al., 1972, 1975; Epstein, 1978).

Torphy (1965), in a comparison of water immersion and bedrest effects on orthostatic tolerance and plasma volume, also observed a significant decrease in plasma volume following both immersion and bedrest. Immersion, both with and without physical activity, however, resulted in a greater decrease in plasma volume than did inactive bedrest. Fluid loss in the urine was larger than determined plasma volume losses, leading to the conclusion that there was a loss of extravascular water as well. These findings, however, have not been borne out by subsequent studies (Epstein, 1978). In a later comparison of the two simulations of weightlessness, Torphy (1966b) noted that inactive immersion resulted in a plasma volume loss of 290 ml, immersion with physical activity in a loss of 284 ml, and inactive bedrest in a loss of 146 ml—as compared with a loss during normal activity (office work) of 144 ml.

Vanyushina (1963), in a comparison of the physiological responses of chair rest and immersion, conducted two series of experiments with male subjects (ages 20–22 years). In the first series, six subjects were immobilized for 5.5–10.5 days in armchairs. In the second series, three subjects remained in a tank of water for 5.5–11.5 days. Orthostatic tolerance was determined using tilt and stand tests. After water immersion, extreme tachycardia, accompanied by an increase in pulse rate of 50–74 bpm and a drop in systolic pressure (26 mm Hg), was observed. Diastolic pressure tended to rise, causing a marked decrease in pulse pressure (about 8–12 mm Hg). The response to chair rest was less than half the magnitude of the response to water immersion. Changes in responses to the tilt and stand tests before both chair rest and immersion were negligible (heart rate increase of 10–12 bpm; systolic blood pressure changes of −2 to +8 mm Hg). These studies again point up the more exaggerated responses seen after water immersion compared with those after immoblization.

In a later study comparing water immersion and bedrest responses, Vanyushina and co-workers (1966) found that blood taken from the subjects after both water immersion and bedrest had a norepinephrinelike effect when tested on frog hearts (exhibited a decreased chronotropic effect and an increased inotropic effect), but no specific measures were taken to evaluate such possibilities either during the test or afterward.

In another study that again compared the physiological effects of immersion and bedrest, White and co-workers (1966) exposed 10 subjects to alternate 10-day periods of bedrest and immersion in fluid silicone. The investigators found that both bedrest and immersion resulted in significant cardiovascular deconditioning. Plasma, blood, and extracellular fluid volumes were reduced; maximum oxygen consumption decreased; and postural equilibrium was somewhat impaired. The subjects also exhibited higher heart rates and lower pulse pressures with immersion as compared with bedrest. Extracellular fluid decreased by 3% after 5 days of immersion and by 2% after the same duration of bedrest. After 10 days the net decrease in fluid was 5% for immersion and 7% for bedrest. Changes in blood volume paralleled those of plasma volume. Although the changes occurred more rapidly with immersion, the net loss after 10 days was approximately the same for both approaches.

Arborelius and co-workers (1972) tested 10 subjects seated in neutral temperatures in air (28°C) or immersed with head above water (35°C) both with and without oxygen breathing. Measurements were made of cardiac output (dye dilution method) and right atrial and brachial arterial pressures. In three air-breathing subjects, central blood volume and pulmonary arterial pressure were also measured. During immersion and air breathing, cardiac output increased by 1.8 liters/min (32%); stroke volume increased by 26 ml (35%); but heart rate was almost unchanged. Right atrial and pulmonary arterial transmural pressure gradients increased in the immersed subjects by about 13 mm Hg. Systemic vascular resistance decreased by 30%. During immersion, central blood volume increased by about 0.7 liters. The subjects exhibited extra systoles at times during the first minutes of immersion. The relative changes in circulatory parameters measured during oxygen breathing were not significant compared with those noted during air breathing.

More recently, Begin and co-workers (1976), using acetylene rebreathing techniques to study the central circulation of subjects during 4 hr of immersion, confirmed the magnitude of the acute findings of a significant increase in cardiac output and demonstrated their persistence over the period of study. A potential reduction in venous tone as a primary or secondary explanation for the marked susceptibility to orthostatic collapse was investigated by Gauer and co-workers on two occasions (Echt et al., 1974; Kaiser and Gauer, 1966). In the first set of experiments venous occlusive plethysmography was used to determine changes that occurred in the forearm. In the second set of experiments, during a 3-hr immersion exposure, right atrial, esophagal, and forearm venous pressures were recorded, including occlusive plethysmography. A significant (30%) decrease in venous tone was demonstrated, as were significant increases in recorded and transmural central venous pressure (mean CVP of 3.4 mm Hg rising at once to 15.2 mm Hg). These findings verified data previously reported by Arborelius and co-workers (1972). Following immersion, return to normal took several hours. Gauer felt that the loss of tone represented a reflex response directed toward diminishing central engorgement and that it persisted because of a loss of general sympathetic tone caused by the reduction in total peripheral flow resistance during immersion. In contrast to these findings, Campbell and co-workers (1969) found that total immersion for only a few minutes resulted in a 61% ± 43% increase in forearm vascular resistance and an associated 29% ± 15% reduction in forearm blood flow.

Tilt table, centrifuge, and heat chamber studies (Graveline and Barnard, 1961) showed that significant cardiovascular deterioration occurs even after only 6 hr of immersion. Symptoms become progressively more severe with 12-hr and 24-hr immersion. Urinary output during the first 6 hr was not excessive, but tended to increase with immersion time. Hemodilution was found to be prevalent at 6 hr, followed by hemoconcentration at 24 hr.

Evidence of hemodilution during 4- to 6-hr immersion has been reported by a number of investigators (Behn *et al.,* 1969; Crane and Harris, 1974; Kaiser *et al.,* 1963; McCally, 1964), but not consistently (Epstein, 1978).

Changes in epinephrine and norepinephrine with immersion have not been significant. Torphy (1966b) studied five subjects after 6 hr of normal activity, bedrest, and immersion. The subjects were tilted at 44° following exposure to each test condition. Urinary excretion of epinephrine and norepinephrine showed the same expected rise following each state. The findings demonstrated that the vasoconstrictive response to orthostasis, as evidenced by norepinephrine excretion, was not impaired by 6 hr of immersion.

In a study of urinary catecholamine responses to water immersion, McCally and Graveline (1963) measured urinary excretion of adrenaline and noradrenaline by bioassay in 16 subjects during 6 hr of complete water immersion. Adrenaline excretion increased moderately and may have been related to the subjects' anxiety over immersion. Noradrenaline excretion, on the other hand, decreased significantly ($P < 0.01$) during immersion. Following immersion, six subjects observed during passive vertical tilt exhibited significant orthostatic intolerance, which differed markedly from their control (preimmersion) responses.

The original observation made by Graybiel and Clark (1961) that work capacity is significantly reduced after immersion has been confirmed by other investigators (Stegemann *et al.,* 1969; Ulmer *et al.,* 1972). Stegemann and co-workers, in a study of four endurance-trained and four nontrained subjects after 6 hr of immersion, found that aerobic work capacity decreased by 10% in the untrained subjects and by 20% in the trained group. The performance–heart rate index rose by about 14% in the untrained subjects and by 28% in the trained subjects. No significant changes in maximal voluntary force were observed. In contrast to these findings, Denison and co-workers (1972) compared exercise responses in air and water. Respiratory gas exchange, end-tidal gas tensions, alveolar ventilation, respiratory frequency, cardiac output, and pulse rate were measured in four healthy male subjects at rest and during mild and moderate exercise ($V_{O_2} = 0.2$–2.0 liter/min) in air (18°–22°C) and under water (35°–35.5°C). The subjects respired at normal pressures from the same breathing circuit throughout the study. Sixty-four determinations were made of each variable for each study environment. Immersion was associated with a 10% increase in pulse rate and cardiac output at all levels of exercise. No changes were observed in end-tidal CO_2 tension, alveolar ventilation, or work capacity. The investigators concluded that subjects performing mild and moderate exercise in warm water show the same responses as those exercising in air.

A number of investigators have sought to develop countermeasures to cardiovascular deconditioning with exposure to weightlessness and have used immersion studies toward this end. Hunt (1967) compared the effects of vasopressin and positive pressure breathing in reversing cardiovascular deconditioning following water immersion. In this study six USAF airmen were exposed for 6 hr to the following conditions: (1) routine daily activity, (2) confinement in a deckchair in a semirecumbent position, (3) semirecumbent confinement immersed to the neck in 33°–34° water, and (4) immersion with 20 mm Hg positive pressure breathing. The first three conditions were also used to compare the effects of vasopressin versus a saline placebo. Following exposure to each experimental environment, the subjects were given a tilt-table test consisting of a 10-min baseline period, followed by 15 min of 70° tilt. Pulse rate and blood pressure were recorded every other minute. Water immersion increased diuresis and decreased tilt-table tolerance. Positive pressure breathing inhibited diuresis by 70% and improved tilt tolerance. Vasopressin reduced saline diuresis by 50%, but did not improve tilt tolerance. Neither countermeasure totally reversed immersion diuresis. Tilt tolerance was better among the subjects exposed to positive pressure breathing.

Six hours of head-out immersion at a neutral temperature produces significant orthostatic tachycardia and hypotension during 70° tilt (McCally, 1964). The condition may be related to plasma volume contraction during immersion diuresis, alterations in capacitance vessel reactivity, or disturbance of catecholamine metabolism. McCally and co-workers (1966a) evaluated four techniques to determine whether they would be useful in preventing postimmersion orthostatic intolerance: (1) use of extremity venous occlusive tourniquets, (2) injection of antidiuretic hormone (ADH), (3) use of positive pressure breathing (15 mm Hg), and (4) wearing of an elastic gradient leotard. The leotard, which was donned after immersion and just prior to tilt, provided significant protection ($P < 0.01$) and restored tilt-table responses to control levels. Venous tourniquets, which were inflated to 80 mm Hg, 1 min on and 1 min off, provided partial protection. Positive pressure breathing and ADH prevented immersion diuresis but did not significantly alter postimmersion orthostatic intolerance.

Vogt (1965, 1967a,b; Vogt and Johnson, 1967) has used intermittently inflated extremity cuffs as a countermeasure to cardiovascular deconditioning following immersion. In the first of such studies, he studied the tilt-table tolerance of four healthy young males in two water immersion experiments of 6 hr duration. During the first experiment the subjects were unprotected; during the second, cuff tourniquets were applied to the four extremities and inflated to a pressure of 60 mm Hg, 1 min off and 1 min on. After the first immersion experiment, three of the four subjects experienced syncope during tilt-table testing, and all exhibited marked changes in heart rate and blood pressure during tilting after immersion. The cuffs afforded a degree of protection, since none of the three subjects experienced syncope or showed the marked changes in heart rate and blood pressure observed previously. In these studies and another (Vogt and Johnson, 1967), cuff tourniquets were found to be partially effective.

Heat acclimatization in conjunction with exercise training has also been studied as a countermeasure (Shvartz et al., 1977). These investigators subjected five male volunteers (ages 18–26 years) to exercise training in a heated environment (39.8°C, relative humidity of 50%). The subjects were acclimatized for 8 days prior to immersion; during acclimatization they exercised for 2 hr a day on upright bicycle ergometers at 50% of their $V_{O_2 max}$. Five control subjects performed the same exercise regimen, but did so in a cool environment (23.8°C). At the end of the acclimatization period, all subjects were administered 70° head-up tilt and $\dot{V}_{O_2 max}$ tests. The following day they were immersed in water (34.5°C) for 8 hr. The tilt tests were again administered after immersion. Heat acclimatization appeared to provide substantial protection against the adverse effects of water immersion deconditioning; exercise training under cool conditions also had an effect, but to a much lesser degree.

3. Countermeasures

A variety of protective measures, as shown in Table IX, have now been evaluated to prevent a "deconditioned state" after bedrest or weightlessness. No reasonably reliable or totally effective countermeasure has been found to date. The greatest attention has been placed on periodic exercise regimens (isotonic and isometric), which have been used extensively during space flight (Beregovkin et al., 1969, 1976; Thornton et al., 1977) and bedrest (Balakhovskiy et al., 1972; Beregovkin and Kalinichenko, 1974; Birkhead et al., 1963a, 1966; Brannon et al., 1963; Cardus, 1966; Georgiyevskiy et al., 1973; Korolev, 1968a; McCally et al., 1968; Miller et al., 1964a). It was initially anticipated that heavy exercise with attendant physical conditioning would increase intravascular volumes, decrease heart rate, and improve general skeletal muscle strength and tone. Although some evidence is available that such effects occur during bedrest, various regimens have failed to prevent orthostatic intolerance (Birkhead et al., 1963a; McCally et al., 1968; Miller et al., 1964a; Triebwasser et al., 1970) or loss of acceleration tolerance (Greenleaf et al., 1975). Bungee cord exercises (principally isometric) used during the 8- and 14-day Gemini missions (Berry et al., 1966) and during bedrest (Vogt, 1966) did not provide protection. Astronauts and cosmonauts participating in the longer-duration Skylab and Soyuz missions have praised the use of isotonic exercise in providing a sense of well-being during flight, but orthostatic intolerance was still pre-

TABLE IX

Countermeasures: Bedrest–Induced Cardiovascular Deconditioning

Exercise
Isotonic — Mild, Moderate, Heavy
Isometric
Fluid Replacement — Oral or Drug
Drugs
9-alphafluorohydrocortisone, DOCA, Angiotensin, Amphetamines
Nerobol, Propranalol
Centrifugation or Load Suits
G-Suits
Oscillating Bed or Trampoline
Lower Body Negative Pressure
Together with —
Fluid Ingestion
Exercise
Venous Occlusion — Suits, Cuffs
Hypoxia

sent among them despite the heavy use of exercise (Johnson *et al.,* 1977). Future study in this area appears to be indicated to determine whether exercise is really necessary and whether it will be effective for shortening the readaptation period following flight.

The effects of venous pooling in the extremities as a means of preventing orthostatic intolerance have also received considerable attention. Such pooling was postulated to improve venomotor tone and decrease central venous pressure and volume. Techniques have varied from the use of periodically inflated cuffs (McCally *et al.,* 1968; Vogt and Johnson, 1967) to the wearing of a reverse gradient garment (Annis, 1974). Proximally placed cuffs have been used on the legs alone (Cardus, 1966; Pestov *et al.,* 1969; Vogt, 1966; Vogt and Johnson, 1967) or on both the legs and arms (Graveline, 1962; McCally *et al.,* 1968; Vogt and Johnson, 1967). After initial positive findings by Graveline (1962) and Vogt and Johnson (1967), subsequent configurations have neither prevented plasma volume losses nor offset loss of tolerance during LBNP and tilt (Cardus, 1966; McCally *et al.,* 1968; Stevens, 1966; Vogt, 1966, 1967a; Vogt and Johnson, 1967). In-flight cuffs used in Gemini IV and Gemini VII failed to affect postflight deconditioning in any of the flight crew (Dietlein and Judy, 1966).

A reverse gradient suit has been used during simulation of weightlessness to provide counterpressure to venous return so as to pool blood in the extremities exactly as occurs when in the upright posture (Annis, 1974).

Use of this technique, however, failed to return heart rate and blood pressure during LBNP to prebedrest levels or to improve degraded acceleration tolerance at +3.0 G_z (Convertino *et al.*, 1978; Sandler *et al.*, in preparation).

Exposure to LBNP has also been tested as a means of reversing postbedrest orthostatic intolerance and as a means of rehydration of body fluids lost during recumbency. Musgrave and co-workers (Henry *et al.*, 1962) were the first to demonstrate that 40 mm Hg suction approximated the peripheral pooling effect seen during an upright stance or 70° passive tilt. A number of subsequent studies have now demonstrated that negative pressure of this level applied over protracted periods of time (up to 4–6 hr each day) can either prevent or restore decreases in plasma volume and lost orthostatic tolerance during bedrest (Asyamolov *et al.*, 1973; Beregovkin and Kalinichenko, 1974; Birkhead *et al.*, 1966; Cramer, 1971; Gilbert and Stevens, 1966; Hyatt and West, 1977; Lamb *et al.*, 1965a; McCally *et al.*, 1966a; Miller, 1965; Stevens *et al.*, 1966c,d). Although the use of LBNP as a countermeasure is feasible during ground-based studies, the need for long-term treatment periods makes it impractical for space flight. Russian investigators seem to have solved part of this problem, however, through the design and use of a lower body negative pressure suit (from the waist down) that is worn throughout the flight day (Barer *et al.*, 1975). Reentry acceleration tolerance is also improved by requiring each individual to drink approximately 1 liter of saline solution immediately prior to reentry, in conjuction with wearing the suit. Specific results on responses of subjects wearing and not wearing the suits and the suit's effect on postflight readaptation have not yet been published. Orthostatic intolerance is known to occur, however, postflight despite the use of such suits (Gazenko *et al.*, 1976).

Support for the combined use of LBNP and fluid injestion comes from studies by Hyatt and West (1977). The investigators applied −30 mm Hg LBNP for 4 hr a day, with the subjects also consuming 1,000 ml of beef bouillon containing 154 mEq of sodium. With this regimen subjects bedrested for 1 week showed significant improvement in plasma volume levels and orthostatic tolerance. Consumption of a saline solution alone had a lesser effect. Greenleaf and co-workers (1973a,b) reported a similar response to saline injestion—after bedrest and the injestion regimen, subjects were better able to tolerate +G_z acceleration.

Periodic centrifugation has also been used to readapt the cardiovascular system to orthostatic stress after bedrest. White and co-workers (1966) reported that four 7.5-min daily rides on a short-radius (7-ft) centrifuge prevented orthostatic syncope after 10 days of bedrest. Such exposures, however, failed to readjust other cardiovascular variables, including weight, plasma volume, and red cell mass to prebedrest values. Similar findings have been reported by Russian investigators (Shulzenko *et al.*, 1976) for two subjects during 56 days of water immersion. The use of an on-board centrifuge, however, seems remote at present because of cost, weight, power, and volume requirements. Results from the foregoing investigators nonetheless have contributed importantly toward suggesting the use of artificial gravity during flight. They have also provided useful data toward determining the level of gravity needed to prevent cardiovascular deconditioning.

Several innovative procedures that do not require a centrifuge to induce accelerative forces have also been tested during bedrest studies. Periodic bouncing exercises on a railed bed between two trampolines to induce $+G_z$ (along the long axis of the body) were found to be ineffective in preventing orthostatic intolerance (Chase *et al.*, 1966). Battacharya and co-workers (1978), on the other hand, induced a programmed level of acceleration by restraining subject horizontally on a mechanically driven table so that they received acceleration along the spine ($+G_z$). The subjects were exposed to 70° passive tilt before and after bedrest and 6 hr of head-down tilt and again in each state after 20 min of whole body acceleration. Findings indicate that syncope can be prevented as well as the postbedrest increased heart rate with 70° passive tilt. Acceleration profiles were similar to those measured during upright jumping on a trampoline or a hard surface. Repetition rate of the imposed forces was 1 G_z, and peak table acceleration was $+1.5$ G_z.

Positive pressure breathing, as indicated earlier, has been used in water immersion studies to prevent cardiovascular deconditioning by preventing fluid shifts to the chest (Hunt, 1967). Its use as a countermeasure during bedrest has not been investigated. However, periodic Flak maneuvers (Valsalva procedures) were tested in one bedrest study (Vogt, 1965) and failed to prevent tilt intolerance.

Because many of the physiologic responses to hypoxia are the reverse of those seen with weightlessness, investigators have exposed bedrested subjects to altitudes of 10,000–20,000 feet in chambers (Korol'kov and Mirrakhimov, 1976; Lamb, 1965; Lynch *et al.*, 1967; Makarov, 1970; Stevens, 1966). The resultant mild hypoxia prevented the loss of red cell mass but did not significantly alter orthostatic intolerance.

The most effective countermeasure to date has been a lower body pressure garment (anti-G suit) or leotard (Buyanov *et al.*, 1967; McCally *et al.*, 1968; Miller *et al.*, 1964a). In an extensive bedrest study lasting 2–4 weeks, Miller and co-workers (1964a,b) successfully protected subjects from orthostatic intolerance after bedrest by the use of G-suits. Subjects were placed in a totally vertical (90°) body position using a parachute harness and were held there passively for 20 min. G-suits have also been effective in restoring orthostatic tolerance after water immersion (McCally *et al.*, 1966a,b). The external pressure provided by the suit acts to prevent excessive blood pooling and fluid loss to the lower body and abdomen when the individual is in the standing position (Gauer and Thron, 1963). This method has been used successfully to prevent fainting in individuals suffering from postural hypotension, particularly when the condition results from autonomic insufficiency (Ibrahim *et al.*, 1975). Two studies have demonstrated its effectiveness in reversing physiological changes during acceleration (Chambers and Vykukal, 1972; Jacobson *et al.*, 1974). Conventional or modified G-suits have been worn regularly by American and Russian space crews to provide protection against syncopal reactions in the immediate postflight period (Hordinsky, 1977).

The use of most drugs as countermeasures has been ineffective to date. Although the administration of 2 mg daily of 9-fluorohydrocortisone for 2–4 days following 6, 43, 53, or 74 days of bedrest returned plasma volume to normal, it did not prevent orthostatic intolerance (Bohnn *et al.*, 1970; Hyatt, 1971; Stevens, 1966; Stevens and Lynch, 1965). A dose of 0.2 mg of 9α-fluorohydrocortisone given daily during a 14-day study (Hyatt, 1971) or 0.4 mg given daily over a 10-day study (Bohnn *et al.*, 1970; Hyatt, 1971) had identical effects. The drug caused nausea in several subjects and did not prevent orthostatic intolerance (Stevens, 1966). Similarly, pitressin administered to subject during water immersion or bedrest prevented the diuresis and associated decrease in plasma volume but did not affect the loss of orthostatic tolerance (Hunt, 1967; McCally *et al.*, 1968; Parin *et al.*, 1971). Soviet investigators have also used a variety of pharmacologic agents, including adrenal steroids (deoxycorticosterone) (Parin *et al.*, 1971), central nervous system stimulants (amphetamine, caffeine, and strychnine) (Pestov, 1968; Pestov *et al.*, 1969), and androgens (nerobol) (Grigor'yev *et al.*, 1976; Parin *et al.*, 1971). These medications have had partial, but incomplete, restorative effects on cardiovascular and fluid-electrolyte changes and muscle degeneration. Recently, Melada and co-workers (1975) have demonstrated promising results with the β-adrenergic blocker, propranolol. Exaggerated metabolic and circulatory responses to tilt were reduced or abolished following intravenous infusion of this drug (0.15–0.2 mg/kg over 5 min. followed by 0.04 mg/kg every 20 min). Although the results are promising, the findings need to be verified and the oral administration of this drug further investigated.

V. Conclusions

The similarities of cardiovascular changes seen during space flight and bedrest have been well documented. The most striking findings are related to orthostatic intolerance and changes in fluid and electrolyte balance. The precise mechanisms that cause these changes in man, however, have yet to be determined. Fluid shift to the chest associated with postural change or weightlessness clearly plays a role. As originally described by Gauer (1950), such changes trigger the intrathoracic low-pressure mechanoreceptors to alter the renal handling of water and electrolytes, primarily through the inhibition of antidiuretic hormone secretion and secondarily through decreased aldosterone production. Alterations in central nervous system activity resulting from a change in the thresholds or metabolism of neurotransmitter substances, as well as loss of cardiac muscle mass, have not been adequately studied to date. Information for these latter possibilities has come from recent work with nonhuman primates who were totally immobilized for up to 6 months. The inability to find an acceptable animal model for ground-based studies has severely limited investigative programs, since man has had to serve as the primary experimental subject, which accounts for the large number of bedrest studies that have been conducted since the onset of the space program.

Over the past several years, both American and Russian investigators have begun to emphasize the use of head-down bedrest ($-2°$ to $-12°$) because of reports by cosmonauts that the head-down body position better replicates their feelings during weightlessness. The ability to confirm or refute the effectiveness of this technique will depend on appropriate, definitive cardiovascular measurements made during future manned space flights. In addition to critical experiments that will provide data to be used in defining the mechanisms by which the body adapts to weightlessness, consideration must be given to cardiovascular changes that will inhibit man's free participation in space as scientist and worker. In the near term, such studies should concentrate on determining whether weightlessness affects processes that will accelerate or ameliorate cardiovascular disease. Some useful data will be provided postflight from careful study of the physical condition of all flight crews. The small number of individuals from both the United States and Russia who have been exposed to weightlessness to date will make this task difficult. (Less than 70 individuals have flown in space, and only 15 of them have experienced weightlessness for three weeks or longer.) Collection of the needed data, however, will be facilitated by the advent of more frequent flights. In this regard, carefully planned and executed animal flights concerned with epidemiology will provide the most information.

To the present time, no acceptable countermeasure has been found to offset the deconditioning resulting from space flight and hypodynamia. This area will require considerable attention over the next several years. Soviet investigators have used LBNP garments during flight, combined with fluid injection just prior to reentry, to offset postflight orthostatic changes.

G-suits have also been used postflight by both countries. As more extensive information becomes available concerning the mechanisms that trigger the changes observed in the past, there will be a greater possibility for devising and utilizing specific protective procedures. In the past, countermeasures that have proved effective during space flight have also been effective during bedrest studies. Consequently, bedrest studies and particularly water immersion exposure, both of which simulate the weightless condition, will be important ground-based tools for evaluating any devised countermeasures before they are actually used in flight.

References

Adey, W. R., and Hahn, P. M. (1971). *Aerosp. Med.* **42**, 271–336.

Aleksandrov, A. N., and Kochetov, A. K. (1974). *Space Biol. Aerosp. Med.* **8**(1), 104–105.

Anashkin, O. D. (1969). *Space Biol. Med.* **3**(1), 148–156.

Annis, J. F. (1974). *Aerosp. Med. Assoc. Prepr.* pp. 96–97.

Arborelius, M. Jr., Balldin, U. I., Lilja, B., and Lundgren, C. E. G. (1972). *Aerosp. Med.* **43**, 590–592.

Asyamolov, B. F., and Voskresenskiy, A. D. (1968). *Space Biol. Med.* **2**, 33–37.

Asyamolov, B. F., Panchenko, V. S., Pestov, I. D.. and Tikhonov, M. A. (1973). *Space Biol. Med.* **2**(6), 80–87.

Balakhovskiy, I. S., Bakhteyva, V. T., Beleda, R. V., Biryukov, Ye. I., Vinogradova, L. A., Grigor'yev, A. I., Zakharova, T. A., Dlusskaya, I. G., Kiselev, R. K., Kislovskaya, T. A., Kozrevskaya, G. I., Noskov, V. B., Orlova, T. A., and Sokolova, N. M. (1972). *Space Biol. Med.* **6**(4), 110–116.

Baranski, S., Baranska, W., and Kujawa, M. (1975). *Int. Astronaut. Congr., Proc.* **26**, 39.

Barer, A. S., Savinov, A. P., Severin, G. I., Stroklitskiy, A. Yu., and Tikhomirov, Ye. P. (1975). *Space Biol. Med.* **9**(1), 41–47.

Bartok, S. J., Carlson, L. D., and Walters, R. F. (1968). *Aerosp. Med.* **39**, 1157–1162.

Battacharya, A., Knapp, C. F., McCutcheon, E. P., Kearney, J., and Cornish, A. (1978). *Int. Conf. Mech. Med. Biol. 1st* (abstr.)

Begin, R., Dougherty, R.. Michaelson, E. D., and Sacker, M. A. (1976). *Aviat., Space, Environ. Med.* **47**(9), 937–941.

Behn, C., Gauer, O. H., Kirsch, K., and Eckert, P. (1969). *Pfllüegers Arch.* **313**, 123–125.

Belaya, N. A., Amirov, R. Z., Shaposhnikov, Ye. A., Lebedeva, I. P., and Sologob, B. S. (1975). *Vopr. Kurortol., Fizioter. Lech. Fiz. Kul't.* **40**(3), 238–241.

Belkaniya, G. S. (1978). *Usp. Fiziol. Nauk* **9**(2), 103–128.

Belkaniya, G. S., Rasumeyev, A. N., and Lapin, B. A. (1973). *Space Biol. Aerosp. Med.* **8**(5), 17–27.

Benevolenskaya, T. V., Korotayev, M. M., Krupina, T. N., Maslov, I. A., Mikaylovskiy, G. P., Petrova, T. A., Smirnov, K. V., and Yakoleva, I. Ya. (1967). *Int. Congr., Astronaut. Proc.* **18**, 81–87.

Beregovkin, A. V., and Kalinichenko, V. V. (1974). *Space Biol. Aerosp. Med.* **8**, 72–77.

Beregovkin, A. V., Buyanov, P. V., Galkin, A. V., Pisarenko, N. V., and Sheludyakov, Ye. (1969). *Probl. Space Biol.* **13**, 221–227.

Beregovkin, A. V., Vodolazov, A. S., Georgiyevskiy, V. S., Kalinichenko, V. V., Korelin, N.

V., Mikhaylov, V. M., Pometov, Yu. D., Shchigoov, V. V., and Katkovskiy, B. S. (1976). *Space Biol. Aerosp. Med.* 5(5), 30–38.

Berl, T., and Schrier, R. W. (1973). *J. Clin. Invest.* 52, 463–471.

Bernauer, E. M.. Adams, W. C., and Fuller, J. H. (1968). "The Effect of Nine Days of Recumbency, with and without Exercise, on the Redistribution of Body Fluids and Electrolytes, Renal Function and Metabolism," NASA CR-73664. Human Performance Laboratory, University of California, Davis.

Berry, C. A., Coons, D. O., Catterson, A. D., and Kelly, G. F. (1966). "Man's Response to Long Duration Flight in the Gemini Spacecraft," Gemini Midprogram Conf., NASA SP-121, pp. 235–263. NASA, Washington, D.C.

Bevegard, S., Johnson, B., and Karlof, I. (1962). *Acta Med. Scand.* 172, 623–636.

Birkhead, N. C., Blizzard, J. J., Daly, J. W., Haupt, G. J., Issekutz, B., Jr., Myers, R. N., and Rodahl, K. (1963a). "Cardiodynamic and Metabolic Effects of Prolonged Bedrest," Rep. No. AMRL-TDR-63-37. Wright-Patterson AFB, Ohio.

Birkhead, N. C., Haupt, G. J., Blizzard, J. J., Lachance, P. A., and Rodahl, K. (1963b). *Physiologist* 6, 140.

Birkhead, N. C., Haupt, C. J., Issekutz, B., Jr., and Rodahl, K. (1964). *Am. J. Med. Sci.* 247, 243.

Birkhead, N. C., Blizzard, J. J., Issekutz, B., Jr., and Rodahl, K. (1966). "Effects of Exercise, Standing, Negative Trunk and Positive Skeletal Pressure on Bed Rest-Induced Orthostasis and Hypercalciura," Rep. No. AMRL-TR-66-6. Wright-Patterson AFB, Ohio.

Blomquist, G., Mitchell, J. H., and Saltin, B. (1971). *In* "Hypogravic and Hypodynamic Environments" (R. H. Murray and M. McCally, eds.), NASA SP-269, pp. 171–176. NASA, Washington, D.C.

Bobkova, N. N., and Grinio, L. P. (1971). *Curr. Probl. Space Biol. Med.* pp. 19–20.

Bohnn, B. J., Hyatt, K. H., Kamenetsky, L. G., Calder, B. E., and Smith, W. M. (1970). *Aerosp. Med.* 41, 495–499.

Bokhov, B. B., Kornilova, L. N., and Yakovleva, I. Ya. (1975). *Space Biol. Aerosp. Med.* 9(1), 82–89.

Boldov, V. A. (1971). *Curr. Probl. Space Biol. Med.* pp. 26–27.

Bourne, G. H. (1977). *Yerkes Newsl.* 14(2), 3–13.

Brannon, E. W., Rockwood, C. A., Jr., and Potts, P. (1963). *Aerosp. Med.* 34, 900–906.

Browse, N. L. (1965). "Physiology and Pathology of Bed Rest," pp. 44–45 and 148–152. Thomas, Springfield, Illinois.

Buderer, M. C., Rummel, J. A., Michel, E. L.. Maulden, D. C., and Savin, C. F. (1976). *Aviat., Space, Environ. Med.* 47, 365–372.

Bugrov, B. G., Gorlov, O. G., Petrov, A. V., Serov, A. D., Yugov, Ye. M., and Yakovelev, V. I. (1962). *Aerosp. Med.* 33, 1056–1068.

Buhr, P. A. (1963). *Helv. Med. Acta* 30, 156–175.

Buyanov, P. V., Beregovkin, A. V., and Pisarenko, N. V. (1967). *Space Biol. Med.* 1(1), 95–100.

Buznik, I. M., and Kamforina, S. A. (1973). *Space Biol. Med.* 7, 60–64.

Bychkov, V. P., Markaryan, M. V., and Khokhlova, O. S. (1976). *In* "Life Sciences and Space Research XIV" (P. N. A. Sneath, ed.), pp. 281–284. Akademie-Verlag, Berlin.

Campbell, L. B., Gooden, B. A., and Horowitz, J. D. (1969). *J. Physiol. (London)* 202, 239–250.

Cardus, D. (1966). *Aerosp. Med.* 37, 993–999.

Cardus, D., Vallbona, C., Vogt, F. B., Spencer, W. A., Lipscomb, H. S., and Eik-Nes, K. B. (1965). *Aerosp. Med.* 36, 524–528.

Chambers, A., and Vykukal, H. C. (1972). "The Effect of Bed Rest on Crew Performance during Simulated Shuttle Re-Entry," Vol. I, NASA TN-D-7503, pp. 1–29. NASA, Washington, D.C.

Chapman, L. W. and Henry, J. P. (1973). *Physiologist* **16(2)**, 194–201.

Chase, C. A., Grave, E., and Rowell, L. B. (1966). *Aerosp. Med.* **37**, 1232–1238.

Chavarri, M., Ganguly, A., Leutscher, J. A., and Zager, P. G. (1977). *Aviat., Space, Environ. Med.* **48**, 633–636.

Chazov, Ye. I., and Ananchenko, V. G. (1963). *In* "Aviation and Space Medicine" (V. V. Parin, ed.), pp. 414–415. Akad. Med. Nauk, Moscow.

Cherepakhin, M. A. (1968). *Space Biol. Med.* **2**(1), 52–59.

Cherepakhin, M. A. (1970). *Space Biol. Med.* **4**(3), 103–110.

Chobanian, A. V., Little, R. D., Tercyak, A., and Blevins, P. (1974). *Circulation* **49**, 551–559.

Chung, A. T.-C. (1966). Master of Science Thesis, Texas Woman's University, Denton (unpublished).

Clamann, H. G. (1961). "Biological Experiments with Space Probes," Lect. Aerosp. Med., Sect. 19, pp. 1–15. U.S. School of Aviation Medicine.

Clarke, N. P., and Leverett, S. D. (1976). *AGARD Conf. Proc.* **189**, 1–80.

Convertino, V. A., Stremel, R. W., Bernauer, E. M., and Greenleaf, J. E. (1975). *Aerosp. Med. Assoc. Prepr.* pp. 238–239.

Convertino, V. A., Sandler, H., and Webb, P. (1978). *Aerosp. Med. Assoc. Prepr.* pp. 148–149.

Cramer, D. B. (1971). "Modification of Orthostatic Tolerance with Periodic Lower Body Negative Pressure," AIAA Pap. No. 71–859. Am. Inst. Aeronaut. Astronaut., New York.

Crane, M. G., and Harris, J. J. (1974). *J. Clin. Endocrinol. Metab.* **23**, 359–368.

Deitrick, J. E., Whedon, G. D., Shorr, E., Toscani, V., and Davis, V. B. (1948). *Am. J. Med.* **4**, 3–35.

de Marees, H., Kunitsch, G., and Barbey, K. (1974). *Basic Res. Cardiol.* **69**(4), 462–478.

Denison, D. M., Wagner, P. D., Kingaby, G. J., and West, J. B. (1972). *J. Appl. Physiol.* **33**, 426–430.

DiBona, G. F. (1978). *Fed. Proc., Fed. Am. Soc. Exp. Biol.* **37**, 1214–1217.

Dietlein, L. F. (1977). *In* "Biomedical Results from Skylab" (R. S. Johnson and L. F. Dietlein, eds.), NASA SP-377, pp. 408–418. NASA, Washington, D.C.

Dietlein, L. F., and Judy, W. V. (1966). *In* "Gemini Mid-Program Conference," NASA SP-121, pp. 381–392. NASA, Washington, D. C.

DiGiovanni, C., Jr., and Birkhead, N. C. (1964). *Aerosp. Med.* **35**(3), 225–228.

Dlusskaya, I. G., Vinogradov, L. A., Noskov, V. B., and Balakhovskiy, I. S. (1973). *Space Biol. Med.* **7**(3), 61–68.

Dolkas, C., and Greenleaf, J. (1977). *J. Appl. Physiol.* **43**, 1033–1038.

Dolkas, C., and Sandler, H. (1974). *Aerosp. Med. Assoc. Prepr.* pp. 169–170.

Donald, D. E., and Shepherd, J. T. (1963). *Am. J. Physiol.* **205**, 393.

Donald, D. E., Milburn, S. E., and Shepherd, J. T. (1964). *J. Appl. Physiol.* **19**, 849.

Donaldson, C. L., Hulley, S. B., Rosen, S. N., Friedman, R. J., and Vogel, J. M. (1970). *Clin. Res.* **18**, 453.

Dorchak, K. J., and Greenleaf, J. E. (1976). "The Physiology and Biochemistry of Total Body Immobilization in Animals: A Compendium of Research," NASA TM X-3306, pp. 1–50. NASA, Washington, D.C.

Drozdova, N. T., and Grishin, Ye. P. (1972). *Space Biol. Med.* **6**(4), 74–78.

Echt, M., Lange, L., and Gauer, O. H. (1974). *Pflüegers Arch.* **352**, 211–217.

Ellis, J. P., Welch, B. E., and Prescott, J. M. (1972). *Aerosp. Med.* **43**, 22–27.

Ellis, J. P., Jr., Lecocq, F. R., Garcia, J. B., Jr., and Lipman, R. L. (1974). *Aerosp. Med.* **45,** 15–18.

Epstein, M. (1970). *Aerosp. Med. Assoc. Prepr.* pp. 71–72.

Epstein, M. (1971). *J. Appl. Physiol.* **30,** 366–369.

Epstein, M. (1978). *Physiol. Rev.* **58,** 529–581.

Epstein, M., Duncan, D., and Fishman, L. M. (1972). *Clin. Sci.* **43,** 275–287.

Epstein, M., Pins, D. S., Arrington, R., Denunzio, A. G., and Engström, R. (1975). *J. Appl. Physiol.* **39,** 66–70.

Epstein, S. E., Beiser, G. D., Stampfer, M., and Braunwald, E. (1968a). *J. Clin. Invest.* **47,** 139–152.

Epstein, S. E., Stampfer, M., and Busie, G. D. (1968b). *Circulation* **37,** 524–533.

Farhi, L. E., Hesarjh, M. S., Olszoroka, J., Metilda, L. A., and Ellis, A. K. (1976). *Respir. Physiol.* **28,** 141–159.

Fedorov, B. M., Tkachev, V. V., Timova, L. A., and Kul'kov, E. N. (1976). *Hum. Physiol.* **2**(5), 588–593.

Federova, I. V., and Shurova, I. F. (1973). *Space Biol. Med.* **7**(2), 17–21.

Folkow, B. (1955). *Physiol. Rev.* **35,** 629–663.

Folkow, B. (1960). *Physiol. Rev.* **40,** Suppl. 4, 93–99.

Friman, G., and Hamrin, E. (1976). *Upsala J. Med. Sci.* **81**(2), 79–83.

Galkin, A. M., Gorlov, O. G., Kotova, A. R., Kosov, I. I., Petrov, A. V., Serov, A. D., Chernov, V. N., Yakolev, V. I., and Popov, V. I. (1962). *Aerosp. Med.* **33,** 1056–1068 (as cited by J. P. Henry).

Galle, R. R., Usachev, V. V., Gavrilova, L. N., Yelkina, L. G., Yelkin, P. A., Krikun, I. S., Ovechkin, V. G., and Ustyushin, B. V. (1976). *Space Biol. Aerosp. Med.* **10**(4), 49–57.

Gatts. J. D., and Beard, D. A. (1967). "Human Factors Suitability of the Gravitational Acceleration Simulation Suit (GASS)," Final Rep. Fairchild Hiller Corp., Framingdale, New York.

Gauer, O. H. (1950). "The Physiological Effects of Prolonged Acceleration in German Aviation Medicine, World War II," Vol. I, pp. 534–583. Dept. of the Air Force, Washington, D. C.

Gauer, O. H. (1971). *In* "Hypogravic and Hypodynamic Environments" (R. H. Murray and M. McCally, eds.), NASA SP-269, pp. 345–355. NASA, Washington, D.C.

Gauer, O. H., and Thron, H. L. (1963). *In* "Handbook of Physiology" (W. F. Hamilton and P. Dow, eds.), Sect. 2, Vol. III, pp. 2409–2439. Williams & Wilkins, Baltimore, Maryland.

Gauer, O. H., and Zuidema, G. D. (1961). "Gravitation Stress in Aerospace Medicine." Little, Brown, Boston, Massachusetts.

Gauer, O. H., Henry, J. P., and Behn, C. (1970). *Annu. Rev. Physiol.* **32,** 547–596.

Gayevskaya, M. S., Veresotskaya, N. A., Kolganova, N. S., Kolchina, Ye. V., Kurkina, L. M., and Nosova, Ye. A. (1976). *Space Biol. Aerosp. Med.* **2**(5), 49–53.

Gazenko, O. G., Il'in, Ye. A., and Parfenov, G. P. (1974). "Biological Research in Space (Some Conclusions and Prospects)," NASA TTF-15, 961, pp. 1–26. NASA, Washington, D.C.

Gazenko, O. G., Fedorov, B. M., Pikus, V. G., Tarannikova, V. A., and Sinitsyna, T. M. (1976). *Dokl. Akad. Nauk SSSR* **230**(5), 1240–1241.

Genin, A. M., and Kakurin, L. I. (1972). *Space Biol. Med.* **6**(4), 26–28.

Genin, A. M., Sorokin, P. A., Gurvich, G. I., Dzhamgarov, T. T., Panov, A. G., Ivanov, I. I., and Pestov, I. D. (1969). *Probl. Space Bio.* **13,** 256–262.

Georgiyevskiy, V. S., and Mikhaylov, B. M. (1968). *Space Biol. Med.* **2**(3), 73–77.

Georgiyevskiy, V. S., Kakurin, L. I., Katkovskiy, B. S., and Senkevich, Yu. A. (1966). *In* "The

Oxygen Regime of the Organism and Its Regulation" (N. V. Lauer and A. Z. Kolchinskaya, eds.), pp. 181–184. Naukova Dumka, Kiev, USSR.

Georgiyevskiy, V. S., Gornago, V. A., Divina, L. Ya., Kalmykova, V. M., Plakhatnyuk, V. I., Pometov, Yu. D. Smyshlyayeva, V. V., Vikharev, N. D., and Katkovskiy, B. S. (1973). *Space Biol. Med.* **7** (6), 88–97.

Gilbert, C. A., and Stevens, P. M. (1966). *J. Appl. Physiol.* **21**, 1265–1272.

Goetz, K. L., Bond, G. C., and Bloxham, D. D. (1975). *Physiol. Rev.* **55**, 157–205.

Golarz, M. N., and Bourne, G. H. (1972). *Aviat. Space Med., Proc. Int. Congr.,* (abstract).

Golarz, M. N., Bourne, G. H., McClure, H., and Keeling, M. (1973). *Aerosp. Med. Assoc. Prepr.* p. 295–296.

Golarz, M. N., Bourne, G. H., McClure, H. M., and Keeling, M. (1974). *Proc. Int. Congr. Primatol., 5th. 1974* p. 508.

Golarz, M. N., Stone, H. L., Bourne, G. H., Sandler, H., and McClure, H. (1977). *Aerosp. Med. Assoc. Prepr.* p. 213.

Goldwater, D., Sandler, H., Rositano, S., and McCutcheon, E. P. (1977). *Aerosp. Med. Assoc, Prepr.* pp. 240–241.

Gowen, R. J., Montgomery, L. D., McCutcheon, E. P., and Sandler, H. (1977). *Aerospace Med. Assoc. Prepr.* pp. 158–159.

Graveline, D. E. (1962). *Aerosp. Med.* **33**(3), 297–302.

Graveline, D. E., and Barnard, G. W. (1961). *Aerosp. Med.* **32**, 726–736.

Graveline, D. E., and Jackson, M. M. (1962). *J. Appl. Physiol.* **17**, 519–524.

Graveline, D. E., Balke, B., McKenzie, R. E., and Hartman, B. (1961). *Aerosp. Med.* **32**, 387–409.

Graybiel, A., and Clark, B. (1961). *Aerosp. Med.* **32**, 181–196.

Graybiel, A., Holmes, R. H., Beischer, D. E., Champlin, G. E., Pedigo, G. P., Hixson, C., Davis, T. R. A., Barr, N. L., Kistler, W. G., Niven, J. I., Wilbarger, E., Stullken, D. E., Augerson, W. D., Clarke, R., and Berrian, J. H. (1959). *Aerosp. Med.* **30**, 871–931.

Greenleaf, J. E., Van Beaumont, W., Bernauer, E. M., Haines, R. F., Sandler, H., Staley, R. W., Young, H. L., and Yusken, J. W. (1973a). *Aerosp. Med.* **44**, 715–722.

Greenleaf, J. E., Young, H. L., Bernauer, E. M., Armbruster, R. H., Sagan, L. A., Staley, R. W., Juhos, L., Van Beaumont, W., and Sandler, H. (1973b). *Aerosp. Med. Assoc. Prepr.* pp. 23–24.

Greenleaf, J. E., Haines, R. F., Bernauer, E. M., Morse, J. T., Sandler, H., Armbruster, R., Sagan, L., and Van Beaumont, W. (1975). *Aviat., Space, Environ. Med.* **46**, 671–678.

Greenleaf, J. E., Greenleaf, C. J., Van Derveer, D., and Dorchak, K. J. (1976). "Adaptation to Prolonged Bed Rest in Man: A Compendium of the Research," NASA TMX-3307, pp. 1–150. NASA, Washington, D.C.

Greenleaf, J. E., Bernauer, E. M., Young, H. L., Morse, J. T., Staley, R. W., Juhos, L. T., and Van Beaumont, W. (1977a). *J. Appl. Physiol.* **42**, 59–66.

Greenleaf, J. E., Stinnett, H. O., Davis, G. L., Kollias, J., and Bernauer, E. M. (1977b). *J. Appl. Physiol.* **42**, 67–73.

Greenleaf, J. E., Bernauer, E. M., Juhos, L. T., Young, H. L., Morse, J. T., and Staley, R. W. (1977c). *J. Appl. Physiol.* **43**, 126–132.

Greenleaf, J. E., Brock, P. J., Haines, R. F., Rositano, S. E., Montgomery, L. D., and Keil, L. C. (1977d). *Aviat. Space, Environ. Med.* **48**, 693–700.

Grigor'yev, A. I. (1971). *Curr. Probl. Space Biol. Med.* pp. 31–32.

Grigor'yev, A. I. (1978). *Space Biol. Aerosp. Med.* **12**(3), 38–43.

Grigor'yev, A. I., Pak, Z. P., Koloskova, Yu. S., Kozyrevskaya, G. I., Korotayev, M. M., and Bezumova, Yu. Ye. (1976). *Space Biol. Aerosp. Med.* **10**(4), 83–89.

Gurovskiy, N. N., and Kiselev, A. A. (1973). "Physiological Problems of Prolonged Weightlessness," NASA TT-F-14672, pp. 1–14. NASA, Washington, D.C.

Gurvich, G. I., and Yefimenko, G. D. (1967). *Space Biol. Med.* 1(3), 97–102.

Gurvich, G. I., Marishchuk, V. L., Tishchenko, M. I., Yefimenko, G. D., and Khvoynov, B. S. (1967). *Space Biol. Med.* 1(4), 114–118.

Haines, R. F. (1973a). *Aerosp. Med.* 44(4), 425–432.

Haines, R. F. (1973b). *Aerosp. Med. Assoc. Prepr.* pp. 17–18.

Haines, R. F. (1973c). *J. Appl. Physiol.* 34, 329–333.

Henry, J. P., and Mosely, J. D. (1963). *In* "Results of the Project Mercury Balistic and Orbital Chimpanzee Flights," NASA SP-39, pp. 1–71. NASA, Washington, D.C.

Henry, J. P., Augerson, W. S., Belleville, R. E., Douglas, W. K., Grunzke, M. K., Johnston, R. S., Laughlin, P. C., Mosely, J. D., Rohles, F. H., Voas, R. B., and White, S. C. (1962). *Aerosp. Med.* 33, 1056–1068.

Herron, R. E., and Keys, C. W. (1977). "JSC/Methodist Hospital 28-Day Bedrest Study," Vol. II, NAS 9–14578. Johnson Space Center, Houston, Texas.

Hoffler, G. W., and Johnson, K. I. (1975). *In* "Biomedical Results of Apollo," NASA SP-368, pp. 227–264. NASA, Washington, D.C.

Hoffler, G. W., Wolthuis, R. A., and Johnson, R. L. ((1971). *Aerosp. Med. Assoc Prepr.* pp. 174–175.

Hoffler, G. W., Bergman, S. A., Johnson, R. L., Nicogossian, A. E., and Jackson, M. M. (1976). "Report of a 14-Day Bedrest Simulation of Skylab," NASA CR-147758. Texas Methodist Hospital, Houston.

Hoffler, G. W., Baker, J. T., Johnson, R. L., and Crosier, W. (1977). "JSC/Methodist Hospital 28-day Bedrest Study," Vol. II, NAS 9–14578. Johnson Space Center, Houston, Texas.

Homick, J. L., Reschke, M. F., Moore, M. J., and Anderson, D. J. (1977). "JSC/Methodist Hospital 28-Day Bedrest Study," Vol. II, NAS 9–14578. Johnson Space Center, Houston, Texas.

Hordinskiy, J. R. (1977). *In* "Biomedical Results from Skylab" (R. S. Johnson and L. F. Dietlein, eds.), NASA SP-377, pp. 30–35. NASA, Washington, D.C.

Howard, P. H. (1965). *In* "Textbook of Aviation Physiology" (J. A. Gillies, ed.), pp. 551–688. Pergamon, Oxford.

Hunt, N. C. (1967). *Aerosp. Med. Assoc. Prepr.* pp. 52–53.

Hyatt, K. H. (1970). "A Study of the Role of Extravascular Dehydration in the Production of Cardiovascular Deconditioning by Simulated Weightlessness (Bedrest)," Parts 1 and 2, Final Rep. U.S. Public Health Service Hospital, San Francisco, California.

Hyatt, K. H. (1971). *In* "Hypogravice and Hypodynamic Environments" (R. H. Murray and M. McCally, eds.), NASA SP-269, pp. 197–199. NASA, Washington, D.C.

Hyatt, K. H., and West, D. A. (1976). *USPHS Prof. Assoc. Prepr.* p. 38.

Hyatt, K. H., and West, D. A. (1977). *Aviat., Space, Environ. Med.* 48, 120–124.

Hyatt, K. H., Kamenetsky, L. G.. and Smith, W. M. (1969). *Aerosp. Med.* 40(6), 644–650.

Hyatt, K. H., Johnson, P. C., Hoffler, G. W., Rambaut, P. C., Rummel, J. A., Hulley, S. B., Vogel, J. M., Huntoon, C., and Spears, W. R. (1973). *Aerosp. Med. Assoc. Prepr.* pp. 100–101.

Hyatt, K. H., Jacobson, L. B., and Schneider, V. S. (1975). *Aviat., Space, Environ. Med.* 46, 801–806.

Ibrahim, M. M., Tarazi, R. C., and Dustan, H. P. (1975). *Am. Heart J.* 90, 513–520.

Ioffe, L. A., Stoyda, Yu. M., and Vasil'yeva, T. D. (1966). *Probl. Aerosp. Med.* pp. 237–238.

Ioffe, L. A., Abrikosova, M. A., and Stoyda, Yu. M. (1968). *Teor. Prakt. Fiz. Kul't.* 2, 33–40.

Isabayeva, V. A., and Ponomareva, T. A. (1973). *Space Biol. Med.* 7(1), 84–91.

Iseyev, L. R., and Katkovskiy, B. S. (1968a). *Space Biol. Med.* **2**, 67–72.

Iseyev, L. R., and Katkovskiy, B. S. (1968b). *Space Biol. Med.* **2**(4), 117–124.

Iseyeva, L. R., and Nefedov, Yu. G. (1968). *Space Biol. Med.* **2**(1), 60–65.

Ivanov, L. A. (1972). *Space Biol. Med.* **6**(1), 123–129.

Ivanov, L. A., and Orlov, P. A. (1973). *Byull. Eksp. Biol. Med.* **76**(7), 35–37.

Jacobson, L. B., Hyatt, K. H., Sullivan, R. W., Cantor, S. A., and Sandler, H. (1973). "Evaluation of +G_z Tolerance Following Simulated Weightlessness (Bedrest)," NASA TM X-62311, pp. 1–91. NASA-Ames Res. Cent., Moffett Field, California.

Jacobson, L. B., Hyatt, K. H., and Sandler, H. (1974). *J. Appl. Physiol.* **36**, 745–752.

Johnson, P. C., and Driscoll, T. (1977). "JSC/Methodist Hospital 28-Day Bedrest Study," Vol. II, NAS 9–14578. Johnson Space Center, Houston, Texas.

Johnson, P. C., Fisher, C. L., and Leach, C. (1971a). *In* "Hypogravic and Hypodynamic Environments" (R. H. Murray and M. McCally, eds.), NASA SP-269, pp. 27–34. NASA, Washington, D.C.

Johnson, P. C., Driscoll, T. B., and Carpentier, W. R. (1971b). *Aerosp. Med.* **42**, 875–878.

Johnson, R. L., Hoffler, C. W., Nicogossian, A. E., Bergman, S. A., Jr., and Jackson, M. M. (1977). *In* "Biomedical Results from Skylab" (R. S. Johnson and L. F. Dietlein, eds.), NASA SP-377, pp. 284–312. NASA, Washington, D.C.

Kaiser, D., and Gauer, O. H. (1966). *Pflüegers Arch. Gesamte Physiol. Menschen Tiere* **289**, 76–77.

Kaiser, D., Eckert, P., Gauer, O. H., and Linkenbach, H. J. (1963). *Pflüegers Arch. Gesamte Physiol. Menschen Tiere* **278**, 52–53.

Kaiser, D., Linkenbach, H. J., and Gauer, O. H. (1969). *Pflüegers Arch.* **308**, 166–173.

Kakurin, L. I. (1968). *Space Biol. Med.* **2**(2), 85–91.

Kakurin, L. I. (1976). *US/USSR Conf. Space Biol. Med., 8th, 1975* NASA TT-F 17285, pp. 1–32.

Kakurin, L. I. (1978). Intercosmos Council, Academy of Sciences, USSR, NASA TM-75075, pp. 1–26. NASA, Washington, D.C.

Kakurin, L. I., Katkovskiy, B. S., Kozlov, A. N., and Mukharlyamov, N. M. (1963). *In* "Aviation and Space Medicine" (V. V. Parin, ed.), pp. 192–194. Akad. Med. Nauk, Moscow.

Kakurin, L. I., Akhrem-Akhremovich, R. M., Vanyushina, Yu. V., Vartbaronov, R. A., Georgiyevskiy, V. S., Katkovskiy, B. S., Kotovskaya, A. R., Mukharlyamov, N. M., Panferova, N. Ye., Pushkar', Yu. T., Senkevich, Yu. A., Simpura, S. F., Cherepakhin, M. A., and Shamrov, P. G. (1966). *In* "Materials from a Conference on Space Biology and Medicine" (A. V. Lebedinsiy, Yu. G. Nefedov, and I. M. Khazen, eds.), pp. 110 117. Akad. Med. Nauk, Moscow.

Kakurin, L. I., Yegorov, B. B., Il'ina, Ye. I., and Cherepakhin, M. A. (1976). *In* "Int. Symp. Basic Environ. Prob. Man in Space" (A. Graybiel, ed.), pp. 241–247. Pergamon, Oxford.

Kakurin, L. I., Katkovskiy, B. S., Georgiyenskiy, V. S., Purakin, Yu. N., Cherepakhin, M. A., Mikhaylov, V. M., Petukhov, B. N., and Biryukov, Ye. N. (1970). *Vopr. Kurortol. Fizioter. Lech. Fiz. Kul't.* **35**(1), 19–24.

Kakurin, L. I., Lobachik, V. I., Mikhaylov, V. M., and Senkevich, U. A. (1976). *Aviat., Space, Environ. Med.* **47**(10), 1083–1086.

Kakurin, L. I., Katkovskiy, B. S., Tishler, V. A., Kozyrevskaya, V. S., Shashkov, V. S., Georgiyevskiy, V. S., Grigor'yev, A. I., Mikhaylov, V. M., Anashkin, O. D., Machinskiy, G. V., Savilov, A. A., and Tikhomirov, Ye. P. (1978a). *Space Biol. Aerosp. Med.* **12**(3), 23–31.

Kakurin, L. I., Arzamazov, G. S., and Grigor'yev, A. I. (1978b). *Space Biol. Aerosp. Med.* **12**(4), 14–20.

Karapu, V. Ya., and Ferents, A. I. (1978). *Arkh. Anat., Gistol. Embriol.* **1**, 28–37.

Katkovskiy, B. S. (1966). *In* "The Oxygen Regime of the Organism and Its Regulation" (N. V. Lauer and A. Z. Kolchinskaya, eds.), pp. 231–235. Naukova Dumka, Kiev, USSR.

Katkovskiy, B. S. (1967). *Space Biol. Med.* 1(5), 100–107.

Katkovskiy, B. S., and Pometov, Yu. D. (1971a). *Space Biol. Med.* 5(3), 105–113.

Katkovskiy, B. S., and Pometov, Yu. D. (1971b). *Space Biol. Med.* 5(3), 69–74.

Katkovskiy, B. S., and Pometov, Yu. D. (1976). *In* "Life Sciences and Space Research XIV" (P. N. A. Sneath, ed.), pp. 301–305. Akademie-Verlag, Berlin.

Katkovskiy, B. S., Pilysvskiy, O. A., and Smirnova, G. I. (1969). *Space Biol. Med.* 3(2), 77–85.

Katkovskiv, B. S., Georgiyevskiy, V. S., Cherepakhin, M. A., Purakhin, Yu. N., Kakurin, L. I., Vysotskiy, V. G., Petukhov, B. N., Mikhaylov, V. M., Machinskiy, G. V., Pometov, Yu. D., Ivanov, P. P., Laricheva, K. A., and Ushakov, A. S. (1971). *Vopr. Pitan.* 4, 55–59.

Katkovskiy, B. S., Machinskiy, G. V., Toman, P. S., Danilova, D. I., and Demida, B. F. (1974). *Space Biol. Aerosp. Med.* 8(4), 62–68.

Katz, F. H. (1964). *Aerosp. Med.* 35(9), 849–851.

Kiselev, R. K., Balakhovskiy, I. S., and Virovets, O. A. (1975). *Space Biol. Aerosp. Med.* 9(5), 130–136.

Kolenchenko, V. V., Asyamolov, B. F., and Zhernakov, A. F. (1976). *Space Biol. Aerosp. Med.* 10(5), 18–23.

Kollias, J., Van Derveer, D., Dorchak, K. J., and Greenleaf, J. E. (1976). "Physiologic Responses to Water Immersion in Man: A Compendium of the Research," NASA TM X-3308, pp. 1–87. NASA, Washington, D.C.

Kolpakhov, M. G., Tarasevich, V. P., and Markel', A. L. (1970). *Space Biol. Med.* 4(4), 52–56.

Korobkov, A. V., Ioffe, L. A., Abriksova, M. A., and Stoida, Yu. M. (1968). *Space Biol. Med.* 2(3), 48–57.

Korolev, B. A. (1968a). *Space Biol. Med.* 2(5), 79–85.

Korolev, B. A. (1968b). *Space Biol. Med.* 2(6), 127–134.

Korolev, B. A. (1969). *Space Biol. Med.* 3(5), 96–101.

Korol'kov, V. I., and Mirrakhimov, M. M. (1976). *Space Biol. Aerosp. Med.* 10(6), 26–52.

Korol'kov, V. I., Savilov, A. A., and Lunev, I. Y. (1973). *Space Biol. Med.* 6(6), 94–100.

Korol'kov, V. I., Mirrakhimov, M. M., Dzhaylobayev, A. D., Nerbekov, O. N., Yusupova, N. Ya., and Verigo, V. V. (1976). *Space Biol. Aerosp. Med.* 10(1), 39–45.

Korol'kov, V. I., Kovalenko, Ye. A., Krotov, V. P., Ilyusho, N. A., Kondrat'yeva, V. A., and Kondrat'yev, Yu. I. (1977). *Pathol. Fiziol. Eksp. Ter.* 6, 32–35.

Kotovskaya, A. R., Kakurin, L. I., Konnova, N. I., Simpura, S. F., and Grishina, I. S. (1965). *Probl. Space Biol.* 4, 333–342.

Kotovskaya, A. R., Vartbaranov, R. V., and Simpura, S. F. (1969). *Probl. Space Biol.* 13, 248–255.

Kovalenko, E. A. (1976). *Space Biol. Aerosp. Med.* 10(1), 3–15.

Kovalenko, E. A., and Krotov, V. P. (1975). *Patol. Fiziol. Eksp.* 19(5), 64–68.

Krasnykh, I. G. *Voen.-Med. Zh.* 12, 54–56.

Krasnykh, I. G. (1974). *Space Biol. Aerosp. Med.* 8(1), 98–103.

Krotov, V. P., and Romanovskaya, L. L. (1975). *Bull. Exp. Biol. Med.* (*Engl. Transl.*) 79(2), 116–118.

Krotov, V. P., Kovalenko, Ye. A., and Katuntsev, V. P. (1976). *Byull. Eksp. Biol. Med.* 81(3), 279–281.

Krotov, V. P., Titov, A. A., Kovalenko, Ye. A., Bogomolov, V. V., Stazhadze, L. I., and Masenko, V. P. (1977). *Space Biol. Aerosp. Med.* 11(1), 42–49.

Krupina, T. M., and Federov, B. M. (1977). *Fiziol. Chel.* 3(6), 997–1005.

Krupina, T. N., Tizul, A. Ya., Boglevskaya, N. M., Baranova, B. P., Matsnev, E. I., and Chertovskikh, Ye. A. (1967). *Space Biol. Med.* 1(5), 91–99.

Krupina, T. N., Federov, B. M., Benevolenskaya, T. V., Boykova, O. I., Nevstruyeva, V. S.,

Kul'kov, Ye. N., Morozov, R. S., and Romanov, V. S. (1971). *Space Biol. Med.* 5(2), 111–119.

Krupina, T. N., Fedorov, B. M., Filatova, L. M., Tsyganova, N. I., and Matsnev, E. I. (1976). *In* "Life Sciences and Space Research XIV" (P. N. A. Sneath, ed.), pp. 285–287. Akademie-Verlag, Berlin.

Kuz'min, M. P. (1973). *Space Biol. Med.* 7(2), 98.

LaFevers, E. V., Booher, C. R., Crozier, W. N., and Donaldson, J. (1977). "JSC/Methodist Hospital 28-Day Bedrest Study," Vol. II, NAS-9–14578. Johnson Space Center, Houston, Texas.

Lamb, L. E. (1964). *Aerosp. Med.* 35, 313–319.

Lamb, L. E. (1965). *Aerosp. Med.* 36(2), 97–100.

Lamb, L. E., and Stevens, P. M. (1965). *Aerosp. Med.* 36, 1145–1151.

Lamb, L. E., Johnson, R. L., Stevens, B. M., and Welch, B. E. (1964a). *Aerosp. Med.* 35, 420–428.

Lamb, L. E., Johnson, R. L., and Stevens, P. M. (1964b). *Aerosp. Med.* 35, 646–649.

Lamb, L. E., Stevens, P. M., and Johnson, R. L. (1965). *Aerosp. Med.* 36, 755–763.

Lancaster, M. D., and Triebwasser, J. H. (1971). *In* "Hypogravic and Hypodynamic Environments" (R. H. Murray and M. McCally, eds.), NASA SP-269, pp. 225–248. NASA, Washington, D.C.

Lange, I., Lange, S., Echt, M., and Gauer, O. H. (1974). *Pflüegers Arch.* 352, 219–226.

Leach, C. S., Johnson, P. C., and Driscoll, T. B. (1972). *Aerosp. Med.* 43(4), 400–402.

Leach, C. S., Hulley, S. B., Rambaut, P. C., and Dietlein, L. F. (1973). *Space Life Sci.* 4, 415–423.

Leverett, S. D., Jr., Shubrooks, S. J., and Shumate, W. (1971). *Aerosp. Med. Assoc. Prepr.* pp. 90–91.

Linden, R. J. (1973). *Circulation* 48, 463–480.

Lubin, A., Hord, D. J., Tracy, M. L., and Johnson, L. C. (1976). *Psychophysiology* 13(4), 334–339.

Lutwak, L., and Whedon, G. D. (1959). *Clin. Res.* 7, 143–144.

Lynch, T. N., Jensen, C. L., Stevens, R. M., Johnson, R. L., and Lamb, L. E. (1967). *Aerosp. Med.* 38, 10–20.

McCally, M. (1964). *Aerosp. Med.* 30, 130–132.

McCally, M. (1967). *Science J.* 3(11), 39–43.

McCally, M., and Graveline, D. E. (1963). *N. Engl. J. Med.* 269, 508–596.

McCally, M., and Wunder, C. C. (1971). *In* "Hypogravic and Hypodynamic Environments" (R. H. Murray and M. McCally, eds.), NASA SP-269, pp. 323–344. NASA, Washington, D.C.

McCally, M., Piemme, T. E., and Murray, R. H. (1966a). *Aerosp. Med.* 37, 1247–1249.

McCally, M., Thompson, L. J., and Heim, J. W. (1966b). *Fed. Proc., Fed. Am. Soc. Exp. Biol.* 25, 461.

McCally, M., Pohl, S. A., and Sampson, P. A. (1968). *Aerosp. Med.* 39, 722–734.

McCally, M., Kazarian, H. E., and von Gierke, H. E. (1971). *Proc. Int. Congr. Astron., Proc.* 21, 264–282.

McCutcheon, E. P., and Sandler, H. (1975). *Aerosp. Med. Assoc. Prepr.* pp. 163–164.

McDonald, C. D., Burch, G. E., and Walsh, J. J. (1971). *Ann. Intern. Med.* 74, 681–691.

McDonald, C. D., Burch, G. E., and Walsh, J. J. (1972). *Am. J. Med.* 52, 41–50.

McDonald, J. K., Reilly, T. J., Zeitman, B. B., Greenleaf, J. E., Sandler, H., and Ellis, S. (1974). *Aerosp. Med. Assoc. Prepr.* pp. 167–168.

Mack, P. B., Alford, B. B., Pyke, R. E., Klapper, A., and English, S. N. (1965). "Fundamental Investigation of Losses of Skeletal Mineral In Young Adult Human Males and Collaterally in Young Adult Male Pigtail Monkeys (Macacus Nemestrima) through Immobilization for Varying Periods of Time, Coupled with a Study of Methods of Preventing or Reducing Mineral Loss," NASA CR-63993. Texas Woman's University, Denton.

Makarov, G. F. (1970). *Space Biol. Med.* 4, 64–67.

Maksimov, D. G., and Domracheva, M. V. (1976). *Space Biol. Aerosp. Med.* 10(5), 72–80.

Maksimov, V. A., Vyazitskiy, P. O., Slyusar, I. B., and Ivanov, S. L. (1978). *Voen.-Med. Zh.* 2, 73–75.

Meehan, J. P., and Jacobs, H. (1959). "Relation of Several Physiological Parameters to Positive G," Tech. Doc. 58–665. NASA, Washington, D.C.

Meehan, J. P., and Henry, J. P., Brunjes, S., and de Vries, H. (1966). "Investigation to Determine the Effects of Long-Term Bed Rest on G-Tolerance and on Psychomotor Performance," NASA CR-62073. University of Southern California, Los Angeles.

Melada, G. A., Goldman, R. H., Leutscher, J. A., and Zager, P. G. (1975). *Aviat., Space, Environ. Med.* 46(8), 1049–1055.

Menninger, R. P., Mains, R. C., Zechman, F. W., and Piemme, T. A. (1969). *Aerosp. Med.* 40, 1323–1326.

Michel, E. L., Rummel, J. A., Sawin, C. F., Buderer, M. C., and Lem, J. D. (1977). *In* "Biomedical Results from Skylab" (R. S. Johnson and L. F. Dietlein, eds.), NASA SP-377, pp. 372–387. NASA, Washington, D.C.

Mikhaylov, V. M., and Georgiyevskiy, V. S. (1976). *Space Biol. Aerosp. Med.* 10(6), 56–63.

Mikhaylovskiy, G. P., Benevolenskaya, T. V., Petrova, T. A., Yakoleva, I. Ya., Boykova, O. I., Kuzmin, M. P., Savilov, A. A., and Solov'yeva, S. N. (1967). *Space Biol. Med.* 1(5), 86–90.

Miller, P. B. (1965). *Tex. J. Med.* 61, 720–724.

Miller, P. B., and Leverett, S. D., Jr. (1963). "Tolerance to Transverse ($+G_x$) and headward ($+G_z$) Acceleration after Prolonged Bed Rest," School of Aerospace Medicine, Brooks AFB, Texas.

Miller, P. B., and Leverett, S. D., Jr. (1965). *Aerosp. Med.* 36, 13–15.

Miller, P. B., Hartman, B. O., Johnson, R. L., and Lamb, L. E. (1964a). *Aerosp. Med.* 35, 931–939.

Miller, P. B., Johnson, R. L., and Lamb, L. E. (1964b). *Aerosp. Med.* 35(12), 1194–1200.

Miller, P. B., Johnson, R. L., and Lamb, L. E. (1965). "Effects of Moderate Physical Exercise during Four Weeks of Bed Rest on Circulatory Function in Man," SAM-TR-65-263. Brooks AFB, Texas.

Montgomery, L. D., Kirk, P. J., Payne, R. A., Gerber, R. L., Nerton, S. D., and Williams, B. A. (1977). *Aviat., Space, Environ. Med.* 48, 138–145.

Morse, B. S. (1967). "Erythrokinetic Changes in Man Associated with Bed Rest," Lect. Aerosp. Med. (6th ser.), NTIS No. AD-665–107, pp. 240–254. School of Aerospace Medicine, Brooks AFB, Texas.

Musgrave, F. S., Zechman, F. W., and Mains. R. C. (1969). *Aerosp. Med.* 40, 602–606.

Musgrave, F. S., Zechman, F. W., and Mains, R. C. (1971). *Aerosp. Med.* 42, 1065–1069.

Myasnikov, A. L., Akhrem-Akhremovich, R. M., Kakurin, L. I., Pushkar', Yu. T., Mukharlyamov, N. M., Georgiyevskiy, V. S., Tokarev, Yu. N., Senkevich, Yu. A., Katkovskiy, B. S., Kalinina, A. N., Cherepakhin, M. A., Chichkin, V. A., Filosofov, V. K.. and Shamrov, P. G. (1963). *In* "Aviation and Space Medicine" (V. V. Parin, ed.), pp. 316–318. Akad. Med. Nauk SSSR, Moscow.

Newsom, B. D., Goldenrath, W. L., Winter, W. R., and Sandler, H. (1977). *Aviat., Space, Environ. Med.* 48, 327–331.

Nicogossian, A. (1977). "The Apollo-Soyuz Test Project," NASA SP-411, pp. 1–129. NASA, Washington, D.C.

Nixon, J. V., Murrary. R. G., Bryant, C., Johnson, R. L., Mitchell, J. H., Holland, O. B., Gomez-Sanchez, C., Vergne-Marini, P., and Blomquist, C. G. (1979). *J. Appl. Physiol.* **46**, 541–548.

Novikov, I. I., and Vlasov, V. B. (1976). *USSR East. Eur. Sci. Abstr., Biomed. Behav. Sci.* **59**, 9.

Oberfield, R. A., Ebaugh, F. G., Jr., O'Hanlon, E. P., and Schoaf, M. (1968). *Aerosp. Med.* **39**, 10–13.

Olree, H. D., Corbin, B., Dugger, G., and Smith, C. (1973). "An Evaluation of the Effects of Bed Rest, Sleep Deprivation, and Discontinuance of Training on the Physical Fitness of Highly Trained Young Men," NASA CR-134044. Harding College, Searcy, Arkansas.

Oganov, V. G. (1977). "Dynamics and Certain Mechanisms of the Changes of Skeletal Muscular Systems of Man under Bed Rest Conditions," NASA TM-75073, pp. 1–40. NASA, Washington, D. C.

Pace, N., Grunbaum, B. W., Kodama, A. M., and Price, D. C. (1974). "In Vivo Measurement of Human Body Composition," NASA CR-143375, SASR-5, Rep. No. 5. White Mountain Research Station, University of California, Berkeley.

Pace, N., Grunbaum, B. W., Kodama, A. M., Price, D. C., and Newsom, B. D. (1975). *Aerosp. Med. Assoc. Prepr.* pp. 143–144.

Pak, Z. P., Kozyrevkaya, G. I., Koloskova, Yu. S., Grigor'yev, A. I., Bezumova, Yu. Ye.,, and Biryukov, Ye. N. (1973). *Space Biol. Med.* **7**(4), 86–91.

Panferova, N. Ye. (1972). *Space Biol. Med.* **6**(2), 74–79.

Panferova, N. Ye., Tishler, V. A., and Popava, T. G. (1967). *Space Biol. Med.* **1**(6). 111–122.

Panov, A. G., and Lobzin, V. S. (1968). *Space Biol. Med.* **2**(4), 103–116.

Parin, V. V., Krupina, T. N., Mikhaylovskiy, G. P., and Tizul, A. Ya. (1971). *Space Biol. Med.* **4**(5), 91–98.

Pekshev, A. P. (1969). *Probl. Space Biol.* **13**, 43–51.

Pelletier, C. L., and Shepherd, J. T. (1973). *Circ. Res.* **33**, 131–138.

Pestov, I. D. (1968). *Int. Astron. Congr., Proc.* **19**, in English, NTIS No. N69–14025, pp. 1–13.

Pestov, I. D., and Asyamolov, B. F. (1972). *Space Biol. Med.* **6**(4), 95–102.

Pestov, I. D., Tishchenko, M. I., Korolev, B. A., Asyamolov, B. F., Simonenko, V. V., and Baykov, A. Ye. (1969). *Probl. Space Biol.* **13**, 238–247.

Pestov, I. D., Panchenko, V. S., and Asyamolov, B. F. (1974). *Space Biol. Aerosp. Med.* **8**(4), 75–80.

Pometov, Yu. D., and Katkovskiy, B. S. (1972). *Space Biol. Med.* **6**(4), 62–73.

Portugalov, V. V., Ivanov, A. A., and Shvets, V. N. (1976). *Space Biol. Aerosp. Med.* **10**(2), 84–86.

Prokhazka, I., Khavkina, V., and Barbashova, Z. I. (1973). *Fiziol. Zh. SSSR in I. M. Sechenova* **59**(8), 1237–1241.

Pruss, G. M., and Kuznetsov, V. I. (1972). *Space Biol. Aerosp. Med.* **8**(6), 45–49.

Purakhin, Yu., Kakurin, L. I., Georgiyevskiy, V. S., Petukhov, B. N., and Mikhaylov, V. M. (1972). *Space Biol. Med.* **6**(6), 74–82.

Rambaut, P. C., Heidelbaugh, N. D., and Smith, M. C., Jr. (1973). *Aerosp. Med. Assoc. Prepr.* pp. 96–97.

Reck, G., Beckerhoff, R., Vetter, W., Armbruster, H., and Siegenthaler, W. (1975). *Klin. Wochenschr.* **53**(20), 955–959.

Remington, J. W., and Wood, E. H. (1956). *J. Appl. Physiol.* **9**, 433–442.

Rinks, D. (1977). *In* "JSC/Methodist Hospital 28-Day Bedrest Study" (P. C. Johnson and C. Mitchell, eds.), Vol. II, NAS 9–14578. Johnson Space Center, Houston. Texas.

Rokotova, N. A., Bogina, I. D., Bolotina, O. P., Kucherenko, T. M., Rogovenko, Ye. S., and Shevkin, R. L. (1962). *Probl. Space Biol.* **2**, 424–434.

Romanov, V. S. (1976). *Space Biol. Aerosp. Med.* **10**(4), 74–82.

Roth, E. M., Teichner, W. G., and Craig, R. L. (1968). "Compendium of Human Responses to the Aerospace Environment," Vol. II, NASA CR-1205. NASA, Washington, D.C.

Rummel, J. A., Swain, C. F., and Michel, E. L. (1975). "Biomedical Results of Apollo," NASA SP-368, pp. 265–275. NASA, Washington, D.C.

Rushmer, R. F. (1959). *Physiol. Rev.* **39,** 41.

Rushmer, R. F. (1970). "Cardiovascular Dynamics," 3rd ed., pp. 89–98. Saunders, Philadelphia, Pennsylvania.

Rushmer, R. F., and Smith, O. A., Jr. (1959). *Physiol. Rev.* **39,** 41–68.

Saltin, B., and Steinberg, J. (1964). *J. Appl. Physiol.* **19,** 833.

Saltin, B., Blomquist, G., Mitchell, J. H., Johnson, R. L., Jr., Wildenthal, K., and Chapman, C. B. (1968). *Circulation* **38,** Suppl. 7, 1–78.

Sandler, H. (1976). *In* "Progress in Cardiology" (P.N. Yu and J. F. Goodwin, eds.), pp. 227–270. Lea and Febiger, Philadelphia, Pennsylvania.

Sandler, H. (1977). *In* "The Use of Nonhuman Primates in Space" (R. Simmonds and G. H. Bourne, eds.), NASA Conf. Pub. 005, pp. 3–21. NASA, Washington, D.C.

Sandler, H., and Winter, D. L. (1978). "Physiological Responses of Women to Simulated Weightlessness: A Review of the Significant Findings of the First Female Bed-Rest Study," NASA SP-430, pp. 1–87. NASA, Washington, D.C.

Sandler. H., Greenleaf, J. E., Young, H. L., Bernauer, E. M., Morse, J. T., Staley, R. W., Haines, R. F., and Van Beaumont, W. (1973). *Aerosp. Med. Assoc. Prepr.* pp. 21–22.

Sandler, H., Rositano, S. A., and McCutcheon, E. P. (1976). *Int. Astronaut. Congr., Proc.* **27,** IAF-76-034, pp. 1–7.

Sandler, H., Popp, R., and McCutcheon, E. P. (1977). *Aerosp. Med. Assoc. Prepr.* pp. 242–243.

Sandler, H., Webb, P., Annis, J. F., and Newsom, B. D. In preparation.

Schmid, P. G., Shaver, J. A., McCally, M., Bensy, J. J., Pawlson, L. G., and Piemme, T. E. (1968). *Aerosp. Med. Assoc. Prepr.* p. 104

Schmid, P. G., McCally, M., Piemme, T. E., and Shaver, J. A. (1971). *In* "Hypogravic and Hypodynamic Environments" (R. H. Murray and M. McCally, eds.), NASA SP-269, pp. 211–224. NASA, Washington, D.C.

Schneider, V. S., Hulley, S. B., Donaldson, C. L., Vogel, J. M., Rosen, S. N., Hartman, D. A., Lockwood, D. R., Seid, D., Hyatt, K. H., and Jacobson, L. B. (1974). "Prevention of Bone Mineral Changes Induced by Bed Rest," NASA CR-141453. Public Health Service Hospital, San Francisco, California.

Schønheyder, F., and Christensen, P. J. (1957). *Scand. J. Clin. Lab. Invest.* **9,** 107–108.

Shepherd, J. T. (1966). *Circulation* **33,** 484.

Shtykhno, Yu. M., and Udovichenko, V. I. (1978). *Vestn. Akad. Med. Nauk SSSR* **2,** 68–71.

Shulzhenko, E. B., Vil'-Vil'yams, I. F., Khudiakova, M. A., and Grigor'yev, A. I. (1976). *Life Sci. Space Res.* **14,** 289–294.

Shurygin, D. Ya., Sidorov, K. A., Mazurov, V. I., and Alekseyeva, N. M. (1976). *Mil. Med. J.* **12,** 55–58.

Shvartz, E., Battacharya, A., Brock, P., Greenleaf, J., Haines, R. F., Keil, L., Kravik, S., Morse, J., and Sciaraffa, D. (1977). "The Effects of Heat Acclimatization and Exercise Training on Deconditioning Following Water Immersion," Intern. Rep., pp. 1–20. NASA-Ames Research Center, Moffett Field, California.

Simonenko, V. V. (1969). *Probl. Space Biol.* **13,** 34–42.

Sjöstrand, T. (1955). *Physiol. Rev.* **33,** 202–228.

Smirnova, G. I. (1971). *Curr. Probl. Space Biol. Med.* pp. 97–98.

Smith, R. F., Stoop, K., Brown, D., Jansuz, W., and King, P., (1977). *In* "Biomedical Results from Skylab" (R. S. Johnson and L. F. Dietlein, eds.), NASA SP-377, pp. 339–350. NASA, Washington, D.C.

Smith, W. M., Hyatt, K. H., and Kamenetsky, L. G. (1966). *Aerosp. Med. Assoc. Prepr.* pp. 166–167.

Sokolkov, V. I. (1971). *Probl. Space Biol.* (abstract).

Sorokin, P. A., Simonenko, V. V., and Korolev, B. A. (1969). *Probl. Space Biol.* **13**, 15–25.

Spealman, C. R., Bixby, E. W., Wiley, J. L., and Newton, M. (1948). *J. Appl. Physiol.* **1**, 242–253.

Spears, W. R., Hyatt, K. H., Vetter, W. R., and Sullivan, R. W. (1973). *Aerosp. Med. Assoc. Prepr.* pp. 102–103.

Speckman, E. W., Smith, K. J., Offner, K. M., and Day. J. L. (1965). "Physiological Status of Men Subjected to Prolonged Confinement." AMRL-TR-65–141. Aerosp. Med. Res. Lab., Wright-Patterson AFB, Ohio.

Stegemann, J., von Framing, H. D., and Schiefling, M. (1969). *Pflüegers Arch.* **312**, 129–138.

Stepantsov, V. I., Tikhonov, M. A., and Yermin, A. V. (1972). *Space Biol. Med.* **6**(4), 103–109.

Stevens, P. M. (1966). *Am. J. Cardiol.* **17**, 211–218.

Stevens, P. M., and Lynch, T. N. (1965). *Aerosp. Med.* **36**, 1151–1156.

Stevens, P. M., Lynch, T. N., Gilbert, C. A., Johnson, R. L., and Lamb, L. E. (1966a). *Aerosp. Med. Assoc. Prepr.* pp. 160–161.

Stevens, P. M., Lynch, T. N., Johnson, R. L., and Lamb, L. E. (1966b). *Aerosp. Med.* **37**, 1049–1056.

Stevens, P. M., Miller, P. B., Gilbert, C. A., Lynch, T. N., Johnson, R. L.. and Lamb, L. E. (1966c). *Aerospace Med.* **37**, 357–367.

Stevens, P. M., Miller, P. B., Lynch, T. N., Gilbert. C. A., Johnson, R. L., and Lamb, L. E. (1966d). *Aerosp. Med.* **37**(5), 466–474.

Stevenson, F. H. (1952). *J. Bone Jt. Surg., Bi. Vol.* **34**, 256–265.

Stremel, R. W., Convertino, V. A., Bernauer, E. M., and Greenleaf, J. E. (1976). *J. Appl. Physiol.* **41**(6), 905–909.

Suvorov, P. M. (1974). *Space Biol. Aerosp. Med.* **8**(1), 93–97.

Syzrantsev, Yu. K. (1967). *Probl. Space Biol.* **7**, 317–322.

Taylor, H. L., Erickson, L., Henschel, A., and Keys, A. (1945). *Am. J. Physiol.* **144**, 227–232.

Taylor, H. L., Henschel, A., Brozek, J., and Keys, A. (1949). *J. Appl. Physiol.* **2**, 223–239.

Tenney, S. M. (1959). *J. Appl. Physiol.* **14**, 129–132.

Texas Woman's University (1970). "Bone Density Studies of Bed Rest Subjects at the Public Health Service Hospital in San Francisco, by the Texas Woman's University Radiographic Method," NASA CR-114784. Texas Woman's University, Denton.

Thornton, W. E., Hoffler, G. W., and Rummel, J. A. (1977). *In* "Biomedical Results from Skylab" (R. S. Johnson and L. F. Dietlein, eds.), NASA SP-377, pp. 330–339. NASA, Washington, D.C.

Tkachev, V. V., and Kul'kov, Ye. (1975). *Space Biol. Aerosp. Med.* **9**(1), 135–142.

Torphy, D. E. (1965). *Aerosp. Med. Assoc. Prepr.* pp. 271–272.

Torphy, D. E. (1966a). *Aerosp. Med.* **37**, 119–124.

Torphy, D. E. (1966b). *Aerosp. Med.* **37**, 383–387.

Triebwasser, J. H., Fasola, A. F., Stewart, A., and Lancaster, M. C. (1970). *Aerosp. Med. Assoc. Prepr.* pp. 65–66.

Triebwasser, J. H., Johnson, R. L., Jr., Burpo, R. P., Campbell, J. C., Reardon, W. C., and Blomquist, C. G. (1977). *Aviat., Space, Environ. Med.* **48**, 203–209.

Udalov, Yu. F., Kudrova, R. V., Kuznetsov, M. I., Lobzin, P. O., Petrovykh, V. A., Popov, I. G., Romanova, I. A., Syzrantsev, Yu. K., Terilovskiy. A. M., Rogatina, L. N., and Chelnokova, N. A. (1967). *Probl. Space Biol.* **7**, 348–354.

Ulmer, H. V., Böning, D., Stegemann, J., Meier, U., and Skipka, W. (1972). *Z. Kreislaufforsch.* **61**, 934–946.

Umapathy, M. K. (1967). Doctoral Dissertation, Texas Woman's University, Denton (unpublished).

Ushakov, A. S., and Vlasova, T. F. (1976). *Life Sci. Space Res.* **14**, 257–262.

Ushakov, A. S., Ivanova, S. M., and Brantova, S. S. (1977). *Aviat., Space, Environ. Med.* **48**(9), 824–827.

Vallbona, C., Cardus, D., Vogt, F. B., and Spencer, W. A. (1965). "The Effect of Bedrest on Various Parameters of Physiological Function. Part VIII, NASA (CR-178. Texas Institute for Rehabilitation and Research, Houston.

Van Beaumont, W., Greenleaf, J. E., and Juhos, L. (1972). *J. Appl. Physiol.* **33**(1), 55–61.

Van Beaumont, W., Greenleaf, J. E., and Davis, J. (1974a). *Aerosp. Med. Assoc. Prepr.* p. 61.

Van Beaumont, W., Greenleaf, J. E., Young, H. L., and Juhos, L. (1974b). *Aerosp. Med.* **45**, 425–430.

Vanyushina, Yu. V. (1963). *In* "Aviation and Space Medicine" (V. V. Parin, ed.), pp. 92–94. Akad. Med. Nauk SSSR, Moscow.

Vanyushina, Yu. V. Ger, M. A., and Panferova, N. Ye. (1966). *In* "Problems of Space Medicine," pp. 88–89. Ministry of Health of the USSR, Moscow.

Vasil'yev, P. V., and Kotovskaya, A. R. (1965). *Int. Aeron. Congr., 16th,* p. 1–15.

Vatner, S. F. (1975). *In* "The Peripheral Circulation" (R. Zeli, ed.), pp. 211–237. Grune & Stratton, New York.

Vaysfel'd, I. L., and Il'icheva, R. F. (1972). *Space Biol. Med.* **6**(5), 88–98.

Verney, E. B. (1946). *Lancet* **2**, 739–744.

Vernikos-Danellis, J., Leach, C. S., Winget, C. M., Rambaut, P. C., and Mack, P. B. (1972). *J. Appl. Physiol.* **33**, 644–648.

Vernikos-Danellis, J., Winget, C. M., Leach, C. S., and Rambaut, P. C. (1974). "Circadian, Endocrine, and Metabolic Effects of Prolonged Bedrest: Two 56-day Bedrest Studies," NASA TMX-3051, p. 145. NASA-Ames Research Center, Moffett Field, California.

Vetter, W. R., Sullivan, R. W., and Hyatt, K. H. (1971). *Aerosp. Med. Assoc. Prepr.* pp. 56–57.

Vikhert, A. M., Metelitsa, V. I., Baranova, V. D., and Galakhov, I. Ye. (1972). *Kardiologiya* **12**, 143–146.

Vlasova, T. F., Miroshnikova, Ye. B., and Ushakov, A. S. (1978). *Space Biol. Aerosp. Med.* **12**(4), 29–34.

Vogt, F. B. (1965). *Aerosp. Med.* **36**(5), 442–447.

Vogt, F. B. (1966). *Aerosp. Med.* **37**, 943–947.

Vogt, F. B. (1967a). *Aerosp. Med.* **38**(5), 460–464.

Vogt, F. B. (1967b). "Use of Extremity Cuffs as a cardiovascular Reflex Conditioning Technique," NASA CR-90248. Texas Institute for Rehabilitation and Research, Houston.

Vogt, F. B. (1967c). *Aerosp. Med.* **38**, 564–568.

Vogt, F. B., and Johnson, P. C. (1967). *Aerosp. Med.* **38**, 21–25.

Vogt, F. B., Mack, P. B., and Johnson, P. C. (1967a). *Aerosp. Med.* **38**, 1134–1137.

Vogt, F. B., Mack, P. B., and Johnson, P. C., and Wade, L., Jr. (1967b). *Aerosp. Med.* **38**, 43–48.

Vogt, F. B., Cardus, D., Vallbona, C., and Spencer, W. A. (1965). "The Effect of Bedrest on Various Parameters of Physiological Function," Part VI. NASA CR-176. Texas Institute for Rehabilitation and Research, Houston.

Volicier, L., Jean-Charles, R., and Chobanian, A. V. (1977). *Aviat., Space, Environ. Med.* **47**, 1065–1068.

Vorob'yev, Ye. I., Gazenko, O. G., Gurovskiy, N. N., Nefedov, Yu, G., Yegorov, B. B., Bayevskiy, R. M., Bryanov, I. I., Genin, A. M., Degtyarev, V. A., Yegorov, A. D., Yeremin, A. V., and Pestov, I. D. (1976). *Space Biol. Aerosp. Med.* **10**(5), 3–18.

Voskresenskiy, A. D., Yegorov, B. B., Pestov, I. D., Belyashin, S. M., Tolstov, V. M., and Lezhin, I. S. (1972). *Space Biol. Med.* 6(4), 45–51.

Vyazitskiy, P. O., and Kumanichkin, S. D. (1970). *Mil. Med. J.* 7, 38–40.

Weissler, A. M., Warren, J. V., Ester, H. E., Jr., McIntosh, H. D., and Leonard, J. J. (1957). *Circulation* 15, 875.

White, P. D., Nyberg, J. W., Finney, L. M., and Shite, W. J. (1966). "Influence of Periodic Centrifugation on Cardiovascular Functions of Men During Bed Rest," NASA CR-65422. Douglas Aircraft Co., Inc., Santa Monica, California.

Widdowson, E. M., and McChance, R. A. (1950). *Lancet* 258, 539.

Williams, B. A., and Resse, R. D. (1972). *Aerosp. Med. Assoc. Prepr.* pp. 8–11.

Wolthuis, R. A., LeBlanc, A., Carpentier, W. A., and Bergman, S. A., Jr. (1975). *Aviat., Space, Environ. Med.* 46, 697–702.

Wurtman, R. J. (1965). *N. Engl. J. Med.* 273, 637–646.

Yakoleva, I. Ya. (1971). *Space Biol. Med.* 5(3), 91–97.

Yakoleva, I. Ya., Baranova, V. P., Kornilova, L. N., Nefedova, M. V., Lapayev, E. V., and Raskatova, S. R. (1972). *Space Biol. Med.* 6(4), 79–87.

Yefimenko, G. D. (1969). *Probl. Space Biol.* 13, 121–132.

Yegorov, P. I., Dupik, V. S., Yermakova, N. P., Korotayev, M. M., Kochina, Y. E., Mikhaylovskiy, G. P., Neumyvakin, I. P., Petrova, T. A., Reutova, M. B., Filatova, L. M., Tsyganova, I. I., and Yakovleva, I. Ya. (1966). *Probl. Kosm. Med.* pp. 162–163.

Yegorov, P. I., Smirnov, K. V., Korotayev, M. M., and Lukasheva, M. V. (1967). *Space Biol. Med.* 1(2), 106–110.

Zav'yalov, Ye. S., and Mel'nik, S. G. (1967). *Space Biol. Med.* 1(3), 89–96.

Zelis, R., ed. (1975). "Normal Circulation." Grune & Stratton, New York.

Zhdanova, A. G. (1965). *Arkh. Anat., Gistol. Embriol.* 49, 29–34.

Ziegler, M. G., Lake, C. R., and Kopin, I. J. (1977). *N. Engl. J. Med.* 296, 293–297.

Zubek, J. (1968). *J. Abnorm. Psychol.* 73, 223–225.

Zvonarev, G. P. (1971). *Space Biol. Med.* 5(4), 71–76.

11

Chemical and Nervous Control of the Coronary System

Germano Marchetti

I. Hemodynamics of Coronary Circulation

Coronary blood flow is determined by perfusion pressure and vascular resistance. However, blood is supplied intermittently to the myocardium, because flow is noticeably reduced by the contraction of the muscular mass surrounding the coronary channels. The effects of extravascular compression also affect the pattern of coronary flow; the flow curve decreases during systole, with this period accounting for about 20% of the total flow (Gregg and Fisher, 1963). The highest values are attained during diastole, when the myocardium relaxes.

At the beginning of isometric contraction there is a sudden fall in coronary flow in the left ventricle to the extent that backflow sometimes occurs. However, during systole there is generally a moderate forward flow in coronary vessels, which increases quickly as aortic pressure rises and drops in late systole (Fig. 1). At the onset of isometric relaxation there is a marked rise in coronary flow which reaches its highest level during early diastole after which it gradually falls. A late negative diastolic wave is always present at approximately the time of atrial systole and immediately before isometric contraction.

The cardiac systole thus acts to impede coronary flow through the ventricular wall; in effect, coronary blood flow increases considerably during ventricular asystole induced by peripheral vagal stimulation (Gregg and Fisher, 1963).

The coronary flow during asystole is about 50% higher than the control flow, and this demonstrates the extent of the mechanical throttling effect of muscular contraction in reducing the flow to the myocardium (Gregg and Fisher, 1963; Rubio and Berne, 1975). This effect, however, does not affect all the layers of the ventricles to the same extent. It is stronger in the subendocardial layers of the left ventricle, where intramural pressure reaches considerably higher levels than aortic pressure (Kirk and Honig, 1964), but it is less in outer layers of the left ventricle and in the wall of the right, in which intramural pressure is lower than aortic pressure throughout all the cardiac cycle (Gregg and Fisher, 1963). Consequently, subendocardial layers in the left ventricle receive coronary blood only during diastole and have a very large number of open capillaries, whereas subepicardial layers are also nourished during systole and the number of open capillaries in them is lower. The tone of the subendocardial vessels is always very low and this reduces the capacity for further vasodilation that can be obtained if metabolic needs increase (Rubio and Berne, 1975).

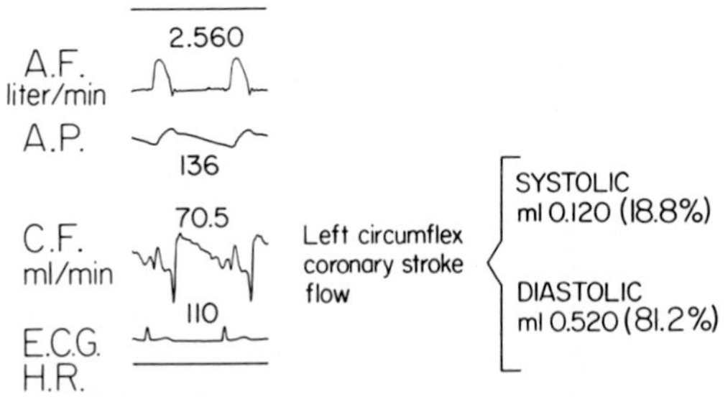

Fig. 1.   Flow in the left coronary artery. Tracing recorded in a conscious dog showing the normal pattern of phasic coronary (CF) and aortic (AF) flows and aortic pressure (AP). Flows were recorded by electromagnetic probes applied chronically around the circumflex branch of the left coronary artery and aortic root, respectively. HR = heart rate, mean coronary resistance can be calculated by the ratio AP/CF = 1.93, and total peripheral resistance = AP/AF = 0.053. The recordings were performed 14 days after implantation, when the dog had completely recovered from surgery. (From Marchetti, 1971, by permission of S. Karger, Publisher.)

The mean flow in the left ventricle is lower than that in other tissues; consequently, the O_2 A-V difference is very high. This difference is larger in the heart than in any other organ, and it frequently exceeds 12–14 vol $\%O_2$. (Gregg and Fisher, 1963a). During enhanced myocardial metabolic activity or reduced O_2 supply it can fall to levels as low as 1 vol $\%O_2$ ml of blood (Scott, 1961).

Thus about 75% of the O_2 in the arterial blood is extracted during its passage through the myocardium of the left ventricle irrespective of changes in stress. Increasing metabolic requirements during muscular work can be covered mainly by the increase in coronary blood flow.

In the arterial blood, P_{O_2} is 70–100 mm Hg and in the mixed venous blood P_{O_2} is 40–60 mm Hg, whereas in the subepicardial region and coronary sinus P_{O_2} are always very low, on the order of 18–20 mm Hg (Moss and Johnson, 1970; Opie, 1968, 1969; Bing, 1965; Fabel, 1968).

In the subendocardial inner zone there is a significantly ($P < 0.001$) lower oxygen tension on the order of 10 mm Hg (Moss, 1968). Probably in the myocardial cell, near the mitochondria, P_{O_2} is even lower (1–2 mm Hg) (Wittenberg, 1970).

However, even in the absence of stress, the left ventricular myocardial cell works at a very low O_2 tension. This situation, which seems to be unfavorable, can have a logical explanation. It is therefore possible that lack of O_2 might increase the regional uniformity of capillary distribution as well as the total number and regularity of open capillaries in the myocardium. In moderate hypoxia the number of open capillaries should thus be greater and O_2 supply to the myocardium might accordingly increase (Gregg and Fisher, 1963).

In the right ventricle the flow pattern resembles the aortic pressure curve as intraventricular and intramyocardial pressure are invariably much lower than aortic pressure (Gregg and Fisher, 1963). Systolic flow in the right coronary artery is constantly higher than that during diastole and flow is almost continuous, because aortic and right coronary perfusing pressure always exceeds myocardial resistance (Fig. 2).

It is therefore likely that coronary flow/100 g of the right ventricular myocardium is higher than that in the left ventricle. In effect, in the right ventricle, the O_2 A-V difference is much lower than that in the left ventricle and O_2 content in the anterior cardiac vein blood is considerably higher than that in coronary sinus blood (Marchetti, 1971) (Fig. 3).

The difference is probably the result of mechanical factors that play an active role in regulating coronary blood flow. Extravascular compression during ventricular systole is considerably lower in the right side of the heart than in the left, and therefore the right coronary flow is less impaired than the flow in the left coronary artery (Gregg, 1963a). This view is supported

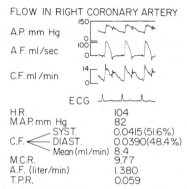

FLOW IN RIGHT CORONARY ARTERY

A.P. mm Hg	150 / 0
A.F. ml/sec	100 / 0
C.F. ml/min	14 / 0

ECG

H.R.	104
M.A.P. mm Hg	82
C.F. ⟨ SYST.	0.0415 (51.6%)
DIAST.	0.0390 (48.4%)
Mean (ml/min)	8.4
M.C.R.	9.77
A.F. (liter/min)	1.380
T.P.R.	0.059

Fig. 2. Blood flow in the right coronary artery in a conscious dog. AP = aortic pressure, AF = aortic flow, CF = coronary blood flow, HR = heart rate, MAP = mean aortic pressure, MCR = mean coronary resistance, TPR = total peripheral resistance. (From Marchetti, 1971, by permission of S. Karger, Publisher.)

by the observation that blood O_2 content in the anterior cardiac vein decreases markedly until it approaches that in coronary sinus, when the hemodynamic load on the right ventricle is suitably increased by raising its systolic pressure (Marchetti *et al.*, 1969; Gregg *et al.*, 1972).

II. Regulation of Coronary Resistance

The increase in myocardial O_2 consumption and coronary blood flow chiefly results in a reduction in coronary resistance (Gregg, 1963b). A significant correlation was in effect also demonstrated between coronary

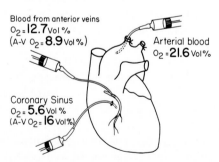

Blood from anterior veins
$O_2 = 12.7$ Vol %
(A-V $O_2 = 8.9$ Vol %)

Arterial blood
$O_2 = 21.6$ Vol %

Coronary Sinus
$O_2 = 5.6$ Vol %
(A-V $O_2 = 16$ Vol %)

Fig. 3. Oxygen content in the arterial blood, in venous blood from coronary sinus, which drains mainly from the left ventricle, and in venous blood returning from the anterior cardiac veins, which flows mainly out of the right ventricle. Arteriovenous differences are also shown. (From Marchetti, 1971, by permission of S. Karger, Publisher.)

resistance and O_2 consumption in the myocardium in the conscious dog (Fig. 4.).

The regulation of coronary resistance comes about through several mechanisms, the most important of which are the local metabolic control systems (Rubio and Berne, 1975; Gregg, 1963b).

The factors external to the heart, such as sympathetic and parasympathetic drive to the heart, hormones, and changes in blood electrolytes, do not seem very effective in modulating coronary blood flow (Rubio and Berne, 1975).

Regulation of the diameter of coronary precapillaries and thus of the nutritional blood flow can be easily demonstrated during myocardial hypoxia (Olsson and Gregg, 1965).

In the dog's coronary vessels, reactive hyperemia ensues after a transient occlusion. This can be shown by using an electromagnetic flowmeter and placing a probe and a snare or pneumatic cuff around the coronary artery, a few millimeters beyond the site of the flowmeter. Zero blood flow can thus be determined by momentary artery occlusion. The intensity of the reactive hyperemia that follows the reopening of the vessel depends on the duration of myocardial ischemia. If the occlusion is prolonged for 5–10 sec, a dilation

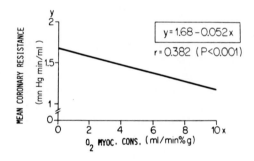

Fig. 4. Relation between O_2 myocardial consumption and mean coronary resistance. Experiments were performed in conscious dogs in which previously an electromagnetic probe had been implanted surgically around the circumflex branch of the left coronary artery, while catheters were chronically implanted into the coronary sinus through the wall of the right atrium and into the aortic lumen through the carotid artery. Coronary resistance was calculated by the mean arterial pressure/mean coronary flow ratio. O_2 myocardial consumption was calculated by multiplying the O_2 A-V difference across the heart by the coronary flow per minute. O_2 content in arterial and coronary sinus blood was measured by Van Slyke's method. The regression line was calculated on 171 couples of data.

can be achieved without changes in blood pressure, heart rate, or cardiac work (Fig. 5).

Peak flow response can be as high as 400–500% or more above base flow (Olsson and Gregg, 1965). The flow response occurs not only in the heart *in situ,* but also in isolated heart and heart–lung preparation (Gregg and Fisher, 1963).

Flow debt, reactive hyperemic flow, and repayment of flow debt can be calculated according to Coffman and Gregg (1960):

Flow debt = control flow rate × duration of occlusion

Reactive hyperemic flow = integral of the flow curve during reactive hyperemia) – (control flow rate × duration of reactive
hyperemia)

Percent repayment of flow debt = (reactive hyperemic flow/flow debt)
× 100

The volume of reactive hyperemia blood flow increases with lengthening periods of coronary artery occlusion up to about 120 sec. The theoretical blood flow "debt" is always considerably overpaid (Gregg and Fisher, 1963; Olsson, 1975; Giles and Wilcken, 1977).

After 8 sec occlusion with unrestricted inflow in the coronary arteries, repayment of the flow debt was about 600% compared to control flow (Giles and Wilcken, 1977). But if the arterial inflow is restricted for a short period, after release of a brief coronary arterial occlusion, the degree of reactive hyperemia is markedly reduced, not exceeding about 300%, though it prolongs the duration of the response (Giles and Wilcken, 1977).

These data confirm the earlier statement that the reactive hyperemia is greatly in excess of metabolic requirements (Eikens and Wilcken, 1974; Bache *et al.*, 1974).

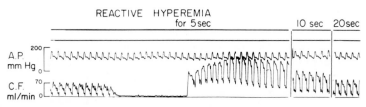

Fig. 5. Reactive hyperemia after 5-sec occlusion of the circumflex branch of the left coronary artery in a dog with flowmeters chronically implanted. (From Marchetti, 1971, by permission of S. Karger, Publisher.)

However, during restricted reactive hyperemia a change of endocardial–epicardial blood supply ensues and a relative endocardial ipoperfusion and ischemia take place (Olsson, 1975); in effect, the fraction of flow distributed to the epicardium increased by 20% and that distributed to endocardium decreased by 26%. An "overpayment" of the oxygen debt is therefore probably required for a number of reasons, such as increase in heart rate, elevation of coronary flow, which can by itself stimulate oxygen consumption (Gregg, 1963a); ischemia in the deeper layers of the myocardium; and release of catecholamines (Olsson, 1975).

III. Mechanism of Myocardial Reactive Hyperemia

Complete depletion of myocardial oxygen stores is probably attained in a few seconds after coronary occlusion (Olsson, 1975). Myocardial anoxia ensues and thus reactive hyperemia is thought to be due to accumulation of vasodilator metabolites during the period of coronary occlusion (Lewis and Grant, 1925–1926; Olsson and Gregg, 1965). This hypothesis is supported by the findings of Pauly et al. (1973), which provide evidence that the volume of myocardial reactive hyperemia in dogs is greatly influenced by interventions that can change myocardial O_2 consumption. In effect, an augmentation in cardiac metabolic activity obtained in the dog by paired pacing or increasing heart rate during the period of occlusion leads to an increase in the integral of the flow curve during reactive hyperemia, probably because the accumulation of vasodilator metabolites in the tissue is increased. The lowering of cardiac O_2 requirements obtained by administering β-blockers or by cooling the heart produces an opposite effect. Besides, in conscious dogs with coronary sinus chronically cannulated and a flowmeter around a coronary artery, 3 to 5 sec occlusion produces an appreciable hyperemic response without any demonstrable lactic acid production (Olsson and Gregg, 1965). However, a 10 sec period of coronary occlusion is followed by a discharge of lactate and increased production of pyruvate (Table I) and then by some clear alterations in cardiac metabolism (Marchetti et al., 1971). Thus only occlusions longer than 5–10 sec are able to modify myocardial metabolism and produce a lactate discharge and probably accumulation of some vasodilator substance.

According to Frölich (1965), several intermediary products of oxidative metabolism, such as acetate, citrate, fumarate, malate, α-ketoglutarate, oxalacetate, and succinate, given at submaximal dosage produce a significant vasodilation and thus can be included among these agents termed "vasodilating metabolites," which can contribute to the local regulation of blood flow like adenosine and inosine.

TABLE I

Modifications of Cardiac O_2, Lactate, and Pyruvate Metabolism[a,b]

| | Basal occlusion | 10 sec | 40 sec | 1 min | After release pneumatic cuff | | | | |
					3 min	5 min	15 min	30 min
Coronary flow (ml/min)	54.4	157.7	96.3	69.3	56.9	58.4	52.7	56.3
O_2 Consumption (ml/min)	5.70	11.96	8.61	6.49	5.90	6.09	5.46	5.67
Pyruvate (mg%)								
A	0.660	0.523	0.513	0.536	0.485	0.489	0.536	0.409
V	0.937	0.969	1.085	1.029	0.963	0.881	0.861	0.937
Consumption (mg/min)	−0.163	−0.718	−0.472	−0.353	−0.283	−0.241	−0.183	−0.287
Lactate (mg%)								
A	5.11	4.78	4.82	5.11	4.99	5.27	5.58	5.34
V	4.63	7.51	5.22	4.00	4.17	4.49	4.76	4.42
Consumption (mg/min)	−0.20	−3.58	−0.19	−0.94	−0.44	−0.46	−0.45	−0.63

[a] After a 10 or 20-sec occlusion of the circumflex branch of the left coronary artery. Mean values of experiments performed in eight conscious dogs with a flow probe chronically implanted around the circumflex branch and the coronary sinus chronically cannulated.

In these animals the concentrations of lactate and pyruvate in blood reaching and leaving the myocardium was studied. The normal pattern is that lactate is consumed by the heart (the level in arterial blood is higher than in coronary sinus blood), whereas pyruvate is produced.

After the release of the pneumatic cuff there is a sudden increase in coronary blood flow and myocardial O_2 consumption. Pyruvate blood levels do not change, whereas lactate is discharged by the heart for about 40 sec. One minute after the release of the artery, lactate begins to be consumed again by the heart.

[b] Reprinted from Marchetti et al., 1971, with modifications. By permission of S. Karger, Publisher.

According to Rubio and Berne (1975), when O_2 myocardial consumption increases or coronary blood supply declines, myocardial ischemia ensues, thereby enhancing the release of adenosine and inosine by the cardiac cell into the interstitial fluid.

When ATP is degraded successively to ADP and AMP, it cannot be regenerated, because of the lack of O_2. The decrease in ATP increases the activity of 5-nucleotidase, the enzyme that catalyzes the hydrolysis of AMP to adenosine and inosine. The 5-nucleotidase is bound to external cell membranes and then adenosine and inosine form and are released into the extracellular space, where they cause the coronary channels to dilate, thus increasing coronary blood flow and O_2 myocardial supply toward normal. Consequently, the concentration of adenosine and inosine decreases in the interstitial fluid because the nucleotides return to the cardiac cells or diffuse into capillaries, and the myocardial level in AMP, ADP, and ATP is enhanced following the higher availability of O_2. Coronary blood flow is thus once again reduced toward a level at which myocardial O_2 balance is maintained (Rubio and Berne, 1975).

This sequence of events was demonstrated to be consistent with the existence of a vasodilator that accumulates in the myocardium during the period of coronary occlusion and its disappearance during the reactive hyperemia follows exponential kinetics (Olsson, 1964). The measurements of myocardial adenosine content during reactive hyperemia showed that adenosine increases following 5–15 sec of left coronary artery occlusion and falls exponentially to control levels thereafter, accounting for the way coronary flow changes during this response (Olsson et al., 1978).

Adenosine and its degradation products have been recovered from coronary venous blood during ischemic perfusion (Jacob and Berne, 1960; Katori and Berne, 1966), reactive hyperemia (Rubio et al. 1969), and pacing-induced ischemia in man (Fox et al., 1974).

The role of adenosine has recently been questioned by investigations showing that methylxanthines can inhibit the vasodilating effect of adenosine on coronaries in oxygenated hearts (Afonso, 1970), whereas they are almost ineffective on myocardial reactive hyperemia (Juhran et al., 1971; Curnish et al., 1972). It is therefore possible that the responsiveness of the coronary arteries to adenosine is enhanced during the period of ischemia (Olsson et al. 1978). Furthermore, the lack of oxygen is also able to relax directly the coronary arterial wall (Gellai et al. 1972), and the combined effect of adenosine and hypoxia could overcome methylxanthine inhibition.

Besides adenosine and inosine, other metabolic factors can probably contribute to the regulation of resistance in the coronary vessels, namely, histamine (Giles et al., 1977), carbon dioxide (Case et al., 1978), catecholamines, hydrogen and potassium ions, lactic acid, increased osmolarity, potassium, bradykinin, and serotonin (Berne, 1964).

The possibility that the endogenous vasoactive prostaglandins* or their precursors may influence the coronary response to hypoxia cannot be ruled out (Block et al., 1975; Alexander et al., 1975). However, recent studies do not seem to confirm the role of prostaglandins in mediating the coronary vasodilation that accompanies anoxia. After cessation of coronary perfusion for several minutes, isolated rabbit hearts show coronary vasodilation and release of prostaglandinlike material proportional to the duration of ischemia. Indomethacin eliminates the prostaglandin release, whereas it has no effect on vasodilation (Needleman et al., 1975, 1977).

Myogenic relaxation of coronary smooth muscle cells during the period of occlusion can also contribute to reactive hyperemia. The intravascular pressure distal to occlusion drops for a few seconds to figures on the order of 2–15 mm Hg (Elliott et al., 1968) and increases suddenly when the artery is released. The following reactive hyperemia could reflect myogenic relaxation occurring during the period of occlusion. Even very brief occlusions lasting one or two beats (Eikens and Wilcken, 1974) can elicit a clear hyperemic response. In this case it is unlikely that significant myocardial ischemia occurs, and the reactive hyperemia may thus be myogenic.

In conclusion, reactive hyperemia in the myocardium is a complex response due to mechanical and metabolic determinants. There is evidence that in this response there is the intervention of some vasodilatory metabolites, such as adenosine, but also the loss of myogenic tone during the interval of coronary occlusion and possibly also the effects of oxygen deprivation in vascular smooth muscle (Olsson et al., 1978).

The surgical denervation of the heart obtained by left stellectomy increased the volume of reactive hyperemia by 31% (Schwartz and Lowell Stone, 1976). These results confirm that the cardiac sympathetic nerves exert a tonic influence on coronary circulation (Feigl, 1975) and their activity represents a limiting factor for reactive hyperemia (Schwartz and Lowell Stone, 1976).

Reactive hyperemia can also be decreased or eliminated by massive dilation of the coronary bed, as in dogs submitted to hemodilution (Bagger, 1978). Progressive hemodilution produces an increase in flow and a decline in resistance in coronary vessels because the blood capacity to carry oxygen decrease more and more until the maximum dilation of the coronaries is reached. At this degree of hemodilution, the increase in systolic and diastolic coronary flow is sixfold and threefold, respectively, and the reactive

---

*For more extensive and detailed information about this field refer to Chapter 2 by Wennmalm, "Prostaglandins and the Heart."

hyperemia response to 10 sec occlusion of the circumflex branch disappeared completely. In these conditions a relative endocardial hypoperfusion ensues (Bagger, 1978), along with alterations of the electrocardiogram.

Reactive hyperemia was attenuated by 25% by preventing the fall in intravascular pressure associated with coronary artery occlusion. This was obtained by infusion of saline or plasma distal to occlusion that could remove vasodilating substances from myocardium or impede reflex vasodilation (Bittar *et al.*, 1975) or myogenic relaxation of coronary channel walls.

IV. Coronary Reserve in Normal and Hypertrophic Hearts

The peak flow during reactive hyperemia increases with the duration of the occlusion until 20–30 sec. With longer occlusions peak flow does not increase further and that means that the maximum dilation of the coronary bed has been attained. In this way it is possible to measure the dilatory ability of the coronary circulation and thus the coronary reserve in normal and diseased hearts.

In normal hearts the coronary reserve is about 300% above that of controls. In some dogs figures of 500% higher than those in controls were noted.

In dogs with experimental cardiac hypertrophy the mass of myocardial fibers increases, whereas the coronary bed remains almost unchanged (Linzbach, 1960). However, coronary blood flow at rest has to increase considerably in order to supply adequate nourishment for the enlarged mass while the "coronary reserve" decreases.

When myocardial O_2 consumption increases, as in muscular exercise, coronary blood flow can only increase to a very limited degree, consequently, an imbalance between O_2 supply and myocardial demand may arise (Marchetti *et al.*, 1973; Holz *et al.*, 1977; O'Keefe *et al.*, 1978; Mueller *et al.*, 1978).

V. Autoregulation of Coronary Flow

If perfusion pressure is either increased or decreased suddenly, coronary blood flow initially changes in the same direction, but in a short time, after having attained the peak level, it tends to return toward the previous figure. This has been defined as "autoregulation" and means that coronary flow tends to remain constant even in the presence of modifications in perfusion pressure (Berne, 1964).

Autoregulation is likely to be explained by the myocardial cells producing vasodilator metabolites when their O_2 requirements are not satisfied (Berne, 1964) and also by a myogenic mechanism. Hence a decrease in perfusion pressure, and thus in flow, would be accompanied by the release of vasodilator metabolites, which in turn would induce a vasodilation and an increase in flow and O_2 supply toward normal.

An increase in strain in the coronary smooth vascular fibers, induced by an increase in perfusion pressure could stimulate the smooth fibers to contract, and the following vasoconstriction should again bring blood flow back toward control levels (Olsson, 1975). As a result of the autoregulation mechanism, coronary resistance can probably adapt itself in such a way that coronary supply can precisely fulfil the metabolic requirements of the myocardium at varying levels of cardiac work irrespective of changes in systemic circulation.

VI. Coronary Flow Responses to Natural Stresses

The order of magnitude of the vasodilation of which the coronary channels are capable under natural stress conditions is extremely large (Gregg, 1971–1972). The dilatability of coronary circulation during exercise (Khouri et al., 1965) and under the influence of emotion and natural stress could not be thoroughly investigated until it became technically possible to implant miniaturized electromagnetic flowmeters chronically around coronary vessels and experiments were performed on conscious animals (Gregg et al., 1965; Marchetti et al., 1971; Bergamaschi and Longoni, 1973; Caraffa Braga et al., 1973; Newton and Ehrlick, 1969).

Excitement can produce a very considerable increase in coronary blood flow, although generally less than in reactive hyperemia. For instance, when a normal meal was shown and then given to a dog that had been fasting for 24 hr, coronary blood flow and heart rate showed a considerable increase, whereas coronary resistance decreased almost immediately after the dog saw the food (Fig. 6). The circulatory response begins from 6–10 sec after the food is first seen. The greatest changes were reached in a few seconds; then, circulatory modifications tended to prolong during the ingestion. Five minutes after the meal the hemodynamic response was almost completely over. Table II shows the average modifications recorded in nine fasting dogs during the sight of food and eating. At the sight of food there is a significant increase in heart rate (39%), mean arterial pressure (23%), mean coronary flow (60%), aortic flow (16%), and cardiac work (43%). Coronary resistance decreased by 29%, whereas total peripheral resistance increased, al-

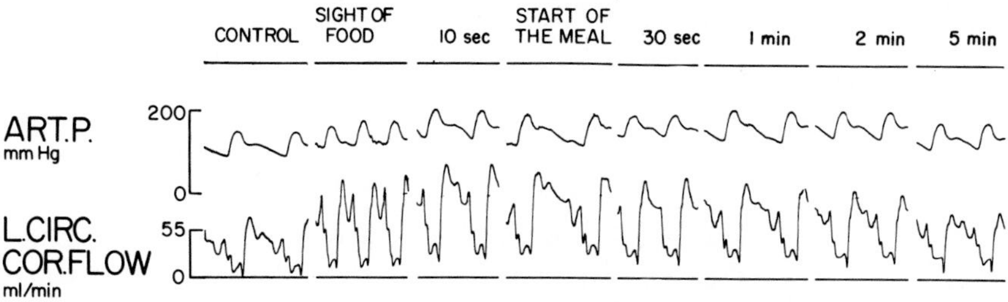

	CONTROL	SIGHT OF FOOD	10 sec	START OF THE MEAL	30 sec	1 min	2 min	5 min
STROKE SYST. FLOW	0.028	0.046	0.065	0.070	0.061	0.067	0.060	0.051
STROKE DIAST. FLOW	0.265	0.212	0.454	0.674	0.304	0.480	0.332	0.271
MEAN COR. FLOW	35.2	57.2	80.0	78.1	62.4	68.3	58.8	48.3
MEAN AORTIC PRESS.	110	133	156	142	159	156	159	133
HEART RATE	120	222	154	105	171	125	150	150
MEAN COR. RES.	3.13	2.32	1.95	1.82	2.55	2.28	2.70	2.75
LATE DIAST. COR.RES.	2	1.1	1.4	1.5	1.7	1.6	1.7	2.2

Fig. 6. Tracings recorded in a fasting conscious dog weighing 17.5 kg, 13 days after the chronic implantation of an electromagnetic probe on the coronary artery and a catheter into the aorta, showing the effect of the sight and ingestion of food on phasic aortic pressure and left circumflex coronary artery flow. After the dog sees the food there is a sudden increase in heart rate, coronary flow, and arterial pressure that persists when the dog starts to eat and then tends to disappear in the course of a few minutes. (From Marchetti *et al.*, 1968, by permission of Springer-Verlag.)

beit not significantly. The response did not change even when stimulations were repeated on different days.

When the dogs started eating, the changes in some hemodynamic parameters became more noticeable. Heart rate and cardiac work increased by a further 20% (a total of 70% from control); mean aortic pressure increased by 12% more (total 35% from control). The difference between the control values and changes observed in heart rate, aortic pressure, and cardiac work on the sight of food and during the meal were significant ($P < 0.01$). Mean coronary blood and average aortic flow did not show any significant differences in either conditions.

The maximal increase in coronary blood flow is about 80% and is thus less than the maximum ability of the coronary circulation to dilate. Aortic pressure and flow generally increase to a less marked degree (15–35%) than coronary flow and heart rate (60–80%). Similar modifications in coronary flow and arterial pressure can be observed in other natural situations, such as in spontaneous excitement or following auditory and light stimulations or in a male dog approaching a bitch in estrus, courting it, and engaging in sexual intercourse (Fig. 7). About the same increase in coronary flow and arterial pressure was recorded when the dog was allowed to approach the bitch but was prevented from attaining coitus.

TABLE II

Effect of Excitement on Hemodynamics^{a,b}

Dogs n°	Heart rate	Mean arterial pressure	Coronary flow (ml/min)	Mean coron. resist.	Aortic flow (l/min)	Card. work (l-atm/min)	Total periph. resist.
Control							
9	107	117	69.5	1.75	2.670	0.415	0.0472
Sight of food							
9	149	144	111.4	1.36	3.090	0.593	0.0498
	**	**	**	**	*	**	
Eating							
9	179	159	120.9	1.33	3.415	0.706	0.0537
	***	***	***	*	*	***	

^{a} Nine conscious dogs with chronic implantation of flowmeters around the aorta and coronary circumflex artery and a catheter into the aorta. The dogs had been fasting for 24 hr and the stimulus was represented by the sight of usual food and actual eating. The following parameters were recorded and measured: heart rate, mean arterial pressure, coronary flow, mean coronary resistance, aortic flow, cardiac work, and total peripheral resistance.

At the sight of food there is an increase in heart rate, mean arterial pressure, mean coronary flow, aortic flow, and cardiac work and a decrease in coronary resistance. When the dogs start eating, the variations in some hemodynamic parameters become more noticeable.

^{b} *P < 0.05, **P < 0.01, ***P < 0.001.

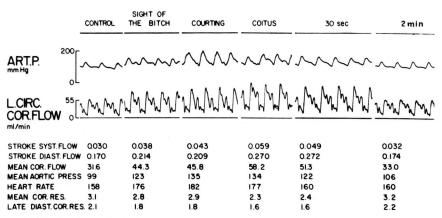

Fig. 7. Tracings recorded in a conscious 21-Kg dog seven days postoperatively, showing the effect of sexual excitement and intercourse on phasic aortic pressure, and left circumflex coronary artery phasic flow. (From Marchetti *et al.*, 1968, by permission of Springer-Verlag.)

It must be stressed that coronary resistance does not show any further decrease in actual eating and sexual intercourse than in the excitement preceding them. Hemodynamic changes obtained with different types of excitement were very similar. However, a number of natural stimuli and physiological actions that occur during the dog's daily life are associated with very considerable changes in coronary blood flow, heart rate, and arterial pressure.

Emotions probably influence the heart rate first, and the resultant elevation in cardiac output is mainly due to tachycardia; at this stage, left ventricle filling and consequently stroke volume tend to diminish. The rise in coronary blood flow is mainly induced by a noticeable reduction in mean and late diastolic coronary resistance; in effect, the modifications in coronary blood flow were not related only to the heart rate variations, as the coronary flow per beat tended to increase.

Total peripheral resistance rose constantly but not significantly. In fact, after emotional stimulation, there is a rapid decrease in vascular resistance, in coronary arteries, and in some other beds, such as the hind limb vessels (Caraffa Braga *et al.* , 1973), whereas considerable vasoconstriction takes place in other circulatory districts, such as mesentery and kidneys. The net effect of circulatory modifications following excitement is an average increase in total peripheral resistance (Caraffa Braga *et al.*, 1973).

Even though it is not possible to identify the mechanism that elicits the coronary response because of the complex reaction brought about by the stimuli, it is reasonable to suggest that at least three mechanisms may be involved:

1. local metabolic control by flood-borne substances, P_{O_2}, and metabolites from tissues.
2. Release of catecholamines from the adrenals into the bloodstream.
3. Excitation of the sympathetic nervous system by stimuli from the central nervous system.

VII. Local Metabolic Control of Coronary Resistance

Coronary blood flow and O_2 supply to the heart must precisely meet the metabolic needs of the myocardium at various levels of cardiac work. The overall metabolic activity of the myocardium as reflected by its oxygen consumption correlates closely with the coronary flow in various stress states (Fig. 8).

When cardiac work increases, coronary blood flow rises, and this augmentation can even reach values on the order of 200–300% higher than control (Alella et al., 1955). The increase in flow is mainly determined by simultaneous rises in arterial pressure and heart rate: the contribution of the increase in cardiac output in determining the elevation in coronary flow is less significant (Alella et al., 1955; Marchetti and Merlo, 1964).

The factors act indirectly on coronary flow by raising O_2 consumption of the myocardium (Fig. 9). The graph, however, shows that the same level of O_2 consumption may correspond to very different figures of cardiac work, probably because pressure development elevates O_2 consumption more than cardiac output. In effect, the correlation coefficient between O_2 consumption and cardiac work is very low ($r = 0.23$). Indeed, it is not possible to calculate exactly the energetic needs of the myocardium by simply multiplying mean arterial pressure times cardiac output. However, both left

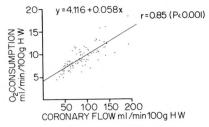

Fig. 8. Relation between coronary flow and oxygen consumption of the myocardium at various levels of cardiac work. Experiments were performed on narcotized dogs with bypass of the right heart. (From Marchetti and Merlo, 1964, by permission of S. Karger, Publisher.)

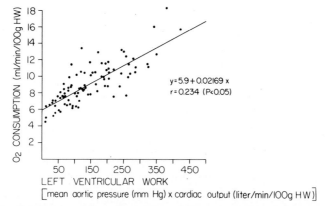

Fig. 9. Relation between cardiac work and O_2 consumption of the myocardium. The cardiac work was calculated by multiplying mean arterial pressure by cardiac output. The experiments were performed on anaesthetized open-chest dogs with bypass of the right atrium and ventricle. Cardiac work was progressively increased by raising either mean arterial pressure or cardiac output or both. (From Marchetti and Merlo, 1964, by permission of S. Karger, Publisher.)

ventricular pressure and volume, according to the statement of Laplace, contribute to determining the tension of the myocardial wall

$$T = \pi r P$$

where T is cardiac wall tension; r, radius of the left ventricular cavity; and P, left ventricular pressure.

Myocardial O_2 consumption is more strictly correlated with T than with the product: mean arterial pressure times cardiac output (Fig. 10). The rate of rise of left ventricular pressure dP/dt is also closely correlated with O_2 myocardial consumption (Fig. 11). The most important determinants of myocardial O_2 consumption, are (Gibbs, 1978) heart rate, cardiac work, wall tension, and contraction velocity dP/dt.

So most of the determinants of O_2 myocardial consumption relate to the mechanical aspects of contraction. However, some of the modifications in O_2 consumption by the myocardial muscle are not necessarily linked to mechanical activity of the heart.

Changes in coronary perfusion pressure in several animal preparations (Gregg, 1963a; Marchetti *et al.*, 1966; Arnold *et al.*, 1968) may induce similar directional changes in O_2 consumption and coronary blood flow in the absence of associated changes in mechanical heart performance. A satisfactory explanation for the increase in O_2 consumption along with coronary perfusion pressure has not been given to date (Gregg, 1963a). Despite this there is no question that coronary blood flow correlates with the metabolic

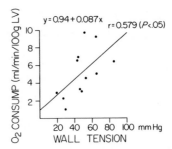

Fig. 10. Relation between O_2 myocardial consumption and tension of the heart walls. Experiments were performed on narcotized dogs in which the following parameters were measured: (a) coronary flow by an electromagnetic flowmeter, (b) left ventricular pressure by a catheter inserted into the left ventricular cavity through the left carotid artery, (c) the end-diastolic volume of left ventricular cavity by the thermodilution method, and (d) O_2 myocardial consumption by multiplying coronary blood flow times the difference between O_2 content in arterial and coronary sinus blood. The radius r of the left ventricular cavity was calculated as well as the tension of the heart walls (T) according to the statement of Laplace. $T = \pi r P$, in which P = systolic pressure in left ventricular cavity.

activity of the myocardium as reflected by its oxygen consumption and is in some manner regulated about a constant myocardial P_{O_2} (Rubio and Berne, 1975).

Several other metabolic factors, however, cooperate with P_{O_2} in regulating coronary resistance.

Bradley (1975) perfused in series two isolated guinea pig hearts with oxygenated saline. Vasodilation was obtained in the first heart by various stimulations, such as catecholamines, histamine and electrical pacing. The saline effluent from the first heart after oxygenation and adding propranolol

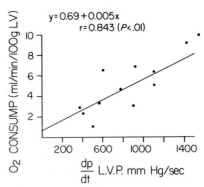

Fig. 11. Relations between O_2 myocardial consumption and the rate of rise of the left ventricular pressure curve dP/dt. The experiments were performed on the same narcotized dogs as in Fig. 10 using a differentiating circuit.

and antihistamine agents was again able to dilate the second heart. The presence of some chemical mediators arising from local metabolic process is implied.

Recent investigations have shown that P_{CO_2} may modulate coronary resistance when coronary sinus P_{O_2} is kept constant. When coronary arterial P_{CO_2} was lowered, coronary vascular resistance increased (Case *et al.*, 1978), showing a linear but opposite effect in comparison with P_{O_2}.

The sensitivity of coronary resistance to P_{O_2} changes is two times that to P_{CO_2} modifications (Case *et al.*, 1978). Thus in the case of a sudden increase in myocardial O_2 consumption, both a transient fall in myocardial P_{O_2} and a transient increase in P_{CO_2} would increase coronary flow, and in the opposite situation would decrease coronary flow. This hypothesis is supported by results obtained in patients with ischemic heart disease in whom coronary blood flow also decreased after voluntary hyperventilation that lowered arterial P_{CO_2} from 33 to 19 mm Hg (Neill and Hattenhauer, 1975). It is well known that changes in arterial P_{CO_2} can considerably influence central blood flow, probably interfering with prostaglandin synthesis (Pickard and MacKenzie, 1973).

Probably a similar mechanism could be operative in the coronary circulation, mainly because the myocardium does not possess extravascular carbonic anhydrase (Zborowska-Sluis *et al.*, 1975) and thus during a period of increased cardiac O_2 consumption, myocardial hypercapnia can be prolonged (Case *et al.*, 1978).

The role of adenosine in coronary metabolic vasoregulation during stresses of everyday life is still under evaluation.

Coronary flow and adenosine concentration in isolated guinea pig hearts in various inotropic states correlate fairly well (Degenring, 1976b). It seems, however, that adenosine release by the heart may be more important with ischemia, as in the case of reactive hyperemia, than when O_2 consumption is increased during efforts or emotions. In effect, sinus coronary blood collected from human subjects during atrial pacing or exercise did not contain measurable concentrations of adenosine except in patients who develope anginal pain during the experiment (Fox *et al.*, 1974). Besides, aminophylline can inhibit most of the coronary vasodilatory response to increased heart pacing rate in dogs, but had no effect on resting coronary flow (Lammerant and Becsei, 1975), as in inhibiting reactive hyperemia (Juhran *et al.*, 1971; Curnish *et al.*, 1972). Adenosine is continuously produced and present in vasodilator concentrations, even in the well-oxygenated heart, and aminophylline blockade might have been expected to induce a vasoconstriction even at rest. It is possible indeed that the positive inotropic effect of aminophylline is accompanied by a metabolic vasodilation overcoming the adenosine blockade (Olsson, 1975).

Prostaglandins may act to reduce the coronary vasodilator response to increased cardiac activity. In isolated perfused cat or rat hearts, catecholamines or calcium increase contractility and coronary flow. Aspirin and Indomethacin enhance the flow response but do not influence contractility (Sen *et al.*, 1976) and infusion of prostaglandin GE_2 reduces the flow responses but not the increase in contractility (Sen *et al.*, 1976). Intracoronary injection of 40 μmol of isotonic KCl produces a decrease in coronary resistance ranging between 34 and 48% (Murray and Sparks, 1978). According to Gellai (1974), the possibility that potassium may contribute to metabolic coronary vasoregulation primarily as a steady-state regulator of coronary blood flow is unlikely. However, Belloni (1979) notes that K^+ seems to act as an imitation of the coronary vascular response to changes in cardiac work.

Intracoronary histamine infusion (5–20 μg/min) produces a dose-related increase in coronary blood flow without changing heart rate or pressure. H_1 and H_2 receptor antagonists Metiamide and Mepyramide (100 μg/min) given simultaneously shift the histamine dose-response curve to the right.

When the two inhibitors are given together, the blockade of the histamine effect is augmented. These results show that histamine-induced coronary vasodilation is mediated by both H_1 and H_2 receptors. However, Mepyramide and Metiamide together had no effect on flow response during reactive hyperemia (Giles *et al.*, 1977).

To summarize, our knowledge of the problems concerning the metabolic regulation of coronary vessels in natural stresses and during a variety of everyday situations is still limited. In the heart, as in other tissues, vascular regulation seems to be accomplished by several different mechanisms and factors, including O_2, adenosine, CO_2, prostaglandins, K, and other metabolites. Evidence suggests that O_2 and adenosine might modulate the effect of all other determinants and regulate coronary flow to maintain the myocardium in oxygen balance. The flow in the coronary capillaries is therefore likely to be controlled by the levels of oxidation in the myocardial cells through the release of metabolites, mainly adenosine.

VIII. Neural Regulation of Coronary Resistance: Sympathetic and Parasympathetic Regulation of Coronary Blood Flow

Both sympathetic and parasympathetic systems innervate the coronary channels. The direct effect of cardiac sympathetic nerve stimulations is coronary constriction (Hamilton and Feigl, 1976) and that of parasympathetic nerve stimulations is vasodilation (Feigl, 1969). This direct action is difficult to observe in intact animals because of the simultaneous changes in cardiac work, frequency, contractility, metabolism, and myocardial external compression on coronary channels. It is possible, however, to separate these effects by stimulating or blocking specific myocardial or coronary receptors. According to Alhquist (1948), it is possible to divide adrenergic receptors into two groups that differ in their response to agonists and block agents. One group, designated as "α", is excited by adrenaline, noradrenaline (Gaal *et al.*, 1966; Zuberbühler and Bohr, 1965), and dopamine (Nayler *et al.*, 1971) and is blocked by several drugs like phenoxybenzamine and benzodioxane (Feigl, 1975). This group mediates vasoconstriction in the entire cardiovascular system. Their constrictive effect on coronary vessels can be better demonstrated after β-blockade with propranolol (Feigl, 1967, 1975; Ross and Mulder, 1969; Ek and Ablad, 1971; McRaven *et al.*, 1971), which blunts the increase in metabolism produced by the stimulation of myocardial β-receptors. In these conditions stimulation of the left stellate ganglion decreases coronary blood flow and oxygen tension in coronary sinus blood, in absence of changes in cardiac metabolism (Mohrman and Feigl, 1978), and the administration of noradrenaline or phenylephrine considerably increases coronary resistance (Morhman and Feigl, 1978; Marchetti *et al.*, 1972). The further administration of an α-blocking agent eliminates the decrease in coronary sinus oxygen tension as well as the increase in coronary resistance (Marchetti *et al.*, 1972; Morhman and Feigl, 1978).

The surgical interruption of sympathetic nerves to the heart is followed by an increase in the volume of reactive hyperemia by 31% (Schwartz and Lowell Stone, 1976) and left ventricular oxygen consumption by 30% (Drake *et al.*, 1978). Hence the removal of a dominant α-receptor constrictor activity would dilate coronary vessels.

Recently Smith *et al.* (1978) performed experiments in dogs in order to ascertain whether activation of adrenergic receptors in the coronary vasculature could modify the time course of the coronary vasodilation accompanying the increase in myocardial metabolic activity. In effect, if the mechanisms that control coronary vascular resistance are closely linked to myocardial metabolism, during transient periods changes in the metabolic process would precede changes in coronary resistance. By injecting noradrenaline or isoproterenol they stimulated concomitantly coronary adrenergic receptors and myocardial activity and metabolism. The results showed that after intracoronary noradrenaline, the decrease in coronary resistance was smaller and slower in relation to the time changes in myocardial O_2 consumption than was the coronary dilation in response to isoproterenol. Hence the coronary resistance change lags behind O_2 consumption change during noradrenaline stimulation to a greater extent than during isoproterenol infusion, and this can be largely ascribed to the α-adrenergic action of noradrenaline.

The results of Mohrman and Feigl (1978), Schwartz and Lowell Stone (1976), Drake *et al.* (1978), and Smith *et al.* (1978) show that the α-receptor constrictor mechanism competes with metabolic vasodilation during sympathetic activation even when there are large increases in myocardial metabolism. However, the net effect of α-receptor constrictor influence is to restrict the metabolically related flow increase by only about 30% (Schwartz and Lowell Stone, 1976; Mohrman and Feigl, 1978; Drake *et al.*, 1978). This competition may actually result in lowering of P_{O_2} in coronary sinus blood (Feigl, 1975) and in some cases a net coronary vasoconstriction may occur (Vatner *et al.*, 1974).

Physiological sympathetic nerve vasoconstriction can be reflexly modulated. In effect, in the dog after β-blockade and vagotomy or treatment with atropine, the increase in sympathetic activity induced by bilateral common carotid artery occlusion causes coronary vasoconstriction, whereas a reflex decrease in sympathetic tone by stimulation of the carotid sinus nerve produces vasodilation (Feigl, 1968; Hackett *et al.*, 1972; Vatner *et al.*, 1970).

The β-receptors, which belong to the second group, mediate vasodilation and myocardial inotropic and chronotropic responses. Isoproterenol is the most potent and specific agonist of these receptors, which are blocked by propranolol and allied drugs. The activity of the α-agonists noradrenaline, adrenaline, and dopamine on β-receptors is less than that of isoproterenol. Recently it has been possible to separate the β-receptors into two subgroups, i.e., β_1, responsible for inotropic and chronotropic myocardial responses, and β_2, responsible for bronchodilation and vasodilation.

Propranolol can block myocardial β_1 and vascular β_2 receptors equally, whereas some other β-adrenergic blocking agents like practolol and atenolol can selectively block the effects of isoproterenol on myocardial β_1 receptors, leaving the response to isoproterenol of bronchial and vascular smooth muscle almost unaltered (Feigl, 1968; Malindzak *et al.*, 1978; Ross, 1976). In effect, in dog hearts treated with practolol, intracoronary administration of isoproterenol still produces a decrease in resistance, although smaller than that noted before practolol administration. This vasodilation is completely blocked by propranolol (McRaven *et al.*, 1971; Hamilton and Feigl, 1976).

In conscious dogs intracoronary injection of epinephrine results in coronary vasodilation. Coronary flow begins to increase and coronary resistance to decline 7 sec after the injection, whereas the myocardial effects (increase in contractility and heart rate) first become noticeable after about 10 sec and are clearly manifested after 25 sec (Pitt *et al.*, 1967). All these effects are blocked by propranolol. Hence coronary vasodilation elicited by epinephrine and isoproterenol is a β_2-receptor-mediated vasodilation and cannot be considered only as a secondary effect mediated by an increase in myocardial oxygen consumption (Pitt *et al.*, 1967). However, the physiological importance of β_2-receptors in coronary vessels seems to be very small. In effect, after blockade of α-receptor by phentolamine and β_1 myocardial receptors by Practolol, the stimulation of cardiac sympathetic nerves results either in a small transient coronary vasodilation (Hamilton and Feigl, 1976) or vasoconstriction, whereas vasodilation would always be expected, since the coronary β_2-receptors are intact (McRaven *et al.*, 1971).

Dopamine produces a dose-dependent constriction of isolated coronary arteries (Toda and Goldberg, 1975) and vessels of the arrested or fibrillating dog heart (Nayler *et al.*, 1971). After α-adrenergic blockade by phentolamine this constriction is reversed. In the beating heart dopamine induces vasodilation, sometimes preceded by a brief constriction (Nayler *et al.*, 1971). After α and β_1 and β_2 blockade dopamine still produces a coronary vasodilation in dogs (Vatner *et al.*, 1973) because of stimulation of specific "dopamine receptors" similar to those that have been described in mesenteric and renal arteries (McDonald and Goldberg, 1963).

The coronary vasodilation mediated by "dopamine receptors" is very slight and thus the increase in coronary blood flow observed in dogs given dopamine is mainly due to the increase in cardiac contractility and metabolism induced by myocardial β_1-receptor stimulation. Hence α-, β_1-and β_2-adrenergic receptors and dopamine-specific receptors can all be stimulated by intravenous infusion of dopamine. However, cardiac and vascular β-receptors are excited by low doses only (5–8 μg/kg/min), whereas when higher doses are given (8–40 μg/kg/min) α-receptors are also stimulated. The excitation of specific vasodilator receptors takes place after infusion of all therapeutic doses of dopamine (Goldberg, 1972).

In dogs the intracoronary injection of acetylcholine produces an increase in coronary blood flow and a decrease in resistance that were blocked by atropine but not by propranolol. The coronary dilator response together with a negative inotropic effect are probably mediated through muscarinic receptors (Blesa and Ross, 1970). Coronary vasodilation can also be elicited reflexly in anesthetized dogs by stimulating parasympathetic cardiac receptors by an intracoronary injection of veratridine. The effect was abolished when the reflex arc was interrupted by either vagotomy or atropine administration (Feigl, 1975).

IX. Conclusions

Coronary resistance is regulated by several factors, namely, mechanical, myogenic, neural, humoral, and metabolic (Johnson, 1974). Mechanical influence consists basically of the throttling effect of the myocardium during systole on the coronary channels and acts mainly in the subendocardial layers of the left ventricle. It is possible, however, to differentiate the effects of myocardial extravascular compression from the total coronary vascular resistance by calculating them in the late diastolic period, when the myocardial extravascular compression is minimal or nonexistent (Malindzak *et al.*, 1978). The myogenic factors appears to play a role mainly in the case of reactive hyperemia that takes place after transient myocardial ischemia (Olsson, 1975), whereas it is not clear whether this factor contributes to adjustments of coronary vascular tone (Rubio and Berne, 1975). Neural and humoral influences are concerned with the existence in the coronary vasculature and myocardium of adrenergic receptors α, β_1, and β_2, which can be activated by catecholamines or sympathetic nerve stimulation.

α-Receptor activity can be demonstrated in large conductive coronary arteries by recording the effect of noradrenaline injections on coronary flow and resistance before and after β-blockade or surgical denervation of the heart (Feigl, 1975; Schwartz and Lowell Stone, 1976; Drake *et al.*, 1978). The almost pure α-adrenergic agonist phenilephrine induces constriction that is blocked by an α-adrenergic blocking agent (Zuberbühler and Bohr, 1965; Malindzak *et al.*, 1978; Feigl, 1975). In contrast, smaller arteries (100–500 μm) have functionally very weak α-adrenergic activity; in effect, they are not significantly constricted by noradrenaline or phenilephrine (Bayer *et al.*, 1974), whereas a weak constrictor response can be elicited by β-adrenergic blockade (Bayer *et al.*, 1974; Baron *et al.*, 1972). The evidence of β_2-adrenergic receptors in coronary arteries has been demonstrated, since isoproterenol, noradrenaline, and adrenaline relax both large and small coronary arteries and this relaxation is blocked by β-blocking drugs (Bayer *et al.*, 1974) and potentiated by α-adrenergic blocking agents (Hamilton and Feigl, 1976) in various stress conditions. It is unlikely, however, that sympathetic activation of coronary β_2-receptors has much physiologic importance.

The intravenous injection of noradrenaline and the stimulation of β-receptors with isoproterenol or other adrenergic amines elicit a marked increase in coronary blood flow, which seems to be mainly determined by the β_1 sympathetic increase in myocardial, mechanical, and metabolic activity and to a lesser extent by direct coronary vasodilation because of the excitation of β_2-receptors.

The coronary vasodilation mediated by local metabolic factors either present in the blood or produced by myocardial activity is likely to be the main regulator of blood and oxygen supply to the heart (Rubio and Berne, 1975; Gregg, 1963b). Metabolic activity of the left myocardium as reflected by P_{O_2}, which corresponds to the ratio between oxygen supply and consumption, correlates closely with the left coronary blood flow and resistance. The close coupling between coronary blood flow in the left heart and local metabolic activity, which in turn depends on myocardial contractility, myocardial wall tension, and heart rate, is demonstrated by several investigations (Gregg, 1971–1972; Berne, 1964; Scott, 1961; McGregor and Fam, 1965; Rubio and Berne, 1975), whereas the nature of the biochemical process linking coronary blood flow with metabolic needs in the myocardium is not clearly understood (Rubio and Berne, 1975).

Several substances arising from local metabolic activity are known to affect coronary blood flow either through a primary coronary vasodilating action or through effects secondary to changes in myocardial activity. These include catecholamines, kinins, adenosine, inosine, H^+, prostaglandins, increase in P_{CO_2}, decrease in P_{O_2}, K^+, and presumably many others not yet identified (Rubio and Berne, 1975).

The resistance in the small coronary arteries seems to be controlled mainly by the metabolic activity of the myocardium as well as by humoral and neural factors. The resistance in the large conductive coronary vessels does not seem to be influenced by the metabolic activity of the myocardium (Malindzak *et al.*, 1978). However, in the presence of enhanced sympathetic activity or intracoronary norepinephrine infusion, coronary vessels are simultaneously subjected to an α-receptor constrictor influence (Mohrman *et al.*, 1978; Schwartz and Lowell Stone, 1976; Drake *et al.*, 1978; Smith *et al.*, 1978) and a metabolic vasodilator influence (Morhman and Feigl, 1978). Net vasodilation results but the increase in coronary blood flow is generally insufficient to meet precisely the increased metabolic needs of the myocardium.

A functional competition between local metabolic and sympathetic control of the coronary circulation exists and if sympathetic drive to the hearts is elevated, the α-receptor constrictor influence limits the coronary blood flow and thus induces an increase in O_2 myocardial extraction and a decrease in O_2 content in venous coronary sinus blood. This restricts O_2 supply to the myocardium to about 30% below the increased metabolic needs during cardiac effort.

References

Afonso, S. (1970). Inhibition of coronary vasodilating action of dipyridamole and adenosine by aminophylline in the dog. *Circ. Res.* **26**, 743–752.

Alella, A., Williams, F. L., Bolene Williams, C., and Katz, L. N. (1955). Interrelation between cardiac oxygen consumption and coronary blood flow. *Am. J. Physiol.* **183**, 570–582.

Alexander, R. W., Kent, K. M., Pisano, J. J., Keiser, H. R., and Cooper, T. (1975). Regulation of postocclusive hyperemia by endogenously sinthetized prostaglandins in the dog heart. *J. Clin. Invest.* **55**, 1174–1181.

Alhquist, R. P. (1948). A study of the adrenotropic receptors. *Am. J. Physiol.* **153**, 586–600.

Arnold, G., Koshe, F., and Miessner, E. (1968). The importance of the perfusion pressure in the coronary arteries for the contractility and the oxygen consumption of the heart. *Pflüegers Arch. Gesamte Physiol. Menschen Tiere* **299**, 339–356.

Bache, R. J., Cobb, F.R., and Greenfield, J. C., Jr. (1974). Limitations of the coronary vascular response to ischemia in the awake dog. *Circ. Res.* **35**, 527–535.

Bagger, A. (1978). Distribution of maximum coronary blood flow in the left ventricular wall of anesthetized dogs. *Acta Physiol. Scand.* **104**, 48–60.

Baron, G. D., Speden, R. N., and Bohr, D. F. (1972). Beta-adrenergic receptors in coronary and skeletal muscle arteries. *Am. J. Physiol.* **223**, 878–881.

Bayer, B. C., Mentz, P., and Forster, W. (1974). Characterization of the adrenoceptors in coronary arteries of pigs. *Eur. J. Pharmacol.* **29**, 58–65.

Belloni, F. L. (1979). The local control of coronary blood flow. *Cardiovasc Res.* **13**, 63–85.

Bergamaschi, M., and Longoni, A. M. (1973). Cardiovascular events in anxiety: Experimental studies in the conscious dogs. *Am. Heart J.* **86**, 385–394.

Berne, R. M. (1964). Regulation of coronary blood flow. *Physiol. Rev.* **44**, 1–29.

Bing, R. J. (1965). Cardiac metabolism. *Physiol. Rev.* **45**, 171–213.

Bittar, N., Pauly, T. J., and Koke, J. R. (1975). Changes in ischemic coronary vasodilatation produced by blood plasma and saline infusion. *Recent Adv. Stud. Card. Struct. Metab.* **10**, 475–482.

Blesa, M. I., and Ross, G. (1970). Cholinergic mechanism on the heart and coronary circulation. *Br. J. Pharmacol.* **38**, 93–105.

Block, A. J., Feinberg, H., Herbaxzynska-Cedro, K., and Vane, J. R. (1975). Anoxia induced release of prostaglandins in rabbits isolated hearts. *Circ. Res.* **36**, 34–42.

Bradley, K. J. (1975). The release of a coronary vasodilator metabolite from the guinea-pig isolated perfused heart stimulated by cathecolamines, histamine and electrical pacing and by exposure to anoxia. *Br. J. Pharmacol.* **58**, 89–100, 1975.

Caraffa Braga, F., Granata, L., and Pinotti, O. (1973). Changes in blood-flow distribution during acute emotional stress in dogs. *Pflüegers Arch.* **339**, 203–216.

Case, R. B., Felix, A., Wachter, M., Kyriakidis, G., and Castellana, F. (1978). Relative effect of CO_2 on canine coronary vascular resistance. *Circ. Res.* **42**, 410–418.

Coffman, J. D., and Gregg, D. E. (1960). Reactive hyperemia characteristics of the myocardium. *Am. J. Physiol.* **199**, 1143–1149.

Curnish, R. R., Berne, R. M., and Rubio, R. (1972). Effect of aminophylline on myocardial reactive hyperemia. *Proc. Soc. Exp. Biol. Med.* **141**, 593–598.

Degenring, F. H. (1976a). The effects of acidosis and alkalosis on coronary flow and cardiac nucleotides metabolism. *Basic Res. Cardiol.* **71**, 287–290.

Degenring, F. H. (1976b). Cardiac nucleotides and coronary flow during changes of cardiac inotropy. *Basic Res. Cardiol.* **71**, 291–296.

Drake, A. J., Stubbs, J., and Noble, M. I. M. (1978). Dependence of myocardial blood flow and metabolism on cardiac innvervation. *Cardiovasc. Res.* **12**, 69–80.

Eikens, E., and Wilcken, D. E. L. (1974). Reactive hyperemia in the dog heart: Effects of temporary restricting arterial inflow and of coronary occlusions lasting one and two cardiac cycles. *Circ. Res.* **35**, 702–712.

Ek, L., and Åblad, B. (1971). Effects of three beta-adrenergic receptor blockers on myocardial oxygen consumption in the dog. *Eur. J. Pharmacol.* **14**, 19–28.

Elliott, E. C., Jones, E. L., Blood, C. M., Leon, A. S., and Gregg, D. E. (1968). Day to day changes in coronary haemodynamics secondary to constriction of circumflex branch of left coronary artery in conscious dogs. *Circ. Res.* **22**, 237–250.

Fabel, H. (1968). Normal and critical oxygen-supply of the heart. In "Oxygen Transport in

Blood and Tissue" (D.W. Lübbers, U. C. Luft, G. Thewa, and E. Witzleb, eds.), pp. 159–171. Thieme, Stuttgart.

Feigl, E. O. (1967). Sympathetic control of the coronary circulation. *Circ. Res.* **20**, 262–271.

Feigl, E. O. (1968). Carotid sinus reflex control of coronary flow. *Circ. Res.* **23**, 223–237.

Feigl, E. O. (1969). Parasympathetic control of the coronary blood flow in dogs. *Circ. Res.* **25**, 509–519.

Feigl, E. O. (1975). Control of myocardial oxygen tension by sympathetic coronary vasoconstriction in the dog. *Circ. Res.* **37**, 88–95.

Fox, A. C., Reed, G. E., Glassman, E., Kaltman, A. J., and Silk, B. B. (1974). Release of adenosine from human hearts during angina induced by rapid atrial pacing. *J. Clin. Invest.* **53**, 1447–1457.

Fröhlich, E. D. (1965). Vascular effects of the Krebs intermediate metabolites. *Am. J. Physiol.* **208**, 149–153.

Gaal, P. G., Kattus, A. A., Kolin, A., and Ross, G. (1966). Effect of adrenaline and noradrenaline on coronary blood flow before and after β-adrenergic blockage. *Br. J. Pharmacol. Chemother.* **26**, 713–722.

Gellai, M., Norton, J. M., and Detar, R. (1972). Effect of aminophylline on myocardial reactive hyperemia. *Proc. Soc. Exp. Biol. Med.* **141**, 593–598.

Gibbs, C. L. (1978). Cardiac energetics. *Physiol. Rev.* **58**, 174–254.

Giles, R. W., and Wilcken, D. (1977). Reactive hyperemia in the dog heart: Interrelations between adenosine, ATP and aminophylline and the effects of indomethacin. *Cardiovasc. Res.* **11**, 113–121.

Giles, R. W., Heise, G., and Wilcken, D. E. L. (1977). Histamine receptors in the coronary circulation of the dog. Effects of mepyramine and metiamide on responses to histamine infusion. *Circ. Res.* **40**, 541–546.

Goldberg, L. I. (1972). Cardiovascular and renal actions of Dopamine. Potential clinical application. *Pharmacol. Rev.* **24**, 1–29.

Gregg, D. E. (1963a). Effect of coronary perfusion pressure or coronary flow on oxygen usage of the myocardium. *Circ. Res.* **13**, 497–500.

Gregg, D. E. (1963b). The George E. Brown Memorial lecture. Physiology of the coronary circulation. *Circulation* **27**, 1128–1137.

Gregg, D. E. (1971–1972). Relationship between coronary flow and metabolic changes. *Cardiology* **56**, 291–301.

Gregg, D. E., and Fisher, L. C. (1963). Blood supply to the heart. *In* "Handbook of Physiology" (W. F. Hamilton and F. Dow, eds., Sect. 2, Vol. II, pp. 1517–1583. Williams & Wilkins, Baltimore, Maryland.

Gregg, D. E., Khouri, E. M., and Rayford, C. R. (1965). Systemic and coronary energetics in the resting unanaesthetized dog. *Circ. Res.* **66**, 102–113.

Gregg, D. E., Lowensohn, H. S., and Khouri, E. M. (1972). The effect of chronic pulmonic stenosis in the right coronary circulation in the conscious dog. *In* "Myocardial Blood Flow in Man" A. Maseri, ed., pp. 5–9. Minerva Medica, Torino.

Hackett, J. G., Abbond, F. M., Mark, A. L., Schmid, P. G., and Heistad, D. D. (1972). Coronary vascular response to stimulation of chemoreceptors and baroreceptors. *Circ. Res.* **31**, 8–17.

Hamilton, F. N., and Feigl, E. O. (1976). Coronary vascular sympathetic beta-receptor innervation. *Am. J. Physiol.* **230**, 1569–1576.

Holtz, J., vonRestorff, W., Bard, P., and Bassenge, E. (1977). Transmural distribution of myocardial blood flow and of coronary reserve in canine left ventricular hypertrophy. *Basic Res. Cardiol.* **72**, 286–292.

Jacobs, M. I., and Berne, R. M. (1960). Metabolism of purine derivative by the isolated cat heart. *Am. J. Physiol.* **198**, 322–326.

Johnson, P. C. (1974). The microcirculation and local and humoral control of the circulation. *In* "Cardiovascular Physiology" (A. C. Guyton and C. E. Jones, eds., pp. 163–195. Butterworth, London.

Juhran, W., Voss, E. M., Dietmann, K., and Schaumann, W. (1971). Pharmacological effects on coronary reactive hyperemia in conscious dogs. *Naunyn-Schmiedebergs Arch. Pharmakol.* **269**, 32–47.

Katori, M., and Berne, R. M. (1966). Release of adenosine from anoxic hearts. Relationship to coronary flow. *Circ. Res.* **19**, 420–425.

Khouri, E. M., Gregg, D. E., and Rayford, C. R. (1965). Effect of exercise on cardiac output, left coronary flow and myocardial metabolism in the unanaesthetized dog. *Circ. Res.* **17**, 427–437.

Kirk, E. S., and Honig, C. R. (1964). An experimental and theoretical analysis of myocardial tissue pressure. *Am. J. Physiol.* **207**, 661–668.

Lammerant, J., and Becsei, I. (1975). Inhibition of pacing induced coronary dilation by aminophylline. *Cardiovasc. Res.* **9**, 532–537.

Lewis, T., and Grant, R. (1925–26). Observations upon reactive hyperemia in man. *Heart* **12**, 73–110.

Linzbach, A. J. (1960). Heart failure from the point of view of quantitative anatomy. *Am. J. Cardiol.* **5**, 370–382.

McDonald, R. H., and Goldberg, L. I. (1963). Analysis of cardiovascular effects of dopamine in the dog. *J. Pharmacol. Exp. Ther.* **140**, 60–66.

McGregor, M., and Fam, W. M. (1966). Regulation of coronary blood flow. *Bull. N.Y. Acad. Med.* [2] **42**, 187–950.

McRaven, D. R., Mark, A. L., Abbond, F. M., and Mayer, H. E. (1971). Responses of coronary vessels to adrenergic stimuli. *J. Clin. Invest.* **50**, 773–778.

Malindzak, G. S., Kosinski, E. J., Green, H. D., and Yarborough, G. W. (1978). The effects of adrenergic stimulation on conductive and resistive segments of the coronary vascular bed. *J. Pharmacol. Exp. Ther.* **206**, 248–258.

Marchetti, G. (1971). Physiology of the coronary circulation. *Physiol. Blood Lymph Vessels, Symp. Angiol. Santoriana, 3rd,* 1970 Part II, pp. 1–26 (157–182).

Marchetti, G., and Merlo, L. (1964). Modifications of the coronary blood flow, oxygen consumption of the myocardium and cardiac efficiency as related to variations of dog heart work. *Cardiologia* **44**, 366–391.

Marchetti, G., Merlo, L., and Noseda, V. (1966). Flow and O_2 content of the blood return from the myocardium to the coronary sinus and other cardiac vessels. *Pflüegers Arch. Gesamte Physiol. Menschen Tiere* **287**, 99–110.

Marchetti, G., Merlo, L., and Noseda, V. (1968). Response of coronary blood flow to some natural stresses of excitement in the conscious dog. *Pflügers Arch.* **298**, 200–212.

Marchetti, G., Merlo, L., and Noseda, V. (1969). Coronary sinus outflow and O_2 content in anterior cardiac vein blood at different levels of right ventricular performance. *Pflüegers Arch.* **310**, 116–127.

Marchetti, G. V., Merlo, L., and Noseda, V. (1971). Modification in myocardial metabolism of lactate and pyruvate following temporary occlusion in the conscious dog. *Cardiology* **56**, 354–357.

Marchetti, G., Merlo, L., and Noseda, V. (1972). Mechanism of the decrease in coronary blood flow after β-blockade in conscious dogs. *Cardiovasc. Res.* **6**, 532–540.

Marchetti, G. V., Merlo, L., Noseda, V., and Visioli, O. (1973). Myocardial blood flow in experimental cardiac hypertrophy in dogs. *Cardiovasc. Res.* **7**, 519–527.

Mohrman, D. E., and Feigl, E. O. (1978). Competition between sympathetic vasoconstriction and metabolic vasodilation in the canine coronary circulation. *Circ. Res.* **42**, 79–86.

Moss, A. J. (1968). Intramyocardial oxygen tension. *Cardiovasc. Res.* **3**, 314–318.

Moss, A. J., and Johnson, J. (1970). Effects of oxygen inhalation on intramyocardial oxygen tension. *Cardiovasc. Res.* **4**, 436–440.

Mueller, T. M., Marcus, M. L., Kerber, R. E., Young, J. A., Barnes, R. W., and Abbond, F. M. (1978). Effect of renal hypertension and left ventricular hypertrophy on the coronary circulation in dogs. *Circ. Res.* **42**, 543–549.

Murray, P. A., and Sparks, H. U. (1978). The mechanism of K^+ induced vasodilation of the coronary vascular bed of the dog. *Circ. Res.* **42**, 35–42.

Nayler, W. G., McInnes, I., Stone, J., Carson, V., and Lowe, T. E. (1971). Effect of dopamine on coronary vascular resistance and myocardial function. *Cardiovasc. Res.* **5**, 161–168.

Needleman, P., Key, S. L., Isakson, P. C. and Kulkarni, P. S. (1975). Relationship between oxygen tension, coronary vasodilatation and prostaglandin biosynthesis in the isolated rabbit heart. *Prostaglandins* **9**, 123–134.

Needleman, P., Kulkarni, P. S. and Raz, A. (1977). Coronary tone modulation: Formation and action of prostaglandins, endoperoxides and thromboxanes. *Science* **195**, 409–412.

Neill, W. A., and Hattenhauer, M. (1975). Impairement of myocardial O_2 supply due to hyperventilation. *Circulation* **52**, 854–858.

Newton, J. E. O., and Ehrlich, W. (1969). Coronary blood flow in dogs: Effect of a person. *Cond. Reflex* **4**, 81–88.

O'Keefe, D., Hoffman, J. I. E., Cheitlin, R., O'Neill, M., Allard, J. R. and Shapkin, E. (1978). Coronary blood flow in experimental canine left ventricular hypertrophy. *Circ. Res.* **43**, 43–51.

Olsson, R. A. (1964). Kinetics of myocardial reactive hyperemia blood flow in the anaesthetized dog. *Circ. Res., Suppl.* **1**, I-81–I-86.

Olsson, R. A. (1975). Myocardial reactive hyperemia. *Circ. Res.* **37**, 263–270.

Olsson, R. A., and Gregg, D. E. (1965). Myocardial reactive hyperemia in the unanaesthetized dog. *Am. J. Physiol.* **208**, 224–230.

Olsson, R. A., Snow, J. A., and Gentry, M. K. (1978). Adenosine metabolism in canine myocardial reactive hyperemia. *Circ. Res.* **42**, 358–362.

Opie, L. (1968). Metabolism of the heart in health and disease. Part 1. *Am. Heart J.* **76**, 685–698.

Opie, L. (1969). Metabolism of the heart in health and disease. Parts 2 and 3. *Am. Heart J.* **77**, 100–122 and 383–410.

Pauly, T. J., Zarnstorff, W. C., and Bittal, N. (1973). Myocardial metabolic activity as a determinant of reactive hyperemia responses in the dog heart. *Cardiovasc. Res.* **7**, 90–94.

Pickard, J. D., and MacKenzie, E. T. (1973). Inhibition of prostaglandin synthesis and the response of baboon cerebral circulation to carbon dioxide. *Nature (London), New Biol.* **245**, 187–188.

Pitt, B., Elliott, E. C., and Gregg, D. E. (1967). Adrenergic receptor activity in the coronary arteries of the unanaesthetized dog. *Circ. Res.* **21**, 75–84.

Ross, G. (1976). Adrenergic response of the coronary vessels. *Circ. Res.* **39**, 461–465.

Ross, G., and Mulder, D. G. (1969). Effects of right and left cardio-sympathetic nerve stimulation on blood flow in the major coronary arteries of the anesthetized dog. *Cardiovasc. Res.* **3**, 22–29.

Rubio, A., Berne, R. M., and Katori, M. (1969). Release of adenosine in reactive hyperemia of the dog heart. *Am. J. Physiol.* **216**, 56–62.

Rubio, R., and Berne, R. M. (1975). Regulation of coronary blood flow. *Prog. Cardiovasc. Dis.* **18**, 105–122.

Schwartz, P. J. and Lowell Stone, H. (1976). Tonic influence of the sympathetic nervous system on myocardial reaction hyperemia and on coronary blood flow distribution in dogs. *Circ. Res.* **41,** 51–58.

Scott, J. C. (1961). Myocardial coefficient of oxygen utilization. *Circ. Res.* **9,** 906–910.

Sen, A. K., Sunahara, F. A., and Talesnik, J. (1976). Prostaglandin E_2 and cyclic AMP in the coronary vasodilatation due to cardiac hyperactivity. *Can. J. Physiol. Pharmacol.* **54,** 128–139.

Smith, R. E., Belloni, F. L., and Sparks, H. V. (1978). Coronary vascular resistance and myocardial oxygen consumption dynamics in response to catecholamine infusion. *Cardiovasc. Res.* **12,** 391–400.

Toda, N., and Goldberg, L. I. (1975). Effects of dopamine on isolated canine coronary arteries. *Cardiovasc. Res.* **9,** 384–389.

Vatner, S. F., Franklin, D., Van Citters, R. L., and Braunwald, E. (1970). Effects of carotid sinus nerve stimulation on the coronary circulation of the conscious dog. *Circ. Res.* **27,** 11–21.

Vatner, S. F., Millard, R. W., and Higgins, C. B. (1973). Coronary and myocardial effects of dopamine in the conscious dog: Parasympatholytic augmentation of pressor and inotropic actions. *J. Pharmacol. Exp. Ther.* **187,** 280–295.

Vatner, S. F., Higgins, C. B., and Braunwald, E. (1974). Effects of norepinephrine on coronary circulation and left ventricular dynamics in the conscious dog. *Circ. Res.* **34,** 812–823.

Wittenberg, J. B. (1970). Myoglobin-facilitated oxygen diffusion: Role of myoglobin in oxygen entry into muscle. *Physiol. Rev.* **50,** 559–636.

Zborowska-Sluis, D. T., L'Abbata, A., Mildenberg, R. R., and Klassen, G. A. (1975). The effect of acetazolamide on myocardial carbon dioxide space. *Respir. Physiol.* **23,** 311–316.

Zuberbühler, R. C., and Bohr, D. F. (1965). Response of coronary vascular smooth muscle to catecholamines. *Circ. Res.* **16,** 431–440.

Index

A

AA, *see* Arachidonic acid
Acceleration tolerance, after bedrest, 492–495
Accentuated antagonism, 196
Acetate, vasoactivity, 531
Acetylcholine, 162
  cardiocardiac reflexes and, 200
  cyclic nucleotide levels and, 198, 429
  effect on cardiac electrical activity, 215, 220
  exercise training and, 403, 405, 406
  in hyperthyroidism studies, 115–116, 129
  inhibitor, of norepinephrine release, 196, 197, 198
  prostaglandin release and, 57–58
  release, prostaglandins and, 76–77, 83
  stimulator, of catecholamine release, 174
  vasoactivity, 547
Acetylcholinesterase, 196, 403
Acetylstrophanthidin, 18, 133
cis-Aconitate, in hypoxic metabolism, 359
ACTH, *see* Adrenocorticotropin
Actinomycin D, 122, 124
Actomyosin ATPase, exercise training and, 395–397
Acylhydrolase, 61
Adaptation, emotional stress and, 281–282
Adaptation stage, 296
Adenine nucleotides, prostaglandin biosynthesis and, 51, 55
Adenosine
  chronotropic effects, 206
  prostaglandins and, 72, 78
  vasoactivity, 72, 207, 461, 531, 533, 534, 543–544
S-Adenosylmethionine, 171, 174

Adenylate cyclase
  activity, in denervated heart, 214
  in adrenergic response, 178, 180, 182–183
  glucagon and, 13–14, 15
  hypothyroidism and, 144
  prostaglandins and, 71
  role in cardiac hypertrophy, 426–430
  thyroid hormone and, 112, 117–120
ADH, *see* Vasopressin
Adrenal cortical steroid, *see* Corticosteroid
Adrenalectomy
  angiotensin II effect and, 24
  effect on adrenergic receptor, 181
Adrenal gland hormones, in chronic hypoxia, 376
Adrenaline, *see* Epinephrine
Adrenal medulla, catecholamine content, 174
Adrenal regeneration hypertension, 317–318
Adrenergic neuron, definition, 164
Adrenergic receptors, 175–187, *see also*
  Catecholamines; Epinephrine; Isoproterenol; Norepinephrine; Sympathetic nervous system
  in coronary circulation, 185–187
  hyperthyroidism and, 113–115
  hypothyroidism and, 142–143
  in myocardium, 181–185
  prostaglandin effects on, 74–76, 81–83
  responses, in cardiac electrical activity, 216
  thyroid hormone and, 112–113, 135–136
  types and functions, 175, 545–546
  vasoactivity, 545–549
α-Adrenergic blocking agents, stimulators, of
  norepinephrine release, 169
α-Adrenergic receptors
  agonists, 176, 177
  antagonists, 176, 177
  PG effects and, 57, 71

TCH CARDIOLOGY

TCH CARDIOLOGY

TCH CARDIOLOGY